AF843391

Cancer Research Guidance for Clinicians and Researchers

Jeffrey Huang • Heather S.L. Jim
Editors

Cancer Research Guidance for Clinicians and Researchers

Springer

Editors
Jeffrey Huang
Anesthesiology and Critical Care
Moffitt Cancer Center
Tampa, FL, USA

Heather S.L. Jim
Health Outcomes and Behavior
Moffitt Cancer Center
Tampa, FL, USA

ISBN 978-3-032-19174-8 ISBN 978-3-032-19175-5 (eBook)
https://doi.org/10.1007/978-3-032-19175-5

This Springer imprint is published by the registered company Springer Nature Switzerland AG
The registered company address is: Gewerbestrasse 11, 6330 Cham, Switzerland

Preface

Cancer stands as one of the most formidable health challenges of our age, having accounted for 17% of all deaths in 2021 and solidifying its place as the second-leading cause of death across all ages in the United States—and the leading cause for individuals younger than 85. Yet, amid these sobering statistics, there is clear evidence of progress: the 5-year survival rate for all cancers has increased from just 49% in the mid-1970s to 69% between 2013 and 2019, a remarkable 20% rise over the past 50 years. Globally, improvements in both treatment and diagnosis have driven survival rates up from 50% to approximately 60%, demonstrating the immense value that sustained research brings to patients and communities.

Despite this global progress, a silent divide persists in how cancer research is advanced and applied. More than half of all cancer treatments in the United States take place in community hospitals. For some cancers, rates are much higher. For example, a recent study found that up to 83% of women diagnosed with uterine cancer received their initial treatment in a community setting *(Gynecol Oncol*, 2022; 164:325–332). Only a small percentage of patients at community hospitals are enrolled in cancer research studies or clinical trials in these community environments, while the majority of leading-edge research remains concentrated at major academic and NCI-designated cancer centers.

This book was born out of both promise and need. Approximately 40–50% of residency programs are based at community hospitals, and these programs require their faculty and trainees to participate in scholarly activities, including clinical research. However, practical guidance for conducting robust, impactful cancer research in these settings is often lacking.

"Cancer Research Guidance for Clinicians and Researchers" aims to bridge that gap. It is designed to serve clinicians, trainees, and research staff working in community hospital contexts, providing them with pragmatic research knowledge, actionable frameworks, and up-to-date best practices. The aspiration is not only to enhance the quality of research in community settings but also to empower clinicians to make direct contributions to the advancement of cancer care and, ultimately, to improved patient outcomes. Through supporting research where most patients actually receive their care, we hope to advance equity, scientific discovery, and the shared mission to defeat cancer.

This book is organized into two major parts.

The first part presents core research methodologies to help readers understand study design and data analysis, while also guiding them in developing rigorous interventional studies tailored to community hospital settings. Recognizing the growing role of technology in cancer research, this part also features chapters on mathematical modeling and artificial intelligence.

The second part provides a comprehensive review of current cancer research across major tumor types and supporting disciplines. Each subspecialty professional will find a dedicated chapter discussing research related to their field. This part serves as a practical guide for all clinicians seeking to initiate their own research projects.

This book serves as an invaluable resource for all cancer specialties, including oncologic surgeons, medical oncologists, radiologists, pathologists, anesthesiologists, certified registered nurse anesthetists, certified anesthesiologist assistants, oncology nurse practitioners, oncology physician assistants, oncology nurses, researchers, social workers, residents, fellows, and medical students.

Tampa, FL, USA Jeffrey Huang
Tampa, FL, USA Heather S.L. Jim

Acknowledgments

The journey of creating this book has been both challenging and rewarding—from finding the right contributors to bringing each chapter to completion. But together, we did it.

I would like to express my deepest gratitude to my family for their unwavering support and confidence in me throughout this process. Their encouragement has been my greatest motivation and strength.

I am equally grateful to my colleagues and collaborators, whose expertise and passion for advancing cancer research have been a constant source of inspiration.

To all the authors who contributed their time, knowledge, and passion to this project—thank you for your collaboration, commitment, and shared belief in the importance of this work.

Tampa, FL, USA — Jeffrey Huang

Contents

Part III Special Topics

Part I

Clinical Research Designs

In Vitro (Cell-Based) Studies

1

Nicol Mecozzi, Zulaida Soto-Vargas, Kaizhen Wang, Neel Jasani, and Xiaonan Xu

Introduction

Cancer remains one of the leading causes of morbidity and mortality worldwide. In the United States, cancer is the second most common cause of death, with an estimated 2 million new cases and approximately 611,000 deaths projected for 2024 [1]. Globally, cancer is responsible for nearly 10 million deaths annually. The most prevalent cancer types include lung, breast, colorectal, and prostate cancers, with risk factors ranging from aging and genetic predisposition to environmental exposures and lifestyle choices. Despite significant advances in early detection, preventive measures, and the development of targeted therapies and immunotherapies, treatment outcomes and prognosis for many cancer types remain suboptimal. The complexity of cancer pathogenesis, characterized by intrinsic cellular heterogeneity, plasticity, and the influence of extrinsic factors from stromal cells and extracellular matrix (ECM), contributes to the development of adaptive resistance to therapy in numerous cancer patients, leading to therapeutic failure [2]. As a result, the development of combination therapies targeting novel and druggable pathways is urgently needed to improve patient outcomes. However, how to promptly identify the key driver genes and validate their cellular functions remains a challenge.

This chapter provides an overview of various in vitro methodologies to assess the candidate genes in modulating cancer cell phenotypes, including cell cycle regulation, proliferation, survival, apoptosis, migration, and invasion. These approaches together provide a comprehensive evaluation of the therapeutic potential of candidate genes and will assist physician-scientists in prioritizing targets for subsequent in vivo investigations and drug development. Regarding drug development, advancements in computational modeling and synthetic chemistry have facilitated the rapid design and synthesis of small molecular inhibitors targeting specific genes. However, the effective screening of large libraries of candidate inhibitors remains a significant challenge. In this chapter, we also summarize several strategies for assessing cancer cell responses to inhibitors, enabling physician-scientists to select the most promising candidates for further in vivo studies.

Cell Viability Assays

Cell viability assays are practical tools in biological research to measure cell growth and survival in vitro. These assays provide insights into cellular responses to stimuli, drug treatments, and genetic modifications [3–6], which are crucial for understanding cancer cell biology, disease mechanisms, and therapeutic interventions. Commonly used methods to measure cell viability include cell proliferation assays, low-density colony formation assays, and anchorage-independent growth assays (see Fig. 1.1). These assays emphasize different aspects of cell viability. They are powerful tools to identify critical genes or pathways regulating cell proliferation and survival, and also to evaluate the inhibitory effects of new drugs.

Cell proliferation assays measure the ability of cells to divide and grow over time. It focuses on short-term growth, usually over 4–7 days. It quantifies total cell numbers as an indicator of cell proliferation. Advantages of this assay include an easy setup and quick results. Disadvantages include the following: (1) the plate needs to be processed every day if Incucyte is not available, (2) the assay detects cell proliferation only in relatively normal conditions, and (3) cell morphology changes may affect the final result. Therefore, this assay is a good fit if the researcher wants preliminary data for a large number of samples in a short time.

Authors Nicol Mecozzi, Zulaida Soto Vargas, Kaizhen Wang and Neel Jasani have equally contributed to this chapter.

N. Mecozzi · Z. Soto-Vargas · K. Wang · N. Jasani · X. Xu (✉)
Department of Molecular Oncology, H. Lee Moffitt Cancer Center and Research Institute, Tampa, FL, USA
e-mail: xiaonan.xu@moffitt.org

J. Huang, H. S.L. Jim (eds.), *Cancer Research Guidance for Clinicians and Researchers*,
https://doi.org/10.1007/978-3-032-19175-5_1

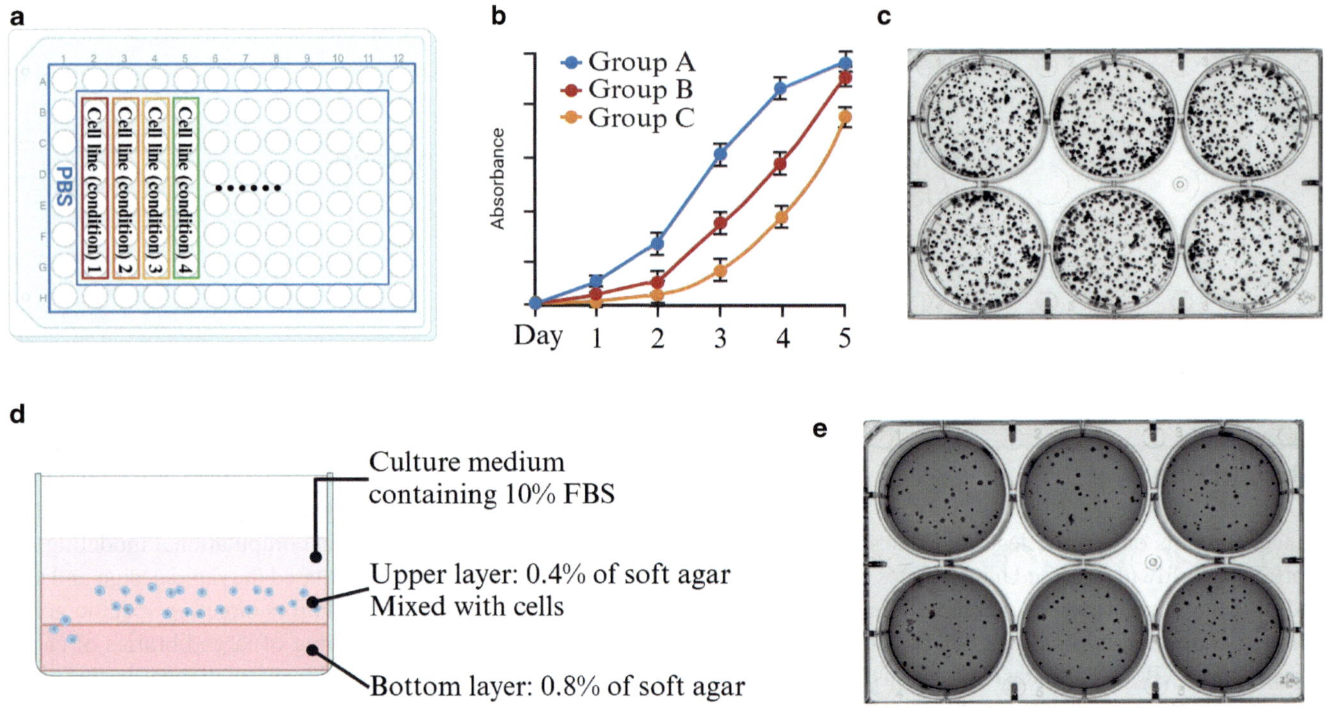

Fig. 1.1 Cell viability assays. (**a**) Arrangement of cell proliferation assay on a 96-well plate. 6 replicates were plated for each cell line. (**b**) Example of growth curve for cell proliferation assay. Absorbance for each cell line was measured each day and mean ± SD were presented. (**c**) Example of scanned plate in low-density focus formation assay. (**d**) Schematic diagram of anchorage-independent growth assay plated in a 6-well plate. (**e**) Example of a scanned plate with colonies at optimal sizes

The low-density colony formation assay evaluates the ability of single cells to grow into colonies when plated at low density. It measures clonogenic potential, indicating the ability of a single cell to proliferate and form a colony. Advantages of this assay include an easy setup and detection of both cell survival (colony number) and cell proliferation (colony size) at the same time. Disadvantages include the following: (1) 2–3 weeks before results are available, (2) not every cell line can grow from a single cell, and (3) some cell lines migrate so quickly that the margin of colony is hard to determine. This assay is a good fit when researcher wants to determine the tumorigenic potential of cancer cell.

The anchorage-independent growth assay measures the survival ability of cancer cells when detached from other cells or extracellular matrix (ECM). This process, in which normal cells usually enter anoikis, is a type of programmed cell death (a form of apoptosis) that occurs when cells detach from the ECM. In this assay, cells are embedded in a semi-solid agar medium, in which only transformed or cancerous cells can form colonies [7]. An advantage of the anchorage-independent growth assay is that it can determine the survival ability of cancer cells in an adverse environment by detecting the colony number and size. However, it is procedurally complex, requiring proper training. It can take 2–4 weeks to acquire results. In addition, only a minority of cell lines can grow in soft agar. This assay is best for studies focused on cancer metastasis, because it recaptures the process of cancer cells surviving in the circulation.

Cell Cycle and Apoptosis

Cell viability is summation of cell growth and cell death. For example, increased cell viability could be due to an increase of cell proliferation, or a decrease of cell death, or both. This section summarizes the main approaches to investigate mechanisms of change in cell viability, in which cell cycle analysis mainly characterizes cell proliferation, and apoptosis analysis mainly characterizes cell death.

Cell cycle analysis is a critical tool for understanding cellular behavior, particularly in the contexts of growth and division. In fact, dysregulation of cell cycle pathways is one of the initial steps of carcinogenesis [8]. Identification of changes in progression through the cell cycle is important for evaluating drug efficiency and identifying potential targets of cancer treatment [9]. By staining cells with a DNA dye (such as PI4,6-diamidino-2-phenylindole (DAPI), Hoechst 33258, or Hoechst 33342) and utilizing flow cytometry, scientists can measure the DNA content of individual cells, enabling the determination of the proportion of cells in different phases of the cell cycle. Throughout their life cycle, cells progress through various phases (Fig. 1.2a):

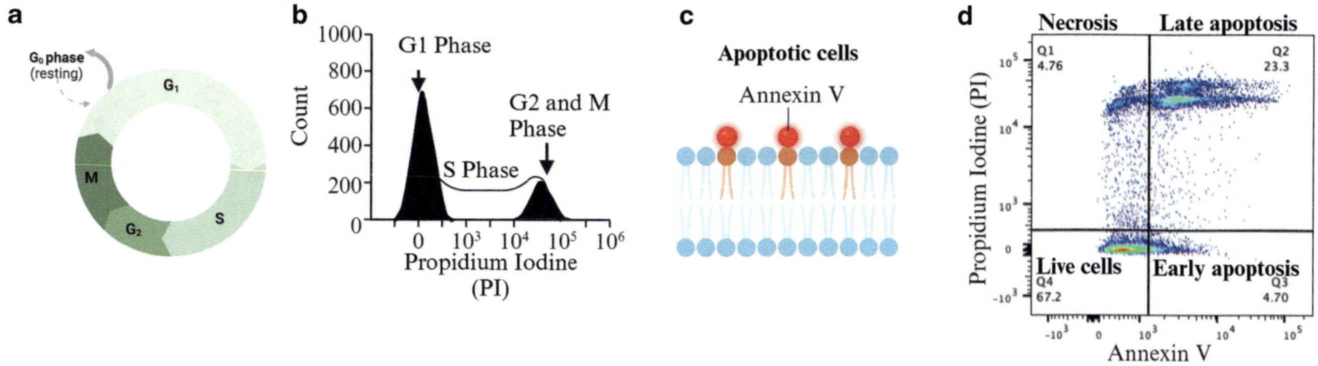

Fig. 1.2 Cell cycle and apoptosis. (**a**) Principle of cell cycle phases. (**b**) Schematic diagram of flow cytometry result of cell cycle analysis. (**c**) Principle of annexin V staining. (**d**) Example of flow cytometry result of annexin V staining to determine cell apoptosis

- G0/G1 Phase: Cells are in the resting or initial growth phase, characterized by a diploid DNA content. For the majority of normal cells, 60 ~ 70% are typically in the G0/G1 phase, whereas cancer cells are usually characterized by a decreased proportion of those in G0/G1 phase, indicating a faster cell cycle.
- S Phase: Cells are actively synthesizing DNA, showing intermediate fluorescence intensity due to partial DNA replication. In normal cells, approximately 15% are in the S phase at any given time, whereas cancer cells usually are characterized by an increased proportion in S phase, indicating active DNA replication.
- G2/M Phase: Cells are in the second growth phase or undergoing mitosis, with double the DNA content compared to the G0/G1 phase. Approximately 10–20% of normal cells are typically in the G2/M phase, whereas the proportion of cancer cells in G2/M phase is likely to be varied and context dependent.
- Sub-G0 Phase: This phase represents apoptotic cells with fragmented or degraded DNA, indicated by fluorescence signals lower than those in the G0/G1 phase.

Apoptosis assays are widely used to measure the number of cells undergoing programmed cell death, a process essential for understanding cancer biology. These assays play a critical role in evaluating the effects of therapeutic drugs and advancing the development of treatments aimed at promoting the efficient elimination of cancer cells through apoptosis [10]. One of the most commonly used approaches for assessing apoptosis involves staining cells with an annexin V-conjugated antibody and a DNA dye such as propidium iodide, followed by flow cytometry analysis [11]. This method is based on the principle that normal cells are hydrophobic and maintain phosphatidylserine on the inner leaflet of the plasma membrane (facing the cytoplasm). During apoptosis, the cell membrane undergoes a "flip-flop," exposing phosphatidylserine on the outer membrane. Annexin V specifically binds to this exposed phosphatidylserine, marking apoptotic cells (Fig. 1.2c). Propidium iodide is a widely used fluorescent dye that binds to DNA by intercalating into the DNA double helix. Its fluorescence intensity is proportional to the DNA content of the cell. Propidium iodide is impermeable to live cells and only stains DNA when the plasma membrane is compromised [12]. As a result, propidium iodide stains necrotic cells, which have lost membrane integrity, allowing the dye to access and bind to their DNA. This dual staining approach enables the clear differentiation between viable, apoptotic, and necrotic cells. The annexin V apoptosis assay is a powerful approach for target identification and drug discovery. Firstly, it can identify pro-apoptotic or anti-apoptotic genes, proteins, and signaling pathways. Secondly, it can evaluate the efficiency of a drug by testing whether the drug can induce cell apoptosis. However, it should be noted that both cell cycle assay and apoptosis assay are highly relied on flow cytometry, which requires either a proper training for the physician-scientist or a strong core facility. Also, the annexin V apoptosis assay is not very efficient for high-throughput drug screening.

Cell Migration and Invasion

Cancer metastasis is the process by which cancer cells spread from a primary tumor to distant organs, leading to secondary tumors. This multistep process includes detachment from the original tumor, migration through surrounding tissues, invasion into blood or lymphatic vessels, and survival in new environments. Migration and invasion assays are instrumental in studying the metastatic potential of cancer cells, offering significant insights into how cells move, interact with their environment, and invade tissues [13]. Here we introduce multiple approaches to comprehensively determine cell migration and invasion in vitro. The wound healing assay (i.e., scratch assay) measures the

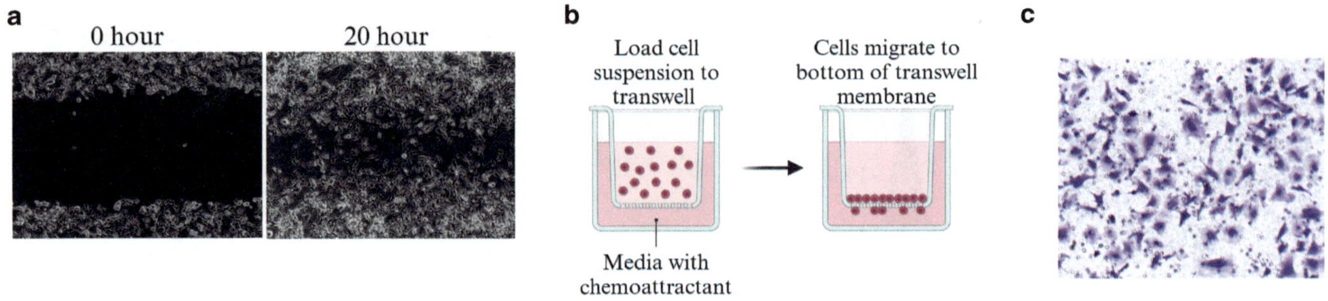

Fig. 1.3 Cell migration and invasion. (**a**) Example image of wound healing assay. (**b**) Schematic diagram (B) and example image (**c**) of transwell assay

migration speed of the cell. The transwell migration assay measures the deformability to squeeze through a pinhole (Fig. 1.3b). The transwell invasion assay is similar to transwell migration assay, but also builds a 3D matrix to measure the capability of degrading the ECM in cancer cells (Fig. 1.3b). These assays are important approaches to identify and validate genes, proteins, and signaling pathways related to cytoskeletal regulation, cell adhesion, ECM remodeling, and other aspects of cell migration and invasion. Moreover, these assays can test if a drug can affect cell motility, adhesion, cytoskeletal rearrangement, or proteolytic activity, and also help researchers study the mechanism of drug resistance.

Several factors must be considered when conducting migration and invasion assays such as selection of appropriate cell lines, which have distinct migration and invasion characteristics, and ensuring the cells are in optimal health and growth phases. Experimental controls are crucial, with positive controls known to migrate or invade well and negative controls used to block migration or invasion pathways. The choice of ECM components is important in invasion assays, as different matrices may affect cell behavior differently. Additionally, proper cell culture conditions, including the type of medium, growth factors, and the density of cells, should be optimized.

Summary and Perspectives

In vitro assays are fundamental tools in cancer biology research, providing a wide variety of techniques to explore key cellular behaviors and mechanisms relevant to tumorigenesis and therapeutic response. These include cell viability assays, such as cell proliferation, low-density colony formation, and soft agar growth that assess cellular growth, clonogenic potential, and anchorage-independent proliferation, respectively. Cell cycle analysis elucidates disruptions in regulatory checkpoints, while apoptosis assays reveal the molecular pathways governing programmed cell death. Migration and invasion assays reveal the cell mobility and invasiveness, indicating their metastatic potential. Drug response studies enable detailed evaluation of therapeutic efficacy and mechanisms of resistance at the cellular level. Together, these approaches offer a robust framework for identifying novel therapeutic targets and dissecting the fundamental processes underlying cancer progression, which pave the way for developing new therapeutic strategies.

Future directions in this field will focus on enhancing the physiological relevance of in vitro models through the adoption of advanced technologies. For example, 3D organoid cultures and patient-derived tumor spheroids offer a more accurate representation of the tumor microenvironment and its complex cellular interactions [14]. High-throughput screening platforms, coupled with CRISPR-based genome editing and multi-omics approaches, will facilitate the identification of novel therapeutic targets and biomarkers [15, 16]. Additionally, live-cell imaging and real-time analysis are poised to provide dynamic insights into cellular processes, capturing temporal events such as metastasis, drug-induced apoptosis, and cell cycle transitions with unparalleled resolution [17]. The integration of these methodologies with machine learning and artificial intelligence will further enable the analysis of large, complex datasets, paving the way for predictive modeling of cancer biology and drug responses. By bridging these innovations with conventional assays, future in vitro studies will be focused on unraveling sophisticated questions in cancer biology, such as tumor heterogeneity, immune-tumor interactions, and adaptive resistance mechanisms, ultimately advancing precision oncology and accelerating the development of next-generation cancer therapies (Fig. 1.4).

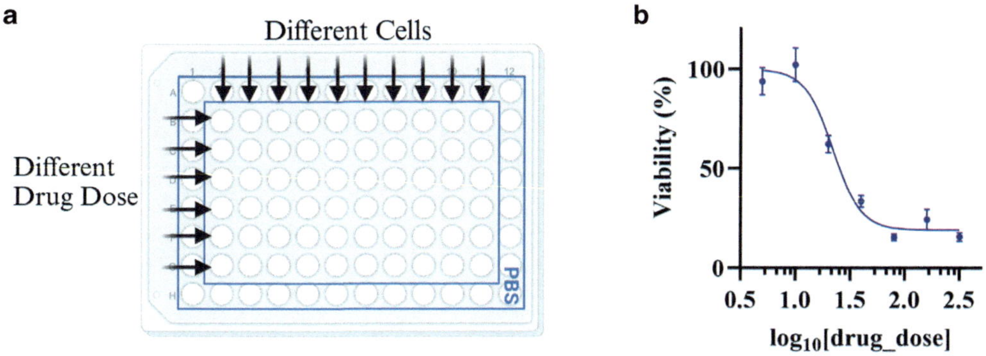

Fig. 1.4 Cell response to drug.(**a**) Arrangement of drug response assay on a 96-well plate.(**b**) Example of cell viability curve of cell response to drug, fitting curve were shown, IC50 = 21.99 nM

References

1. Siegel RL, Giaquinto AN, Jemal A. Cancer statistics, 2024. CA Cancer J Clin. 2024;74(1):12–49.
2. Hanahan D. Hallmarks of cancer: new dimensions. Cancer Discov. 2022;12(1):31–46.
3. Bai L, Zhou H, Xu R, Zhao Y, Chinnaswamy K, McEachern D, et al. A potent and selective small-molecule degrader of STAT3 achieves complete tumor regression in vivo. Cancer Cell. 2019;36(5) 498–511:e17.
4. Escobar-Hoyos LF, Penson A, Kannan R, Cho H, Pan CH, Singh RK, et al. Altered RNA splicing by mutant p53 activates oncogenic RAS signaling in pancreatic cancer. Cancer Cell. 2020;38(2):198–211 e8.
5. Bok I, Vera O, Xu X, Jasani N, Nakamura K, Reff J, et al. A versatile ES cell-based melanoma mouse modeling platform. Cancer Res. 2020;80(4):912–21.
6. Xu X, Bok I, Jasani N, Wang K, Chadourne M, Mecozzi N, et al. PTEN lipid phosphatase activity suppresses melanoma formation by opposing an AKT/mTOR/FRA1 signaling Axis. Cancer Res. 2024;84(3):388–404.
7. Cai J, Li R, Xu X, Zhang L, Lian R, Fang L, et al. CK1alpha suppresses lung tumour growth by stabilizing PTEN and inducing autophagy. Nat Cell Biol. 2018;20(4):465–78.
8. Krabbe LM, Margulis V, Lotan Y. Prognostic role of cell cycle and proliferative markers in clear cell renal cell carcinoma. Urol Clin North Am. 2016;43(1):105–18.
9. Ligasova A, Frydrych I, Koberna K. Basic methods of cell cycle analysis. Int J Mol Sci. 2023;24(4):3674.
10. Carneiro BA, El-Deiry WS. Targeting apoptosis in cancer therapy. Nat Rev Clin Oncol. 2020;17(7):395–417.
11. Kari S, Subramanian K, Altomonte IA, Murugesan A, Yli-Harja O, Kandhavelu M. Programmed cell death detection methods: a systematic review and a categorical comparison. Apoptosis. 2022;27(7–8):482–508.
12. Crowley LC, Scott AP, Marfell BJ, Boughaba JA, Chojnowski G, Waterhouse NJ. Measuring cell death by Propidium iodide uptake and flow cytometry. Cold Spring Harb Protoc. 2016;2016(7)
13. Xu X, Wang K, Vera O, Verma A, Jasani N, Bok I, et al. Gain of chromosome 1q perturbs a competitive endogenous RNA network to promote melanoma metastasis. Cancer Res. 2022;82(17):3016–31.
14. Porter RJ, Murray GI, McLean MH. Current concepts in tumour-derived organoids. Br J Cancer. 2020;123(8):1209–18.
15. Mayoh C, Mao J, Xie J, Tax G, Chow SO, Cadiz R, et al. High-throughput drug screening of primary tumor cells identifies therapeutic strategies for treating children with high-risk cancer. Cancer Res. 2023;83(16):2716–32.
16. Bock C, Datlinger P, Chardon F, Coelho MA, Dong MB, Lawson KA, et al. High-content CRISPR screening. Nat Rev Methods Primers. 2022;2(1):9.
17. Alieva M, Wezenaar AKL, Wehrens EJ, Rios AC. Bridging live-cell imaging and next-generation cancer treatment. Nat Rev Cancer. 2023;23(11):731–45.

In Vivo Study Designs (Animal Model)

2

Margaret A. Park

Background/Introduction

All models are wrong, but some are useful. George E.P. Box, Journal of the American Statistical Association, 1976 [1]

The idea that even imperfect models can be used to investigate facets of the universe is not new and indeed predates the quotation above. Although it was first put into words by a statistician, this concept can be applied to models of all types including animal models of cancer which are discussed in this chapter. Given the fact that no models perfectly recapitulate the real world, care must be taken in model design, model selection, and interpretation of data from these models. The question that a physician-scientist should ask is not: "Is my model true?". It is instead: "Is my model appropriate for the question I would like to answer?"

Most models have advantages (and disadvantages) over other models. For example, the model organism *Drosophila melanogaster* has a very fast breeding time, is inexpensive, and does not require lengthy Institutional Animal Care and Use Committee (IACUC) approvals—a boon that all scientists can appreciate. Nevertheless, their primitive immune and circulatory systems make them an inappropriate model for many tumor microenvironment or metastasis studies. Although there are single-celled organism models of cancer (e.g., yeast), organisms that do not possess organ systems are usually used for potential proto-oncogene/tumor suppressor gene identification [2–4]. These models will not be the focus of this chapter, as they are not considered animals and we wish to focus on translational/clinical models for our clinician audience. We will thus discuss invertebrate models of cancer, followed by vertebrate, nonmammalian models of cancer, and finally mammalian models focusing on rodents.

M. A. Park (✉)
Department of GI Oncology, Department of Biostatistics and Bioinformatics, Moffitt Cancer Center,
Tampa, FL, USA
e-mail: Margaret.park@moffitt.org

Invertebrate Models

C. elegans, *Caenorhabditis elegans*, a soil nematode, is a multicellular worm with a well-characterized genome, making it an attractive model for gene discovery. In addition, this organism has a convenient generation time (~3.5 days) [5], a short lifespan (2–3 weeks), a large number of progeny (300–1000), a transparent body (making it easy to image), and an invariable and fully characterized number of cells in each individual with traceable lineages [5, 6]. Furthermore, *C. elegans* has homologs for ~60–80% of human genes and can be used to study 10 of the 14 "hallmarks of cancer" described by Hanahan and Weinberg (2000) and updated in 2022 [7, 8].

Groups have most often used *C. elegans* as a model of aging as its lifespan and health span are very well defined. Indeed, MTOR, FOXO, ABL1, and the SIRT genes have all been studied in the context of cancer and aging in this organism [9–12]. Nevertheless, *C. elegans* is not an appropriate model for the study of many clinical outcomes due to its simple life cycle, nor is it suitable for studies of tumor size and metastasis. In summary, *C. elegans* is a powerful and convenient model, especially for models where imaging or known cell lineages are important, but is not well-suited for studies that necessitate multi-organ systems.

Drosophila melanogaster The humble fruit fly *D. melanogaster* is a powerful tool for genetic research and has been instrumental in seminal studies that elucidate mechanisms of inheritance and the genetic underpinnings of organism development, two key processes which are also important in cancer progression and initiation [13–15]. Advantages of these animals are that they are convenient, cost- and time-effective, and well-studied. Further enhancing their value as a model is the ease with which genetic mosaics can be generated and visualized (Fig. 2.1) [16, 17].

Genetic mosaicism (a model system where some cells display the mutation or "knockout" and some cells do not) is

J. Huang, H. S.L. Jim (eds.), *Cancer Research Guidance for Clinicians and Researchers*,
https://doi.org/10.1007/978-3-032-19175-5_2

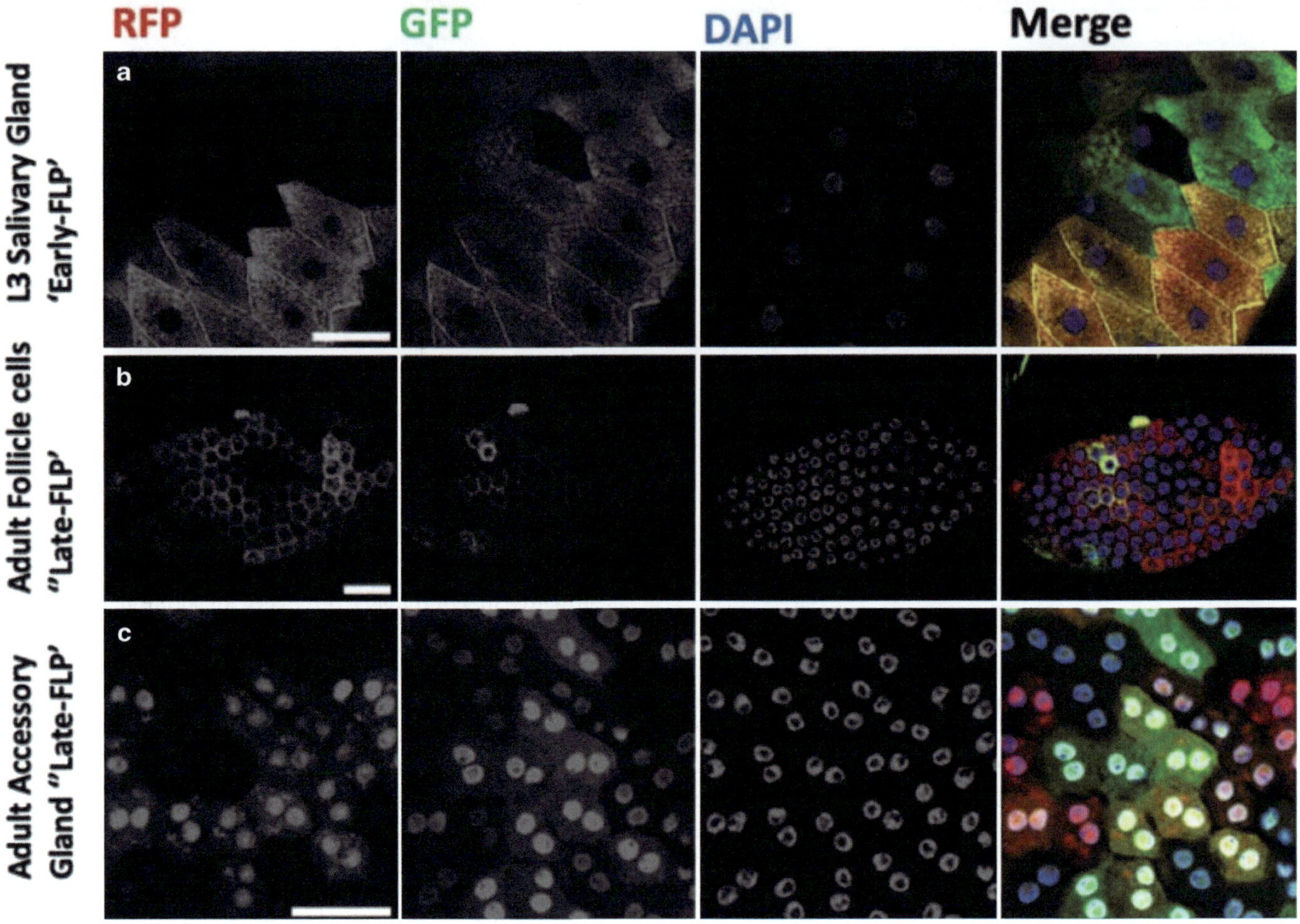

Fig. 2.1 The "CoinFLP" system can label known polyploid cells in *D. melanogaster* larvae as well as adults. (**a**) Larval polytene salivary gland labeled with "early-FLP." (**b**) Adult endocycling vesicles in the female and (**c**) binucleate accessory gland cells in the male labeled with "late-FLP." Scale bars = 100 uM. (Adapted from Nandakumar and Buttitta [17])

somewhat similar to tissue-specific "knockouts" in mice, in the sense that only a targeted subset of the cells in the organism display the genetic change of interest. Mosaicism can occur naturally in both humans and *Drosophila*; however, through the use of the targeted knockout approaches such as the FLP-FRT site-specific recombinase system, mosaics can be induced via the tissue- or cell-specific induction of FLP recombinase expression. Flp is a yeast DNA recombinase that targets specific DNA sequences (FRT sites) for the induction of double-strand breaks and recombination, thereby enabling site-, condition-, and/or cell type-specific knockout of a target gene (see Fig. 2.2). For example, when FLP is put under a heat-shock inducible promotor such as HSP70, recombination can be easily induced via heat shock [16] and can thus be used to induce a genetic change in a desired timeframe. Indeed, many other systems are in use to induce mosaicism in *D. melanogaster*. For example, the Gal4-UAS system (a binary expression system that makes use of the Gal4 transcriptional activator coupled to an upstream activating sequence (UAS) to induce gene expression) can be used for gene-inactivating studies, and the mosaic analysis with repressible cell marker (MARCM, whereby a ubiquitous Gal4-UAS marker is put under the control of an inducible FLP-Frt system which is used to suppress Gal4 only after mitosis—thereby expressing markers in a lineage-specific fashion) system has been utilized extensively for lineage analysis [18]. In the context of research, mosaicism is a powerful way to genetically manipulate an organism such that "wild-type" and "mutant" cells exist in the same organism, allowing researchers to study "knockouts" of genes that would otherwise be lethal.

Another useful aspect of the *D. melanogaster* model is the fact that stocks (lines of *D. melanogaster* which are commonly used for genetic manipulation (e.g., a line carrying FLP under a useful promoter)) and genetic mutants are readily available to the wider research community [19]. Flybase (https://flybase.org/) [20] is a rich resource of available stocks and mosaics, reagents, taxonomy, expression patterns, homologs, and other tools for *D. melanogaster* researchers. Overall, fruit flies can be a useful model to generate a large

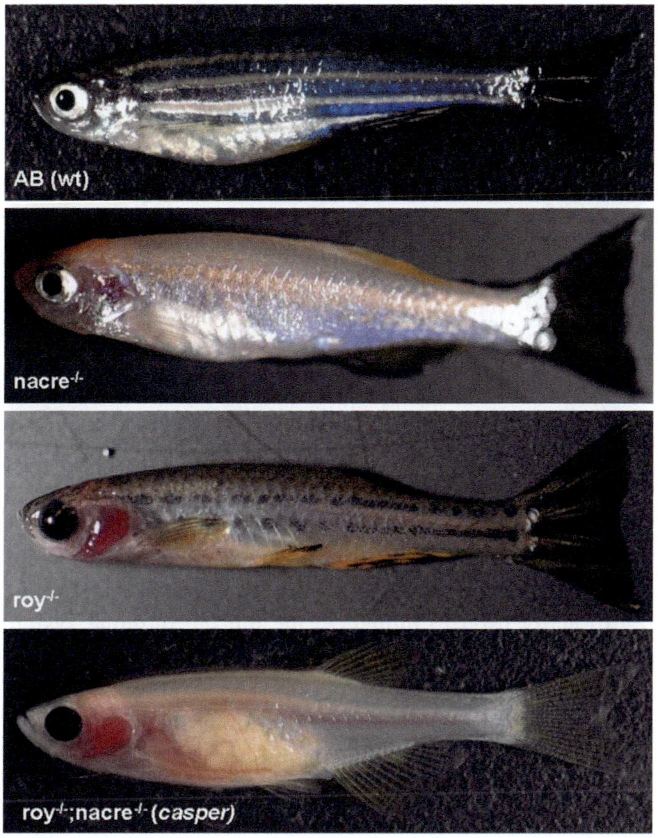

Fig. 2.2 Overview of the Flp-FRT system for a conditional knockout of a gene of interest

amount of data regarding gene function and/or expression in a short time.

Vertebrate Models (Nonmammalian)

***Danio rerio* (Zebrafish)** Similar to more primitive organisms, *Danio rerio* are very amenable to genetic manipulation, are inexpensive to maintain, and have high fecundity, allowing population or phenotype studies to be performed in a short time span (Fig. 2.3). Approximately 82% of disease-related human genes have at least one orthologue in *D. rerio*, making this organism useful for many disease processes including cancer [21]. Although zebrafish are not mammals, they nevertheless have many (albeit rudimentary) organ systems which are similar to humans such as a circulatory system, liver, pancreas, and testicles, which can all develop cancer phenotypes [22]. In addition, similar to *C. elegans*, the "casper" strain of zebrafish is not only transparent at the embryonic and larval stages but also maintains this transparency throughout adulthood [23, 24]. This trait can be useful for imaging fluorescently labeled tissues to assess tumor growth, neovascularization, and metastasis. Further, since *D.*

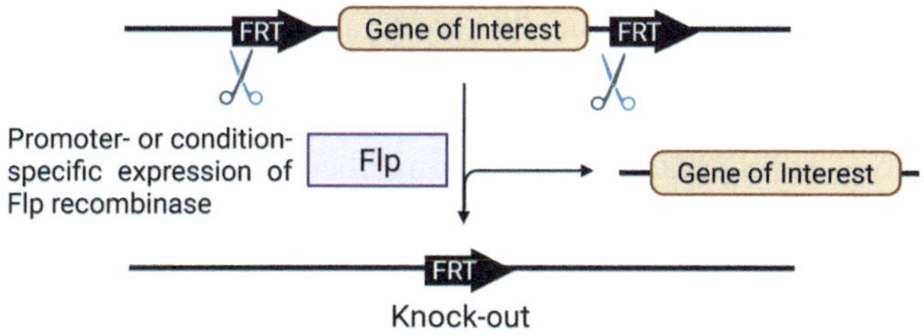

Fig. 2.3 Zebrafish pigmentation mutants exhibit defects in specific neural crest-derived populations. A wild-type zebrafish demonstrates alternating patterns of deeply pigmented stripes comprised largely of melanocytes. The interstripe regions, devoid of melanocytes, contain primarily reflective iridophores and yellowish xanthophores. The *nacre−/−* shows a loss of embryonic and adult melanocytes. The *roy orbison* (roy−/−) mutant shows a severe disruption of melanocyte numbers/patterning, and a complete loss of the iridophore layer. The compound *roy;nacre* double homozygous mutant, *casper*, shows the effect of combined melanocyte and iridophore loss, in which the body of the adult fish is largely transparent due to loss of light absorption and reflection. (Adapted from Fig. 2.1, White et al.)

rerio has an immune system with some similar components to humans, it can be used in tumor microenvironment studies and indeed has been used to assess immune evasion in human/zebrafish xenografts [25]. Due to their high fecundity and the fact that xenograft implantation is possible in this organism, *D. rerio* have also been used in high-throughput screens for precision therapeutics in breast and colon cancer models [26]. Although these screens are recent, they allow for the possibility of this nonmammalian invertebrate to serve as a more ethical replacement for rodents in these types of studies. Some drawbacks of using *D. rerio* as a model are that they are poikilothermic fish and have a preferred temperature of 28 °C, instead of the 32 °C optimal temperature for human cells. Furthermore, their small size limits the available tumor tissue, which may be an issue if downstream analysis requires large amounts of starting material. Overall, *D. rerio* may be an optimal model if high throughput is required.

Xenopus laevis This amphibian has been used as a model for embryonic developmental processes for decades [27]. Like *D. rerio*, *X. laevis* is a fecund and economic model, requires little upkeep, and has a fast breeding cycle. *X. laevis* has been crucial to the discovery and characterization of the neural crest, which can develop melanoma later in life [28]. Because of its short lifespan and its ability to produce numerous offspring, this species has also been used to model neurodevelopmental outcomes after environmental exposure [29]. Finally, this species has a well-defined spatiotemporal apoptotic pattern during embryogenesis and has thus been used extensively to characterize programmed cell death [27]. Although *X. laevis* has many applications in oncology research, there are several drawbacks to using it as a model organism. For example, this species has a tetraploid genome, and it is thus more difficult to create a knockout system than in diploid organisms [27]. To date, xenografts of human tissues have not been successful; thus, other organisms are more appropriate for tumor microenvironment studies. Nevertheless, *X. laevis* continues to make contributions to cancer research as a model organism, especially in the characterization of development and the interactions between development and cancer progression.

Mammalian Models (Rodent)

If any animal can be called "the king of models" in cancer research, it is that of the house mouse *Mus musculus*. This species and its multiple derivative strains continue to be widely utilized as models for almost all phases of cancer initiation and progression. From a practical standpoint, advantages of this species include its relatively small size and fast breeding cycle. From a scientific perspective, mammalian models are in many ways superior to nonmammalian models as they more closely mimic conditions in humans. In general, mouse (and, to a certain extent, rat) models can be divided into two broad and sometimes overlapping subgroups, each with its own advantages and disadvantages. These are xenograft models and genetically engineered mouse models (GEMMs).

Xenograft Models The term xenograft comes from the Greek "xeno-" meaning "foreign" and graft, which refers to inserting a piece of living tissue into another piece of living tissue, originally a way to propagate trees. These powerful models usually make use of an immunocompromised host (the mouse) and either patient-derived tissue or cell lines [30, 31]. Some patient-derived tissue xenograft (PDX) models use a small piece of tumor tissue from a human cancer patient and insert it subcutaneously.

Alternatively, tissue or dissociated cells from a patient of interest can be injected or sutured to an organ of interest, which is called an orthotopic model. These models have the advantage that the tumor grows at a clinically relevant site. However, they can be more technically challenging and expensive than flank models (in which a tumor or cell line is implanted to grow in the flank of the mouse), usually requiring a survival surgery to implant the tumor. The nature of the surgery will depend on the site of interest, but one example of an orthotopic model is that of a lung cancer model developed in 2023 whereby cancer cells of interest are injected into the lung parenchyma [32].

Xenograft models have the advantage of using human tissue or cells, which are more clinically relevant than using rodent cancer tissues. However, they have the drawback of needing the rodent to be immunocompromised in order to successfully implant foreign tissue. A second drawback is the time and effort for regulatory approval required for rodent work. Finally, for patient-derived xenografts, another challenging area is the sometimes low success rate of human tumor engraftment. For example, the success rate of estrogen receptor positive-breast cancer models is reported to be ~50% [33]. Thus, both the monetary and resource costs of these models can be quite high. Furthermore, bias may be introduced as the characteristics of tumors which implant successfully may be different than those which are unsuccessful.

If the clinician/researcher is interested in murine models of immuno-oncology, one way to overcome this limitation is to use "humanized mice." These murine models are usually severely immunodeficient, but have been engrafted with or been genetically modified to contain human immune system components [34]. Either human hematopoietic stem cells (HSCs) or peripheral blood mononuclear cells (PBMCs) are traditionally used to humanize the murine immune system [35]. The use of PBMCs can quickly lead to graft-versus-host disease and is fatal, which limits the experimental timeline for these models. On the other hand, use of HSCs usually requires extensive preconditioning to deplete the host's endogenous immune cells. Variability in donor immune cells can affect experimental outcomes for these models [35], and they have the disadvantage that they lack thymic selection of T-cell populations. However, they have been used in the past to model many aspects of onco-immunology. The most complex method of human immune engraftment involves the implantation of human fetal liver $CD34^+$ HSCs and fetal thymus tissue into severe combined immunodeficiency (SCID) mice, generating the bone marrow, liver, and thymus (or "BLT" mouse), which at least partially overcomes the lack of T-cell selection [35, 36]. Overall, xenograft models, either in immunocompromised or in humanized mice, can be useful tools to model various tumor processes.

Genetically Engineered Mouse Models (GEMMs) The xenograft models discussed in the previous section are an outstanding way to model many aspects of cancer but have the drawback that the disease does not usually have a natural progression in the host. If the clinician-scientist would like to model the genetic and/or environmental underpinnings of disease, then a genetically engineered mouse model (GEMM) may be useful [37]. Mice are usually genetically altered in one of the three ways: (1) retroviral infection during embryonic development; (2) genetic manipulation of murine embryonic stem cells by the use of a construct, a piece of DNA designed to contain a gene or gene fragment of interest and other components which are necessary for that gene to be transcribed and translated into a protein of interest; and (3) microinjection of Cas9 or other constructs into the pronucleus of a fertilized female mouse (see Fig. 2.4); CRISPR

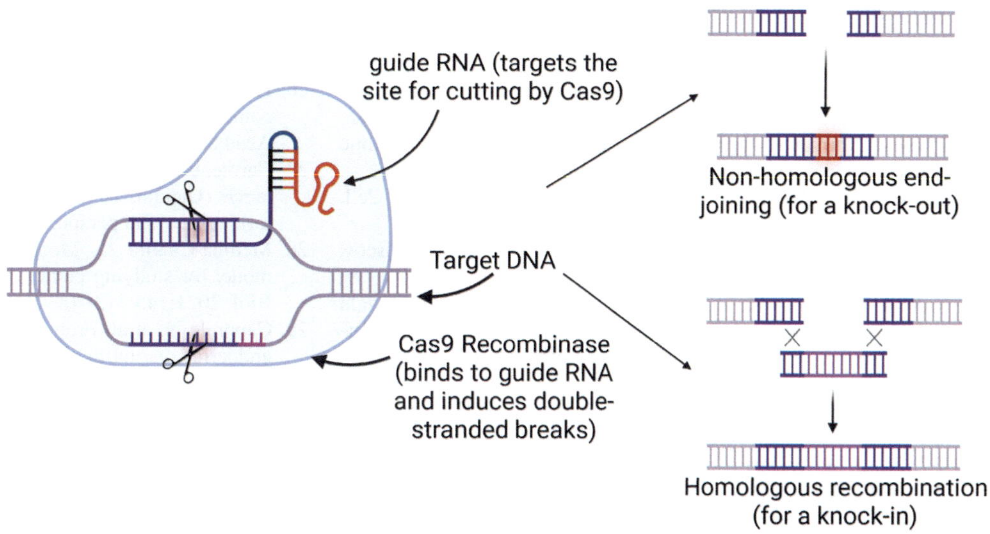

Fig. 2.4 Diagram of the CRISPR-Cas9 system for inducing genetic changes in cells (generated in BioRender)

(clustered regularly interspaced short palindromic repeats)/Cas9 is a relatively easy and precise way to target mutations of deletions of genes in cells instead of entire organisms using enzymes which are part of the bacterial immune system. After genetic manipulation, embryonic stem cells are then injected into a pseudopregnant mouse [38] (a mouse that has been injected with hormones to simulate pregnancy, but that has not been in contact with male mice). Constructs often will be targeted toward a particular organ or cell type using Cre-LoxP (which is very similar to the FLP-Frt system but uses LoxP sequences which are targeted by Cre recombinase) or other targeting systems to ensure development of the cancer type of interest.

In contrast to many xenograft models, GEMMs develop tumors in an immune-competent environment. Thus, they can capture both tumor-specific and environmental factors which influence tumor initiation, development, and progression. Indeed, GEMMs are especially useful when trying to model evolutionary aspects of tumor biology since the murine tumors, like those in humans, arise from a single cell that may undergo many genetic alterations before successful neoplastic transformation [37]. GEMMs are a particularly useful tool to model response to therapy for interventions targeted toward a particular genetic subset of cancer patients [39]. For example, KRAS-driven murine models have been shown to recapitulate human therapeutic response in pancreatic cancers [39], but other drivers and cancer types are more complex to model. Murine drug metabolism is also very different than human and must be taken into consideration when planning these experiments.

Care should be taken to choose the genetic model wisely however, as GEMMs do have some drawbacks. For example, since they arise from a controlled genetic alteration and since tumor growth rate is accelerated in these models, they usually do not display the high mutational burden that human cancers do [40], though some progress has been made in newer models [41]. Thus, researchers who wish to focus on mutational burden in cancer may wish to consider other models such as orthotopic models. Additional drawbacks of GEMMs include the fact that, for cancers with multiple important mutational events during initiation/progression, these do not occur simultaneously in humans, but for a GEMM, all mutations are usually present at birth. Furthermore, the high cost in effort, time, and money to generate, characterize, and validate murine models is a consideration if a new GEMM is being proposed. Nevertheless, GEMMs remain a valuable tool in our arsenal and are ideal for many studies.

Summary and Conclusions

Overall, there are no "perfect" models for cancer research. Cost, effort required, accuracy of the model, and the ability of the model to mimic the mechanism in question are all fair concepts to take into account when choosing a model. As seen in this chapter, a variety of organisms and approaches are available, and the clinician-scientist would be best served by carefully considering multiple models to find the one best suited to their scientific question.

References

1. Box GEP. Science and statistics. J Am Stat Assoc. 1976;71:791–9.
2. Barbari SR, Kane DP, Moore EA, Shcherbakova PV. Functional analysis of cancer-associated DNA Polymerase epsilon variants in Saccharomyces cerevisiae. G3 (Bethesda). 2018;8:1019–29.
3. Li Y, et al. A programmable fate decision landscape underlies single-cell aging in yeast. Science. 2020;369:325–9.

4. Murakumo Y, Sakurai Y, Kato T, Hashimoto H, Ichinoe M. REV7 in cancer biology and management. Cancers (Basel). 2023;15:1721.
5. Kyriakakis E, Markaki M, Tavernarakis N. Caenorhabditis elegans as a model for cancer research. Mol Cell Oncol. 2015;2:e975027.
6. Jones M, Norman M, Tiet AM, Lee J, Lee MH. C. elegans germline as three distinct tumor models. Biol (Basel). 2024;13:425.
7. Hanahan D, Weinberg RA. The hallmarks of cancer. Cell. 2000;100:57–70.
8. Hanahan D. Hallmarks of cancer: new dimensions. Cancer Discov. 2022;12:31–46.
9. Vidovic T, Dakhovnik A, Hrabovskyi O, MacArthur MR, Ewald CY. AI-predicted mTOR inhibitor reduces cancer cell proliferation and extends the lifespan of C. elegans. Int J Mol Sci. 2023;24(9):7850.
10. Sporbeck K, et al. The ABL-MYC axis controls WIPI1-enhanced autophagy in lifespan extension. Commun Biol. 2023;6:872.
11. Qi Z, et al. Sulforaphane promotes C elegans longevity and healthspan via DAF-16/DAF-2 insulin/IGF-1 signaling. Aging (Albany NY). 2021;13:1649–70.
12. Chen C, Zhou M, Ge Y, Wang X. SIRT1 and aging related signaling pathways. Mech Ageing Dev. 2020;187:111215.
13. Charron F, Stein E, Jeong J, McMahon AP, Tessier-Lavigne M. The morphogen sonic hedgehog is an axonal chemoattractant that collaborates with netrin-1 in midline axon guidance. Cell. 2003;113:11–23.
14. Lobo IS, Shaw K. Thomas Hunt Morgan, genetic recombination, and gene mapping. Nat Educ. 2008;1(1):205.
15. Martinez Arias A, Baker NE, Ingham PW. Role of segment polarity genes in the definition and maintenance of cell states in the drosophila embryo. Development. 1988;103:157–70.
16. Germani F, Bergantinos C, Johnston LA. Mosaic analysis in drosophila. Genetics. 2018;208:473–90.
17. Nandakumar S, Buttitta L. Using mosaic cell labeling to visualize Polyploid cells in the drosophila brain. Methods Mol Biol. 2023;2545:413–25.
18. Wong DC, et al. Postembryonic lineages of the drosophila brain: II. Identification of lineage projection patterns based on MARCM clones. Dev Biol. 2013;384:258–89.
19. https://flybase.org/.
20. https://flybase.org/. Accessed 6 Nov 2025
21. Astell KR, Sieger D. Zebrafish in vivo models of cancer and metastasis. Cold Spring Harb Perspect Med. 2020;10(8):a037077.
22. Hason M, Bartunek P. Zebrafish models of cancer-new insights on modeling human cancer in a non-mammalian vertebrate. Genes (Basel). 2019;10:935.
23. White RM, et al. Transparent adult zebrafish as a tool for in vivo transplantation analysis. Cell Stem Cell. 2008;2:183–9.
24. Chen X, Li Y, Yao T, Jia R. Benefits of zebrafish xenograft models in cancer research. Front Cell Dev Biol. 2021;9:616551.
25. Povoa V, et al. Innate immune evasion revealed in a colorectal zebrafish xenograft model. Nat Commun. 2021;12:1156.
26. Fior R, et al. Single-cell functional and chemosensitive profiling of combinatorial colorectal therapy in zebrafish xenografts. Proc Natl Acad Sci USA. 2017;114:E8234–43.
27. Carotenuto R, Pallotta MM, Tussellino M, Fogliano C. Xenopus laevis (Daudin, 1802) as a model organism for bioscience: a historic review and perspective. Biol (Basel). 2023;12:890.
28. Medina-Cuadra L, Monsoro-Burq AH. Xenopus, an emerging model for studying pathologies of the neural crest. Curr Top Dev Biol. 2021;145:313–48.
29. Caporale N, et al. From cohorts to molecules: adverse impacts of endocrine disrupting mixtures. Science. 2022;375:eabe8244.
30. Singhal SS, et al. Recent advancement in breast cancer research: insights from model organisms-mouse models to zebrafish. Cancers (Basel). 2023;15:2961.
31. Liu Y, et al. Patient-derived xenograft models in cancer therapy: technologies and applications. Signal Transduct Target Ther. 2023;8:160.
32. Wilson AN, Chen B, Liu X, Kurie JM, Kim J. A method for orthotopic transplantation of lung cancer in mice. Methods Mol Biol. 2022;2374:231–42.
33. Landis MD, Lehmann BD, Pietenpol JA, Chang JC. Patient-derived breast tumor xenografts facilitating personalized cancer therapy. Breast Cancer Res. 2013;15:201.
34. Chupp DP, et al. A humanized mouse that mounts mature class-switched, hypermutated and neutralizing antibody responses. Nat Immunol. 2024;25:1489–506.
35. Chuprin J, et al. Humanized mouse models for immuno-oncology research. Nat Rev Clin Oncol. 2023;20:192–206.
36. Lockridge JL, et al. Mice engrafted with human fetal thymic tissue and hematopoietic stem cells develop pathology resembling chronic graft-versus-host disease. Biol Blood Marrow Transplant. 2013;19:1310–22.
37. Hill W, Caswell DR, Swanton C. Capturing cancer evolution using genetically engineered mouse models (GEMMs). Trends Cell Biol. 2021;31:1007–18.
38. Lampreht Tratar U, Horvat S, Cemazar M. Transgenic mouse models in cancer research. Front Oncol. 2018;8:268.
39. Singh M, et al. Assessing therapeutic responses in Kras mutant cancers using genetically engineered mouse models. Nat Biotechnol. 2010;28:585–93.
40. McFadden DG, et al. Mutational landscape of EGFR-, MYC-, and Kras-driven genetically engineered mouse models of lung adenocarcinoma. Proc Natl Acad Sci USA. 2016;113:E6409–17.
41. Chung WJ, et al. Kras mutant genetically engineered mouse models of human cancers are genomically heterogeneous. Proc Natl Acad Sci USA. 2017;114:E10947–55.

Case Report and Case Series

3

Lindsey Ammann, Claudia D. Andl, Taseen S. Desin, and Hatem Kaseb

Introduction

In medical research, understanding the spectrum of study designs is crucial for interpreting findings and determining the strength of evidence. In evidence-based medicine, a hierarchy of evidence has been well established (Fig. 3.1). Though multiple versions of an evidence pyramid have been created, each pyramid displays case reports/series at the bottom, case-control and cohort studies in the middle, randomized controlled trials above them, and finally systematic reviews and meta-analysis at the top [1].

Case reports are a "time-honored tradition" with this approach utilized in both old and modern medicine [2, 3]. Many of the diseases we know today were originally reported as case reports with AIDS and Parkinson's disease being classical examples [2]. Case reports/case series are typically recognized as the first step in the field of clinical research. They are primary studies rather than secondary studies. Primary studies typically present firsthand research, while secondary studies focus on analyzing and drawing conclusions. Most of the time clinicians like to present case reports/case series with some form of medical literature review; typically the objective is to highlight how the presented study adds to the current understanding of the disease. High-quality case reports/series should aim to contribute to the expansion of current medical knowledge [2, 3].

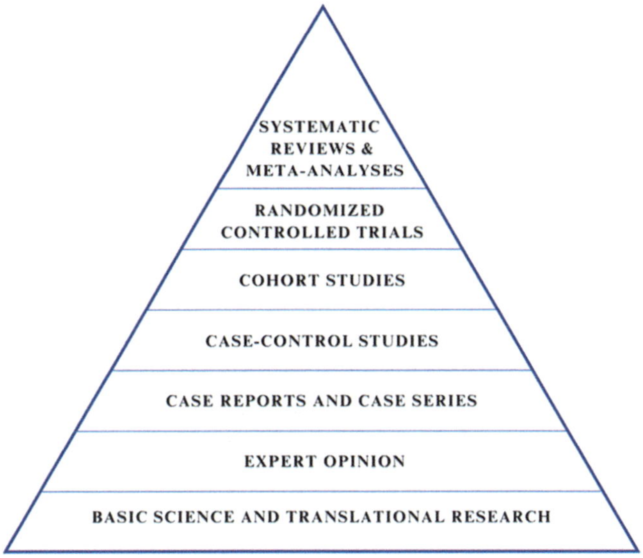

Fig. 3.1 Evidence pyramid [1]

Case reports and case series are recognized as weak scientific evidence, because they mainly report observations [3]. In general, conclusions drawn cannot be applied to clinical practice/clinical intervention; in addition the majority of case reports and series are rarely cited [4, 5]. Another important drawback of case reports/series is publication bias, with the majority of articles focusing on successful rather than failed interventions [6]. However, case reports and case series have several advantages and continue to be published and considered by the majority of medical journals [6]. Firstly, the amount of detail that can be addressed in case reports and case series is significantly more than other types of research such as case/control studies or cross-sectional studies [7]. Secondly, case reports and series are simple and easily understood by trainees, early career scientists, and

L. Ammann
University of Central Florida College of Medicine, Orlando, FL, USA

C. D. Andl
Burnett School of Biomedical Sciences, University of Central Florida College of Medicine, Orlando, FL, USA

T. S. Desin
Department of Medical Education, College of Medicine, UCF, Orlando, FL, USA

H. Kaseb (✉)
Department of Clinical Sciences, Pathology, University of Central Florida College of Medicine, Orlando, FL, USA

Department of Pathology, University of Central Florida Lake Nona Hospital, Orlando, FL, USA
e-mail: hatem.kaseb@ucf.edu

J. Huang, H. S.L. Jim (eds.), *Cancer Research Guidance for Clinicians and Researchers*,
https://doi.org/10.1007/978-3-032-19175-5_3

Table 3.1 Some examples of the role of clinical case reports/series in medical oncological literature

Describe a new phenotype or genotype of disease	Somatic mutations in UBA1 and severe adult-onset autoinflammatory disease leading to discovery of VEXAS [9]
Recognize a known or common manifestation of a rare neoplasm	Identification of rare squamous cell carcinoma in the breast of two individuals using mammography [10]
Recognize a rare manifestation of a common neoplasm	Malignant melanoma arising from a spinal nerve root [11]
Describe a new pathogen (microbe, virus, or environmental exposure) associated with a neoplasm	Detection of Merkel cell carcinoma polyomavirus in mucosal Merkel cell carcinoma [12]
Describe unknown adverse effect of an existing drug	Pembrolizumab-induced giant cell arteritis in the setting of urothelial carcinoma [13]
Describe a novel treatment for a known neoplasm	A new promising treatment for pulmonary sarcomatoid carcinoma—tislelizumab and anlotinib combined with local radiotherapy [14] The use of the use of pembrolizumab in cutaneous SCC [15]
Elucidate the mechanism of a neoplasm	ERCC2-mutated lung adenocarcinoma at the center of a family history of cancer [16] Novel k-ras mutation in colorectal cancer [17] A triple-negative breast cancer diagnosed in a RAD51D mutation carrier [18]

even the general public. This enhances the educational impact of these articles [5]. Thirdly, they can be produced rapidly and are cost-effective relative to other types of research where data collection, analysis, and integrations typically takes several months to years resulting in high costs. Fourthly, case reports and case series remain the main approach for reporting new interventions in rare disorders because randomized clinical trials (RCT) are difficult in this setting [8] (Table 3.1).

Case Reports

Case reports are recognized as the first step in clinical research; they are considered as an integral part of the evidence hierarchy in evidence-based practice [1, 2, 6] (Fig. 3.1). Indeed, case reports are a "time-honored tradition" with this approach utilized in both old and modern medicine [2]. Many of the diseases we know today were originally reported as case reports with sickle cell trait being an excellent example [19]. Despite being in an era marked by discovery and randomized clinical trials, reporting case reports can still have big impacts especially in rare diseases and certain settings such as drug side effects [20, 21]. Case reports are still the basis of case-based conferences, an important approach utilized in graduate medical education today [22]. Overall, case reports have completely different objectives and value than other types of research such as randomized clinical trials [23].

Case reports can generally be classified into two main categories: "diagnosis-related" and "management-related" [3]. The typical objective of a case report/study is to present some unusual/unexpected finding/presentation in an already known disease that should not have been published previously [2]. Other objectives of case reports include new insight on laboratory/radiological diagnosis, pathogenesis, treatment response, and treatment side effects [5]. Currently, the majority of case report focus on highlighting new treatments, rare adverse reactions to treatment, and/or introducing a new use of an available treatment [6]. To hypothesize the possibility of a new disease, a case series would certainly be the first step rather than just a case report.

Writing case reports is a good introductory experience for students, trainees, early healthcare providers, and younger faculty who are learning and exploring the world of clinical research. The main factor that makes a case report unique is the amount of detail that is conveyed in a short format [6]. Additionally, it is essential for authors to regularly review the different factors that serve as guidelines for a high-quality case report [6] (Table 3.3). Among the many guidelines for case reports include the Institution Review Board (IRB) approval especially if this involves an unusual treatment protocol that may or may not require informed consent [3]. Likewise, it is important to highlight that certain institutions require that researchers get an IRB exemption prior to starting the research process. Nevertheless, ensuring patient confidentiality must always remain an important priority [5].

Like all other types of clinical research, a case report should clearly address the three general research questions: (1) Why was the study needed? (2) What was the research design? (3) Was the research design appropriate to the question? [7]. Of these three questions, "Why was the study needed?" should be addressed clearly in the introduction and sometimes even in the title of the paper; the reader should be able to clearly identify the test hypothesis from reading the introduction. Having a clear introduction explaining the current status of the disease and how the study answers or adds to the current literature through the testing of the hypothesis should be evident. Moreover, like other types of clinical research, a case report/case study could address more than one test hypothesis. Traditionally research papers are presented as follows: introduction, methods, results, and discussion sections (IMRAD) [20]. However, case reports are typically presented as a story with the following typical components: introduction, case description/presentation, and a discussion [5] (Table 3.2). A case report should discuss in detail the patient's presentation, management, and outcome [24]. Starting with the article title, it should be concise and informative; long detailed titles should be avoided [3]. The word "case report" should be included in the title to increase visibility on medical database search engines [3]. The abstract should be focused and concise (preferably under 350 words or in accordance with journal requirements) and should clearly introduce the clinical question/problem [5]. The introduction section should provide background to the current knowledge and understanding of the disease/condition in the context of the research question, supported by a focused relevant literature review [2, 3, 5]. The case presentation section is a critical component of any case report. It should be detailed and in chronological order; authors should not omit information and then discuss it in the discussion section to make the case interesting. Clear and detailed patient demographics, clinical history, physical examination findings, laboratory/radiological results, differential diagnosis, management, follow-up, and final diagnosis should be presented [3, 5]. Like other types of articles, the discussion section is the most important part of the article and should focus on why the case report is innovative, how it answers the question of the study, and how it contrasts to our current knowledge [2, 5]. Connecting the results to the current literature is perhaps the most important aspect that should be addressed in the discussion. The discussion section is also a great place to include any case limitations if any that should be considered [5]. Overall, having a fluent story in enough detail and chronological order with a well-structured discussion section is the basic component of a case report/study.

In 2011–2012, an international panel of experts, including clinicians, researchers, and journal editors, created the CAse REport (CARE) Statement and Checklist, a consensus-based guideline designed to enhance the transparency and thoroughness of published case reports [25]. This guideline offered a structured format for reporting patient cases, ensuring that relevant details such as the clinical presentation, diagnostic methods, treatment, and outcomes are clearly documented. By standardizing these reports, CARE facilitates better communication between healthcare professionals, supports evidence-based practice, and helps integrate individual patient cases into broader medical research, which is particularly valuable for rare diseases or unique presentations. Factors that could help in improving the quality of the case report include having a clear clinical message, having enough educational content, employing appropriate tables/figures when necessary, being concise and focused, and doing an extensive literature review before starting the writing process (Table 3.3) [5, 21]. Additionally, the researcher should determine whether this condition or new finding has been reported before. If the case has been reported, the researcher should not proceed and consider other educational/research opportunities. Trainees and younger faculty should not just proceed with writing a case report because of the increased pressure to publish; this is indeed a significant issue [23]. The graduate educators should guide novice writers to expand skills aligned with the six competencies set forth by the American College of Graduate Medical Education and consequently improve the quality of case reports. Case reports should advance medical knowledge and at the same time provide significant education value as the writers apply skills in areas of critical thinking, problem-solving, as well as communication in general [26].

Case reports can be considered a "hybrid narrative," serving dual medical and humanistic importance [26]. Cancer medications, unlike other treatments, can be approved with minimal clinical trial data, such as Phase II or non-randomized trials, and they may also receive "conditional" approval, subject to additional evidence from Phase III trials [27]. For cancer and certain patient groups, case reports might represent the only available evidence until post-marketing surveillance is carried out or larger observational studies are completed after randomized controlled trials [28]. An important example of how case reports can be valuable in the field of oncology is how the use of pembrolizumab was

Table 3.2 Highlights of a case report

Title should be brief, concise, specific, and descriptive
Case reports are written in "introduction, case presentation, and discussion" format
Introduction: Describe the disease/condition and the hypothesis
Case description/presentation: Should be detailed and in chronological order
Discussion section should connect the results to the current literature
Quality case reports definitely could contribute to the medical knowledge about the disease

Table 3.3 Important factors for writing high-quality case reports

Thorough detail	Include clear patient demographics, clinical history, examination findings, diagnosis, investigations, management, and if available follow-up
Structured format	Follow CARE guidelines: Abstract, introduction, case presentation, discussion
Relevant literature review	Compare findings to existing studies and explain their significance
Educational content	Focus on the educational value for trainees and professionals
Ethical considerations	Ensure informed consent and patient confidentiality
Concise writing	Avoid unnecessary details; focus on clinical and educational relevance
Use of figures/ tables	Include clear visuals to improve clarity and highlight key points
Innovation	Highlight unique findings, treatments, or associations that contribute to knowledge

expanded. Pembrolizumab was a first-in-class programmed death protein 1 (PD-1) inhibitor initially approved by the US Food and Drug Administration (FDA) for unresectable melanoma; a case report on its off-label use in an unresectable cutaneous squamous cell carcinoma highlighted the potential for further clinical trials of pembrolizumab in other cases of cutaneous squamous cell carcinoma [15]. This case report successfully inspired further clinical trials for use of pembrolizumab in squamous cell cancer and is now listed as an approved FDA indication. This case report and others show how treatment options can be broadened and how similar research can shape future therapeutic strategies.

Currently, several journals seem hesitant to publish case reports since it is the weakest form of scientific evidence and can even lead to a reduction in the journal impact factor because case reports are rarely cited [5, 6, 20, 23]; thereby many journals consider a case series as the minimum clinical research that could have potential value for its readers; this was associated with the creation of many journals that focus on case reports. For example, the American College of Gastroenterology (ACG) spectrum of journals still includes ACG case reports in its list of journals. Unfortunately, the gap and the need for case reports in journals has been filled by numerous "predatory/questionable" journals that focus on publication fees [23]. These journals are typically open access, with more than half of them not indexed in PubMed or assigned a Thomson Reuters impact factor [23]. Many medical schools and medical training programs still encourage there trainees to write case reports as an evidence of research productivity [20]. Taken together, it appears that requesting students and new trainees to collaborate and work together to write a systematic review may be more beneficial toward a preliminary start to their research career rather than engaging in a case report that is suboptimal in quality.

Case Series

A case series continues to be, and will remain, a vital approach in clinical research and was certainly the backbone of medical literature in the twentieth century where a lot of medical diseases were described [8, 29, 30]. While case reports and case series share a similar methodology mainly focusing on generating new hypothesis, a case series is typically reserved when cases reported are more than three [8]. Certainly the value of case series is stronger than case reports, because in case series, a narrative or quantitative synthesis is possible [30]. Case series are commonly published for reporting rare diseases, novel treatments, and minority health issues, as well as in situations like drug side effects and health crises, such as the coronavirus pandemic, where rapid dissemination of information is critical [4, 8, 21]. Furthermore, the value of case series has been and remains significant as many of the major diseases we know today began as case series. For instance, the genetic basis of leukemias was first described by Nowell in 1967 when he reported that leukemia exhibited abnormal chromosomes [31]. Dr. Janet Rowley, a young cytogeneticist at the time, later built on these findings and published a case series confirming that leukemias, such as chronic myeloid leukemia (CML), are caused by genetic translocations [32]. The combined efforts of these two groups launched the field of cancer genetics and were the first in establishing the role of genetics in neoplasms and malignancies in general. Therefore, it is imperative that we recognize how the aforementioned case series were the basis for major outcomes and advancements in the field of medicine. Likewise, a recent example that illustrates the value of a case series in reporting new diseases is the report by Beck et al., where the group presented VEXAS syndrome, a new prototype of "hematoinflammatory diseases" by presenting it in a case series of 25 patients [9]. Taken together, this further demonstrates that case series continue to play a promising role in the medical research.

While case series design may overlap with some other types of clinical research, there is some inconsistency of what constitutes a case series in medical literature, because of the similarity to some cohort studies and/or quasi-experimental designs, such as before-and-after studies; however, there is a consensus that these studies are "observational, descriptive and non-comparative and typically lack randomization or experimental interventions" [29]. Like case reports, case series are descriptive, but they involve broader patient populations and can help identify patterns or associations between exposure and outcome [33]. In general, a case series expands on the case report by including multiple patients (>3) with similar clinical presentations, diagnoses, or treatments without a control group. These cases are typically collected retrospectively based on prevalence without randomization; however, a consecutive inclusion criterion is generally favored [29, 30, 33]. Case series are typically initiated when a pattern emerges across several patients. They are especially valuable when randomized controlled trials are impractical, due to either the rarity of the condition or ethical considerations [29].

Case series are valuable in early-stage research, providing preliminary data that can form the basis for more robust studies like cohort studies or clinical trials. They can reveal trends in disease progression or response to treatment. Like case reports, case series are valuable for studying rare diseases and publishing early signals that can alert the medical community to watch for similar cases [8]. When high-quality experimental studies, such as randomized controlled trials, are scarce, case series can serve as the best available evidence to guide clinical practice, as they offer valuable insights into the effectiveness and safety of interventions [29].

An ideal case series will have a clear methodology, well-articulated study protocol, and consistent data collection across all cases (Table 3.4) [8]. The case collection should have clear inclusion criteria, standardized reliable measurement criteria, and clear acceptable approach for disease diagnosis and/or management [29]. It should also provide an analysis of the similarities and differences among the cases and be transparent about potential biases. Authors should always put attention to de-identify individuals to protect the patient's privacy [8]. A suboptimal case series might present inconsistent or incomplete data, lack analysis, or draw inappropriate conclusions about causality without sufficient evidence. In general, case series tend to have some disadvantages that include selection bias, insufficient follow-up period, and limited prospects of generalizability [8]. Yet, they are particularly useful for novel observations and publishing early signals that can inform the medical community to be vigilant for similar cases. An important example of how case series can be valuable in the field of oncology is how breast-associated anaplastic lymphoma with lymph node metastasis was examined by Ferrufino-Schmidt et al. [34]. The study looked carefully at this cohort describing clearly the patterns of metastasis and the prognosis [34]. This study was well designed with clear outcome points assessed and limited bias [34]. Another important example of how case series can be valuable in the field of oncology is how lymphoepithelioma-like carcinoma (LELC) was discovered in 1991 [35]. Scientists when assessing some undifferentiated gastric carcinomas identified a rare type of carcinoma resembling nasopharyngeal cancer, with nearly all tested samples showing Epstein-Barr virus (EBV) positivity [35]. This case series of eight patients with undifferentiated gastric carcinoma and EBV positivity was reclassified as lymphoepithelioma-like carcinoma (LELC). These findings highlight how case series can help in establishing new disease categories/entities, uncover disease associations in cancer, and help guide further research into disease mechanisms and treatment strategies in oncology research. Case series like this are crucial for identifying novel risk factors, mechanisms, or trends that may otherwise be overlooked in larger studies.

Table 3.4 Important factors for writing high-quality case series [33]

Clear study objective/question Well-defined study protocol	Define the study's purpose/research questions explicitly
Clear inclusion/exclusion criteria	Clear and reasonable
Sampling	Clear and specified Specify sampling method Specified time interval for patient recruitment Consecutive patient enrollment
Selection of variables of interest with sufficient clinical detail	Clearly defined and clinically relevant interventions, complications, adverse events, and outcomes Clinically relevant outcomes Prospective outcome data collection High follow-up rate
Systematic collection of data and robust analysis	Relevant statistical analysis and clear discussion section

Summary

Case reports and case series are essential components of medical literature, particularly in the field of oncology. Case reports/series still play an essential role in the dissemination of knowledge in medicine [24]. They document individual patient cases, allowing clinicians to observe rare cancers, unique presentations, and unexpected responses to treatments. Case reports/series typically present weak evidence because changes in clinical practice typically need larger and/or multicentric studies. However, they still offer many advantages especially in identifying rare side effects and/or in identifying new uses of some current medications [6]. In oncology, where treatment approaches are increasingly personalized, case reports can provide valuable insights into the effectiveness of therapies for specific patient populations. They can highlight novel therapeutic strategies, reveal unexpected side effects, and help refine existing treatment protocols. By offering detailed patient histories and clinical outcomes, case reports and series inform clinical decision-making and stimulate further research. Ultimately, the findings from case reports and case series can lead to the formulation of new hypotheses and pave the way for larger clinical trials, making them foundational for advancing cancer research and improving patient care. In the setting of evidence based learning, case reports and case series present an opportunity to acquire experience in competencies such as critical thinking, problem-solving, and decision-making. In conclusion, these types of studies will remain a vital part of our research literature, particularly when they are well-articulated and adhere to the highest standards of medical writing quality.

Competing Interests and Funding None

References

1. Murad MH, Asi N, Alsawas M, Alahdab F. New evidence pyramid. Evid Based Med. 2016;21(4):125–7.
2. Rison RA. A guide to writing case reports for the journal of medical case reports and BioMed central research notes. J Med Case Rep. 2013;7:239.
3. Erol A. Basics of writing case reports. Noro Psikiyatr Ars. 2023;60(1):1–2.

4. Suvvari TK. Are case reports valuable? Exploring their role in evidence based medicine and patient care. World J Clin Cases. 2024;12(24):5452–5.
5. Sun Z. Tips for writing a case report for the novice author. J Med Radiat Sci. 2013;60(3):108–13.
6. Albrecht J, Werth VP, Bigby M. The role of case reports in evidence-based practice, with suggestions for improving their reporting. J Am Acad Dermatol. 2009;60(3):412–8.
7. Greenhalgh T. How to read a paper: the basics of evidence-based medicine. In: How to read a paper: the basics of evidence-based medicine. Blackwell Publishing; 2010.
8. Colwill M, Baillie S, Pollok R, Poullis A. Using clinical cases to guide healthcare. World J Clin Cases. 2024;12(9):1555–9.
9. Beck DB, Ferrada MA, Sikora KA, Ombrello AK, Collins JC, Pei W, et al. Somatic mutations in UBA1 and severe adult-onset autoinflammatory disease. N Engl J Med. 2020;383(27):2628–38.
10. Yoneto T, Hasumi K, Yoshimoto T, Takahashi N, Takeda Y. Case report: two cases of extremely rare primary pure squamous cell carcinoma of the breast. Medicine (Baltimore). 2018;97(37):e12340.
11. Naing A, Messina JL, Vrionis FR, Daud AI. Uncommon manifestations of common malignancies: case 3. malignant melanoma arising from a spinal nerve root. J Clin Oncol. 2004;22(15):3194–5.
12. Wu KN, McCue PA, Berger A, Spiegel JR, Wang ZX, Witkiewicz AK. Detection of Merkel cell carcinoma polyomavirus in mucosal Merkel cell carcinoma. Int J Surg Pathol. 2010;18(5):342–6.
13. Miano DI, Cosgrove R, Sherman J, Balaraman S, Sherman M. Pembrolizumab-induced Giant cell arteritis in the setting of urothelial carcinoma. Neuroophthalmology. 2023;47(2):93–9.
14. Cai R, Liu Y, Sha H, Yu J, Fang Y, Zhou G, Shen B. A case report: a new promising treatment for pulmonary sarcomatoid carcinoma – Tislelizumab and Anlotinib combined with local radiotherapy. Heliyon. 2023;9(11):e21902.
15. Chang AL, Kim J, Luciano R, Sullivan-Chang L, Colevas AD. A case report of Unresectable cutaneous squamous cell carcinoma responsive to Pembrolizumab, a programmed cell death protein 1 inhibitor. JAMA Dermatol. 2016;152(1):106–8.
16. Liu L, Cui J, Liu S, Pan E, Sun L. Case report: lung adenocarcinoma associated with germline ERCC2 frameshift mutation. Front Oncol. 2023;13:1177942.
17. Palmirotta R, Savonarola A, Formica V, Ludovici G, Del Monte G, Roselli M, Guadagni F. A novel K-ras mutation in colorectal cancer. a case report and literature review. Anticancer Res. 2009;29(8):3369–74.
18. Baker JL, Schwab RB, Wallace AM, Madlensky L. Breast cancer in a RAD51D mutation carrier: case report and review of the literature. Clin Breast Cancer. 2015;15(1):e71–5.
19. Herrick JB. Peculiar elongated and sickle-shaped red blood corpuscles in a case of severe anemia. Arch Intern Med (Chic). 1910;VI(5):517–21.
20. Weinstein R. Writing scientific case reports for top-line journals. J Clin Apher. 2021;36(3):465–9.
21. Bhattacharrya S, Miller J, Ropper AH. The case for case reports. Ann Neurol. 2014;76(4):484–6.
22. Pierson DJ. How to read a case report (or teaching case of the month). Respir Care. 2009;54(10):1372–8.
23. Akers KG. New journals for publishing medical case reports. J Med Libr Assoc. 2016;104(2):146–9.
24. Chait R, Donini G, Flynn MG. A guide to writing quality case reports. HCA Healthc J Med. 2023;4(1):61–8.
25. Gagnier JJ, Kienle G, Altman DG, Moher D, Sox H, Riley D. The CARE guidelines: consensus-based clinical case reporting guideline development. Glob Adv Health Med. 2013;2(5):38–43.
26. Sayre JW, Toklu HZ, Ye F, Mazza J, Yale S. Case reports, case series – from clinical practice to evidence-based medicine in graduate medical education. Cureus. 2017;9(8):e1546.
27. Gracia-Ramos AE. Writing case reports and series: tricks, traps, and triumphs! Indian J Rheumatol. 2022;17(Suppl 2):S306–S13.
28. Packer CD, Katz RB, Iacopetti CL, Krimmel JD, Singh MK. A case suspended in time: the educational value of case reports. Acad Med. 2017;92(2):152–6.
29. Munn Z, Barker TH, Moola S, Tufanaru C, Stern C, McArthur A, et al. Methodological quality of case series studies: an introduction to the JBI critical appraisal tool. JBI Evidence Synthesis. 2020;18(10):2127–33.
30. Murad MH, Sultan S, Haffar S, Bazerbachi F. Methodological quality and synthesis of case series and case reports. BMJ Evid Based Med. 2018;23(2):60–3.
31. Nowell P, Hungerford D. A minute chromosome in human chronic granulocytic. Leukemia Sci. 1960;132:1497.
32. Rowley JD. Letter: a new consistent chromosomal abnormality in chronic myelogenous leukaemia identified by quinacrine fluorescence and Giemsa staining. Nature. 1973;243(5405):290–3.
33. Torres-Duque CA, Patino CM, Ferreira JC. Case series: an essential study design to build knowledge and pose hypotheses for rare and new diseases. J Bras Pneumol. 2020;46(4):e20200389.
34. Ferrufino-Schmidt MC, Medeiros LJ, Liu H, Clemens MW, Hunt KK, Laurent C, et al. Clinicopathologic features and prognostic impact of lymph node involvement in patients with breast implant-associated anaplastic large cell lymphoma. Am J Surg Pathol. 2018;42(3):293–305.
35. Shibata D, Tokunaga M, Uemura Y, Sato E, Tanaka S, Weiss LM. Association of Epstein-Barr virus with undifferentiated gastric carcinomas with intense lymphoid infiltration. Lymphoepithelioma-like carcinoma. Am J Pathol. 1991;139(3):469–74.

Observational Studies: Cross-sectional, Longitudinal Designs, Case-Control, and Cohort Studies

4

Ranjita Poudel

Background

Observational studies are non-interventional studies where the investigator records, but does not manipulate, study variables in real-world settings [1]. Observational studies are widely used in medical research to generate hypotheses and/or to examine patterns and associations between variables. However, they cannot establish a cause-and-effect relationship (Table 4.1). Different types of observational studies include cross-sectional, case-control, longitudinal, and cohort studies (Table 4.1 and Fig. 4.1). In cross-sectional studies, investigators simultaneously assess the dependent variable (e.g., outcome) and the independent variable (e.g., exposure) in the study participants and examine the relationship between them [2]. Similarly, in a case-control design, the participants are selected based on their outcome status and compared with participants without outcome status (referred to as cases [i.e., with outcome] and controls [i.e., without outcome]) to evaluate the association between exposure and outcomes [3]. Likewise, longitudinal studies assess the relationship between the risk factor and the outcome (e.g., disease development) by recording repeated measures from the same participants over time [4]. Lastly, cohort studies are special cases of longitudinal studies that examine the incidence, cause, or prognosis among participants with similar characteristics by following them over time [5].

Observational studies can be instrumental in cancer research with their utility ranging from identifying cancer etiologies to describing patient outcomes [6]. They can be used to examine the risk factors of various cancers (e.g., what genetic, environmental, and lifestyle factor is associated with an increased likelihood of developing cancer?) as well as to assess the prevalence and incidence of cancer in a particular group (e.g., race, gender, geography, age group) [7]. Observational designs can also determine the prognostic factors, including biomarkers or comorbidities, to predict cancer progression or risk stratification [8]. Another important use case of the observational method is investigating real-world drug efficacy by examining treatment outcomes for standard or off-label drugs [9]. Additionally, behavioral and psychosocial studies use these designs to explore the quality of life (QOL) and psychological effects of cancer diagnosis and long-term treatment effects on survivors [10, 11].

While randomized controlled trials (RCTs) are considered the gold standard for evaluating the safety and causal efficacy of an intervention, observational designs can investigate the real-world application (i.e., long-term effects, population dynamics), complementing clinical trials process in all phases (phases I–IV) [12, 13]. For phase I, observational designs can be used to obtain data to inform trial design and patient selection by providing baseline epidemiological data, disease progression, and identification of patient populations that may benefit from the treatment. Phase II studies are designed to assess preliminary efficacy and adverse effects. Observational studies can be used to describe adverse effects associated with an intervention and identify subgroups with differential responses to inform stratification. They can also be used to determine the prognostic factors by exploring the association with biomarkers and participant characteristics.

Phase III of a clinical trial aims to determine rare side effects and long-term outcomes in the real world as a foundation for regulatory approval that may not be apparent in a controlled environment. Observational studies are critical during phase III to bridge the gap between the controlled setting and real-world application. Additionally, observational designs are less prone to selection bias and are crucial for assessing treatment outcomes in populations often underrepresented in the RCTs (e.g., specific age groups, minority populations, and race) [6, 14]. Phase IV clinical trials detect rare

R. Poudel (✉)
Department of Health Outcomes and Behavior, Moffitt Cancer Center, Tampa, FL, USA
e-mail: ranjita.poudel@moffitt.org

J. Huang, H. S.L. Jim (eds.), *Cancer Research Guidance for Clinicians and Researchers*,
https://doi.org/10.1007/978-3-032-19175-5_4

adverse events, assess long-term outcomes, and evaluate efficacy in routine clinical practice. Phase IV is conducted post-regulatory approval, and observational studies are critical in monitoring adverse effects that are especially long-term and not obvious during earlier phases [15]. Moreover, observational studies can explore patterns of real-world intervention use (e.g., adherence, variation in dosing, etc.) and assess cost-effectiveness and healthcare utilization to inform optimal resource allocation and care delivery [16, 17].

Observational studies are widely applied in various domains beyond therapeutic interventions, including prevention, screening, and supportive care. Regarding cancer prevention, observational studies can evaluate the effectiveness of behavioral interventions or vaccines [18] in the real world in diverse populations. Likewise, real-world uptake, accuracy, and prognosis can be established using these designs to provide evidence-based guidelines for cancer screening [19]. They can also explore the impact of interventions on symptom management, QOL, and palliative care that address the needs of cancer patients, survivors, and caregivers [20, 21]. This chapter will further discuss types of observational studies in detail.

Cross-Sectional Studies

Cross-sectional studies simultaneously measure the dependent variable (i.e., outcome) and independent variable (i.e., exposure/risk) and evaluate the relationship between them. This design can only provide a measure of association between the variables and cannot establish a causal relationship. Participant selection is based on study inclusion and exclusion criteria, unlike in case-control (i.e., participants are selected based on outcome status) and cohort studies (i.e., participants are selected based on exposure status) (Table 4.1). Cross-sectional studies can either be descriptive or analytical. Descriptive cross-sectional studies characterize the prevalence of one or multiple health outcomes/diseases in a specified population. In contrast, analytical cross-sectional studies examine the relationship between exposure and outcome and provide preliminary evidence of causal relationships [2].

If data are collected in the same target population at different time points, then the subtype of the cross-sectional study is called a repeated (or serial) cross-sectional study (Fig. 4.1). Unlike in the longitudinal study (i.e., repeated

Table 4.1 Comparison of observational studies

Category	Cross-sectional	Case-control	Longitudinal/cohort
Participants	Selection is based on study inclusion/ exclusion criteria	Selection is based on the presence/ absence of the outcome	Selection is based on presence/absence of exposure
Design	The exposure and outcome are simultaneously measured	Exposure in both case and control groups is assessed	Repeated measures are collected over time; types include: Prospective Retrospective
Analysis	Prevalence rate Odds ratio Logistic regression models	Odds ratio Logistic regression models	Incidence ratio and rate ANOVA/MANOVA Advanced modeling methods – cox regression, survival analysis, fixed and random effects models
Strengths	Low cost and temporal requirement Can be used as a baseline in cohort studies Hypothesis-generating Ethical constraints are limited	Relatively low cost and temporal need compared to cohort studies (prospective) Useful to study rare outcomes and outcomes with long latent periods Study multiple exposures in the same outcome Hypothesis-generating	The temporality between exposure and outcome is well-defined Study multiple exposures and outcomes Study rare exposure Hypothesis-generating High generalizability
Limitations	Cannot establish a causal relationship Biases: selection, survival	Not useful to study rare exposures Cannot estimate incidence or prevalence Choice of a control group can be difficult Biases: selection, recall	Time-consuming and costly Not efficient for rare outcomes Biases: selection, attrition
Reporting	Strengthening the Reporting of Observational Studies in Epidemiology (STROBE) Transparent Reporting of a Multivariable Prediction Model for Individual Prognosis or Diagnosis (TRIPOD)	Strengthening the Reporting of Observational Studies in Epidemiology (STROBE)	Strengthening the Reporting of Observational Studies in Epidemiology (STROBE) Critical Appraisal Skills Programme (CASP) Consolidated Standards of Reporting Trials (CONSORT)

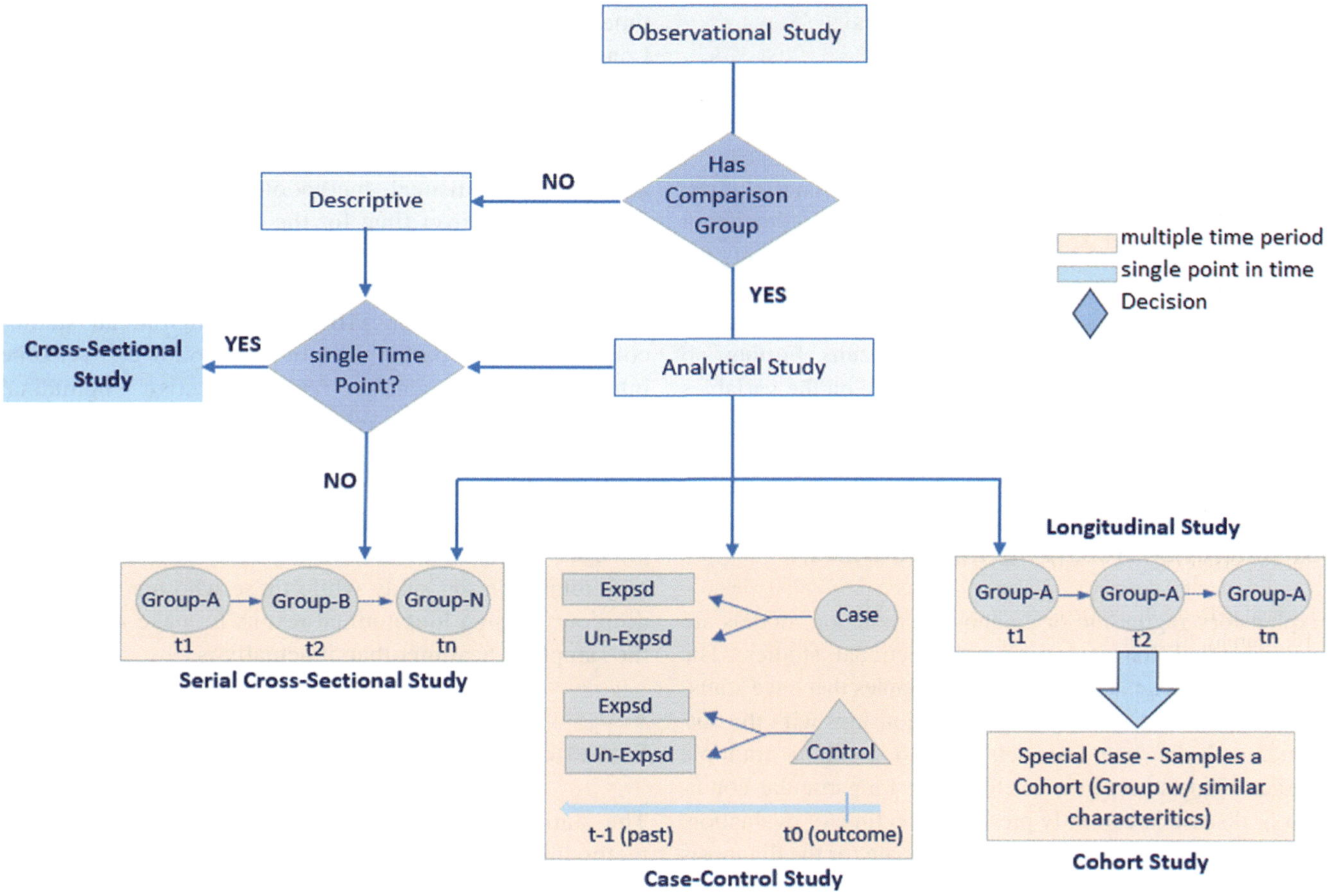

Fig. 4.1 Overview of observational studies

measure is collected from the same individual over time), data is collected from different individuals in the target population at each time point. Thus, repeated or serial cross-sectional studies can be used to analyze change over time in a given population.

Statistical Analysis (Cross-Sectional Studies)

Cross-sectional study designs can be used for population-based surveys, to estimate the prevalence in clinical studies, and to calculate odds ratios (ORs) [2, 22]. In cross-sectional studies, it is common to use descriptive and bivariate analyses, such as chi-square tests, *t*-tests, and correlations, to explore associations between variables. Similarly, analytical cross-sectional studies seek to simultaneously evaluate the relationship between an independent variable (exposure) and a dependent variable (outcome) in a specific population. The participants are initially selected from a population based on the inclusion and exclusion criteria established in the study without considering exposure (independent variable) or outcome status (dependent variable). Once the study population is assembled, exposure and outcomes are evaluated simultaneously and classified for analysis. The measures of association called prevalence odds ratio (POR) and prevalence ratio (PR) are calculated. The mathematical calculations for the POR and PR are the same as those for the OR and risk ratio (RR). However, the interpretation differs, given that this design measures the prevalence or "proportion of cases" within the sample rather than the actual risk of disease development over time [2, 22].

Strengths of Cross-Sectional Studies

Cross-sectional studies are usually faster and inexpensive and can be conducted as a baseline in a cohort study. They are best suited to generate hypotheses and may provide information about the prevalence of outcomes and exposure that may inform study design. They can also study the associations of multiple exposures and outcomes. Since the subjects are rarely exposed or treated, ethical constraints are limited.

Weakness of Cross-Sectional Studies

Cross-sectional studies are prone to biases which are incorrect estimates of the true effect of an exposure or risk on an outcome. Selection and information biases are broad categories of biases [22] inherent to the cross-sectional studies. Selection bias is a distortion of the measure of association when the sample used in the study no longer represents the overall population. Similarly, information bias (e.g., recall and detection) occurs due to inaccurate measurement of study variables and/or interpretation of results. Further, no information regarding the influence of time on the variables measured is available for these designs.

Ethical, Methodologic, and/or Statistical Considerations (Cross-Sectional Studies)

Explanatory regression or diagnostic prediction models are recommended for analytical cross-sectional studies. The explanatory model aims to identify variables that have statistically significant and meaningful relationships with the outcome, and diagnostic models aim to combine multiple predictors to estimate the likelihood that a particular condition or disease is currently present at the time of evaluation, essentially providing a probability estimate for the diagnosis [22]. When a large number of variables are present, and variable selection methods are needed, backward elimination with the Akaike information criteria is recommended for cross-sectional studies [23]. However, stepwise selection methods and P value-based criteria are discouraged because their results may be unique to a given sample (i.e., overfitting) and uncharacteristic of the larger population (i.e., ungeneralizable). Some form of validation (e.g., cross-validation in a new sample or bootstrapping by randomly dividing the original sample into smaller subsamples) is recommended for diagnostic prediction models [24].

It is recommended that cross-sectional studies are reported following the Strengthening the Reporting of Observational Studies in Epidemiology (STROBE) statement containing a checklist of 22 items [25] to improve the assessment of its strengths, weaknesses, and generalizability. Similarly, the Transparent Reporting of a Multivariable Prediction Model for Individual Prognosis or Diagnosis (TRIPOD) statement is recommended if a diagnostic prediction model is used (Table 4.1) [23, 24].

Longitudinal Observational Studies

Longitudinal study designs evaluate continuous or repeated measures data from the same participants over a period of time without any external influence (Fig. 4.1) [4]. Longitudinal designs are primarily observational in nature, but they can also be experimental. They are useful for examining the relationship between risk factors, disease development, and/or health outcomes over time. Appropriate statistical methodologies are required to address change over time for the whole group as well as for particular individuals within longitudinal studies [26]. These studies can be broadly classified into prospective and retrospective [27]. Prospective longitudinal studies collect data from participants that are followed over time into the future. In contrast, for retrospective longitudinal studies, data relating to relevant events or outcomes have already been collected [27]. Since participant follow-up is crucial in longitudinal studies, missing data and bias due to attrition is a major limitation. For example, among longitudinal samples of cancer patients, healthier patients may remain in the study while those who are sicker may drop out, biasing longitudinal results to make it seem that the sample is healthier than it actually is.

Statistical Analyses (Longitudinal Studies)

The statistical analysis of longitudinal studies requires methodologies that take into consideration several factors, including the correlation between repeated measures collected from the same participant, the coexistence of fixed and dynamic variables, and the presence of missing data. Analysis of variance/multivariate analysis of variance (ANOVA/MANOVA), mixed-effect regression models, and generalized estimating equation (GEE) models are some of the commonly applied statistical approaches to analyze data from longitudinal studies [28]. ANOVA/MANOVA compares means (obscuring individual-level variability), assuming equal interval lengths and normal data distribution in all groups. In contrast, the mixed-effect regression model is an individual-level approach that focuses specifically on how continuous outcomes change over time while considering individual differences taking into account fixed effects (i.e., factors that apply to the entire population) and random effects (i.e., individual-level variability). Similarly, GEE is a population-level approach that provides population-averaged estimates of independent variables and dichotomous outcomes. This method is useful when the primary interest is in the population-average exposure effect and is less restrictive, compared to mixed models, regarding the correlation structure between repeated measures [29]. Other statistical considerations for longitudinal analysis include time-to-event analysis and Cox proportional hazards regression [30].

Strengths of Longitudinal Studies

Longitudinal studies allow researchers to follow changes over time in particular individuals in the population, capturing the development and progression of disease. Additionally, when conducted prospectively, the temporality between exposure and outcome is well-defined, which helps determine the sequence of events and potential causal relationships between variables. Similarly, prospective studies also exclude recall bias among participants.

Weaknesses of Longitudinal Studies

Longitudinal study designs are inherently associated with numerous challenges, such as increased financial and temporal demand associated with this approach [4] Another major challenge includes missing data as a result of incomplete and interrupted follow-up and attrition over time. Similarly, the potential for inaccuracy in addressing the intraindividual correlation of measures exists. It is difficult to separate the reciprocal impact of exposure and outcome, typically considering the potentiation between the two and when the induction period between the exposure and onset is extended.

Ethical, Methodologic, and/or Statistical Considerations (Longitudinal Studies)

Given the protracted nature of the longitudinal studies, one of the major challenges associated with these studies is missing data as a result of loss to follow-up and attrition [31]. Statistical techniques including multiple imputations or maximum likelihood estimation are widely used to address missing data [32]. Similarly, controlling for potential confounding variables through adjustment in the statistical model is crucial in observational studies. In a longitudinal analysis, inaccuracies also commonly arise if repeated hypothesis testing is employed as in cross-sectional studies. Repeated testing could lead to an underutilization of available data and underestimation of variability, which results in an increased likelihood of type II errors (false negative) [33].

Several tools are recommended for critical appraisal of longitudinal studies to ensure the believability and usefulness of a particular study [34]. The Critical Appraisal Skills Programme (CASP) [35] offers a series of tools and checklists designed to facilitate the evaluation of the scientific quality of given literature that may be extrapolated to critically assess a proposed study design. Additional depth of quality assessment is available through the use of various tools developed alongside the Consolidated Standards of Reporting Trials (CONSORT) guidelines [36], including structured 33-point guidelines for reporting observational longitudinal studies (Table 4.1) [37].

Longitudinal research has extensive financial and temporal needs. In multisite longitudinal studies, identical and standardized methods across sites are required to facilitate the accuracy of collected data. Numerous confounding variables must be considered and adequately controlled, including factors related to the population and their environment. Stability in terms of geographical mobility and distribution, coupled with an ability to continue to follow up remotely in case of displacement, is crucial. Specific ethical and consent considerations are needed to minimize attrition and ensure maximal participant retention.

Case-Control Observational Studies

In case-control studies, participant selection is based on the outcome status, and participants either have the outcome (referred to as cases) or do not have the outcome (referred to as controls). Exposure is then assessed in both these groups, and the association between exposure and outcome is examined. When defining cases in this design, the criteria for determining a disease and/or outcome should be as specific as possible. Furthermore, the control group should be matched explicitly from the same study base as the cases. Matching is a sampling technique where the cases and controls are selected from an underlying cohort such that they have the same or similar distributions of some characteristics [38]. Compared to prospective cohort studies, case-control studies can be conducted relatively faster and are inexpensive. While these designs could be specifically useful to study rare outcomes with long latent periods, they are not very useful for studying rare exposures. Selection bias and recall bias are the major limitations of case-control designs.

Selection of Cases and Controls

The selection of the cases and controls is an important part of case-control studies. Recommendations on the selection of control include that all comparisons are made within the study base, the comparison of effects of exposure on risk of disease should not be distorted by the effect of other factors (deconfounding), and any errors in measurement of exposure should be nondifferential between cases and controls (comparable accuracy) [39–41].

The cases should be defined as specifically as possible. Study inclusion and exclusion criteria must be predefined before selecting cases to ensure data homogeneity. If a case is determined based on multiple criteria, all these criteria should be explicitly stated. While selecting controls, a critical aspect is that they should be from the same "study base" as the cases. That is, the pool of population from which the cases and controls will be enrolled should be the same. Moreover, the measurement of exposure in cases and controls should be conducted similarly or equivalently.

Controls can be selected from various groups, including the general population, relatives or friends, and hospital patients. Population controls can be easily recruited from the state or hospital registry list. Various sampling methods (e.g., random multistage sampling and random digit dialing) are used to recruit population controls. While the population controls can be expensive, time-consuming, and not inclined to participate (i.e., low response rate), a main advantage is that these controls satisfy the "study base" as recommended by Wacholder and colleagues [39–41]. Patients attending the hospital for disease rather than the outcome of interest can be used as hospital controls. Hospital controls are easy to recruit and are more likely to have similar clinical characteristics. Relative and friend controls are comparatively easy to recruit. They can be particularly useful to ensure that some measurable and nonmeasurable confounders (such as demographics, socioeconomic status, or genetic factors) are equally distributed in cases and controls. However, they are also more likely to have similar behaviors (alcohol use, smoking, etc.); thus, it may not be prudent to use these as controls if we want to study the effect of these exposures on the outcomes.

Statistical Analyses (Case-Control Studies)

Case-control studies typically utilize the logistic regression method and OR to determine how strongly an event/exposure is associated with the outcome [42]. Unmatched case-control studies are typically analyzed using a Mantel-Haenszel method or unconditional logistic regression. In a matched case-control study, controlling for the matching should be considered during the analysis [43].

Matching in Case-Control Studies

Matching is a sampling technique used in case-control studies to ensure that the cases and controls have similar distributions of some characteristics. Matching is useful for increasing the efficiency of the study by avoiding confounding and improving the statistical and cost efficiency [38]. The limitations of matching include increased temporal and financial demands of finding a matching control, selection bias as a result of inappropriate matching, and requirement of statistical methods that can account for actual matching protocol and residual confounding effects [44].

Strengths of Case-Control Studies

Compared to prospective cohort studies, case-control studies have relatively low financial and temporal requirements. Case-control studies are helpful to study rare outcomes and outcomes with long latent periods as well as to study multiple exposures in the same outcome [45].

Weakness of Case-Control Design Studies

These designs are not suitable for studying rare exposures. Additionally, the incidence or prevalence cannot be estimated in a case-control design since the investigators predetermined the number of cases and controls. The proportion of cases may not be representative of the proportion in the population [38]. For instance, the proportion will be determined by the ratio of matching (e.g., if 50 cases were matched with 50 controls, the prevalence of a condition in the cases would be 50%) and does not represent true prevalence. Likewise, case-control studies are prone to recall and selection bias. Recall bias may occur when participants cannot recall all exposures accurately. Similarly, selection bias occurs if the cases and controls are not selected similarly from the study base.

Ethical, Methodologic, and/or Statistical Considerations (Case-Control Studies)

Given the retrospective nature of the case-control studies where participants already have the outcome, the primary ethical consideration is to ensure data is collected fairly (i.e., informed consent where possible) and without bias. Similarly, statistical analysis and methodological tools that address the biases (e.g., selection and recall bias), appropriately match cases and controls, and control for potential confounding variables in the analysis, including controlling for matching, should be selected. Reporting of Observational Studies in Epidemiology (STROBE) is recommended for reporting case-control observational studies (Table 4.1) to improve the transparency of the methods and facilitate critical appraisal of the study [46].

Cohort Studies

A cohort study is a special case of longitudinal study where a cohort is followed over time (Fig. 4.1). A cohort is a group of individuals who share similar characteristics or experiences and are included in the study based on the researcher's definition (e.g., a cohort of people of certain ages, a cohort of people who smoke, etc.). In a cohort study design, participants are selected based on their exposure status at the time of study initiation and followed over time to evaluate the occurrence of the outcome. It is an efficient method to study the relationship between exposure and outcomes in rare exposure to provide evidence suggesting causality [5]. Though the participants do not have an outcome at the time of assignment, the temporality of exposure and outcome is well-defined in this study design. Over the follow-up period, the outcome of interest between the exposed and unexposed groups is compared. In the cohort study, statistical analysis involves measuring incidence rate, cumulative incidence, relative risk, and hazard ratio using advanced modeling techniques (fixed and random effects models) [5]. Attrition and loss to follow-up are some of the biases implicit in cohort studies.

Cohort studies can be prospective, retrospective, or both. In a prospective cohort study, data are collected prospectively. First, the cohort population is defined, followed by a measurement of the potential exposure of interest. The participants are then classified as exposed or unexposed and followed up over time. At baseline and during follow-up, outcome variables and other variables (e.g., confounding variables) are collected. Outcome variables may only occur once (e.g., death) and/or may occur multiple times (e.g., hospitalization, cancer diagnosis). On the other hand, a retrospective cohort study utilizes preexisting data from records to examine the relationship between exposure and outcome. While the outcomes have already occurred, the study design would be the same. The investigator first identifies a cohort with shared characters and divides the cohort into an exposed and non-exposed group. The exposure and other variables are measured at baseline, and the outcome is determined during the follow-up period. However, in some cases, there may not be a clear distinction between prospective and retrospective directions. Retrospective data can be analyzed for a group of people while also collecting prospective data from the same participants.

Other types of cohort studies include multiple cohort studies and nested case-control studies. Multiple cohort study is helpful when we need to compare the outcomes in two or more groups of individuals. Exposure, outcome, and other variables must be measured similarly in both the study and the comparison groups. Similarly, a nested case-control study is a case-control study within a cohort study. At the beginning of the study, cohort members are assessed for risk factors. Subsequently, cases and controls are identified at time t1. The control group is selected from cohort members who do not meet the case definition at t1. This procedure maintains the temporal strength of the cohort study.

Statistical Analysis (Cohort Studies)

Statistical methods for cohort studies primarily aim to calculate incidence rates while allowing the calculation of cumulative risk, hazard ratios, and relative risks. Various statistical methods, including regression models and Cox proportional hazard models for time-to-event data, are utilized to analyze cohort study data. Prognostic or predictive models can be used to establish the association between exposure and outcomes. Statistical methods for cohort studies must also take into consideration the biases that are inherent to this design. A major source of bias in the cohort studies is the loss of follow-up, which impacts the internal validity of the study. An acceptable rate of loss to follow-up depends on the population being studied but ideally should be 20% or less of the total sample [5]. Another challenge in a cohort study is confounding, and appropriate statistical methods such as restriction, stratification, multivariable regression analysis, and propensity score methods should be utilized to control for confounding variables [5].

Strengths of Cohort Studies

Cohort design is instrumental for studying rare exposure, as it can efficiently study the relationship between exposure and outcomes. Since participants do not have an outcome of interest at the study initiation, the temporality between exposure and outcomes is well-defined. A cohort study can be useful for multiple outcomes in the same exposure. In a prospective cohort study, the exposure variable, other variables (confounding), and outcomes may be measured more accurately, which maintains uniformity in exposure and outcome measurements. These designs are also less prone to bias such as recall bias. Compared to a prospective study, a retrospective cohort study is helpful in studying rare exposures, is time-efficient and cost-effective, and has fewer ethical concerns. They can be more efficient for diseases with long latency periods (e.g., unusual occupational exposures).

Weakness of Cohort Studies

Prospective cohort design can be time-consuming and costly. Cohort studies may be inefficient in studying rare outcomes. Biases related to losses to follow-up can skew the measure of association. For a retrospective cohort study, the exposure and outcome variables are collected before the study has been initiated; therefore, the measurements may not be accurate or meet the study's requirements (e.g., exposures may have been assessed differently for various cohort members). Similarly, inadequate data may be available regarding exposure and other confounding factors.

Ethical, Methodologic, and/or Statistical Considerations (Cohort Studies)

Follow-up of the study participants is very important in a cohort study, and losses are an important source of bias. Some patients are lost to follow-up in large cohorts; however, if the proportions are high (>20%), this impacts the validity of the results [5]. Lost to follow-up becomes more important if it relates to the exposure or outcome of interest. Thus, managing follow-ups and minimizing losses are important components of a cohort study design.

Reporting of the cohort studies is recommended following the Strengthening the Reporting of Observational Studies in Epidemiology (STROBE) statement containing 22 items that are considered essential for reporting observational studies [46]. In case of the development of multivariate prognostic models, reporting should follow Transparent Reporting of a Multivariable Prediction Model for Individual Prognosis or Diagnosis (TRIPOD) statements (Table 4.1) [23, 24].

Example I One of the prominent case-control studies includes the examination of the role of the bacterium (*Helicobacter pylori*) in gastric cancer etiology [47]. This paper utilized a case-control design to study diseases with long latency periods (i.e., gastric cancer). Patients (n = 186) with gastric cancer (cases) were matched according to age, sex, and race with subjects (n = 186) without gastric cancer (control). This study was conducted in a large, well-defined cohort with minimal selection bias. It focused on the serological evidence of past *H. pylori* infection among patients and compared them with controls who did not have the infection. Confounding variables such as age, gender, and socioeconomic status that potentially influence gastric cancer were controlled. This study used appropriate statistical methods to assess the relationship between *H. pylori* infection and gastric cancer, including OR, and performed sensitivity analysis. The findings from this study established *H. pylori* as a risk factor for cancer and catalyzed global efforts to recognize this bacterium as a carcinogen (i.e., WHO's decision to classify *H. pylori* as a Class 1 carcinogen) [48] and led to important changes in public health policies focused on *H. pylori* screening and eradication programs.

Example II The Nurses' Health Study (NHS) is a longitudinal project that investigates the long-term effects of diet and lifestyle factors (diet, physical activity, smoking, and hormone use) on the incidence and mortality rates of cancer. Nurses' Health Study (NHS) and the Nurses' Health Study II (NHS II) are among the largest prospective investigations into the risk factors for major chronic diseases in women, also called one of the most significant studies ever conducted on women's health. The original focus of the study was on contraceptive methods, smoking, cancer, and heart disease. Still, it expanded over time to include research on many other lifestyle factors, including behaviors, personal characteristics, and more than 30 diseases, including cardiovascular disease, type 2 diabetes, osteoporosis, hypertension, obesity, and metabolic syndrome. This study is methodologically strong given the large cohort (started with 121,700 registered nurses) providing ample statistical power. Data are collected from validated and reliable measures such as pathology reports, medical records, validated assessment tools, genetic testing, etc. Given the large sample, the study provides the potential for subgroup analysis control for confounders and increased generalizability. Regarding cancer research and global impact, the NHS has provided some of the most compelling evidence on the role of dietary patterns in cancer development, such as colorectal cancer [49] and established risk factors for breast cancer [50, 51]. The NHS study findings have provided data that influence screening and early detection of cancers (e.g., breast and colorectal cancer) and have been cited in global cancer research, influencing cancer epidemiology and public health policy around the world.

Summary

Observational studies in cancer research are feasible alternatives to RCTs when RCTs are unethical or not feasible. While observational studies are used to generate hypotheses, establish associations, and examine patterns between the variables, they cannot establish causation. Observational study designs include cross-sectional, case-control, longitudinal, and cohort studies. These study designs are widely utilized in a naturalistic setting to infer insights that may not be possible in a controlled environment. Numerous biases are implicit in these designs including selection bias, recall bias, and attrition bias, which impact the validity of these studies. Advanced analytical and methodological techniques are required to address these biases. Further, the use of real-world data (e.g., electronic health records (EHRs), genomic data, behavioral data, and digital health technologies) can be leveraged to improve the validity of these studies. As observational research evolves, adherence to standard reporting frameworks, such as STROBE guidelines, CONSORT framework, and open science practices, is critical for enhancing transparency and reproducibility and advancing their scope and impact.

Acknowledgment RP was supported by Ruth L. Kirschstein Institutional National Research Service Award at H. Lee Moffitt Cancer Center and Research Institute [T32 CA090314; MPIs: S. T. Vadaparampil and V.N. Simmons].

References

1. Gilmartin-Thomas JF, Liew D, Hopper I. Observational studies and their utility for practice. Aust Prescr. 2018;41(3):82.
2. Capili B. Cross-sectional studies. AJN Am J Nurs. 2021;121(10):59–62.
3. Karunarathna I, De Alvis K, Gunasena P, Jayawardana A. Designing and conducting clinical research: methodological approaches. ResearchGate https://www researchgate net/publication …; 2024.
4. Caruana EJ, Roman M, Hernández-Sánchez J, Solli P. Longitudinal studies. J Thorac Dis. 2015;7(11):E537.
5. Wang X, Kattan MW. Cohort studies: design, analysis, and reporting. Chest. 2020;158(1):S72–S8.
6. Visvanathan K, Levit LA, Raghavan D, Hudis CA, Wong S, Dueck A, et al. Untapped potential of observational research to inform clinical decision making: American Society of Clinical Oncology research statement. J Clin Oncol. 2017;35(16):1845–54.
7. Khadhouri S, Gallagher KM, MacKenzie KR, Shah TT, Gao C, Moore S, et al. The IDENTIFY study: the investigation and detection of urological neoplasia in patients referred with suspected urinary tract cancer–a multicentre observational study. BJU Int. 2021;128(4):440–50.
8. Pizzuti L, Krasniqi E, Mandoj C, Marinelli D, Sergi D, Capomolla E, et al. Observational multicenter study on the prognostic relevance of coagulation activation in risk assessment and stratification in locally advanced breast cancer. Outline of the ARIAS trial. Cancers (Basel). 2020;12(4):849.
9. Beaulieu-Jones BK, Finlayson SG, Yuan W, Altman RB, Kohane IS, Prasad V, et al. Examining the use of real-world evidence in the regulatory process. Clin Pharmacol Ther. 2020;107(4): 843–52.
10. Joly F, Ahmed-Lecheheb D, Kalbacher E, Heutte N, Clarisse B, Grellard J, et al. Long-term fatigue and quality of life among epithelial ovarian cancer survivors: a GINECO case/control VIVROVAIRE I study. Ann Oncol. 2019;30(5):845–52.
11. Khorana AA, Tullio K, Elson P, Pennell NA, Grobmyer SR, Kalady MF, et al. Time to initial cancer treatment in the United States and association with survival over time: an observational study. PLoS One. 2019;14(3):e0213209.
12. Price D, Bateman ED, Chisholm A, Papadopoulos NG, Bosnic-Anticevich S, Pizzichini E, et al. Complementing the randomized controlled trial evidence base. Evolution not revolution. Ann Am Thorac Soc. 2014;11(Supplement 2):S92–S8.
13. Le-Rademacher J, Gunn H, Yao X, Schaid DJ. Clinical trials overview: from explanatory to pragmatic clinical trials. In: Mayo Clinic Proceedings. Elsevier; 2023.
14. Sharma M, Nazareth I, Petersen I. Observational studies of treatment effectiveness: worthwhile or worthless? Clin Epidemiol. 2018;11:35–42.
15. Suvarna V. Phase IV of drug development. Perspect Clin Res. 2010;1(2):57–60.
16. Merino Almazán M, Duarte Pérez JM, Marín Pozo JF, Ortega Granados AL, Muros De Fuentes B, Quesada Sanz P, et al. A multicentre observational study of the effectiveness, safety and economic impact of nivolumab on non-small-cell lung cancer in real clinical practice. Int J Clin Pharm. 2019;41:272–9.
17. Gao Y, Goldberg JE, Young TK, Babb JS, Moy L, Heller SL. Breast cancer screening in high-risk men: a 12-year longitudinal observational study of male breast imaging utilization and outcomes. Radiology. 2019;293(2):282–91.
18. Monin L, Laing AG, Muñoz-Ruiz M, McKenzie DR, Del Barrio IDM, Alaguthurai T, et al. Safety and immunogenicity of one versus two doses of the COVID-19 vaccine BNT162b2 for patients with cancer: interim analysis of a prospective observational study. Lancet Oncol. 2021;22(6):765–78.
19. Inturrisi F, Aitken CA, Melchers WJ, van den Brule AJ, Molijn A, Hinrichs JW, et al. Clinical performance of high-risk HPV testing on self-samples versus clinician samples in routine primary HPV screening in the Netherlands: an observational study. Lancet Reg Health Eur. 2021;11
20. Sewtz C, Muscheites W, Grosse-Thie C, Kriesen U, Leithaeuser M, Glaeser D, et al. Longitudinal observation of anxiety and depression among palliative care cancer patients. Ann Palliat Med. 2021;10(4):3836846–3846.
21. Kirk DL, Kabdebo I, Whitehead L. Prevalence of distress and its associated factors among caregivers of people diagnosed with cancer: a cross-sectional study. J Clin Nurs. 2022;31(23–24):3402–13.
22. Wang X, Cheng Z. Cross-sectional studies: strengths, weaknesses, and recommendations. Chest. 2020;158(1):S65–71.
23. Moons KG, Altman DG, Reitsma JB, Ioannidis JP, Macaskill P, Steyerberg EW, et al. Transparent reporting of a multivariable prediction model for individual prognosis or diagnosis (TRIPOD): explanation and elaboration. Ann Intern Med. 2015;162(1):W1–W73.
24. Collins GS, Reitsma JB, Altman DG, Moons KG. Transparent reporting of a multivariable prediction model for individual prognosis or diagnosis (TRIPOD) the TRIPOD statement. Circulation. 2015;131(2):211–9.
25. Von Elm E, Altman DG, Egger M, Pocock SJ, Gøtzsche PC, Vandenbroucke JP. The strengthening the reporting of observational studies in epidemiology (STROBE) statement: guidelines for reporting observational studies. Lancet. 2007;370(9596):1453–7.
26. Fitzmaurice GM, Laird NM, Ware JH. Applied longitudinal analysis. John Wiley & Sons; 2012.
27. Chavez-Rivera AD, Inostroza-Nieves Y, Hemal K, Chen W. Longitudinal study: design, measures, and classic example. In: Translational Surgery. Elsevier; 2023. p. 223–6.
28. Schober P, Vetter TR. Repeated measures designs and analysis of longitudinal data: if at first you do not succeed—try, try again. Anesth Analg. 2018;127(2):569–75.
29. Ito T, Sugasawa S. Grouped generalized estimating equations for longitudinal data analysis. Biometrics. 2023;79(3):1868–79.
30. Le-Rademacher J, Wang X. Time-to-event data: an overview and analysis considerations. J Thorac Oncol. 2021;16(7):1067–74.
31. Rosato R, Pagano E, Testa S, Zola P, di Cuonzo D. Missing data in longitudinal studies: comparison of multiple imputation methods in a real clinical setting. J Eval Clin Pract. 2021;27(1):34–41.
32. Heymans MW, Twisk JW. Handling missing data in clinical research. J Clin Epidemiol. 2022;151:185–8.
33. Liu C, Cripe TP, Kim M-O. Statistical issues in longitudinal data analysis for treatment efficacy studies in the biomedical sciences. Mol Ther. 2010;18(9):1724–30.
34. Cavaleri R, Bhole S, Arora A. Critical appraisal of quantitative research. In: Liamputtong P, editor. Handbook of research methods in health social sciences; 2018. p. 1027–49.
35. CASP C. CASP qualitative checklist. Critical Appraisal Skills Programme 2018.
36. Butcher NJ, Monsour A, Mew EJ, Chan A-W, Moher D, Mayo-Wilson E, et al. Guidelines for reporting outcomes in trial reports: the CONSORT-outcomes 2022 extension. JAMA. 2022;328(22):2252–64.
37. Tooth L, Ware R, Bain C, Purdie DM, Dobson A. Quality of reporting of observational longitudinal research. Am J Epidemiol. 2005;161(3):280–8.
38. Iwagami M, Shinozaki T. Introduction to matching in case-control and cohort studies. Ann Clin Epidemiol. 2022;4(2):33–40.
39. Wacholder S, Silverman DT, McLaughlin JK, Mandel JS. Selection of controls in case-control studies: II. Types of controls. Am J Epidemiol. 1992;135(9):1029–41.
40. Wacholder S, McLaughlin JK, Silverman DT, Mandel JS. Selection of controls in case-control studies: I. Principles. Am J epidemiology. 1992;135(9):1019–28.

41. Wacholder S, Silverman DT, McLaughlin JK, Mandel JS. Selection of controls in case-control studies: III. Design options. Am J Epidemiol. 1992;135(9):1042–50.
42. Labrecque JA, Hunink MM, Ikram MA, Ikram MK. Do case-control studies always estimate odds ratios? Am J Epidemiol. 2021;190(2):318–21.
43. Pearce N. Analysis of matched case-control studies. BMJ. 2016;352
44. Mansournia MA, Jewell NP, Greenland S. Case–control matching: effects, misconceptions, and recommendations. Eur J Epidemiol. 2018;33:5–14.
45. Olsson A, Bouaoun L, Schüz J, Vermeulen R, Behrens T, Ge C, et al. Lung cancer risks associated with occupational exposure to pairs of five lung carcinogens: results from a pooled analysis of case-control studies (SYNERGY). Environ Health Perspect. 2024;132(1):017005.
46. Cuschieri S. The STROBE guidelines. Saudi J Anaesth. 2019;13(Suppl 1):S31–S4.
47. Parsonnet J, Friedman GD, Vandersteen DP, Chang Y, Vogelman JH, Orentreich N, et al. Helicobacter pylori infection and the risk of gastric carcinoma. N Engl J Med. 1991;325(16):1127–31.
48. Kim J, Wang TC. Helicobacter pylori and gastric cancer. Gastrointest Endosc Clin. 2021;31(3):451–65.
49. Yuan C, Wang Q-L, Kim H, Babic A, Zhang J, Wolpin BM, et al. Being breastfed in infancy and risk of colorectal cancer and precursor lesions. Clin Gastroenterol Hepatol. 2024;22(7):1508–17. e11.
50. Brantley KD, Ziegler RG, Craft NE, Hankinson SE, Eliassen AH. Circulating estrogen metabolites and risk of breast cancer among postmenopausal women in the nurses' health study. Cancer Epidemiol Biomarkers Prev. 2024;34(3):OF1–OF10.
51. Wang T, Chai B, Chen WY, Holmes MD, Erdrich J, Hu FB, et al. Metformin and other anti-diabetic medication use and breast cancer incidence in the nurses' health studies. Int J Cancer. 2024;

Randomized Clinical Trials

5

Nathan Parker and Tracey O'Connor

Background/Introduction

Randomized clinical trials (RCTs) form the cornerstone of research and clinical practice in oncology by evaluating the efficacy and safety of new therapies and interventions among human participants. Figure 5.1 illustrates a general study design for RCTs in cancer. At their foundation, RCTs are experiments in which manipulation of a single independent variable—typically receiving a specific treatment or intervention or receiving an appropriate control or comparison condition—is evaluated for its effects on important dependent variables, or outcomes. In these trials, participants undergo random assignment to either a group receiving the experimental treatment or intervention condition or to a comparison or control condition receiving standard care or a placebo, ensuring limited influence of participants' characteristics or investigators' hypotheses and preferences on study outcomes. Randomization also helps ensure that study groups are comparable at the start of the trial and only differ based on receiving the trial's experimental or control conditions, which reduces bias and controls for the effects of confounding variables on treatment or intervention outcomes. Experimental blinding, in which participants (i.e., single-blind trials) or both participants and investigators (i.e., double-blind trials) remain unaware of study group assignments for the duration of the trial, is another important aspect of RCTs. Many RCTs incorporate blinding to minimize bias in treatment or intervention administration and assessment or reporting of outcomes. RCTs typically use well-defined, clinically meaningful endpoints to measure efficacy, including response to the treatment or intervention of interest, progression-free survival, disease-free survival, and overall survival. Depending on the treatment or intervention of interest, RCTs frequently also involve carefully monitoring participants for adverse events. Statistical analysis of RCT data typically aims to determine whether the experimental treatment or intervention offers a meaningful benefit over existing standards, thus providing important foundations for regulatory approvals and incorporation into clinical care pathways. RCTs are considered the gold standard for generating high-quality evidence in oncology research, because their structure minimizes bias and allows investigators to make causal inferences about the effects of experimental treatments or interventions on important outcomes [1–3].

Investigators design RCTs to answer specific, high-priority questions about the effectiveness, comparative effectiveness, safety, and optimal use of cancer treatments and interventions.

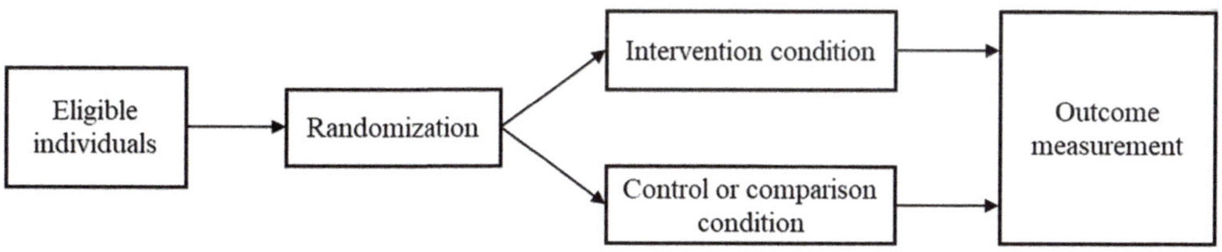

Fig. 5.1 General design of RCTs in oncology

N. Parker (✉)
Department of Health Outcomes and Behavior, Moffitt Cancer Center, FL, USA
e-mail: nathan.parker@moffitt.org

T. O'Connor
Department of Breast Oncology, Moffitt Cancer Center, FL, USA
e-mail: tracey.oconnor@moffitt.org

J. Huang, H. S.L. Jim (eds.), *Cancer Research Guidance for Clinicians and Researchers*, https://doi.org/10.1007/978-3-032-19175-5_5

These trials can determine whether new therapies, such as chemotherapy regimens, immunotherapies, targeted therapies, or surgical techniques, improve patient outcomes compared to placebos or existing treatment standards. RCTs can also help identify optimal dosing patterns, sequences, durations, and treatment combinations to ensure the best possible outcomes for patients and survivors. Finally, RCTs can provide evidence of potential harm or adverse effects from treatments or interventions, guiding clinical and regulatory decisions and informing new treatment standards and guidelines. By minimizing bias through randomization and controlled experimental conditions, RCTs generally provide the most reliable evidence for evaluating therapies and interventions in oncology.

RCTs provide frameworks for testing treatments and interventions across multiple clinical trial phases (Table 5.1). While Phase I trials seldom involve RCT designs, they may occasionally compare the safety, tolerability, and pharmacokinetics of different treatment doses or delivery strategies across small, randomized groups of participants [4]. In Phase II, trials begin to evaluate the efficacy of new treatments and interventions based on outcomes including response rate, progression-free survival, and changes in biomarkers. Phase II RCTs are becoming more common to provide nondefinitive comparisons of experimental regimens, each with independent decision rules informing prioritization of advancement to Phase III [5]. RCTs become central in Phase III clinical trials, where they are the gold standard for determining the comparative effectiveness of new strategies, relative to existing standards of care, in larger groups of participants who meet strict eligibility criteria [6]. Phase III RCTs can establish definitive clinical benefits based on endpoints such as overall survival, disease-free survival, and quality of life. These trials provide the evidence required for regulatory approvals and thereby inform subsequent changes in clinical decision-making. Further investigation in Phase IV may follow regulatory approval for new treatments and interventions and tends to focus on evaluating long-term safety and outcomes in real-world settings, frequently involving broader participant populations who may not have met Phase III eligibility criteria. Phase IV RCT designs can also enhance information about optimizing delivery and implementation of new treatments and interventions [7]. Across all phases, RCTs ensure rigorous evaluation and generate high-quality evidence to inform policy, practice, and future research in oncology.

RCTs also provide frameworks for testing treatments and interventions across the cancer continuum (Table 5.1). RCTs play major roles in research involving primary cancer

Table 5.1 Application of RCTs to research questions in oncology

Research question in oncology	RCT type	Example RCT design(s)	Example endpoint(s)
How efficacious is a treatment or intervention?	Treatment efficacy trial (Phase III)	New treatment vs. standard of care treatment or placebo New intervention vs. standard of care	Progression-free survival Overall survival Quality of life
How does the real-world effectiveness of one treatment or intervention compare to another?	Comparative effectiveness trial (Phase IV)	Treatment A vs. treatment B Intervention A vs. intervention B	Response rate Progression-free survival Overall survival Patient-reported outcomes
How does the safety or toxicity of one treatment compare to another?	Treatment safety or toxicity trial (Phase I)	Treatment A vs. treatment B	Adverse events Dose-limiting toxicity Discontinuation rate
What is the optimal dose or duration of a treatment?	Dose-finding or optimization trial (Phase II)	Treatment A at dose X vs. treatment A at dose Y Treatment A for X months vs. treatment A for Y months	Adverse events Dose-limiting toxicity Maximum tolerated dose
What is the timing of a treatment relative to other treatments?	Optimization trial (Phase III or IV)	Treatment A before treatment B vs. treatment A following treatment B	Response rate Progression-free survival Overall survival
Does an intervention help prevent cancer?	Prevention trial	Intervention A vs. no intervention	Cancer incidence Biomarkers of cancer risk
Does a screening strategy help diagnose cancer early?	Screening trial	Screening strategy A vs. no strategy	Cancer-specific mortality
Does an intervention help reduce treatment side-effects or improve symptoms?	Supportive or palliative care trial	Intervention A vs. no intervention	Symptom control Quality of life
Does an intervention improve aspects of post-treatment cancer survivorship?	Survivorship trial	Intervention A vs. no intervention	Quality of life Physical functioning Psychosocial well-being Biomarkers indicating risk of cancer recurrence

prevention to understand the effects of lifestyle interventions (e.g., tobacco cessation, diet, physical activity, stress management), medications, and supplements on cancer incidence or biomarkers related to cancer risk [8]. Research involving cancer screening (i.e., secondary cancer prevention) can employ RCT designs to evaluate the efficacy of techniques for cancer detection—such as with imaging or blood tests—to reduce late-stage cancer incidence (i.e., stages III–IV) and cancer-specific mortality [9]. Cancer screening RCTs can also help establish new standards for test sensitivity (low false negatives) and specificity (low false positives) compared to reference standards. Perhaps the most widely appreciated role for RCTs falls in cancer treatment, where they provide gold standard information about the efficacy of treatments and interventions on clinical outcomes (i.e., progression-free and overall survival) and patient-centered outcomes (i.e., symptoms, treatment side effects, and quality of life) [1]. The roles of RCTs in supportive and palliative care contexts can overlap with those in cancer treatment contexts, with RCTs informing new guidelines and strategies for managing symptoms and side effects including pain, nausea, and fatigue [10]. Finally, in post-treatment cancer survivorship, RCTs can evaluate the impacts of behavioral and lifestyle interventions on important outcomes such as biomarkers indicating risk of recurrence, quality of life, physical functioning, and psychosocial well-being [11]. Regardless of its context within the cancer continuum, evidence from RCTs is critical to inform and accelerate improvements in policy and practice and to drive future research.

Types of RCTs in Oncology

RCTs provide effective study designs to answer many important questions in oncology (Table 5.1). This section describes important methodological considerations in these trials, applicable strategies for statistical analysis, and their strengths and limitations.

Cancer Treatment Efficacy Trials

RCTs are critical for evaluating treatment efficacy, and their findings drive advancements in policy and care standards. The primary purpose of treatment efficacy RCTs is to determine whether treatments or interventions, such as anticancer drugs, radiation regimens, combinations of treatments, or behavioral interventions, provide clinically meaningful benefits compared to the existing standards of care [12]. Treatment efficacy trials often focus on clinical endpoints such as progression-free survival, overall survival, and quality of life, and they generate high-quality evidence that can inform regulatory approvals, clinical guidelines, and real-world treatment decisions [1, 13].

Methodological Considerations

RCTs evaluating treatment efficacy use rigorous study designs to minimize bias and confounding [14–16]. The basis of these trials is the randomized allocation of participants to study groups receiving either the treatment or intervention of interest or a control condition (i.e., receiving the standard of care). Treatment efficacy RCTs also frequently incorporate stratification and blinding to improve rigor. Stratification based on prognostic or demographic factors (e.g., disease stage, performance status, biomarkers, age, sex) helps ensure balance in baseline characteristics and potential confounding variables between study groups. Blinding, or masking, helps improve the validity of RCT findings by keeping participants and researchers unaware of participants' study group assignments during the study observation period. Masking participants (i.e., single-blind studies) reduces potential biases such as excess dropout and pursuit of additional treatments among participants assigned to control conditions. Masking participants and researchers (i.e., double-blind studies) further reduces potential bias by preventing differential influences, whether conscious or subconscious, on actual participant outcomes and how they are assessed. Treatment efficacy RCTs typically utilize strict eligibility criteria for participants, and these are selected to balance internal validity (i.e., determining a true, causal effect of the treatment or intervention on outcomes) and external generalizability (i.e., applicability of trial findings to other populations or contexts) [17]. Additional considerations in designing treatment efficacy RCTs include optimizing adherence to the study treatment or intervention and limiting or preventing contamination (i.e., control group participants independently or inadvertently receiving experimental treatments or interventions). Participants in cancer treatment efficacy RCTs undergo close monitoring to determine the timing of or evaluate changes in the primary outcome variable. This may include following patients to identify the timing of cancer recurrence or death or employing longitudinal assessments in defined intervals to measure changes in self-reported quality of life.

Statistical Analysis

Statistical analysis in cancer treatment efficacy RCTs typically employs time-to-event methods to estimate treatment effects. These can include Kaplan-Meier survival curves, log-rank tests, and Cox proportional hazards models [18]. Statistical methods to evaluate the efficacy of behavioral interventions on patient-reported outcomes (e.g., quality of life, fatigue) typically involve regression modeling to estimate differences or changes in outcomes by study group and time. Rigorous, intention-to-treat analysis in cancer efficacy RCTs preserves randomization and accounts for all participants based on their group assignments at baseline, though per-protocol and subgroup analyses are often conducted to evaluate the effects of receiving treatments or interventions as intended [19]. Sample size and power calculations are based on expected event rates and effect sizes for changes in study outcomes, and trials may incorporate interim analyses or adaptive designs to determine whether trials will end early or continue based on a priori rules involving treatment efficacy or futility [20]. Handling missing data (i.e., missed assessments, loss to follow-up), allowing or disallowing crossover (i.e., receiving a treatment or intervention after a defined time period in the control condition), and censoring appropriately (i.e., accurately defining and identifying event timing) are also critical for making valid inferences from data in treatment efficacy RCTs.

Strengths and Limitations

As with other RCT designs, the main strength of treatment efficacy RCTs is their potential to establish causal relationships between treatments or interventions on important cancer outcomes due to randomization, which controls for both known and unknown confounders. For this reason, the RCT is considered the gold standard for evaluating the efficacy of treatments and interventions in oncology. However, treatment efficacy RCTs also have limitations [21]. These trials tend to be resource- and time-intensive and may have limited generalizability due to strict eligibility criteria that exclude, for example, older patients or those with comorbidities or lower performance status [13]. Disease progression, recurrence, and symptom regression can occur rapidly in some cancer contexts, presenting important ethical considerations about withholding treatments or interventions that may be effective. Lack of participant blinding in some interventional efficacy RCTs, such as those testing behavioral strategies (e.g., dietary counseling, physical activity promotion), can introduce expectancy bias. Though commonly used as an endpoint in treatment efficacy RCTs due to limited funding and trial durations, improvements in progression-free or recurrence-free survival do not always translate to improvements in overall survival or patient-centered outcomes [22]. Despite these challenges, treatment and intervention efficacy RCTs remain a cornerstone of evidence-based oncology.

Comparative Effectiveness Trials in Oncology

Comparative effectiveness RCTs in oncology are designed to compare how different approved cancer treatments or interventions perform in clinically relevant, real-world settings [23, 24]. Unlike treatment efficacy RCTs that evaluate a new treatment or intervention against a control condition (i.e., standard of care treatment), comparative effectiveness trials compare two or more treatments or interventions that may already constitute standard of care treatment possibilities. Comparative effectiveness RCTs play an important role in oncology by helping clinicians and patients make informed decisions in certain treatment contexts based on the optimal balance of effectiveness, safety, and quality of life.

Methodological Considerations

Comparative effectiveness RCTs in cancer involve unique methodological challenges. The treatments or interventions under evaluation are frequently already used in clinical care, creating potential for preferences among clinicians or patients that can affect trial recruitment and participant adherence [25]. Enhancing generalizability is a key consideration in comparative effectiveness RCTs, and this can be accomplished by incorporating broader eligibility criteria, employing flexible treatment protocols or potential for crossover, and implementing treatments or interventions in real-world clinical settings [25]. Designing comparative effectiveness RCTs to ensure and maintain sufficient statistical power and internal validity can be difficult, particularly with potential for suboptimal adherence or crossover between study conditions. Stratification based on prognostic characteristics or biomarkers is a frequent consideration in comparative effectiveness RCTs to help account for increased heterogeneity in target participant populations. Clinically relevant variables such as treatment or intervention response rates, time-to-treatment failure, progression-free and overall survival, and patient-reported outcomes typically provide the primary endpoints in comparative effectiveness RCTs. Comparative effectiveness RCTs may include superiority, non-inferiority, or equivalence designs [26]. These designs test whether one treatment is favorable compared to another, whether one treatment is not appreciably worse than another, or whether there is no meaningful difference in efficacy between treatments, respectively.

Statistical Analysis

Statistical approaches in comparative effectiveness RCTs must account for real-world complexities in oncology care while still maximizing the validity of study inferences [27]. As in treatment efficacy RCTs, intention-to-treat analysis provides an important standard, but per-protocol and as-treated analyses can help determine the roles of treatment and intervention adherence in improving outcomes. Time-to-event outcomes like overall survival, progression-free survival, and time-to-treatment failure are common and typically analyzed using Kaplan-Meier curves and Cox proportional hazards models. Differences in response rates and patient-reported outcomes between treatments can be compared using logistic and linear regression models, respectively. In comparative effectiveness RCTs with superiority, non-inferiority, or equivalence designs, treatment or intervention effects are typically evaluated using regression models with subsequent comparisons between effect sizes and predefined margins of clinical acceptability.

Strengths and Limitations

One of the most important strengths of comparative effectiveness RCTs is their direct relevance to clinical decision-making in oncology. These trials provide rigorous evidence that is applicable to everyday oncology practice and helps inform treatment guidelines, reimbursement policies, and shared decision-making strategies. However, their weaknesses include challenges with blinding (especially when comparing treatments with different routes of administration or side effect profiles), potential for contamination or crossover between study groups, and difficulties ensuring consistent treatment or intervention delivery and outcome assessments across diverse clinical settings. Despite these limitations and challenges, comparative effectiveness RCTs play an increasingly important role in an era characterized by the rapid expansion of cancer treatment and interventional options and an emphasis on personalized, value-based care.

Dose-Finding or Optimization Trials in Oncology

RCTs focused on identifying optimal treatment doses and durations aim to optimize standard care practices for delivering cancer therapies [28, 29]. These trials may be designed to identify the minimum effective dose or shortest necessary duration of a treatment that maintains efficacy while ensuring safety (i.e., toxicity) and reducing patient burden (i.e., cost and time). These trials are particularly important in cancer care, where treatments are frequently associated with significant side effects and costs. The goals of dose finding and optimization trials include not only improving patient outcomes but also enhancing quality of life and reducing financial burden on patients and healthcare systems. Dose-finding and duration RCTs can be used to evaluate both de-escalation strategies (i.e., reducing dose or shortening duration) and escalation strategies (i.e., intensifying dose or lengthening duration) across different patient groups and treatment contexts.

Dose-finding and optimization trials can also include investigations to determine the optimal timing and sequencing of cancer therapies to maximize clinical benefits while minimizing harm [30]. These RCTs explore critical questions such as whether combinations of chemotherapy and radiation therapy are more effective before cancer surgery (i.e., neoadjuvant therapy) or after cancer surgery (i.e., adjuvant therapy), whether radiation therapy should precede or follow systemic therapy, and how to best sequence emerging therapies like immunotherapy, cellular therapy, and targeted agents. The primary aim of these RCTs typically involves refining delivery of existing treatments by testing the efficacy of different sequences to improve survival outcomes and quality of life—particularly in complex, multimodal treatment settings.

Methodological Considerations

Designing RCTs to refine standard practices regarding treatment doses, durations, and sequences must strike a careful balance between safety and efficacy. Key methodological aspects include identifying appropriate control arms—generally patients receiving doses, durations, or sequences that are currently standard of care—and comparing outcomes to a priori standards that signify non-inferiority or superiority. Treatment de-escalation studies, where new delivery strategies must demonstrate efficacy within a pre-specified margin of the current standard of care, commonly employ non-inferiority designs. RCTs investigating changes to treatment sequences must standardize treatment protocols and timing intervals between study arms to ensure valid comparisons. Additional aspects of treatment delivery, such as anticipated or required recovery time between treatments, delays, or dose reductions due to toxicity, require careful planning and design to optimize adherence to and generate valid comparisons between treatment sequences. Participant selection is also critical in these RCTs, frequently focusing on specific patient groups based on disease stage or risk for adverse treatment outcomes. Furthermore, there must exist clear biological plausibility that the modifications to treatment doses, durations, or sequences under investigation can still lead to clinical benefits. Stratification by prognostic factors, such as tumor burden, biomarkers, and performance status, is often used in dose-finding and optimization trials to limit confounding and ensure balance between study groups.

Statistical Analysis

Statistical analysis for dose and duration RCTs often employs non-inferiority or equivalence testing to determine whether a lower dose or shorter duration results in acceptable outcomes compared to standard treatments [31]. Primary endpoints vary across cancer types and stages but typically include progression-free survival, overall survival, or disease-free survival. Kaplan-Meier estimates, log-rank tests, and Cox proportional hazards models are standard tools, with analyses conducted on an intention-to-treat basis. Power and sample size calculations must be precise, as non-inferiority designs require tight control over type I and II error rates and careful justification of margins indicating non-inferiority.

Timing and sequencing RCTs commonly use time-to-event analyses for endpoints like overall survival, progression-free survival, and recurrence-free survival. Kaplan-Meier survival curves, log-rank tests, and Cox proportional hazards models are standard analytical tools. Pathologic complete response is often used as a surrogate endpoint in neoadjuvant trials. Studies may also employ non-inferiority designs when evaluating whether a more convenient or less intensive sequence maintains comparable efficacy. Subgroup analyses, stratified by tumor subtype or biomarker status, are often planned to identify whether particular patient populations benefit more from specific sequencing strategies. Importantly, analyses must account for treatment compliance and protocol deviations, which can dilute treatment effects [31].

Strengths and Limitations

The major strength of dose-finding and optimization RCTs is their direct applicability to improving patient-centered care by limiting overtreatment in cancer care—and associated burden and costs—without compromising outcomes. Value also stems from employing existing therapies in new ways, often improving patient outcomes and overall healthcare efficiency without requiring the development of new drugs. Results from these trials can change clinical practices, such as by demonstrating the clinical utility of lower doses or shorter durations of systemic therapy, more precise fields for radiation therapy, or different sequences of systemic therapy relative to tumor resection. They can provide actionable insights to integrate multimodal treatments, improve surgical outcomes, and enhance responses to systemic therapy. By balancing efficacy with safety, dose-finding and optimization RCTs can increase rates of treatment adherence and completion while reducing toxicity and costs.

There are also important challenges and limitations associated with dose-finding and optimization RCTs in oncology. Identifying clinically meaningful margins for treatment efficacy that signify non-inferiority and superiority is statistically complex, and suboptimal trial planning and execution can lead to misinterpretation of results [31]. Important differences in treatment efficacy can be quite small, requiring careful consideration of sample size to ensure studies have sufficient power to detect them. RCTs involving treatment sequencing require clinical and research coordination across multiple specialties (e.g., surgery, radiation, medical oncology) and rigorous management of treatment schedules. Deviations from intended treatment doses, durations, and timing can result from treatment toxicities, surgical complications, and delays in recovery, posing threats to the internal validity of findings [32]. Eligibility criteria in dose-finding and optimization RCTs often limit enrollment to patients with well-defined disease stages and good performance status to maintain internal validity, but this can also limit generalizability to broader, real-world clinical contexts. Finally, the need for multidisciplinary clinical investigators to be aware of patients' treatment plans and schedules makes blinding difficult or impossible in treatment sequencing RCTs, which adds risk for bias in assessing clinical outcomes. Despite these limitations, dose-finding and optimization RCTs have an important role in oncology, because they can improve the precision, tolerability, and sustainability of treatments within complex healthcare delivery systems.

Cancer Prevention Trials

RCTs in cancer prevention aim to evaluate the efficacy of various interventions to reduce disease incidence and progression [8]. In primary prevention, trials often involve randomizing individuals who are asymptomatic and have no history of cancer diagnosis to study groups that differ based on receiving or not receiving the intervention of interest. Primary prevention RCTs often focus on populations with comorbid conditions (e.g., obesity, diabetes), behaviors (e.g., tobacco use, physical inactivity, poor diet), or other biological predispositions (e.g., genetic mutations, family history) that increase cancer risk [33–36]. In secondary prevention, trials may target individuals with premalignant conditions or noninvasive cancer (e.g., colon polyps, Barrett's esophagus, cervical dysplasia, ductal carcinoma in situ) to reduce risk of invasive cancer development [37–39]. Cancer prevention RCTs may investigate interventions involving chemoprevention agents (e.g., tamoxifen for breast cancer) [40], vaccines (e.g., HPV vaccine for cervical cancer) [40], and behavioral or lifestyle strategies (e.g., tobacco cessation, physical activity, diet). Primary outcomes in cancer prevention RCTs vary based on the target population, cancer type, and intervention design. These outcomes may be more proximal, such as changes in behaviors, risk factors, or biomarkers of carcinogenesis, or they may be more distal, such as actual cancer incidence. The primary purpose of cancer prevention trials is to provide high-quality evidence to determine whether a specific intervention can lower the risk of cancer development.

Methodological Considerations

Cancer prevention RCTs involve unique methodological considerations. As with other types of RCTs in oncology, randomization to study groups helps to ensure an even distribution of potential confounding variables (e.g., baseline cancer risk, comorbidities, lifestyle factors) between study groups and that observed outcomes can be attributed to the intervention of interest [41]. Large sample sizes and long follow-up periods are generally required for trials that aim to detect meaningful, intervention-related differences in cancer incidence between study groups [42]. Cancer prevention RCTs may require strict eligibility criteria to define the at-risk population and maximize detection of meaningful differences in risk-related outcomes. Longer-term interventions, particularly those promoting changes in lifestyle and behaviors, require careful consideration to optimize participant adherence and retention, because suboptimal adherence and loss to follow-up can threaten validity [42]. Though contamination (i.e., control group participants engaging in intervention-related behaviors independently) is an important consideration in cancer prevention RCTs testing behavioral interventions [43], the ethics of withholding or limiting potentially beneficial preventive measures also factor into intervention and trial design.

Statistical Analysis

Statistical analysis in cancer prevention RCTs varies widely based on intervention design and study outcomes [42]. Comparisons of cancer incidence rates between intervention and control arms in large trials with long follow-up periods typically involve time-to-event analyses such as Kaplan-Meier curves and Cox proportional hazards models. Statistical methods to evaluate the efficacy of interventions on risk-reducing behaviors, risk factors, and biomarkers of cancer risk typically involve regression modeling to estimate differences or changes in outcomes by study group and time [33]. Intention-to-treat analysis in cancer prevention RCTs can be important to preserve randomization and account for all participants based on their group assignments at baseline, regardless of adherence among intervention participants or contamination among control participants. Pre-specified, per-protocol and subgroup analyses are often conducted to evaluate the effects of receiving treatments or interventions as intended and to identify populations who benefit most from the intervention.

Strengths and Limitations

The primary strength of cancer prevention RCTs is their ability to provide definitive evidence about the effectiveness of preventive interventions in reducing cancer risk. These findings can lead to major public health advances, such as the development of vaccination programs and guidelines for lifestyle and behaviors to reduce cancer risk. However, these trials also entail significant limitations. They are often expensive, time-consuming, and logistically complex, and if focused on reducing cancer incidence, results can take many years to mature [42]. Delivering behavioral interventions can require personnel with specialized training and expertise, which can limit generalizability to real-world settings that may lack the same resources. Rare cancer outcomes require large sample sizes, and it can be difficult to maintain strong intervention adherence, limit control group contamination, and retain participants throughout studies with long durations. Additionally, ethical and feasibility concerns may limit the scopes of designing both intervention and control group conditions. Despite these challenges, prevention RCTs remain the cornerstone for establishing evidence-based strategies to reduce cancer incidence at the population level.

Cancer Screening Trials

Cancer screening RCTs are designed to evaluate whether new strategies improve early detection, potentially translating to reductions in advanced or later-stage cancer incidence and reductions in cancer-specific mortality [44]. Randomization in these trials typically allocates participants to a group undergoing the new screening strategy or a group that undergoes no screening or the existing screening standard. Screening strategies have been tested commonly in RCTs involving breast, lung, colorectal, cervical, and prostate cancers. In addition to focusing on primary outcomes including cancer-specific mortality and the incidence and distributions of advanced (i.e., stages III–IV) cancers, cancer screening RCTs can also provide important information regarding the sensitivity (i.e., rate of detecting true positive results, or avoidance of false negatives) and specificity (i.e., rate of identifying true negative results, or avoidance of false positives) of new screening strategies. These are important considerations for new screening strategies in oncology, where it is critical to detect cancer as early as possible but also avoid misdiagnosis and unnecessary burden on individuals and healthcare systems from follow-up testing and procedures.

Methodological Considerations

Methodologically, rigorous randomization procedures are important in cancer screening RCTs to minimize selection bias and ensure comparability between groups [45]. Randomization in these trials frequently incorporates stratification by factors commonly associated with disease incidence, such as age, sex, and cancer-specific risk factors [46]. Clinical and research personnel involved in assessing distal outcomes, such as cancer stage and mortality, can be blinded to help reduce detection bias. Cancer screening RCTs frequently incorporate long follow-up intervals—often a decade or longer—to detect meaningful differences in incidences and distributions of advanced cancers and cancer-specific mortality [46]. Standardized and rigorous protocols detail the types, frequencies, and durations of screening for participants in each study group over time, with emphasis placed on maintaining consistency in all variables except the screening strategy of interest. Control conditions can require careful logistical and ethical consideration to limit contamination, or the pursuit of additional screening outside the trial framework by control arm participants. It is also critical to monitor adherence to screening procedures and losses to follow-up closely. Primary outcomes in cancer screening RCTs often include cancer-specific mortality or stage at diagnosis, while additional outcomes may include overall mortality, quality of life, test sensitivity and specificity, and potential harms and burdens from screening. These trials typically require large sample sizes to achieve sufficient statistical power due to the relative rarity of cancer incidence and mortality among the individuals they enroll and follow.

Statistical Analysis

Statistical analysis in cancer screening RCTs frequently incorporates an intention-to-treat approach to identify group differences regardless of adherence to screening protocols [47]. Intention-to-treat approaches help preserve the reductions in bias and confounding from randomization and yield conservative estimates of screening benefits that are more generalizable to real-world, non-trial settings. Time-to-event analyses such as Kaplan-Meier survival curves and Cox proportional hazards models can help account for differences in follow-up times and censoring between study groups. Although randomization inherently accounts for potential confounding variables, cancer screening RCTs may also employ stratification by or statistical adjustment for baseline characteristics to improve the precision of results. Detailing strategies to account for missing data, such as through imputation strategies or sensitivity analyses, can be particularly important in trials with long follow-up periods and potential for suboptimal screening adherence and losses to follow-up. Subgroup analyses—typically pre-specified to avoid spurious findings—may be conducted across participant groups based on age, sex, and other risk factors to identify specific contexts for screening benefits [47]. Finally, cancer screening RCTs frequently incorporate interim analyses to monitor for early evidence of screening benefits and harms and implement associated stopping rules.

Strengths and Limitations

The primary strength of cancer screening RCTs involves their internal validity and establishment of causal relationships between screening and outcomes. Randomization limits confounding factors and bias, which factor considerably into observational studies examining cancer screening based on individual differences in cancer risk, motivation, and adherence to cancer screening guidelines. Cancer screening RCTs provide robust evidence and have important potential to inform clinical guidelines and public health policies. However, they also have notable limitations. Due to the large sample sizes and lengthy follow-up periods they require [47], cancer screening RCTs can be very expensive. Ethical considerations must be applied to withholding potentially beneficial screening from participants randomized to control groups, and generalizability to broader populations that can benefit from improvements in cancer screening may be limited based on access to screening trials. Lengthy follow-up periods and standardized protocols for screening types, frequencies, and duration pose issues for participant adherence, collecting complete data, and contamination (i.e., control group participants pursuing additional opportunities for screening outside of the study protocol). Cancer screening RCTs focusing on incidence of advanced cancers and mortality outcomes must also involve considerations regarding unique types of bias, such as length-time bias (i.e., better detection of tumors that grow more slowly) and lead-time bias (i.e., earlier cancer detection leading to longer cancer-specific survival without actual prolongment of life) [44, 47]. Though earlier cancer detection and more sensitive screening strategies can lead to important advancements in cancer management and public health, these developments can also create new healthcare challenges from overdiagnosis [48]. For example, new screening strategies may identify nonaggressive tumors that previously would have gone undetected and never require management or treatment, leading to overtreatment and unnecessary impacts on psychosocial well-being and quality of life.

Supportive and Palliative Cancer Care Trials

RCTs in supportive and palliative care aim to improve important outcomes including symptom control and quality of life following a cancer diagnosis, often involving individuals with advanced cancers and limited treatment options to control or cure disease. Unlike treatment trials focused on controlling or curing cancer, supportive and palliative care RCTs may evaluate interventions such as strategies to manage pain or nausea, psychosocial support, nutritional or physical therapy, acupuncture, meditation, yoga, or early integration of palliative care strategies. Though some supportive and palliative care interventions may help prolong survival, survival outcomes are rarely a focus in supportive and palliative care RCTs. Instead, they test the efficacy of interventions to reduce suffering, improve functional status, and provide additional support for patients and caregivers following a cancer diagnosis.

Methodological Considerations

RCTs in supportive and palliative care face unique methodological considerations. Study populations can involve significant heterogeneity with respect to disease stage, treatment experiences, comorbidities, and functional and performance status [49]. Though randomization helps reduce bias and confounding that may otherwise result from this heterogeneity, implementation of control conditions in which patients may not receive desired—and potentially beneficial—supportive and palliative care strategies can raise ethical concerns and pose challenges for recruiting and retaining study participants [49–51]. There is limited potential for participant blinding in trials involving interventions that require their active engagement, such as behavioral and psychological counseling, nutritional and physical therapy, acupuncture, meditation, and yoga, but blinding research personnel conducting outcome assessments can help reduce bias [49]. Implementing placebo control conditions is feasible in some supportive and palliative care RCTs testing pharmacologic treatments. Outcomes in supportive and palliative care RCTs commonly involve subjective, self-reported data such as pain, fatigue, emotional distress, quality of life, and caregiver burden. This requires careful selection of questionnaires to assess patient-reported outcomes, ideally using only those that are well-validated in and clinically meaningful for the target cancer population.

Statistical Analysis

Statistical analysis in supportive and palliative care RCTs typically focuses on evaluating intervention effects on changes in patient-reported outcomes or scores from assessments of symptoms, nutritional status, or functional status assessments. These analyses involving longitudinal changes commonly employ repeated measures or mixed-effects models. Some trials focusing on outcomes such as symptom declines or requirements for hospital admission or hospice care require time-to-event analysis. Survival may be a secondary outcome in many supportive and palliative care RCTs and require time-to-event analysis. Dropout rates can be higher in supportive and palliative care RCTs than in treatment-related RCTs due to disease progression and death, and sample size and power calculations must account for anticipated dropout rates [49, 52]. Intention-to-treat strategies that maintain the benefits of randomization through data analysis are typical in supportive and palliative care RCTs, but additional, pre-specified sensitivity and per-protocol analyses may explore how intervention adherence and completion relate to study outcomes.

Strengths and Limitations

Supportive and palliative care RCTs have direct relevance to improving patient-centered care in oncology. Interventions in these trials are designed to address important concerns that can profoundly impact quality of life [10, 49]. Findings from supportive and palliative care RCTs can improve standard practices and lead to earlier integration of palliative care to improve patients' trajectories following a cancer diagnosis. However, these trials also have notable limitations. Patient-reported outcomes can be difficult to standardize and interpret, and high rates of attrition due to disease progression and death can introduce bias and threaten statistical power to detect improvements in study outcomes. Implementation of supportive and palliative care RCTs in larger, specialized cancer centers and eligibility criteria limiting enrollment based on age and performance status may limit generalizability to broader patient populations [49]. Despite these challenges, supportive and palliative care RCTs are essential for improving patient-centered care in the growing population living beyond a cancer diagnosis.

Cancer Survivorship Trials

RCTs in cancer survivorship generally focus on evaluating interventions designed to improve quality of life and long-term outcomes among people who have completed cancer treatment. Interventions in these trials involve a wide range of health-enhancing strategies, including physical activity and exercise, nutrition, psychosocial support, symptom management, and surveillance methods for recurrent or secondary disease [11, 53–57]. Primary outcomes in cancer survivorship RCTs vary based on the study intervention and cancer context and may include objective measures of fitness, physical functioning, nutrition status, and cognitive function, patient-reported outcomes of symptom burden and quality of life, and longer-term outcomes including progression-free and overall survival. Cancer survivorship RCTs typically aim to address the unique physical, emotional, and social challenges among cancer survivors and optimize their overall quality of life and functional status following treatment.

Methodological Considerations

Cancer survivorship RCTs incorporate careful selection of study populations, typically focusing on individuals who have completed active cancer treatment but are at risk for longer-term effects from treatment or cancer recurrence. Cancer survivor populations can be heterogeneous in terms of cancer type, age, sex, time since diagnosis, and previous cancer treatments, which frequently necessitates identifying specific target populations or stratifying randomization by potential confounding variables [58]. Randomization is essential for limiting bias and ensuring balance between study groups in potential confounding characteristics, allowing for causal inferences regarding intervention effects on study outcomes. Blinding participants is rare in cancer survivorship RCTs due to the incorporation of behavioral and psychosocial interventions that require active participant engagement. However, researchers conducting outcome assessments can be blinded to participants' study arms to help reduce bias. Control groups typically receive usual care, limited interventions (i.e., provision of health education materials), or contact-control conditions to help control for placebo or social effects of engagement with study interventionists [59]. Endpoints in cancer survivorship RCTs often include self-reported outcomes such as quality of life and fatigue, self-reported or objectively measured behavioral outcomes (i.e., improvements in physical activity or diet quality), objectively measured physical functioning, fitness, and body composition, and biomarkers associated with risk of cancer recurrence. Recurrence-free and overall survival can also be primary and secondary endpoints in cancer survivorship RCTs. Study durations and follow-up periods in cancer survivorship RCTs vary depending on the intervention of interest and target outcomes, but these trials generally aim to assess both shorter- and longer-term survivorship outcomes.

Statistical Analysis

Cancer survivorship RCTs typically incorporate intention-to-treat approaches for statistical analysis to maintain randomization integrity and improve generalizability to real-world settings and conditions [60]. Depending on the primary endpoint, analytical approaches can include mixed-effects models for repeated measures or regression models adjusted for baseline characteristics (i.e., for changes in self-reported or objectively measured health outcomes and biomarkers of cancer recurrence risk), or they can include time-to-event analyses to examine recurrence-free and overall survival. Handling missing data is particularly important in survivorship trials due to potential dropout or loss to follow-up over time. Subgroup and sensitivity analyses may explore differential effects based on demographics, cancer type, baseline symptom burden, or intervention adherence. These analyses should be preplanned to reduce the likelihood of finding spurious results.

Strengths and Limitations

Cancer survivorship RCTs rigorously evaluate the efficacy of interventions designed to improve aspects of health and quality of life among survivors. Though high-quality evidence from these trials frequently informs guidelines and practices in survivorship care, there are also limitations. The overall population of cancer survivors is growing in size and diversity, creating challenges for designing, implementing, and evaluating interventions that generalize broadly. Recruitment and retention can be difficult, especially in trials involving longer intervention durations and long-term follow-up to assess survivorship outcomes. Variability in intervention adherence and potential for control group contamination can threaten the validity of results from RCTs involving behavioral and lifestyle interventions [61]. Inter- and intrapersonal characteristics such as motivation and social support for physical activity and dietary change can affect adherence among intervention participants and create contamination among control participants. Blinding participants is rarely feasible in cancer survivorship RCTs involving nonpharmaceutical interventions, leading to potential for bias in subjective outcome measures. Many outcomes in survivorship RCTs, such as quality of life, fatigue, and self-reported behavior, are inherently subjective and may be subject to placebo effects and other influences outside of trial conditions. Finally, survivorship RCTs can be resource-intensive due to large sample size requirements and long follow-up periods to detect meaningful differences in outcomes such as recurrence or late treatment effects.

Ethical Considerations in Oncology RCTs

Planning and conducting RCTs in oncology involve key ethical considerations due to the serious nature of cancer diagnosis, treatment, and survivorship and the unique vulnerabilities of people who have been diagnosed with cancer. Ethical principles guiding biomedical research, such as respect for persons, justice, beneficence, and non-maleficence, must guide the design and conduct of RCTs regardless of their type and context across the cancer continuum [62]. Informed consent is foundational to the ethical design and conduct of RCTs, as participants must have a comprehensive understanding of a trial's purpose, its possible risks and benefits, alternatives to participating, and of their right to withdraw from the study without penalties. All participants must provide informed consent prior to trial enrollment and engagement in any research activities, and it is important that communication about the RCT is clear, compassionate, and appropriate for all potential levels of health literacy.

Additional ethical considerations are common to all RCT types and phases. These include minimization of harm (i.e., non-maleficence), which can be accomplished with vigilant monitoring for adverse events and providing mechanisms by which participants can report trial-related issues and concerns. Vulnerable populations, such as children, older adults, and individuals with cognitive impairments, often require additional safeguards and protections involving informed consent or harm minimization. Institutional review boards (IRBs) or ethics committees oversee trial protocols to ensure that recruitment is equitable, that appropriate safeguards are in place to minimize harm, and that potential benefits outweigh potential risks. RCT protocols must also incorporate rigorous protections to maintain the privacy and confidentiality of participant data. The design and delivery of control conditions in cancer-related RCTs must be fair and ethically justified; control arm participants must not be deprived of usual care for cancer screening, prevention, control, or survivorship, but providing the current standard of care typically meets scientific and ethical standards [63]. Many cancer RCTs provide participants with incentives to compensate them for their time and effort to complete study activities and assessments. However, incentive structures must be equitable, appropriate in scale, and uncoercive.

Several different RCT types and designs involve additional ethical concerns. Though new procedures involved in cancer screening RCTs may benefit participants through earlier detection, potential benefits must balance appropriately with potential harms from overdiagnosis and false positives [48]. Though unintended, these outcomes can cause undue psychological distress and unnecessary follow-up tests, procedures, and treatments. Moreover, long study durations to observe outcomes in cancer screening and prevention RCTs entail concerns about prolonged participant burden and maintenance of informed consent over time.

Phase I–III treatment trials in cancer involve complex ethical issues. Phase I and II treatment efficacy trials frequently evaluate the safety and dosing possibilities of new treatments among patients with advanced (stages III–IV) disease who may have no further options for standard care therapy. The likelihood of clinical benefits from additional treatment can be quite low for these populations, which challenges ethical standards for beneficence and necessitates clear communication about the risks and experimental natures of study treatments. Phase III treatment efficacy trials typically compare clinical outcomes from new treatments to those from current standard care treatments. These trials must meet ethical standards for clinical equipoise, meaning there must be genuine uncertainty about the superiority of one treatment over the other [64]. Predefined and clear procedures governing the interim analysis of emerging data are common in treatment efficacy trials; this helps identify clear superiority or inferiority of new treatments as soon as possible and can lead to early study termination to protect participants and ensure clinical equipoise [65].

Ethical issues in cancer survivorship RCTs center on balancing the autonomy and well-being of individuals who have endured significant emotional and physical challenges from diagnosis and treatment with scientific rigor. Though infrequently incorporated into usual care pathways for cancer survivors, behavioral and supportive care interventions have enormous potential to improve quality of life. There must exist genuine uncertainty about the superiority of new interventions—or new strategies to deliver and support them—to ensure equipoise among participants randomized to intervention and control conditions. Extended durations, high frequencies, and invasiveness of study assessments can exacerbate fatigue and distress among vulnerable cancer survivors, and careful consideration must be given to minimize participant burden. Equitable recruitment is important in cancer survivorship RCTs to include older survivors, those with comorbidities, and those from underserved populations to improve generalizability and access to care [66, 67].

Exemplary RCTs in Oncology

Evidence from RCTs has led to critical advancements in oncology. These trials have provided reliable evidence regarding the safety and efficacy of strategies to improve cancer prevention, screening, treatment, and survivorship. Scientific rigor in randomization, treatment or intervention delivery, and outcome assessment have enabled researchers conducting RCTs to distinguish therapeutic effects from bias and confounding and make valid, causal inferences about efficacy. RCTs have shaped and will continue to shape standard care practices and guidelines that improve outcomes and well-being following cancer diagnosis. This section outlines several RCTs, spanning different cancer diagnoses, trial phases, and cancer continuum stages, which have not only improved survival and quality of life for patients but also set methodological and ethical benchmarks guiding current and future research in oncology.

National Lung Screening Trial

The National Lung Screening Trial (NLST) is an exemplary cancer screening RCT. The NLST compared the efficacy of annual, low-dose computerized tomography (LDCT) scans to that of annual chest X-rays for early lung cancer detection among high-risk individuals at high risk [68]. Participant eligibility focused on high lung cancer risk, including individuals with significant smoking histories and between the ages of 55 and 74. NSLT participants were randomized in a 1:1 ratio to receive either annual LDCT or annual chest X-rays, which were the standard recommendation prior to the NSLT. Recruitment and enrollment took place from 2002 to 2004, with participants undergoing experimental or control imaging for 3 years and followed for a median of approximately 6.5 years for lung cancer specific and overall mortality. A major strength of the NSLT was its exceptionally large study sample (more than 53,000 participants), which was accomplished with multicenter recruitment in diverse regions and populations across the United States. Rigorous randomization procedures, standardized imaging protocols, robust follow-up, and independent verification of cancer detection and mortality outcomes helped minimize variability between study sites and increase the validity of findings. Additionally, the NSLT incorporated ethical safeguards to address concerns about overdiagnosis and false positives, including outlining these potential screening harms explicitly during informed consent. Positive results from LDCT screening triggered carefully tiered pathways for additional diagnostic procedures, emphasizing noninvasive follow-up imaging to avoid unwarranted procedures when possible.

Findings from the NSLT included a 20% reduction in lung cancer mortality and a 6.7% reduction in overall mortality among participants who underwent LDCT compared to chest X-ray [68]. The NSLT provided the first high quality of reduced lung cancer deaths from screening, which motivated changes to national guidelines and worldwide implementation of LDCT screening programs. In addition to clinical impact, the NLST set methodological standards for large-scale cancer screening RCTs by informing balanced, evidence-based public health recommendations based on risk-based eligibility criteria, rigorous randomization and trial design procedures, and ethical attention to unintended harm from cancer screening.

Colon Health and Life-Long Exercise Change (CHALLENGE) Trial

The Colon Health and Life-Long Exercise Change (CHALLENGE) trial represents a recent, landmark RCT in cancer survivorship. The CHALLENGE trial evaluated the effects of a structured exercise program on disease outcomes among colon cancer survivors. Trial participants included stage II–III colon cancer survivors who had recently completed adjuvant chemotherapy [69]. Participants (N = 962) were randomized in a 1:1 ratio to a 3-year aerobic exercise program including both supervised exercise sessions and support for behavior change (experimental group) or a comparison condition that received health education materials focusing on physical activity (control group). Randomization was stratified by study center, disease stage, and body mass index (≤25 vs. >25 kg/m2) to account for potential variations in program delivery and population characteristics across sites and potential confounders in both disease-free survival and intervention response. The primary study endpoint was disease-free survival, and secondary outcomes included objectively measured physical functioning and important survivor-reported outcomes (e.g., quality of life, fatigue). Strengths of the CHALLENGE trial included its large, multicenter structure, long-term follow-up, objective monitoring of exercise and physical activity, and employment of a theory-based approach to promote behavior change and intervention adherence. Targeting a population with high risk for cancer recurrence and incorporating rigorous, standardized procedures to encourage and monitor exercise adherence were also pivotal to the groundbreaking findings from the CHALLENGE trial.

CHALLENGE trial findings demonstrated that the experimental, 3-year aerobic exercise intervention significantly improved disease-free survival, with a 24% reduction in risk for disease recurrence or death observed among intervention participants compared to control participants [69]. The intervention also led to clinically and statistically significant improvements in physical functioning, quality of life, and fatigue. Results from the CHALLENGE trial provide the strongest evidence to date that regular exercise reduces recurrence and mortality risk in a posttreatment cancer survivor population, supporting exercise as a safe, feasible, and potentially life-extending adjunct to standard cancer treatment. CHALLENGE trial investigators carefully considered ethical issues to respect equipoise, autonomy, and non-maleficence among physically and emotionally vulnerable cancer survivors. Ethical considerations included clearly informing participants—prior to consent and enrollment—of the unproven benefits of exercise for preventing cancer recurrence; employing detailed procedures for medical screening and appropriate tailoring of exercise prescriptions; monitoring participants closely for injuries and adverse, intervention-related events; and providing health education materials to participants in the control group as to not withhold well-established benefits from independent physical activity. The CHALLENGE trial established several new benchmarks for RCTs involving lifestyle interventions in oncology and will undoubtedly contribute to the development and reinforcement of guidelines and strategies that improve cancer survival and survivorship. This has important implications for both clinical care (i.e., reinforcing the integration of structured exercise programming and counseling into routine care) and research (i.e., testing the effects of various exercise interventions on clinical outcomes in additional cancer treatment and survivorship contexts).

Improved Outcomes for Patients with Advanced or Metastatic Breast Cancer Receiving Endocrine Therapy and Targeted Therapy (IMPORTANT) Trial

The incidence of breast cancer is high in older women, with approximately 45% of breast cancers diagnosed in women 65 and older. Further, the number of older patients with breast cancer is expected to increase in coming years due to the growing population of older adults. Aging is an independent predictor of adverse treatment outcomes in breast cancer and is associated with increased risk for functional impairment, multimorbidity, and mortality. Unfortunately, older patients have been underrepresented in clinical trials, leading to gaps in published research that can inform tailored treatment approaches. Older patients enrolling in clinical trials are often highly selected with fewer comorbidities compared to real-life matched counterparts. Although evidence from RCTs and observational studies suggests that older patients often derive clinical benefits from cancer therapy, they also face higher risk of treatment-related adverse events, leading to trends in clinical practice toward cautiously initiating therapies at lower doses despite the absence of robust evidence informing these decisions.

The ongoing Improved Outcomes for Patients with Advanced or Metastatic Breast Cancer Receiving Endocrine Therapy and Targeted Therapy (IMPORTANT) trial aims to determine whether combining endocrine therapy with a lower starting dose of CDK4/6 inhibitors (targeted therapy) is as effective as combining endocrine therapy with the full dose of CDK4/6 inhibitors among older women with advanced, hormone receptor (HR)-positive/human epidermal growth factor receptor 2 (HER2)-negative breast cancer [70]. IMPORTANT trial participants include patients who are at least 70 years old, who have not undergone prior treatment for advanced breast cancer, and who are assessed as vulnerable or frail based on comprehensive geriatric assessment (CGA), which has demonstrated reliability for risk stratification and optimizing treatment strategies among older cancer patients. The IMPORTANT trial is a pragmatic, multinational, open-label, Phase II dose optimization RCT.

In the IMPORTANT trial, patients who are categorized as vulnerable or frail based on self-reported CGA comparisons to age-based impairment metrics (N = 346) are randomized in a 1:1 ratio to a lower initial dose or full dose of CDK 4/6 inhibitors combined with endocrine therapy. Stratification factors for randomization in the IMPORTANT trial include the type of CDK4/6 inhibitor patients will receive (i.e., palbociclib, ribociclib, or abemaciclib), the type of endocrine therapy patients will receive (i.e., aromatase inhibitors or fulvestrant), and the level of vulnerability based on CGA (i.e., vulnerable or frail). The primary endpoint in the IMPORTANT trial is time-to-treatment failure, with secondary endpoints including overall treatment utility (i.e., a composite, patient-centered endpoint weighing both treatment efficacy and tolerability), progression-free survival, overall survival, quality of life, and cost-effectiveness [70]. The IMPORTANT trial represents the first RCT incorporating CGA assessment to inform decisions regarding dose optimization among older patients with cancer. IMPORTANT trial findings are anticipated to not only inform standard care clinical practices for the growing population of older cancer patients but also to provide a framework for similar research strategies involving dose optimization for this population.

Investigation of Serial Studies to Predict Your Therapeutic Response with Imaging and Molecular Analysis 2 (I-SPY 2) Trial

Traditional clinical trial and drug approval processes are costly and time-consuming, creating barriers to moving new therapies into the settings where they can most effectively improve clinical outcomes. RCTs in breast cancer treatment have traditionally followed sequential steps for clinical development—first testing agents among patients who have metastatic disease, and if safe and effective, progressing to randomized, Phase III trials in the adjuvant setting. These trials have typically determined treatments and their sequences based on clinical and pathological characteristics rather than more specific, molecular characteristics that may vary widely, even among patients whose clinical and pathological presentations are similar. Primary endpoints of traditional treatment efficacy RCTs, such as recurrence-free survival and overall survival, require large numbers of participants to be randomized and followed for many years.

The original Investigation of Serial Studies to Predict Your Therapeutic Response with Imaging and Molecular Analysis (I-SPY 1) trial, conducted in the early 2000s, provided critical, observational evidence to improve breast cancer treatment [71]. I-SPY 1 employed serial imaging, tissue samples, and genetic profiling to identify tumor biomarkers that predict treatment response among women undergoing neoadjuvant chemotherapy for locally advanced breast cancer. The ongoing, I-SPY 2 trial builds on insights from I-SPY 1 with an adaptive clinical trial platform designed to improve outcomes in high-risk breast cancer patients by testing the efficacy of new drugs in the neoadjuvant setting [72]. The I-SPY 2 trial is an adaptive, Phase II RCT for women undergoing neoadjuvant treatment for high risk, stage II–III breast cancer. In I-SPY 2, breast cancer is categorized into molecular subtypes based on a comprehensive genetic assay as well as HR and HER2 status. The trial classifies breast cancer into ten subtypes based on this information, and patients are randomized to control or experimental arms within strata based on subtypes.

The I-SPY 2 platform has been designed to evaluate new agents (added to standard neoadjuvant chemotherapy) with the primary endpoint of pathologic complete response (pCR).

Though fundamentally a treatment efficacy trial, I-SPY 2 employs an adaptive, Phase II design to identify and select promising therapy combinations for more comprehensive efficacy testing in future, Phase III trials [72]. The I-SPY 2 trial has several innovative design aspects. First, I-SPY 2 builds on a foundation of observational evidence from I-SPY 1 to accelerate the clinical development of promising agents and their combinations based on detailed breast cancer biomarker analysis. Treatment testing in I-SPY 2 follows a biologically guided, precision medicine approach based on molecular biomarkers and hormone and HER2 receptor status. Targeting pCR as an early surrogate endpoint enables more rapid identification of promising agents to accelerate them through the clinical development pipeline. I-SPY 2 also employs Bayesian adaptive randomization, a cutting-edge statistical method that accounts for accumulating trial evidence about treatment efficacy to change the probability of assignment to different treatments. By accelerating endpoint detection, prioritizing more promising treatments, and deprioritizing less promising treatments, I-SPY 2 has potential to demonstrate benefits from new agents and combinations more efficiently than traditional trial designs.

Summary

RCTs are essential for evaluating a wide range of questions in cancer research, from prevention and screening to treatment efficacy, supportive care, and survivorship. RCTs in oncology involve unique endpoints, methodological considerations, and statistical approaches tailored to their specific goals. Methodologically, oncology RCTs emphasize randomization, stratification, and blinding to reduce bias, with careful attention to eligibility criteria, adherence, contamination, and patient monitoring. RCTs have distinct strengths, such as the ability to establish causality, guide clinical decision-making, and improve patient-centered care. However, RCTs can also entail important challenges regarding generalizability, ethical considerations, long follow-up durations, and feasibility constraints. Well-designed RCTs are the cornerstone of evidence-based cancer research, enabling advancements in treatment, prevention, early detection, symptom management, and survivorship care.

References

1. van Amsterdam WAC, Elias S, Ranganath R. Causal inference in oncology: why, what, How and When. Clin Oncol. 2025;38:103616.
2. Sibbald B, Roland M. Understanding controlled trials. Why are randomised controlled trials important? Br Med J. 1998;316:201.
3. Collins R, Bowman L, Landray M, et al. The magic of randomization versus the myth of real-world evidence, Massachusetts medical society. N Engl J Med. 2020;382:674–8.
4. Wong KM, Capasso A, Eckhardt SG. The changing landscape of phase I trials in oncology. Nat Rev Clin Oncol. 2016;13:106–17.
5. Ratain MJ, Sargent DJ. Optimising the design of phase II oncology trials: the importance of randomisation. Eur J Cancer. 2009;45:275–80.
6. Gan HK, You B, Pond GR, et al. Assumptions of expected benefits in randomized phase III trials evaluating systemic treatments for cancer. JNCI J Natl Cancer Inst. 2012;104:590–8.
7. Zhang X, Zhang Y, Ye X, et al. Overview of phase IV clinical trials for postmarket drug safety surveillance: a status report from the ClinicalTrials.gov registry. BMJ Open. 2016;6:e010643.
8. Dewys WD, Malone WF, Butrum RR, et al. Clinical trials in cancer prevention. Cancer. 1986;58:1954–62.
9. Raoof S, Lee RJ, Jajoo K, et al. Multicancer early detection technologies: a review informed by past cancer screening studies. Cancer Epidemiol Biomarkers Prev. 2022;31:1139–45.
10. Hui D, Arthur J, Dalal S, et al. Quality of the supportive and palliative oncology literature: a focused analysis on randomized controlled trials. Support Care Cancer. 2012;20:1779–85.
11. Chan RJ, Nekhlyudov L, Duijts SFA, et al. Future research in cancer survivorship. J Cancer Surviv. 2021;15:659–67.
12. You B, Gan HK, Pond G, et al. Consistency in the analysis and reporting of primary end points in oncology randomized controlled trials from registration to publication: a systematic review. J Clin Oncol. 2012;30:210–6.
13. Tannock IF, Amir E, Booth CM, et al. Relevance of randomised controlled trials in oncology. Lancet Oncol. 2016;17:e560–7.
14. Booth CM, Cescon DW, Wang L, et al. Evolution of the randomized controlled trial in oncology over three decades. J Clin Oncol. 2008;26:5458–64.
15. Breathnach OS, Freidlin B, Conley B, et al. Twenty-two years of phase III trials for patients with advanced non-small-cell lung cancer: sobering results. J Clin Oncol. 2001;19:1734–42.
16. Brown G, Msaouel P, Miller AM, et al. Patient, physician, and assessor blinding in phase III randomized trials in oncology: a meta-epidemiological analysis. Cancer Med. 2025;14:e71097.
17. Srikanthan A, Vera-Badillo F, Ethier J, et al. Evolution in the eligibility criteria of randomized controlled trials for systemic cancer therapies. Cancer Treat Rev. 2016;43:67–73.
18. Péron J, Pond GR, Gan HK, et al. Quality of reporting of modern randomized controlled trials in medical oncology: a systematic review. JNCI J Natl Cancer Inst. 2012;104:982–9.
19. Smith VA, Coffman CJ, Hudgens MG. Interpreting the results of intention-to-treat, per-protocol, and as-treated analyses of clinical trials. JAMA. 2021;326:433–4.
20. Wayant C, Vassar M. A comparison of matched interim analysis publications and final analysis publications in oncology clinical trials. Ann Oncol. 2018;29:2384–90.
21. Di Maio M, Perrone F, Conte P. Real-world evidence in oncology: opportunities and limitations. Oncologist. 2019;25:e746–52.
22. Walia A, Tuia J, Prasad V. Progression-free survival, disease-free survival and other composite end points in oncology: improved reporting is needed. Nat Rev Clin Oncol. 2023;20:885–95.
23. Hahn OM, Schilsky RL. Randomized controlled trials and comparative effectiveness research. J Clin Oncol. 2012;30:4194–201.
24. Chen RC. Comparative effectiveness research in oncology: the promise, challenges, and opportunities. Semin Radiat Oncol. 2014;24:1–4.
25. Meyer A-M, Carpenter WR, Abernethy AP, et al. Data for cancer comparative effectiveness research. Cancer. 2012;118:5186–97.
26. Franklin JM, Gebski V, Poston GJ, et al. Clinical trials of interventional oncology—moving from efficacy to outcomes. Nat Rev Clin Oncol. 2015;12:93–104.
27. Basch E. Methodological standards and patient-centeredness in comparative effectiveness research. JAMA: JAMA J Am Med Assoc. 2012;307
28. Minasian L, Rosen O, Auclair D, et al. Optimizing dosing of oncology drugs. Clin Pharm Therap. 2014;96:572–9.

29. Mathijssen RH, Sparreboom A, Verweij J. Determining the optimal dose in the development of anticancer agents. Nat Rev Clin Oncol. 2014;11:272–81.
30. Huang M, Ramsey S, Xue W, et al. Conceptual framework and methodological challenges for modeling effectiveness in oncology treatment sequence models. PharmacoEconomics. 2022;40:257–68.
31. Fourie Zirkelbach J, Shah M, Vallejo J, et al. Improving dose-optimization processes used in oncology drug development to minimize toxicity and maximize benefit to patients. J Clin Oncol. 2022;40:3489–500.
32. Moon H. FDA initiatives to support dose optimization in oncology drug development: the less may be the better. Transl Clin Pharmacol. 2022;30:71–4.
33. Winzer BM, Whiteman DC, Reeves MM, et al. Physical activity and cancer prevention: a systematic review of clinical trials. Cancer Causes Control. 2011;22:811–26.
34. Greenwald P. Clinical trials in cancer prevention: current results and perspectives for the future. J Nutr. 2004;134:3507S–12S.
35. Greenwald P, Anderson D, Nelson SA, et al. Clinical trials of vitamin and mineral supplements for cancer prevention23. Am J Clin Nutr. 2007;85:314S–7S.
36. Beresford SA, Johnson KC, Ritenbaugh C, et al. Low-fat dietary pattern and risk of colorectal cancer: the Women's Health Initiative randomized controlled dietary modification trial. JAMA. 2006;295:643–54.
37. Bornschein J, Bird-Lieberman EL, Malfertheiner P. The rationale and efficacy of primary and secondary prevention in adenocarcinomas of the upper gastrointestinal tract. Dig Dis. 2019;37:381–93.
38. Frieler M, Moore M, Longacre ML. Primary and secondary prevention interventions to reduce risk factors associated with colorectal cancer in high-risk groups: a systematic literature review. J Cancer Educ. 2023;38:738–51.
39. Kolak A, Kamińska M, Sygit K, et al. Primary and secondary prevention of breast cancer. Ann Agric Environ Med. 2017;24:549.
40. Fisher B, Dignam J, Wolmark N, et al. Tamoxifen in treatment of intraductal breast cancer: National Surgical Adjuvant Breast and bowel project B-24 randomised controlled trial. Lancet. 1999;353:1993–2000.
41. Martínez ME, Marshall JR, Giovannucci E. Diet and cancer prevention: the roles of observation and experimentation. Nat Rev Cancer. 2008;8:694–703.
42. Enserro DM, Gunn HJ, Elsaid MI, et al. Challenges to and considerations of designing cancer prevention trials. JNCI Monogr. 2025;2025:49–55.
43. Cuzick J, Edwards R, Segnan N. Adjusting for non-compliance and contamination in randomized clinical trials. Stat Med. 1997;16:1017–29.
44. Black WC, Haggstrom DA, Gilbert Welch H. All-cause mortality in randomized trials of cancer screening. JNCI J Natl Cancer Inst. 2002;94:167–73.
45. Paci E, Alexander FE. Study Design of Randomized Controlled Clinical Trials of breast cancer screening. JNCI Monographs. 1997;21-25:1997.
46. Vernon SW, Briss PA, Tiro JA, et al. Some methodologic lessons learned from cancer screening research. Cancer. 2004;101:1131–45.
47. Baker SG, Kramer BS, Prorok PC. Statistical issues in randomized trials of cancer screening. BMC Med Res Methodol. 2002;2:11.
48. Croswell JM, Ransohoff DF, Kramer BS. Principles of cancer screening: lessons from history and study design issues. Semin Oncol. 2010;37:202–15.
49. Aktas A, Walsh D. Methodological challenges in supportive and palliative care cancer research. Semin Oncol. 2011;38:460–6.
50. Janssens R, Gordijn B. Clinical trials in palliative care: an ethical evaluation. Patient Educ Couns. 2000;41:55–62.
51. Cherny NI, Abernethy AP, Strasser F, et al. Improving the methodologic and ethical validity of best supportive care studies in oncology: lessons from a systematic review. J Clin Oncol. 2009;27:5476–86.
52. Hui D, Glitza I, Chisholm G, et al. Attrition rates, reasons, and predictive factors in supportive care and palliative oncology clinical trials. Cancer. 2013;119:1098–105.
53. Corbett TK, Groarke A, Devane D, et al. The effectiveness of psychological interventions for fatigue in cancer survivors: systematic review of randomised controlled trials. Syst Rev. 2019;8:324.
54. Finne E, Glausch M, Exner A-K, et al. Behavior change techniques for increasing physical activity in cancer survivors: a systematic review and meta-analysis of randomized controlled trials. Cancer Manag Res. 2018;10:5125–43.
55. Pekmezi DW, Demark-Wahnefried W. Updated evidence in support of diet and exercise interventions in cancer survivors. Acta Oncol. 2011;50:167–78.
56. Chlebowski RT, Reeves MM. Weight loss randomized intervention trials in female cancer survivors. J Clin Oncol. 2016;34:4238–48.
57. Gudenkauf LM, Ehlers SL. Psychosocial interventions in breast cancer survivorship care. Breast. 2018;38:1–6.
58. Moyer A, Sohl SJ, Knapp-Oliver SK, et al. Characteristics and methodological quality of 25 years of research investigating psychosocial interventions for cancer patients. Cancer Treat Rev. 2009;35:475–84.
59. Tock WL, Maheu C, Johnson NA. Considerations of control conditions designs in randomized controlled trials of exercise interventions for cancer survivors. Can J Nurs Res. 2022;54:377–91.
60. Schmitz KH, Holtzman J, Courneya KS, et al. Controlled physical activity trials in cancer survivors: a systematic review and meta-analysis. Cancer Epidemiol Biomarkers Prev. 2005;14:1588–95.
61. Ormel HL, van der Schoot GGF, Sluiter WJ, et al. Predictors of adherence to exercise interventions during and after cancer treatment: a systematic review. Psycho-Oncology. 2018;27:713–24.
62. Kodish E, Lantos JD, Siegler M. Ethical considerations in randomized controlled clinical trials. Cancer. 1990;65:2400–4.
63. Daugherty CK, Ratain MJ, Emanuel EJ, et al. Ethical, scientific, and regulatory perspectives regarding the use of placebos in cancer clinical trials. J Clin Oncol. 2008;26:1371–8.
64. Sargent D. Early Stopping for Benefit in National Cancer Institute–Sponsored randomized phase III trials: the system is working. J Clin Oncol. 2009;27:1543–4.
65. AlHamaly MA, Alzoubi KH, Khabour OF, et al. Review of clinical equipoise: examples from oncology trials. Curr Rev Clin Exp Pharmacol. 2023;18:22–30.
66. Sedrak MS, Freedman RA, Cohen HJ, et al. Older adult participation in cancer clinical trials: a systematic review of barriers and interventions. CA Cancer J Clin. 2021;71:78–92.
67. Parks RM, Holmes HM, Cheung K-L. Current challenges faced by cancer clinical trials in addressing the problem of under-representation of older adults: a narrative review. Oncol Therap. 2021;9:55–67.
68. Team NLSTR. Reduced lung-cancer mortality with low-dose computed tomographic screening. N Engl J Med. 2011;365:395–409.
69. Courneya KS, Vardy JL, O'Callaghan CJ, et al. Structured exercise after adjuvant chemotherapy for colon cancer. N Engl J Med. 2025;393:13–25.
70. Valachis A, Biganzoli L, Christopoulou A, et al. Implementing geriatric assessment for dose optimization of CDK4/6 inhibitors in older breast cancer patients. Future Oncol. 2024;20:2937–48.
71. Esserman LJ, Berry DA, DeMichele A, et al. Pathologic complete response predicts recurrence-free survival more effectively by cancer subset: results from the I-SPY 1 TRIAL—CALGB 150007/150012, ACRIN 6657. J Clin Oncol. 2012;30:3242–9.
72. Wang H, Yee D. I-SPY 2: a neoadjuvant adaptive clinical trial designed to improve outcomes in high-risk breast cancer. Curr Breast Cancer Rep. 2019;11:303–10.

Adaptive Randomized Trials

6

Nyla Dil

Introduction

In the evolving landscape of clinical research, particularly in oncology and immunology, the need for more efficient, flexible, and patient-centered trial designs has never been greater. Traditional randomized controlled trials (RCTs), while considered the gold standard for evaluating therapeutic efficacy, often face limitations such as prolonged timelines, excessive costs, and rigid protocols that may not accommodate emerging data or shifting clinical paradigms. These constraints are especially pronounced in cancer research, where rapid advancements in molecular diagnostics, targeted therapies, and immunotherapies demand adaptive methodologies.

Adaptive randomized trials (ARTs) have emerged as a powerful alternative to conventional RCTs. These trials incorporate pre-specified modifications to key trial parameters, such as sample size, treatment arms, or randomization ratios, based on interim analyses of accumulating data. This flexibility allows researchers to make data-driven decisions during a trial, enhancing efficiency, ethical oversight, and the likelihood of identifying effective treatments.

In the context of cancer research, ARTs are particularly valuable due to the heterogeneity of tumor biology, the need for personalized medicine approaches, and the urgency of identifying effective therapies for aggressive or rare malignancies. Moreover, ARTs have proven instrumental in evaluating monoclonal antibodies (mAbs), a cornerstone of modern immunotherapy, across various indications, including hematologic malignancies, solid tumors, and immune-mediated diseases.

For example, the I-SPY 2 trial, a prominent adaptive platform trial in breast cancer, utilized adaptive randomization to evaluate multiple investigational agents, including monoclonal antibodies, in combination with standard chemotherapy. This trial not only accelerated the identification of promising therapies but also demonstrated the feasibility of adaptive designs in complex, multi-arm oncology studies [1].

Similarly, during the COVID-19 pandemic, adaptive trials such as RECOVERY and REMAP-CAP were pivotal in assessing the efficacy of monoclonal antibodies like tocilizumab (an IL-6 receptor antagonist) and casirivimab/imdevimab, providing rapid, high-quality evidence that informed global treatment guidelines [2, 3].

For community hospital clinicians, understanding and engaging with adaptive randomized trials offers a unique opportunity to contribute to innovative research without the prohibitive barriers often associated with traditional trials. This chapter aims to demystify adaptive trial designs, highlight their applications in cancer and immunotherapy, and

N. Dil (✉)
Department of Medical Education, University of Central Florida-College of Medicine, Orlando, FL, USA
e-mail: Nyla.Dil@ucf.edu

J. Huang, H. S.L. Jim (eds.), *Cancer Research Guidance for Clinicians and Researchers*,
https://doi.org/10.1007/978-3-032-19175-5_6

provide practical guidance for clinicians seeking to implement or participate in such studies.

Historical Context and Rationale

The concept of randomized controlled trials (RCTs) has long been the cornerstone of evidence-based medicine. Since the landmark British Medical Research Council streptomycin trial in 1948, RCTs have provided a rigorous framework for evaluating therapeutic efficacy and safety. However, the traditional fixed design of RCTs, where sample size, treatment arms, and endpoints are predetermined and unchangeable, can be inefficient and inflexible, particularly in rapidly evolving fields like oncology and immunology [4].

Cancer research presents unique challenges: heterogeneous disease biology, variable treatment responses, and the need for personalized approaches. These complexities often render conventional trial designs inadequate, especially when evaluating targeted therapies such as monoclonal antibodies (mAbs). For instance, the development of rituximab, a CD20-targeting mAb for B-cell lymphomas, highlighted the need for trial designs that could adapt to emerging biomarker data and evolving standards of care [5].

Adaptive randomized trials (ARTs) were developed to address these limitations. By allowing pre-specified modifications during the trial, such as adjusting sample sizes, dropping ineffective arms, and enriching populations based on interim findings, ARTs offer a dynamic and responsive approach to clinical research. This flexibility is particularly valuable in oncology, where early signals of efficacy or toxicity can guide trial evolution, potentially accelerating the path to approval and reducing patient exposure to suboptimal treatments [6].

The regulatory landscape has evolved to support adaptive designs. The US Food and Drug Administration (FDA) and the European Medicines Agency (EMA) have issued guidance documents outlining best practices for designing and conducting adaptive trials. These include recommendations for controlling Type I error, ensuring transparency in adaptation rules, and maintaining trial integrity [7, 8].

In recent years, adaptive designs have also gained traction in autoimmune disease research, where heterogeneity in disease presentation and response to biologics like adalimumab and ustekinumab necessitates flexible trial methodologies. Moreover, the urgency of the COVID-19 pandemic catalyzed the widespread adoption of adaptive platform trials, such as REMAP-CAP (A Randomized, Embedded, Multifactorial, Adaptive Platform Trial for Community-Acquired Pneumonia), which evaluated multiple interventions, including mAbs, simultaneously across diverse healthcare settings, including community hospitals [9].

In summary, the historical evolution of adaptive randomized trials reflects a broader shift toward more efficient, patient-centered research. For community hospital clinicians, understanding this trajectory is essential for engaging in modern cancer research and contributing to the development of innovative therapies.

Key Concepts in Adaptive Trial Design

Adaptive randomized trials (ARTs) are defined by their ability to modify trial parameters based on interim data analyses, all within a pre-specified framework that maintains statistical validity and regulatory compliance. These modifications can include changes to sample size, treatment allocation, eligibility criteria, or even the addition or removal of treatment arms. The goal is to make trials more efficient, ethical, and responsive to emerging evidence [6] (Table 6.1).

Table 6.1 Key concepts in adaptive trials

Concept	Description	Example
Types of adaptations		
Adaptive randomization	Adjust treatment allocation probabilities based on interim outcomes	I-SPY 2 trial allocated patients to promising therapies in biomarker-defined subgroups
Group sequential designs	Allows early stopping for efficacy, futility, or safety at predefined interim analyses	RECOVERY trial stopped tocilizumab arm early for efficacy
Sample size re-estimation	Modifies sample size based on interim effect size estimates to maintain power	Used in early-phase mAb trials for lupus and rheumatoid arthritis
Dose-finding designs	Identifies optimal dose using adaptive methods like Bayesian CRM	Phase I oncology trials with nivolumab or daratumumab
Biomarker-adaptive designs	Modifies eligibility or stratifies patients based on biomarker data	Checkpoint inhibitor trials in PD-L1-positive tumors
Seamless phase II/III designs	Combines exploratory and confirmatory phases into one protocol	BATTLE trial in lung cancer evaluated multiple therapies using real-time biomarker data
Statistical considerations		
Error control and unbiased estimates	Requires rigorous planning to control Type I error and ensure unbiased results	Simulation studies evaluate operating characteristics under various scenarios
Bayesian methods	Flexible approach to incorporate prior knowledge and update probabilities	Used in adaptive trials to refine hypotheses and guide decisions

(continued)

Table 6.1 (continued)

Concept	Description	Example
Regulatory perspectives		
Pre-specification of adaptations	Adaptation rules must be defined before trial initiation	FDA guidance emphasizes simulation-based planning
Use of DMCs	Independent committees monitor data and guide adaptations	Ensures trial integrity and safety
Transparency and bias control	Adaptations must be reported clearly and bias minimized	Supported by the FDA and EMA when well-justified

Types of Adaptations

(a) *Adaptive Randomization*

This technique adjusts the probability of assigning patients to different treatment arms based on accumulating outcome data. For example, in the I-SPY 2 trial, adaptive randomization was used to allocate patients to therapies showing early promise in specific biomarker-defined subgroups [1]. This approach is particularly useful in oncology and immunotherapy, where heterogeneity in response to monoclonal antibodies (e.g., trastuzumab and pembrolizumab) can be substantial.

(b) *Group Sequential Designs*

These designs incorporate interim analyses at predefined points, allowing for early stopping due to efficacy, futility, or safety concerns. This method was used in the RECOVERY trial, which evaluated tocilizumab in COVID-19 patients and stopped early for efficacy [2].

(c) *Sample Size Re-estimation*

Based on interim effect size estimates, the sample size can be increased or decreased to maintain adequate power. This is especially relevant in trials with uncertain variance or effect sizes, such as early-phase studies of novel mAbs in autoimmune diseases like lupus and rheumatoid arthritis [7, 10].

(d) *Dose-Finding Designs*

Adaptive dose-finding methods, such as the Bayesian continual reassessment method (CRM), allow for more efficient identification of the optimal dose. These designs are commonly used in phase I oncology trials evaluating mAbs like nivolumab and daratumumab [11].

(e) *Biomarker-Adaptive Designs*

These designs modify eligibility criteria or stratify patients based on biomarker data. For example, adaptive enrichment designs have been used to evaluate checkpoint inhibitors in PD-L1-positive tumors, allowing for targeted recruitment and improved trial efficiency [12].

(f) *Seamless Phase II/III Designs*

These designs combine exploration and confirmatory phases into a single protocol, reducing time and cost. The BATTLE trial in lung cancer used a seamless design to evaluate multiple targeted therapies, including mAbs, based on real-time biomarker data [13].

Statistical Considerations

Adaptive designs require rigorous statistical planning to control Type I error rates and ensure unbiased estimates. Simulation studies are often used to evaluate operating characteristics under various scenarios. Bayesian methods are increasingly employed for their flexibility in incorporating prior knowledge and updating probabilities as data accrue [14].

Regulatory Perspectives

Both the FDA and EMA support adaptive designs, if adaptations are pre-specified and justified. Key regulatory considerations include pre-specification of adaptation rules, use of independent data monitoring committees (DMCs), transparency in reporting adaptations, and control of Type I error and bias. The FDA's 2019 guidance on adaptive designs emphasizes the importance of simulation-based planning and recommends early engagement with regulatory authorities [7].

Advantages and Challenges

Adaptive randomized trials (ARTs) offer a compelling alternative to traditional fixed designs, particularly in fields like oncology and immunology where disease heterogeneity, rapid therapeutic innovation, and ethical considerations demand more flexible approaches. However, the implementation of ARTs also presents unique challenges that must be carefully navigated (Table 6.2).

Table 6.2 Advantages and challenges of adaptive randomized trial

Aspect	Details	Example
Advantages		
Increased efficiency	Fewer patients, shorter duration, optimized resources	I-SPY 2 trial accelerated therapy identification in breast cancer
Ethical benefits	Minimizes exposure to ineffective/harmful treatments	RECOVERY trial stopped tocilizumab arm after benefit observed
Flexibility and responsiveness	Real-time adjustments to biomarkers, dosing, eligibility	Anti-TNF agents vary by genetic/immunologic profiles
Enhanced learning	Iterative refinement of hypotheses and design	Early-phase immunotherapy trials improve dose-response understanding
Challenges		
Statistical complexity	Requires advanced modeling and error control	Simulation-based planning to assess operating characteristics
Operational demands	Needs real-time data systems and trained staff	Community hospitals may need external support
Regulatory scrutiny	Requires detailed pre-specification and justification	Early engagement with FDA/EMA is essential
Resource intensity	High upfront investment in planning and infrastructure	Barrier for smaller or investigator-initiated trials

Advantages

(a) *Increased Efficiency*

Adaptive designs can reduce the number of patients required, shorten trial duration, and optimize resource utilization. For example, the I-SPY 2 trial demonstrated that adaptive randomization could accelerate the identification of effective therapies in breast cancer by preferentially assigning patients to promising treatment arms [15].

(b) *Ethical Benefits*

By allowing early termination for efficacy or futility, ARTs minimize patient exposure to ineffective or harmful treatments. This is particularly important in life-threatening conditions such as metastatic cancer or severe autoimmune diseases. The RECOVERY trial exemplified this by halting enrollment in the tocilizumab arm once clear benefit was observed in COVID-19 patients [16].

(c) *Flexibility and Responsiveness*

ARTs can incorporate emerging biomarker data, adjust dosing strategies, and refine eligibility criteria in real time. This is crucial in immunology, where patient responses to monoclonal antibodies (e.g., anti-TNF agents) can vary widely based on genetic and immunologic profiles [17].

(d) *Enhanced Learning*

Adaptive trials facilitate continuous learning, allowing researchers to refine hypotheses and improve trial design iteratively. This is particularly valuable in early-phase studies of novel immunotherapies, where understanding dose-response relationships and safety profiles is essential.

Challenges

(a) *Statistical Complexity*

Designing and analyzing adaptive trials require advanced statistical expertise. Controlling Type I errors, maintaining blinding, and ensuring unbiased estimates are critical. Simulation-based planning is often necessary to evaluate operating characteristics under various adaptation scenarios [18].

(b) *Operational Demands*

Adaptive trials demand robust infrastructure for real-time data collection, monitoring, and decision-making. Community hospitals may face challenges in implementing such systems without external support or collaboration.

(c) *Regulatory Scrutiny*

Regulatory agencies require detailed pre-specification of adaptation rules and rigorous justification for design choices. Engaging with regulators early in the trial planning process is essential to ensure compliance and avoid delays [7, 8].

(d) *Resource Intensity*

While adaptive designs can be more efficient overall, they often require greater upfront investment in planning, statistical modeling, and data systems. This can be a barrier for smaller institutions or investigator-initiated trials.

Applications for Cancer Research

Adaptive randomized trials have become increasingly prominent in cancer research, offering innovative solutions to the challenges posed by tumor heterogeneity, evolving treatment paradigms, and the need for personalized medicine. These designs are particularly well-suited for evaluating monoclonal antibodies (mAbs), which often target specific molecular pathways and require stratified patient populations for optimal efficacy.

Platform Trials in Oncology

One of the most impactful applications of adaptive designs in oncology is the platform trial, which allows multiple therapies to be evaluated simultaneously within a single, ongoing framework. The I-SPY 2 trial is a landmark example. This trial evaluated various neoadjuvant therapies for breast cancer, including mAbs such as pertuzumab, using adaptive randomization based on biomarker profiles and early response data [1]. The trial's design enabled rapid identification of effective agents and seamless transition to confirmatory studies.

Basket and Umbrella Trials

Adaptive designs also underpin basket and umbrella trials, which stratify patients based on genetic or molecular characteristics rather than tumor histology. For instance, the National Cancer Institute–Molecular Analysis for Therapy Choice (NCI-MATCH) trial used an adaptive approach to assign patients to targeted therapies, including mAbs, based on tumor genomics across multiple cancer types [19]. These designs are particularly valuable for rare cancers or subtypes with limited treatment options.

Dose Optimization and Safety Monitoring

Phase I trials in oncology frequently use adaptive dose-finding designs, such as the Bayesian continual reassessment method (CRM), to identify the maximum tolerated dose of mAbs like daratumumab and nivolumab. These designs allow for real-time adjustment of dosing based on observed toxicities, improving patient safety and trial efficiency [11].

Biomarker-Driven Enrichment

Adaptive enrichment designs enable dynamic modification of eligibility criteria based on interim biomarker analyses. This approach has been used in trials of checkpoint inhibitors (e.g., pembrolizumab, atezolizumab) where PD-L1 expression levels guide patient selection. Such designs enhance the likelihood of detecting treatment effects in responsive subpopulations [12].

Real-World Integration

Adaptive trials are increasingly being conducted in community hospital settings, expanding access to innovative research. The REMAP-CAP trial, although focused on COVID-19, demonstrated the feasibility of deploying adaptive platform trials across diverse clinical environments, including nonacademic centers. This model is now being explored for oncology applications, particularly in evaluating supportive care interventions and immunotherapies [3].

Practical Considerations for Community Hospital Clinicians

While adaptive randomized trials (ARTs) offer numerous advantages, their implementation in community hospital settings requires thoughtful planning and collaboration (Fig. 6.1). Historically, such trials have been concentrated in academic medical centers due to the complexity of design and infrastructure requirements. However, with growing interest in decentralizing research and increasing access to innovative therapies, community hospitals are increasingly participating in adaptive trials, especially in oncology and immunology.

Infrastructure and Resources

Adaptive trials demand robust infrastructure for:

- Real-time data collection and monitoring
- Electronic data capture (EDC) systems
- Statistical support for interim analyses and simulations
- Secure data storage and transfer protocols

Community hospitals may need to partner with academic institutions or clinical research organizations (CROs) to access these resources. For example, the REMAP-CAP trial successfully integrated community hospitals into its adaptive platform by providing centralized data systems and remote monitoring capabilities [3].

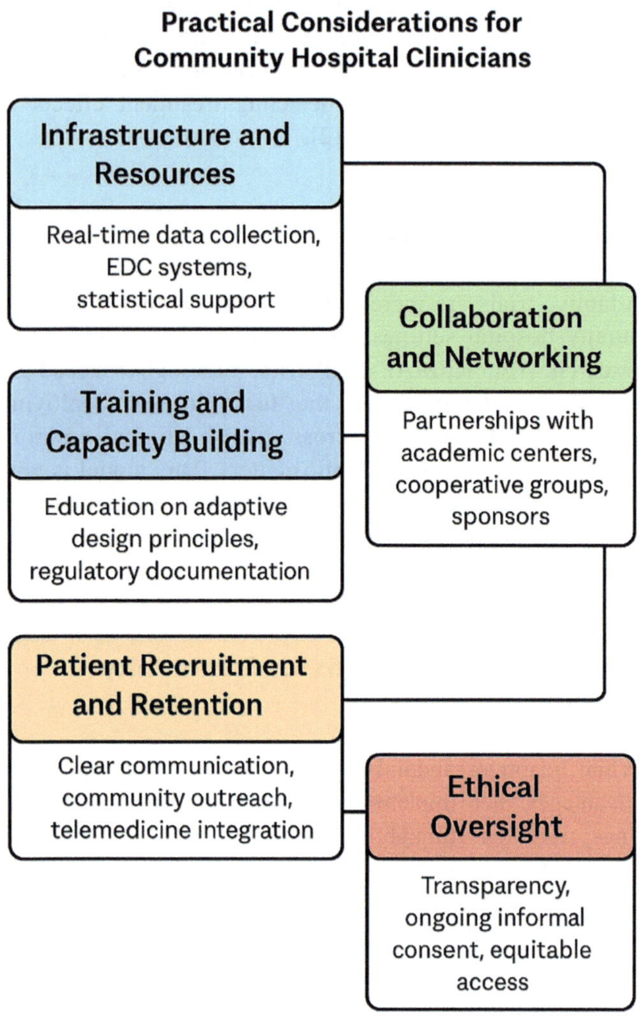

Fig. 6.1 Practical considerations for implementing adaptive randomized trials in community hospitals. Key domains include infrastructure, training, collaboration, patient recruitment, and ethical oversight

Training and Capacity Building

Clinicians and research staff must be trained in:

- Principles of adaptive trial design
- Informed consent processes for adaptive protocols
- Regulatory documentation and reporting
- Use of trial-specific software and platforms

Workshops, online modules, and mentorship from experienced investigators can facilitate capacity building. Institutions like the Clinical Trials Transformation Initiative (CTTI) offer resources tailored to nonacademic settings [20].

Collaboration and Networking

Participation in adaptive trials often requires collaboration with:

- Academic medical centers
- National cooperative groups (e.g., NCI, SWOG)
- Industry sponsors
- Patient advocacy organizations

These partnerships can provide access to trial protocols, funding, and shared infrastructure. For example, community sites involved in the I-SPY 2 trial benefited from centralized biomarker testing and statistical support [1].

Patient Recruitment and Retention

Adaptive trials may involve complex eligibility criteria and dynamic protocols, which can pose challenges for recruitment. Strategies to enhance participation include:

- Clear communication about trial adaptations and potential benefits
- Use of patient navigators and community outreach
- Integration of telemedicine and remote monitoring
- Inclusion of diverse populations to improve generalizability

In trials involving monoclonal antibodies, patient education is critical to address concerns about immunogenicity, side effects, and long-term outcomes.

Ethical Oversight

Adaptive trials require careful ethical oversight, particularly regarding transparency in adaptation rules, ongoing informed consent as trial parameters change, and equitable access to promising therapies. Institutional Review Boards (IRBs) must be engaged early and updated regularly as adaptations occur. Templates for adaptive trial protocols and consent forms are available through regulatory agencies and research networks [7].

Designing an Adaptive Trial: Step-by-Step Guide

Designing an adaptive randomized trial (ART) requires meticulous planning, interdisciplinary collaboration, and a clear understanding of both clinical and statistical principles. For community hospital clinicians, engaging in adaptive trial design may seem daunting, but with the right support and structure, it is entirely feasible. This section outlines a step-by-step approach to designing an ART, with examples relevant to oncology and immunology (Table 6.3).

Step 1: Define the Research Question and Objectives

Start by articulating a clear clinical question. For example:

- Does a novel monoclonal antibody improve progression-free survival in patients with metastatic colorectal cancer?
- Can adaptive enrichment based on PD-L1 expression improve response rates to checkpoint inhibitors?

Define primary and secondary endpoints (e.g., overall survival, tumor response, biomarker modulation) and determine the population of interest.

Step 2: Select Appropriate Adaptive Features

Choose adaptive elements based on the trial's goals and feasibility. Common options include:

- Adaptive randomization to favor promising treatments
- Sample size re-estimation to maintain statistical power
- Interim analysis for early stopping
- Biomarker-based enrichment to target responsive subgroups

For example, in a trial evaluating a new anti-CD38 mAb for multiple myeloma, adaptive randomization could be used to allocate more patients to arms showing early efficacy.

Step 3: Conduct Simulation Studies

Simulations are essential to evaluate the operating characteristics of the adaptive design, including Type I and II error rates, power under various scenarios, and impact of adaptations on trial integrity. Statistical software such as R, SAS, or East can be used for simulation modeling. Collaboration with a biostatistician is highly recommended.

Table 6.3 Steps in designing adaptive randomized trial

Step	Description	Example
1. Define research question and objectives	Identify clinical questions, endpoints, and population	Does a novel mAb improve PFS in metastatic colorectal cancer?
2. Select adaptive features	Choose design elements like adaptive randomization, interim analyses, enrichment	Anti-CD38 mAb trial uses adaptive randomization based on early efficacy
3. Conduct simulation studies	Model trial scenarios to assess power, error rates, and adaptation impact	Use R or SAS to simulate Type I/II error rates
4. Develop protocol and SAP	Define adaptation rules, interim analysis timing, DMC roles, and blinding procedures	SAP includes decision thresholds for early stopping
5. Engage regulatory authorities	Seek early feedback from FDA/EMA on design and simulations	Submit pre-IND with justification and risk mitigation plan
6. Secure ethical approval and consent	Ensure informed consent reflects adaptive nature of trial	IRB reviews contingency plans and adaptation mechanisms
7. Implement trial infrastructure	Set up data systems, analysis platforms, and staff training	Use CROs for real-time data capture and interim analysis
8. Monitor and adapt	Conduct interim analyses, implement changes per protocol, document decisions	DMC reviews safety/efficacy and guides adaptations

Step 4: Develop a Detailed Protocol and Statistical Analysis Plan (SAP)

The protocol must include:

- Clear definitions of adaptation rules
- Timing and frequency of interim analyses
- Role of data monitoring committees (DMCs)
- Procedures for maintaining blinding and data integrity

The SAP should outline how adaptations will be implemented and analyzed, including pre-specified decision rules and thresholds.

Step 5: Engage with Regulatory Authorities Early

Early consultation with regulatory agencies (e.g., FDA, EMA) is critical. Submit a pre-IND or scientific advice request to discuss:

- Justification for adaptive features
- Simulation results
- Risk mitigation strategies
- Plans for maintaining trial validity

Regulators are generally supportive of adaptive designs when they are well-justified and transparently planned [7].

Step 6: Secure Ethical Approval and Prepare Consent Materials

Adaptive trials require special attention to informed consent. Patients must be made aware that:

- Trial parameters may change during the study.
- Their treatment assignment could be influenced by interim results.
- Additional safety monitoring may be required.

IRBs may request detailed explanations of adaptation mechanisms and contingency plans.

Step 7: Implement Trial Infrastructure

Ensure the availability of:

- Real-time data capture systems
- Secure platforms for interim analysis
- Communication protocols for adaptation decisions
- Training for site staff on adaptive procedures

Community hospitals can leverage centralized trial networks or CROs to support these functions.

Step 8: Monitor and Adapt

Once the trial is underway:

- Conduct interim analyses as scheduled.
- Use DMCs to review safety and efficacy data.
- Implement adaptations according to pre-specified rules.
- Maintain documentation of all decisions and changes.

Transparency and adherence to protocol are essential to preserve trial credibility and regulatory compliance.

Data Monitoring and Interim Analyses

Data monitoring and interim analyses are the backbone of adaptive randomized trials (ARTs). These processes ensure that adaptations are implemented safely, ethically, and in accordance with pre-specified rules. For community hospital clinicians, understanding these mechanisms is essential for successful participation in adaptive trials.

Role of Data Monitoring Committees (DMCs)

A data monitoring committee (DMC) is an independent group responsible for reviewing accumulating trial data and making recommendations about continuation, modification, or termination of the study. In adaptive trials, DMCs play a critical role in:

- Evaluating interim efficacy and safety data
- Assessing adherence to adaptation rules
- Maintaining trial integrity and confidentiality

For example, in the REMAP-CAP trial, the DMC oversaw multiple intervention arms and ensured that adaptations (e.g., dropping ineffective treatments) were based on robust evidence [3].

Interim Analyses

Interim analyses are planned evaluations of trial data at predefined points. They serve several purposes:

- Early stopping for efficacy or futility: Prevents unnecessary exposure to ineffective treatments
- Sample size re-estimation: Adjusts enrollment targets based on observed effect sizes
- Adaptive randomization updates: Alters allocation probabilities to favor promising arms

These analyses must be conducted according to a pre-specified statistical analysis plan (SAP) to avoid bias and maintain regulatory compliance [7].

Decision Rules and Transparency

Adaptations should be guided by clear, pre-specified decision rules documented in the protocol and SAP. Examples include:

- Stopping boundaries for efficacy or futility
- Thresholds for biomarker-based enrichment
- Criteria for adding or dropping treatment arms

Transparency is critical. All adaptation decisions should be logged and reported to regulatory authorities and IRBs.

Operational Considerations

Community hospitals participating in adaptive trials should ensure:

- Secure and timely data transfer to centralized monitoring systems
- Training for site staff on interim analysis procedures
- Clear communication channels with the DMC and trial sponsors

Remote monitoring and centralized data platforms can facilitate participation by sites with limited resources.

Ethical and Regulatory Considerations

Adaptive randomized trials (ARTs) introduce unique ethical and regulatory challenges due to their dynamic nature. Unlike traditional fixed designs, ARTs involve pre-specified modifications during the trial, which can impact patient consent, trial integrity, and compliance with international guidelines. For community hospital clinicians, understanding these considerations is critical to ensure patient safety and regulatory approval.

Ethical Principles in Adaptive Trials

Informed Consent Patients must be fully informed that trial parameters may change during the study. Consent forms should clearly explain:

- The possibility of treatment allocation changes based on interim results
- Potential addition or removal of treatment arms
- How these adaptations may affect their participation

Continuous consent or re-consent may be required when significant adaptations occur, such as introducing a new therapy and changing eligibility criteria [21].

(a) *Transparency and Communication*

Ethical conduct demands transparency in adaptation rules and decision-making processes. Investigators should:

- Share adaptation plans with Institutional Review Boards (IRBs).
- Communicate changes promptly to participants and stakeholders.
- Maintain detailed documentation of all adaptations.

Regulatory Framework

Regulatory agencies such as the FDA and EMA support adaptive designs but require rigorous planning and justification. Key requirements include the following.

Pre-specification of Adaptation Rules

All adaptations must be defined in the protocol and statistical analysis plan (SAP) before trial initiation.

Simulation Studies

Sponsors must demonstrate through simulations that the design controls Type I error and maintains statistical validity under various scenarios [7].

Independent Oversight

Use of data monitoring committees (DMCs) is strongly recommended to ensure unbiased interim analyses and adaptation decisions.

Early Engagement with Regulators

Sponsors should seek scientific advice or pre-IND meetings to align design features, adaptation rules, and reporting requirements.

International Guidelines

The ICH E20 Guideline on Adaptive Designs for Clinical Trials (2025) provides harmonized recommendations for adaptive trials globally. It emphasizes:

- Maintaining trial integrity and credibility
- Ensuring patient safety during adaptations
- Transparent reporting of adaptation decisions in publications and regulatory submissions [8]

Special Considerations for Community Hospitals

Community hospitals must:

- Ensure IRBs are familiar with adaptive trial principles.
- Implement robust data security and monitoring systems.
- Collaborate with academic centers or CROs for regulatory compliance and statistical expertise.

Future Directions

Adaptive randomized trials (ARTs) are poised to play an increasingly leading role in clinical research, driven by advances in technology, data science, and global collaboration. For oncology and immunotherapy, these innovations promise to accelerate the development of targeted therapies, including monoclonal antibodies (mAbs), and improve patient outcomes.

Expansion of Platform and Basket Trials

Platform trials like I-SPY 2 and REMAP-CAP have demonstrated the feasibility of evaluating multiple interventions within a single adaptive framework. Future oncology trials will increasingly adopt basket designs to evaluate therapies across tumor types sharing common molecular targets and umbrella designs to evaluate multiple targeted agents within a single cancer type.

These approaches are particularly suited for mAbs targeting immune checkpoints or cytokine pathways, where efficacy may vary across tumor histologies or autoimmune conditions [1].

Decentralized and Hybrid Trial Models

The COVID-19 pandemic accelerated the adoption of decentralized trial models, incorporating telemedicine, remote monitoring, and electronic consent. These innovations will enable greater participation from community hospitals educated patient burden through home-based assessments and real-time data integration for adaptive decision-making. Hybrid models combining on-site and remote procedures will likely become standard for adaptive trials, improving accessibility and diversity in trial populations [20].

Global Harmonization of Regulatory Standards

The ICH E20 Guideline represents a major step toward harmonizing adaptive trial regulations across regions. Future efforts will focus on standardizing simulation requirements, aligning reporting standards for adaptations, and facilitating multinational adaptive trials for rare cancers and immune-mediated diseases [8].

Personalized and Precision Medicine

Adaptive designs will increasingly incorporate genomic, proteomic, and immunologic data to tailor therapies to individual patients. Trials of mAbs targeting specific immune pathways (e.g., PD-1, IL-6, TNF-α) will leverage adaptive enrichment strategies to identify responders early and optimize treatment algorithms [12].

Integration of Artificial Intelligence (AI) and Machine Learning

AI and machine learning algorithms can enhance adaptive trial designs by predicting treatment response based on real-time biomarker and imaging data, optimizing randomization strategies to balance efficacy and safety, and automating interim analyses for faster decision-making. For example, AI-driven models are being explored to refine adaptive enrichment strategies in trials of checkpoint inhibitors, enabling dynamic patient stratification based on evolving molecular profiles.

Summary and Key Takeaways

This chapter provides a comprehensive overview of adaptive randomized trials (ARTs), emphasizing their critical role in advancing cancer research, particularly in oncology and immunotherapy. ARTs represent a powerful tool for optimizing trial design, improving efficiency, and personalizing treatment strategies.

Key Takeaways:

- ARTs offer significant advantages, including increased efficiency, ethical benefits, and enhanced flexibility in response to emerging data.
- Cancer research has been at the forefront of adopting adaptive designs, with successful applications in monoclonal antibody (mAb) trials targeting various tumor and immune pathways.
- Community hospital clinicians can play a crucial role in conducting ARTs by leveraging collaborative networks, investing in training, and adhering to ethical and regulatory guidelines.

References

1. Barker AD, Sigman CC, Kelloff GJ, Hylton NM, Berry DA, Esserman LJ. I-SPY 2: an adaptive breast cancer trial design in the setting of neoadjuvant chemotherapy. Clin Pharmacol Ther. 2009;86(1):97–100.
2. Group RC. Tocilizumab in patients admitted to hospital with COVID-19 (RECOVERY): a randomised, controlled, open-label, platform trial. Lancet. 2021;397(10285):1637–45.
3. Investigators R-C, Gordon AC, Mouncey PR, Al-Beidh F, Rowan KM, Nichol AD, et al. Interleukin-6 receptor antagonists in critically ill patients with Covid-19. N Engl J Med. 2021;384(16):1491–502.
4. Bothwell LE, Greene JA, Podolsky SH, Jones DS. Assessing the Gold Standard--Lessons from the History of RCTs. N Engl J Med. 2016;374(22):2175–81.
5. Coiffier B, Lepage E, Briere J, Herbrecht R, Tilly H, Bouabdallah R, et al. CHOP chemotherapy plus rituximab compared with CHOP alone in elderly patients with diffuse large-B-cell lymphoma. N Engl J Med. 2002;346(4):235–42.
6. Chow SC, Chang M. Adaptive design methods in clinical trials – a review. Orphanet J Rare Dis. 2008;3:11.
7. Federal Drug Administration. Adaptive Design Clinical Trials for Drugs and Biologics Guidance for Industry December 2019. Available from: https://www.fda.gov/regulatory-information/search-fda-guidance-documents/adaptive-design-clinical-trials-drugs-and-biologics-guidance-industry.
8. European Medicines Agency. ICH E20 adaptive designs for clinical trials – Scientific guideline 2025. Available from: https://www.ema.europa.eu/en/ich-e20-adaptive-designs-clinical-trials-scientific-guideline.
9. Angus DC, Derde L, Al-Beidh F, Annane D, Arabi Y, Beane A, et al. Effect of hydrocortisone on mortality and organ support in patients with severe COVID-19: the REMAP-CAP COVID-19 corticosteroid domain randomized clinical trial. JAMA. 2020;324(13):1317–29.
10. Mehta CR, Pocock SJ. Adaptive increase in sample size when interim results are promising: a practical guide with examples. Stat Med. 2011;30(28):3267–84.
11. Neuenschwander B, Branson M, Gsponer T. Critical aspects of the Bayesian approach to phase I cancer trials. Stat Med. 2008;27(13):2420–39.
12. Tu Y, Renfro LA. Latest developments in "Adaptive Enrichment" clinical trial designs in oncology. Ther Innov Regul Sci. 2024;58(6):1201–13.
13. Kim ES, Herbst RS, Wistuba II, Lee JJ, Blumenschein GR Jr, Tsao A, et al. The BATTLE trial: personalizing therapy for lung cancer. Cancer Discov. 2011;1(1):44–53.
14. Granholm A, Jensen AKG, Lange T, Perner A, Moller MH, Kaas-Hansen BS. Designing and evaluating Bayesian advanced adaptive randomised clinical trials: a practical guide. Pharm Stat. 2025;24(6):e70042.
15. Rugo HS, Olopade OI, DeMichele A, Yau C, van't Veer LJ, Buxton MB, et al. Adaptive randomization of Veliparib-carboplatin treatment in breast cancer. N Engl J Med. 2016;375(1):23–34.
16. Salama C, Han J, Yau L, Reiss WG, Kramer B, Neidhart JD, et al. Tocilizumab in patients hospitalized with Covid-19 pneumonia. N Engl J Med. 2021;384(1):20–30.
17. Wang R, Dasgupta A, Ward MM. Predicting probability of response to tumor necrosis factor inhibitors for individual patients with ankylosing spondylitis. JAMA Netw Open. 2022;5(3):e222312.
18. Bhatt DL, Mehta C. Adaptive designs for clinical trials. N Engl J Med. 2016;375(1):65–74.
19. Flaherty KT, Gray R, Chen A, Li S, Patton D, Hamilton SR, et al. The molecular analysis for therapy choice (NCI-MATCH) trial: lessons for genomic trial design. J Natl Cancer Inst. 2020;112(10):1021–9.
20. Initiative CTT. Modernizing Trials Together. https://ctti--clinicaltrials.org/2025.
21. Emanuel EJ, Wendler D, Grady C. What makes clinical research ethical? JAMA. 2000;283(20):2701–11.

Cluster Randomized Trials

7

Ruyi Liu, Monica Taljaard, and Fan Li

Introduction

Randomized controlled trials (RCTs) are considered the gold standard study design for evaluating the effectiveness of medical interventions [1–3]. In a standard RCT, individual participants are randomly assigned to different treatment groups, which will be referred to as intervention or control conditions. Through the process of randomization, observed and unobserved participant characteristics tend to be evenly distributed across the conditions on average so that any observed differences in outcomes between conditions can then be attributed to the intervention. Figure 7.1(a) depicts the generic structure of an RCT with 1:1 randomization.

In a cluster randomized trial (CRT), entire social units or predefined groups of individuals, referred to as clusters, are randomized to different treatment conditions [4, 5], and all individuals within the same cluster are exposed to the same condition; outcomes are then measured on multiple individuals within each cluster. Examples of clusters are wards, hospitals, or primary care clinics [6]. Cluster randomization is employed when individual randomization is impractical (e.g., when the intervention can only be delivered to entire clusters [7]), or when there are substantial risks of contamination when individuals in the same cluster are allocated to differing interventions [8, 9]. CRTs can also be beneficial when providing access to interventions across all participants is costly [10, 11]. Figure 7.1(b) illustrates the generic structure of a CRT with 1:1 randomization.

CRTs are especially useful in public health research where intervention programs are delivered to entire hospitals or geographical regions, such as infection control programs [12] and vaccination campaigns [13]. CRTs are also valuable for evaluating quality improvement initiatives [14] and new models of care delivery in large healthcare systems [15]. In cancer research, CRTs have been used to evaluate diverse types of interventions delivered at cluster level, professional level, or individual level. An example of a cluster-level intervention is implementation of electronic health records in pediatric cancer clinics to improve patient care coordination [16]; an example of a professional-level intervention is notification of physicians of patient nonadherence to colorectal cancer screening to increase screening rates [17]; finally, an example of an individual-level intervention is low-intensity PSA-based screening in prostate cancer to reduce mortality [18]. Regardless of the level of intervention, an important implication of cluster randomization is that, unlike individually randomized trials, the individual outcome measurements are no longer independent within each cluster, leading to a positive intra-cluster correlation coefficient (ICC) that must be adjusted for in both the design and analysis of such trials.

However, CRTs raise additional methodological complexities compared to individually randomized trials, and

R. Liu
Department of Biostatistics, Yale School of Public Health, New Haven, CT, USA

Center for Methods in Implementation and Prevention Science, Yale School of Public Health, New Haven, CT, USA

M. Taljaard
Methodological and Implementation Research, Ottawa Hospital Research Institute, Ottawa, ON, Canada

School of Epidemiology, Public Health and Preventive Medicine, University of Ottawa, Ottawa, ON, Canada

F. Li (✉)
Department of Biostatistics, Yale School of Public Health, New Haven, CT, USA

Center for Methods in Implementation and Prevention Science, Yale School of Public Health, New Haven, CT, USA

Clinical and Translational Research Accelerator, Department of Medicine, Yale School of Medicine, New Haven, CT, USA
e-mail: fan.f.li@yale.edu

J. Huang, H. S.L. Jim (eds.), *Cancer Research Guidance for Clinicians and Researchers*,
https://doi.org/10.1007/978-3-032-19175-5_7

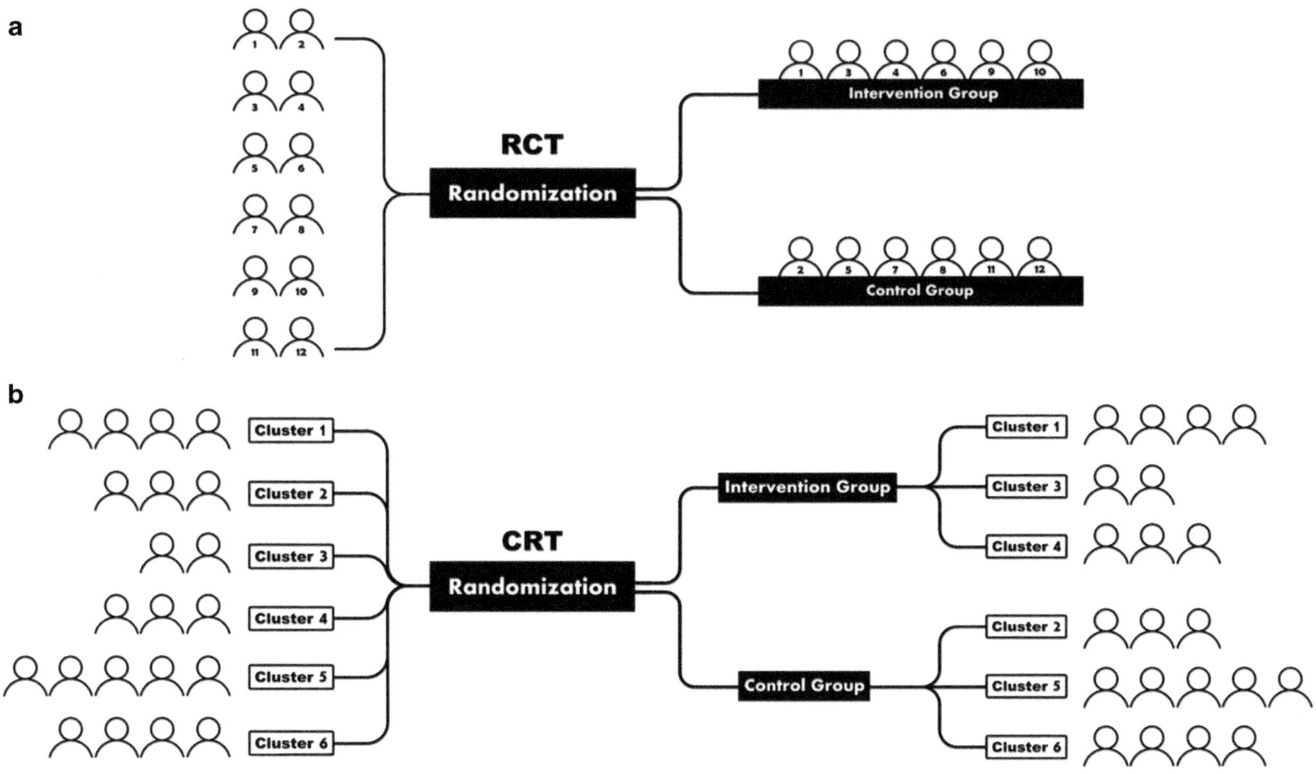

Fig. 7.1 SEQ Figure * ARABIC 1 (**a**) Randomized controlled trial diagram: Participants are individually randomized into either the intervention group or the control group following a 1:1 allocation ratio. (**b**) Cluster randomized trial diagram: Clusters of individuals are randomized rather than individual participants. In this diagram, six clusters are randomized in a 1:1 allocation to either the intervention group or the control group, with three clusters assigned to each arm. All individuals within a cluster receive the same treatment based on the group's assignment

need to be carefully justified [13, 14]. A key concern is the risk of bias from the identification or recruitment of participants within clusters, as most CRTs recruit participants prospectively after clusters have already been randomized; moreover, participants and those recruiting them can often not be blinded so that inclusion in the trial could have been affected by knowledge of the intervention [19, 20]. The implication of such post-randomization selection bias [20] is that, despite cluster-level randomization, the randomization may no long hold at the individual level, leading to biased treatment effect estimates [21–23]. Hemming et al. provided guidelines on designing, conducting, and analyzing CRTs, emphasizing the importance of addressing potential biases, carefully considering sample size, implementing randomization at the lowest possible level, and making statistical adjustments to ensure validity and statistical efficiency [11, 24]. A summary of these guidelines is provided in Table 7.1.

In this chapter, we present examples of CRTs in cancer research, highlighting the rationale for selecting cluster-level randomization over individual-level trial designs. We discuss key considerations in the design and analysis of these trials, including the methods used to calculate sample sizes at the design phase. Furthermore, we examine techniques for improving randomization by addressing chance imbalances, with a focus on covariate-constrained randomization and its practical implementation. Finally, we explore the stepped-wedge trial design, which has gained popularity as an alternative to traditional parallel-arm CRTs. We explain its features, advantages, and challenges, provide an example from cancer research, and review methods for sample size calculation and analysis.

Table 7.1 Key design considerations for cluster randomized trials (CRTs). Following Hemming et al. [11, 24], this table summarizes essential guidelines for designing and analyzing CRTs, including considerations for randomization level, sample size calculations, contamination minimization, and statistical corrections

Considerations	Details
(a) Use cluster randomization only when necessary	1. CRTs require larger sample sizes and are more prone to bias. 2. Individual randomization should be preferred unless contamination or logistical constraints justify cluster randomization.
(b) Randomize at the lowest level whenever possible	Lower-level randomization implies a larger number of available clusters which can improve statistical power and efficiency, but the risk of contamination should be managed.
(c) Account for clustering in sample size calculations	1. Apply a necessary sample size inflation to account for the intra-cluster correlation coefficient (ICC). 2. A further inflation may be required to adjust for cluster size variation.
(d) Consider restricted randomization methods	Use stratified or constrained randomization techniques to reduce the risk of chance imbalance across treatment arms.
(e) Recruit participants before randomization	Pre-randomization recruitment reduces risks of bias but may not be possible. If post-randomization recruitment is necessary, attempt to blind participants and recruiters.
(f) Use strategies to minimize contamination	Consider physical separation of clusters to ensure independent allocation to intervention and control groups is possible.
(g) Use small sample corrections	If the number of clusters is small, use finite-sample corrections such as Kenward-Roger [25] or Satterthwaite [26].

Examples of Cluster Randomized Trials in Cancer Research

CRTs are increasingly used in cancer healthcare delivery research, and we provide two examples before delving into the statistical implications due to cluster randomization. The examples are summarized in Table 7.2. As a first example, a CRT was conducted to evaluate whether a geriatric assessment (GA) intervention can improve communication about aging-related concerns in older patients with advanced cancer [27]. The trial enrolled patients aged 70 years and older with advanced solid tumors or lymphoma, all of whom had at least one impairment in a GA domain. Community oncology practices were randomly assigned to either the intervention group, where oncologists received a tailored GA summary and GA-guided recommendations, or the usual care group, where oncologists were alerted only to potential cognitive or depressive issues [27]. Cluster randomization was used to reduce the risk of contamination by ensuring that all oncologists within a single practice, and hence all patients in the same practice, receive the same condition. Furthermore, randomization at the practice level was considered more logistically feasible than randomization at the patient level and allowed the GA to be evaluated within the context of routine clinical care.

As a second example, studies have shown that mailing fecal immunochemical test (FIT) kits to individuals who are due for colorectal cancer screening can improve screening rates, thus reducing cancer incidence and mortality [28]. In the Stop Colorectal Cancer (STOP CRC) study [29], a CRT was conducted across 26 federally qualified health center clinics to evaluate the effect of a mailed FIT outreach program embedded in electronic health record systems. The primary outcome was the clinic-level proportion of patients who completed a FIT. From an operational standpoint, randomizing at the clinic level facilitated integration of the intervention into existing electronic health record systems and clinic workflows, and simplified the identification of eligible patients for screening and automated delivery of FIT kits. Randomizing individual patients within clinics would also have risked contamination due to possible information sharing between patients within the same clinic.

Table 7.2 Summary of the setting, population, rationale for cluster randomization, and sample size calculations for two cluster randomized trials: (1) the GA intervention study for older cancer patients across community oncology practices and (2) the STOP CRC study evaluating a mailed colorectal cancer screening outreach program in federally qualified health centers

Example 1: Communication with older patients with cancer using geriatric assessment (GA)	
Setting and population	This study is a CRT conducted across 31 community oncology practices, focusing on patients aged 70 years or older with advanced solid tumors or lymphoma, who had at least one impaired domain in a GA, and involving their caregivers to evaluate the impact of providing GA summaries and tailored recommendations on communication outcomes during oncology visits.
Reasoning for cluster randomization	1. Avoid contamination: This use of a CRT design minimizes contamination by ensuring that all oncologists within a single practice follow the same protocol. It prevents the inadvertent sharing of intervention-related strategies or insights between oncologists treating patients in different study arms. 2. Logistical feasibility: It also enhances logistical feasibility, as it is easier to manage the GA intervention for oncologists at the practice level rather than targeting individual patients.
Reported sample size calculation	*"Sample size and power considerations were based on the primary aim of the HCCQ-age to address patient satisfaction with communication about aging-related concerns. This design (8 sites per arm and 31 subjects per site) had 80% power at the 0.05 significance level to detect a difference of 1.3 in HCCQ-age scores, with an intraclass correlation coefficient (ICC) of 0.14, corresponding to an effect size of 0.62. Assuming a withdrawal rate of 5%, the targeted accrual was 528 patients."* [27]
Example 2: Stop Colorectal Cancer (STOP CRC)	
Setting and population	This study is a CRT conducted in 26 federally qualified health center clinics, focusing on adults aged 50–74 years who were overdue for colorectal cancer screening, to evaluate the effectiveness of an electronic health record embedded mailed outreach program using fecal immunochemical tests (FIT).
Reasoning for cluster randomization	1. Operational feasibility: Randomizing clinics allows the intervention to be embedded into the electronic health record (EHR) systems and workflows of entire clinics, streamlining the identification of patients due for screening and the delivery of FIT kits. This clinic-wide integration would not be feasible if individual patients were randomized. 2. Avoid contamination: Since the intervention was integrated into the workflow of clinics and was administered at the clinic level, randomizing individual patients within clinics would have risked contamination.
Reported sample size calculation	*"We assumed equal numbers of subjects per clinic and equal numbers of clinics (n = 13) per group. In practice, the clinic sizes will not be equal, but since almost all clinics have at least 450 active age-eligible patients, we conservatively use this figure for all sites. We based our calculations on the simple paradigm of comparing two binomial proportions with a type I error rate of 5%, and adjusted both for ICC and the reduced degrees-of-freedom for the critical values. Expecting the ICC to be about 0.03, we will have very good power (larger than 91%) to detect absolute differences as small as 10 percentage points even if the FIT completion rate in the usual care arm is as high as 15%."* [29]

Statistical Implications Under Cluster Randomization

A key implication of cluster randomization is that this design is less statistically efficient than an individually randomized design. This is because the outcomes collected from individuals within the same cluster are correlated. A common measure of the degree of similarity between observations in the same cluster is the ICC [8]; a positive ICC reduces the effective sample size, and thus, a larger sample size is required to achieve the same statistical power as an individually randomized trial [30–32]. Accounting for clustering is essential in both the sample size calculation and subsequent analysis [33]. The required sample size, initially calculated under the assumption of individual-level randomization, should be inflated by the design effect (DE) to achieve the same required level of statistical power under cluster randomization. The formula for the DE is

$$DE = 1 + (m-1)\rho \qquad (7.1)$$

where m is the number of individuals per cluster (often assumed equal for simplicity) and ρ is the ICC [34], defined as the proportion of between-cluster variance relative to the overall variance (sum of between-cluster variance and within-cluster variance) of a given outcome. As calculation of the DE requires an advance estimate of the ICC, it has been recommended to report the ICC in completed CRTs to aid investigators planning studies in a similar population [35]. Figure 7.2 illustrates the relationship between the ICC and the DE for a range of cluster sizes m. When the ICC increases, the DE increases more rapidly for larger cluster sizes, illustrating why even a small value for the ICC can lead to a large variance inflation in a common scenario in healthcare delivery research where cluster sizes are large.

In a parallel two-arm CRT design where $100\pi\%$ $(0 < \pi < 1)$ clusters are randomized to intervention, assuming a continuous outcome, the sample size formula based on a two-sided test is calculated as

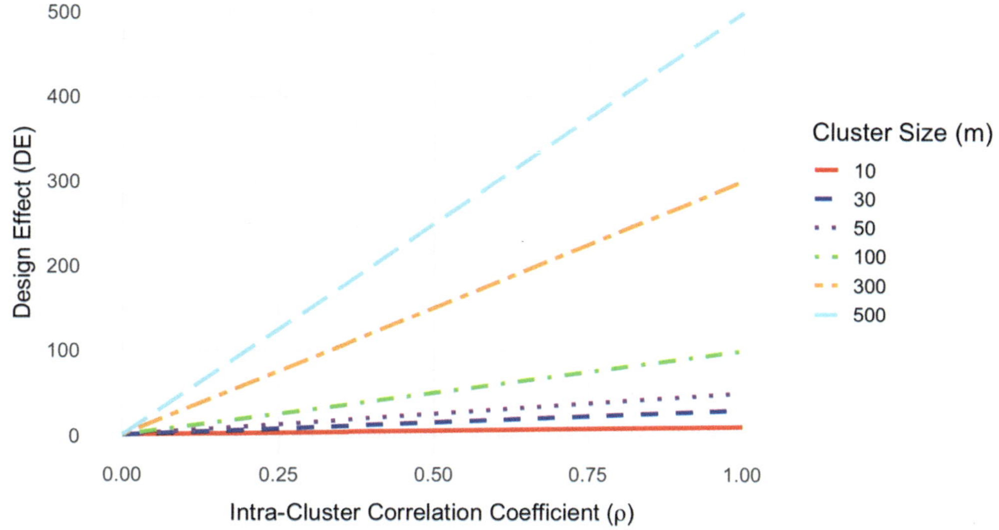

Fig. 7.2 SEQ Figure * ARABIC 2 Relationship between intra-cluster correlation coefficient (ICC) and design effect for different cluster sizes, ranging from 10 to 500. This graph illustrates how the design effect increases as the ICC increases, with larger cluster sizes amplifying the effect

$$n=\frac{\left(Z_{1-\alpha/2}+Z_{1-\beta}\right)^2\sigma^2}{m\Delta^2\pi(1-\pi)}\left[1+(m-1)\rho\right] \qquad (7.2)$$

where Z_x represents the x-th percentile of the standard normal distribution, α is significance level (often taken to be 0.05), β is type II error (corresponding to statistical power $100(1-\beta)\%$), Δ denotes the clinically important mean difference between arms or effect size, σ^2 is the total variance of the outcome, and n is the total number of clusters required [36, 37]. By rearranging the formula, given the sample size, the statistical power $1-\beta$ can be expressed as

$$1-\beta=\Phi\left(\sqrt{\frac{nm\Delta^2\pi(1-\pi)}{\sigma^2\left[1+(m-1)\rho\right]}}-Z_{1-\alpha/2}\right), \qquad (7.3)$$

where Φ denotes the standard normal cumulative distribution function. Consider the sample size calculation for Example 1 (the GA intervention [27]). In this trial, the primary outcome is the patient's score of satisfaction with communication about aging-related concerns. The design parameters are specified in Table 7.2, and we replicate the sample size and power analysis through detailed step-by-step calculations. To optimize statistical power, an equal allocation of patients to the intervention and control arms is applied, i.e., $\pi = 0.5$. With an assumed ICC of 0.14 and 31 individuals per cluster, a total of 14 clusters is required to achieve 80% power at a 0.05 significance level to detect a mean outcome difference of 1.3, corresponding to an effect size of 0.62 [27]. The estimated standard deviation of the outcome was 2.1. Thus, the required sample size can be calculated as

$$\frac{4\times\left(Z_{1-0.05/2}+Z_{0.2}\right)^2\times 2.1^2}{31\times 1.3^2}\left[1+(31-1)\times 0.14\right]=13.74.$$

At a 0.05 significance level, the actual study design of 16 total clusters can achieve $100(1-\beta)\% \approx 85.6\%$ statistical power. Assuming a withdrawal rate of 5% based on observational cohort data [27], 528 patients is the target accrual as reported in the published trial report.

The sample size formula for binary outcomes is similar, but requires one to provide the anticipated prevalence of the outcome under the control and the intervention conditions (thus, the effect size is simply their difference). Formally, the required number of clusters for a two-sided test with type I error rate $100\alpha\%$ and power $100(1-\beta)\%$ is given by

$$n=\frac{\left(Z_{1-\alpha/2}+Z_{1-\beta}\right)^2}{m\Delta^2}\times\left[\frac{P_0(1-P_0)}{1-\pi}+\frac{P_1(1-P_1)}{\pi}\right]\times\left[1+(m-1)\rho\right], \qquad (7.4)$$

where P_1 and P_0 are the expected prevalence of outcome in the intervention and control groups and Δ represents the target difference (or clinically important difference) in proportions between the two groups, calculated as $P_1 - P_0$ [33, 36]. By rearranging the terms, the power for a given sample size can be calculated as:

$$1-\beta=\Phi\left(\sqrt{\frac{nm\Delta^2}{\left[\frac{P_0(1-P_0)}{1-\pi}+\frac{P_1(1-P_1)}{\pi}\right]\times\left[1+(m-1)\rho\right]}}-Z_{1-\alpha/2}\right). \qquad (7.5)$$

Of note, this sample size formula is based on the effect size expressed as an absolute risk difference. If the effect size is expressed as a relative risk, i.e., $\Delta=\frac{P_1}{P_0}$, then the sample size formula becomes:

$$n=\frac{\left(Z_{1-\alpha/2}+Z_{1-\beta}\right)^2}{m\left(log(\Delta)\right)^2}\times\left[\frac{1-P_0}{(1-\pi)P_0}+\frac{1-P_1}{\pi P_1}\right]\times\left[1+(m-1)\rho\right]. \tag{7.6}$$

Finally, when the effect size is expressed as an odds ratio with $\Delta=\frac{\frac{P_1}{1-P_1}}{\frac{P_0}{1-P_0}}$, then the sample size formula is given by [38]:

$$n=\frac{\left(Z_{1-\alpha/2}+Z_{1-\beta}\right)^2}{m\left(log(\Delta)\right)^2}\times\left[\frac{1}{(1-\pi)P_0(1-P_0)}+\frac{1}{\pi P_1(1-P_1)}\right]\times\left[1+(m-1)\rho\right]. \tag{7.7}$$

These three sample size formulas for binary outcomes differ based on the effect size measure they are designed to detect, as well as based on how they model and interpret the effect size. The corresponding power expression for all three sample size formulas can be similarly derived by rearranging the terms.

Consider Example 2, the STOP CRC study [29]. Here, the primary outcome is the clinic-level proportion of patients eligible for CRC screening who complete a FIT within 12 months of being identified as due for screening. Only patients initially identified during the first year of screening are included in the primary outcome analysis. Table 7.2 outlines the design parameters for this study, and we can conduct a step-by-step replication of the sample size calculation and power analysis. To optimize power, this CRT design also assumed equal numbers of individuals per clinic and equal numbers of clinics per arm. Since nearly all clinics have a minimum of 450 active age-eligible patients, this number has been conservatively applied across all clusters for sample size calculation [29]. The baseline completion rate in the control arm is assumed to be 15%. Assuming an ICC of 0.03, a total of 22 clinics is the minimum number of clusters required to achieve 90% power at a 0.05 significance level to detect a 10 percentage point absolute difference in screening completion rates, which represents a meaningful effect size for enhancing standard screening practices [29]. The details of the sample size calculation are given by:

$$\frac{\left(Z_{1-0.05/2}+Z_{0.1}\right)^2}{450\times(0.1)^2}\times\left[\frac{0.15\times(1-0.15)}{0.5}+\frac{0.25\times(1-0.25)}{0.5}\right]\times\left[1+(450-1)\times0.03\right]=21.29.$$

At a 0.05 significance level, the actual study design with 26 clinics can achieve approximately $100(1-\beta)\,\%\approx94.8\%$ power. The target sample size is 26 clinics and 11,700 total patients which is adequate to provide the desired statistical power. If the effect size is expressed as a relative risk, the required number of clusters to achieve 90% power at a 0.05 significance level to detect a $\Delta=\frac{P_1}{P_0}=1.67$ relative risk is

$$\frac{\left(Z_{1-0.05/2}+Z_{0.1}\right)^2}{450\times\left(log(1.67)\right)^2}\times\left[\frac{1-0.15}{0.5\times0.15}+\frac{1-0.25}{0.5\times0.25}\right]\times\left[1+(450-1)\times0.03\right]=22.27.$$

If the effect size is expressed as an odds ratio, the required number of clusters to achieve 90% power at a 0.05 significance level to detect an odds ratio of $\Delta=\frac{\frac{P_1}{1-P_1}}{\frac{P_0}{1-P_0}}=1.89$ is

$$\frac{\left(Z_{1-0.05/2}+Z_{0.1}\right)^2}{450\times\left(log(1.89)\right)^2}\times\left[\frac{1}{0.5\times0.15\times(1-0.15)}+\frac{1}{0.5\times0.25\times(1-0.25)}\right]\times\left[1+(450-1)\times0.03\right]=21.97.$$

The required sample sizes for detecting a risk difference, relative risk, and odds ratio are quite similar when based on the same expected prevalence of the outcome in the intervention and control groups.

Of note, we have so far focused on the simple case where each cluster has approximately the same number of observations. In practice, clusters may vary in size due to the natural differences in their source population [37]. When cluster sizes vary, a common practice is to set m in the design effect to the mean cluster size, but this approach may underestimate the required sample size, especially when the coefficient of variation (CV, defined as the ratio between the standard deviation of cluster sizes and the mean cluster size) becomes large (say greater than 0.5) [39]. A conservative approach that explicitly incorporates the cluster size variation is to consider the following design effect [40]:

$$DE=1+\left\{\left(CV^2+1\right)\overline{m}-1\right\}\rho \tag{7.8}$$

where $\overline{m}$ is the mean cluster size and CV is the coefficient of variation in cluster sizes. Based on this new design effect, the required sample size will increase linearly in the squared value of CV, suggesting an additional loss of statistical efficiency due to variable cluster sizes. When the analysis is performed based on linear mixed models or generalized estimating equations with an exchangeable working correlation structure (methods that estimate ICC as a by-product in their estimation routine), the design effect accounting for variable cluster sizes can be smaller and given by

$$DE = \left\{1 - CV^2 \frac{\bar{m}\rho(1-\rho)}{\{1+(\bar{m}-1)\rho\}^2}\right\}^{-1}, \qquad (7.9)$$

which now has a more subtle relationship with CV [41]. With binary outcomes, Li and Tong [33] presented the comparison between these two design effects, highlighting the importance of estimating the ICC in the primary analysis of CRTs to maximally prevent loss of efficiency due to variable cluster sizes. Based on the design effect formula (7.9), van Breukelen et al. [41] suggested that variable cluster sizes would rarely require more than 10% inflation of the required number of clusters, and Liu and Colditz [42] suggested in an empirical study that variable cluster sizes may lead to approximately 14% efficiency loss in CRTs with large cluster sizes. A survey of sample size formulas with different outcomes and addressing different complexities can be found in Rutterford [37].

Techniques for Improving Randomization

Proper implementation of randomization procedures is integral to securing internal validity of any randomized controlled trial. Baseline balance, i.e., a comparable distribution of key covariates between conditions, is often an indication of internal validity. Chance imbalances not only reduce face validity but also can lead to decreased statistical power and precision. Chance imbalances are less likely with sufficiently large numbers of randomization units. In CRTs, a common practical challenge is that only a limited number of clusters may be available, increasing the risk of imbalance at baseline [43]. Restricted randomization methods are available, but these can be challenging to implement when there are a large number of covariates to balance, and particularly when some covariates are continuous.

Stratification and matching are two conventional strategies for improving baseline balance in CRTs. However, stratification may yield strata with few clusters and becomes increasing challenging to operationalize with larger number of baseline covariates [44]. Pair matching is a variation of stratification with two clusters per stratum, and can be effective in balancing covariates but introduces additional complexities in calculating the ICC [45]. In addition, pair matching may also offer limited benefit in CRTs with few clusters, as weak correlation among matched clusters may mean that any gains in efficiency due to matching are outweighed by losses due to having fewer degrees of freedom in a matched analysis [46, 47]. For this reason, pair matching is not usually recommended for CRTs [48].

Covariate-constrained randomization [49] offers an alternative approach for simultaneously balancing multiple baseline covariates with only a few available clusters [50]. Covariate-constrained randomization is implemented through the following steps [50]. First, suitable covariates to be balanced in the randomization need to be identified; these covariates are typically cluster-level covariates or summaries of individual-level covariates based on historical information and should ideally be correlated with the primary outcome. Second, all possible allocations of clusters to treatment arms are considered (or a random sample when the number of possible allocation is infeasibly large). Third, the subset of allocations that satisfy the predefined covariate balancing criteria, based on a chosen balance metric, is identified. Fourth, from the constrained randomization space, a single allocation is then randomly selected and becomes the final cluster treatment assignment. This approach excludes randomization schemes that yield poor balance and provides the flexibility to balance multiple covariates in the design phase, regardless of whether the covariates are continuous or categorical.

The covariate-constrained randomization design is determined by specifying a balance metric and the size of the randomization space. Different balance metrics can be applied to score the degree of baseline imbalance across arms. In a parallel two-arm CRT, Raab and Butcher introduced an l_2 balance metric [51]. Define S as the number of cluster-level covariates requiring balance at the design stage. The l_2 imbalance score, B_{l_2}, is given by

$$B_{l_2} = \sum_{s=1}^{S} \omega_s \left(\bar{x}_{0s} - \bar{x}_{1s}\right)^2, \qquad (7.10)$$

where ω_s represents a predetermined weight for the s-th covariate and $x\!-_{0s}$ and $x\!-_{1s}$ denote the average of cluster-level variable means within control arm and intervention arm, respectively. The default weight for each covariate is the inverse of the variance of its cluster means, which accounts for the relative influence and priority of each covariate and ensures that the imbalance score can capture an overall covariate balance. Li et al. [50] proposed an alternative l_1 imbalance score, replacing the l_2 metric with the l_1 distance measure, where the default weight is set to the inverse of the standard deviation of cluster means. Both l_2 and l_1 can accommodate continuous and categorical covariates by using dummy variables for multi-category covariates and remains invariant under linear transformations of covariates. In addition, De Hoop et al. [52] introduced an imbalance score, defined as a double sum of squared differences across both cluster-level variables and all levels of each variable, and Li et al. [43] proposed a modified version, expressed as the sum of maximum absolute differences, where the maximum is taken over all levels for each variable. Empirical studies have shown that variations in the balance metrics are less essential compared to the size of the randomization space, for improving baseline balance and statistical power of the final analysis [43, 50, 53]. Thus, these balance metrics may be used interchangeably.

Table 7.3 Allocation of rural and urban clusters across treatment and control arms in a hypothetical trial with 16 clusters. Each row represents a specific allocation type, showing the distribution of rural clusters (in red) and urban clusters (in blue). B_{l_1} represents the l_1 *imbalance score*. The imbalance score ranges from 0 (perfect balance) to 1 (worst balance)

# Rural in Arms	Treatment	Control	# of schemes	B_{l1}
8/0	🔴🔴🔴🔴🔴🔴🔴🔴	🔵🔵🔵🔵🔵🔵🔵🔵	1	1.00
7/1	🔴🔴🔴🔴🔴🔴🔴🔵	🔴🔵🔵🔵🔵🔵🔵🔵	64	0.75
6/2	🔴🔴🔴🔴🔴🔴🔵🔵	🔴🔴🔵🔵🔵🔵🔵🔵	784	0.50
5/3	🔴🔴🔴🔴🔴🔵🔵🔵	🔴🔴🔴🔵🔵🔵🔵🔵	3136	0.25
4/4	🔴🔴🔴🔴🔵🔵🔵🔵	🔴🔴🔴🔴🔵🔵🔵🔵	4900	0.00
3/5	🔴🔴🔴🔵🔵🔵🔵🔵	🔴🔴🔴🔴🔴🔵🔵🔵	3136	0.25
2/6	🔴🔴🔵🔵🔵🔵🔵🔵	🔴🔴🔴🔴🔴🔴🔵🔵	784	0.50
1/7	🔴🔵🔵🔵🔵🔵🔵🔵	🔴🔴🔴🔴🔴🔴🔴🔵	64	0.75
0/8	🔵🔵🔵🔵🔵🔵🔵🔵	🔴🔴🔴🔴🔴🔴🔴🔴	1	1.00

To illustrate, we consider a hypothetical trial with 16 clusters, divided into 8 clusters per arm, and a binary cluster-level covariate indicating whether a cluster is located in a rural ($x = 1$) or urban area ($x = 0$). In this context, the simple randomization space comprises $\binom{16}{8} = 12{,}870$ unique allocation schemes, corresponding to 9 distinct allocation types for the 8 rural and 8 urban clusters, as demonstrated in Table 7.3. Using the l_1 imbalance score, we have $B_{l_1} = \left|\bar{x}_{0s} - \bar{x}_{1s}\right|$. Out of the 12,870 possible allocation schemes, we may constrain the randomization space to a subset of 4,900 schemes with optimal balance, characterized by a balance score of zero, i.e., 4 rural and 4 urban clusters in each arm. By limiting randomization to this balanced subset, constrained randomization with a single binary covariate is akin to stratification; however, continuous covariates can easily be incorporated.

The size of the randomization space, $0 \le q \le 1$, is another key design parameter. Once the balance metric is specified, all possible pairs of allocation schemes and their corresponding imbalance scores are generated, denoted as (I_r, B_r) for $r = 1, \ldots, R$, where I_r represents r-th allocation scheme, B_r is the associated imbalance score, and R is the maximum number of distinct schemes, determined by complete enumeration or random simulation. The constrained space includes only allocation schemes that satisfy the balance threshold. Specifically, the constrained randomization space consists of all allocation schemes I_r for which the imbalance score B_r is less than or equal to $F_B^{-1}(q)$, where F_B^{-1} is the inverse empirical distribution function of the balance metric. This cutoff $F_B^{-1}(q)$ represents the q-quantile of the balance scores across all possible schemes. Thus, $q = 1$ corresponds to simple randomization, because the randomization space includes all possible schemes in the constrained space, and a constrained randomization space is attained with $0 < q < 1$. However, selecting an overly small q may lead to an overly restrictive randomization design, potentially resulting in deterministic allocation and a threat to internal validity. A practical recommendation is to use $q = 0.1$ such that 10% of the schemes are retained for selecting the final allocation.

To illustrate the concept of covariate-constrained randomization further, consider the STOP CRC study. Suppose we would like to balance two clinic-level covariates available at the randomization phase: the baseline National Quality Forum (NQF) score and the health center (HC) classification. The NQF score represents the proportion of the population already compliant with colorectal cancer screening, while the HC identifies the larger administrative networks to which the clinics belong [29, 50]. The NQF score is a continuous variable, whereas the HC is a categorical variable with eight levels. Balancing both a continuous variable and a multilevel categorical variable through stratified randomization is challenging with only 26 clinics; thus, constrained randomization is a more attractive option. Using the B_{l_2} balance metric and constraining to $q = 10\%$ of the simple randomization space, Table 7.4 compares the baseline information between arms under the randomization scheme with best balance, that under the randomization scheme at the boundary of the 10% constrained space (worst possible scheme under constrained randomization), and that under the randomization scheme achieving worst balance had simple randomization been considered. It is evident that constrained randomization can effectively address chance imbalance, as the worst balance under $q = 0.1$ remains generally satisfactory, and significantly improves baseline balance compared to the worst-case scenario under simple randomization.

Although we have discussed the use of covariate-constrained randomization in parallel-arm CRTs, this approach has been extended to more complex designs, including multi-arm [53] and stepped-wedge CRTs [54]. For multi-arm CRTs, imbalance scores, such as the minimum of Kruskal-Wallis test p-values, have been introduced to measure covariate balance across all treatment arms [55]. In a stepped-wedge design (see next section for more informa-

Table 7.4 Comparison of covariate value between arms under the best balance, at the boundary of the 10% constrained space, and under the worst balance within the simple randomization allocation. "Trt" represents intervention arm and "Ctr" represents control arm

		Best		10% Boundary		Worst	
Covariate		Trt	Ctr	Trt	Ctr	Trt	Ctr
National quality forum score – mean		29.9	29.9	28.3	31.5	22.4	37.4
Health center	# of network (1)	1	1	1	1	2	0
	# of network (2)	1	2	1	2	3	0
	# of network (3)	2	1	1	2	3	0
	# of network (4)	2	2	3	1	0	4
	# of network (5)	3	3	3	3	0	6
	# of network (6)	1	1	1	1	2	0
	# of network (7)	2	2	1	3	1	3
	# of network (8)	1	1	2	0	2	0
Balance score		$B_{l_2} = 4.71$		$B_{l_2} = 21.82$		$B_{l_2} = 206.16$	

tion about this design), constrained randomization has been adapted by defining a new balance metric that considers the proportion of participants each cluster contributes to each treatment arm based on its randomized order [54]. These advancements demonstrate the flexibility of covariate-constrained randomization and provide a general framework for improving balance across diverse CRT settings. Finally, it is generally recommended to adjust for the balancing variables in the final analysis for estimating treatment effects. Li et al. [43, 50] and Zhou et al. [53] have demonstrated that failing to adjust for these variables in the analysis can lead to overly conservative standard error estimates and overly wide confidence intervals. For this reason, one should carefully consider the number of covariates to adjust for by constrained randomization in order not to lose limited cluster-level degrees of freedom in small CRTs. In practice, one should use covariate-constrained randomization to balance only the baseline covariates that are expected to be strongly correlated with the primary outcome, such that adjusting for these covariates in the analysis can explain a sufficient amount of outcome variance and hence improve the study power.

Stepped-Wedge Designs

The stepped-wedge cluster randomized trial (SW-CRT) has become a popular alternative to traditional parallel-arm CRTs [56–60]. This design features a sequential crossover of clusters from the control condition to the intervention condition, according to a randomized sequence. Table 7.5 presents an example of a SW-CRT design with six sequences and seven time periods. In practice, each sequence can consist of a single or multiple clusters. Initially, all clusters start the trial in the control condition. At the prespecified time points, the randomly selected cluster (or multiple clusters) switches from the control to the intervention condition. By the final time period, every cluster has transitioned to the intervention condition. Hemming and Taljaard explained four potential rationales for adopting SW-CRTs [61]. First, this design facilitates cluster recruitment when the intervention is perceived to be beneficial by stakeholders, as it guarantees that all clusters will eventually be exposed to the intervention. Second, staggered rollout of the intervention makes this design logistically feasible, especially under resource constraints. Third, it provides a means to conduct a randomized evaluation in cases where complete rollout of intervention is inevitable. Fourth, because it enables both within-cluster and between-cluster comparisons, the design can potentially increase statistical power compared to the traditional parallel-arm CRT.

There are three main types of SW-CRTs depending on how the outcomes are measured [62]. In a cross-sectional SW-CRT, outcomes are taken from different individuals at each time point, meaning that each participant provide data either under the control or the intervention condition, but not both. In a closed-cohort SW-CRT, the same individuals are followed and measured across all time points, allowing each participant to contribute data under both control and intervention conditions. An open-cohort design allows participants to enter or exit the study during the trial, so that the final dataset consists of a mixture of individuals contributing data to either one of the control or intervention conditions or both.

An example of a SW-CRT in cancer research is the Surgery As Needed approach in Oesophageal cancer patients (SANO) trial. The SANO trial was a phase III multicenter study involving patients with locally advanced esophageal cancer who had a clinically complete response after neoadjuvant chemoradiotherapy. The objective was to compare active surveillance to standard esophagectomy [63]. This trial adopted a SW-CRT design to combat logistical constraints and to facilitate the gradual transition of participating centers to the active surveillance strategy over time. The SW-CRT design in the SANO trial is adapted from the diagram in Table 7.5. The SANO trial features the crossover of six sequences, each consisting of two centers. At each time point, occurring every 4.5 months, one sequence (comprising two centers) transitions from the control condition to the intervention condition, continuing until all sequences have completed the transition [63].

Table 7.5 Illustrative diagram of a stepped-wedge cluster randomized trial (SW-CRT) design with six sequences and seven time periods. Each row represents a sequence, and each column represents a time period. Sequences of clusters transition from the control condition (C, shown in blue) to the treatment condition (T, shown in orange) at different time steps, allowing for staggered implementation of the intervention across clusters

	Step 1	Step 2	Step 3	Step 4	Step 5	Step 6	Step 7
Sequence 1	C	T	T	T	T	T	T
Sequence 2	C	C	T	T	T	T	T
Sequence 3	C	C	C	T	T	T	T
Sequence 4	C	C	C	C	T	T	T
Sequence 5	C	C	C	C	C	T	T
Sequence 6	C	C	C	C	C	C	T

Several methods for sample size calculation and analysis of SW-CRTs have been developed in the last decade [64, 65]. The number of clusters required in a SW-CRT to achieve a specified power depends on the number of time periods, the number of participants per time period, the target difference (effect size), and the assumed within-cluster correlation structure [66–69]. The within-cluster correlation structure is more complex in a SW-CRT due to the clustered and longitudinal aspect of this design [70]. Three types of correlation structures commonly used in SW-CRTs include the exchangeable model by Hussey and Hughes [66], the nested or block exchangeable model by Hooper et al. [71] and Girling et al. [72], and the exponential decay model by Kasza [73]. An overview and comparison of sample size methods and software can be found in Ouyang et al. [64]. Methodological research on sample size estimation for SW-CRTs has primarily focused on cross-sectional and closed-cohort designs, although Kasza et al. [74] recently studied sample size methods for open-cohort designs.

Hussey and Hughes [66] introduced a random-intercept model and developed an analytical sample size formula for continuous outcomes in cross-sectional SW-CRTs. This model describes the observed outcome as a combination of several factors: the baseline expected outcome under the control condition, the time effect which accounts for secular trends, the effect of the intervention, and random components capturing the between-cluster variability and the residual error. Inclusion of the time effect is essential to avoid confounding of the intervention effect by secular trends. Between-cluster heterogeneity is induced by a single random intercept term, which models the cluster-specific deviation from the overall average response. However, this deviation is assumed to be homogeneous across all time periods and intervention sequences, implying an exchangeable correlation structure. Under an exchangeable correlation structure, the ICC is defined as the proportion of total outcome variance attributable to the random effect of clusters and is assumed constant over time. Under this model, the sample size formula and design effect are provided in Hussey and Hughes [66].

Hooper et al. [71] and Girling et al. [72] provide an analytical sample size formula for SW-CRTs that allows for different within-period and between-period ICCs. They incorporate an additional random cluster-by-period interaction term into the model to accommodate differences in correlation between outcomes measured within the same period and those measured across different periods. Unlike the Hussey and Hughes [66] model, their model introduces flexibility to capture a slightly more complex correlation pattern, leading to a nested exchangeable correlation structure [75]. The ratio of the between-period ICC to the within-period ICC—called the cluster autocorrelation (CAC)—quantifies the extent of between-period correlation decay. Whereas in the Hooper and Girling model, the between-period ICC remains constant across all time periods, Kasza et al. [73] extended the sample size calculation approach by allowing the between-period ICC to decay over time, leading to the exponential decay model. By incorporating an autoregressive correlation matrix, the between-period ICC is allowed to decay exponentially at a specified rate per period.

Sample size calculation procedures for all three models discussed have been integrated into statistical software packages and web-based applications [64]. For a closed-cohort SW-CRT design, an extra random effect should be incorporated into the models to account for repeated measurements from the same individual within each cluster [70, 75], and leads to an additional within-individual correlation parameter [76].

For each type of correlation model, the ICC is a critical study design parameter and can substantially affect the required sample size. To facilitate the design of SW-CRTs, Korevaar et al. [77] provided a repository of empirical ICC estimates from 29 longitudinal cluster datasets, offering estimates under various correlation structures, including exchangeable, block-exchangeable, and discrete-time decay. These estimates are available via an RShiny app and can help researchers plan SW-CRTs. Ouyang et al. [70] provided a tutorial on estimating ICCs for longitudinal CRTs, offering practical guidance on study planning, code for implementation in R, SAS, and Stata, and a Shiny app for real-time parameter estimation using available trial datasets.

When conducting sample size calculations for an SW-CRT, key features to specify include the outcome type, number of clusters, number of periods, cluster size per period, design structure (e.g., cross-sectional), correlation structure (e.g., exchangeable), allocation strategy, and type of treatment effect. Ouyang et al. [64] reviewed all available software tools for sample size and power calculation for SW-CRTs including SHINYCRT by Hemming et al. [78], SWDPWR by Chen et al. [79], SWCRTDESIGN by Hughes et al. [80], and CRTFASTGEEPWR by Zhang and Preisser [81], comparing their respective strengths and limitations.

While SW-CRTs offer several advantages, they also present challenges. One notable issue is the longer duration of the trial, since the design involves repeated data collection over an extended period. Longer study duration may increase the risk of bias, which can arise from insufficient control of secular trends, external intervention programs, or other unforeseen factors [82]. Moreover, control clusters may struggle to recruit a sufficient number of participants if there is an extended delay before transitioning to the intervention phase. The SW-CRT design may also require careful consideration of complex treatment effect structures, as time-varying effects can pose challenges for valid inference [83]. Although Wang et al. [84] demonstrated that model-robust inference for the treatment effect in SW-CRTs typically requires correct specification of the treatment effect structure, there has been limited guidance to date on how to select treatment effect structures at the design stage. Lastly, small SW-CRTs are prone to risks such as chance imbalances, increased type I and type II errors, reduced generalizability, and limited statistical analysis options [85, 86], although the fixed-effects approach has been shown as a robust option for small SW-CRTs [87]. Therefore, the adoption of a SW-CRT should be carefully evaluated by balancing its advantages against its potential limitations within the context of the specific trial, and researchers should provide a clear and well-supported justification for using this design.

Summary

The literature on CRTs has evolved substantially in recent years, reflecting growing interest in more complex designs, such as multi-arm trials [88] and multi-period designs like stepped-wedge CRTs [74, 78]. These innovative designs provide opportunities to address logistical and ethical challenges in healthcare delivery research, while requiring advanced methods for design and analysis. Collaboration with an experienced statistician is recommended to ensure appropriate sample size calculation and valid analysis. In this chapter, we focused on discussing key considerations for CRTs, justifying the choice of cluster-level randomization, accurately calculating sample sizes, implementing advanced techniques such as covariate-constrained randomization, and exploring more advanced stepped-wedge designs. As CRTs continue to expand into diverse research domains, the development of rigorous methods and accessible software tools will remain a critical area of focus. Researchers are encouraged to leverage existing guidelines [89, 90] to navigate the complexities of these designs.

References

1. Schulz KF, Grimes DA. Generation of allocation sequences in randomised trials: chance, not choice. Lancet. 2002;359:515–9.
2. Clyne B, Boland F, Murphy N, et al. Quality, scope and reporting standards of randomised controlled trials in Irish Health Research: an observational study. Trials. 2020;21:494.
3. Fernainy P, Cohen AA, Murray E, Losina E, Lamontagne F, Sourial N. Rethinking the pros and cons of randomized controlled trials and observational studies in the era of big data and advanced methods: a panel discussion. BMC Proc. 2024;18:1.
4. Hayes RJ, Moulton LH. Cluster randomised trials. Chapman and Hall/CRC; 2017.
5. Donner A, Klar N, Klar NS. Design and analysis of cluster randomization trials in health research. London: Arnold; 2000.
6. Turner EL, Platt AC, Gallis JA, et al. Completeness of reporting and risks of overstating impact in cluster randomised trials: a systematic review. Lancet Glob Health. 2021;9:e1163–8.
7. Bonney A, Metusela C, Mullan J, Barnett S, Rhee J, Kobel C, Batterham M. Clinical and healthcare improvement through my health record usage and education in general practice (CHIME-GP): a study protocol for a cluster-randomised controlled trial. Trials. 2021;22:569.
8. Murray DM. Design and Analysis of Group-Randomized Trials. Oxford University Press; 1998.
9. Wang B, Harhay MO, Tong J, Small DS, Morris TP, Li F. On the mixed-model analysis of covariance in cluster-randomized trials. 2023; https://doi.org/10.48550/arXiv.2112.00832.
10. Taljaard M, Goldstein CE, Giraudeau B, et al. Cluster over individual randomization: are study design choices appropriately justified? Review of a random sample of trials. Clin Trials. 2020;17:253–63.
11. Hemming K, Taljaard M. Key considerations for designing, conducting and analysing a cluster randomized trial. Int J Epidemiol. 2023;52:1648–58.
12. Keil V, Schaumburg T, Buchta F, Luz JK, Kolbe-Busch S, Chaberny IF, von Lengerke T. Improving leadership skills of infection prevention and control teams by psychological empowerment: study protocol for a cluster randomised controlled trial (IP-POWER). BMJ Open. 2024;14:e083806.
13. Patel A, Sims E, Blacklock J, et al. Cluster randomised control trial protocol for estimating the effectiveness and cost-effectiveness of a complex intervention to increase care home staff influenza vaccination rates compared to usual practice (FLUCARE). Trials. 2022;23:989.

14. Sykes M, Copsey B, Finch T, et al. A cluster randomised controlled trial, process and economic evaluation of quality improvement collaboratives aligned to a national audit to improve the care for people with diabetes (EQUIPD): study protocol. Implement Sci. 2023;18:37.
15. Weinfurt KP, Hernandez AF, Coronado GD, et al. Pragmatic clinical trials embedded in healthcare systems: generalizable lessons from the NIH Collaboratory. BMC Med Res Methodol. 2017;17:144.
16. Escoffery C, Gilleland Marchak J, Haardörfer R, Meacham L, Williamson Lewis R, Udelson H, Edwards P, Mertens AC. Scalability of cancer SurvivorLink™: a cluster randomized trial among pediatric cancer clinics. Contemp Clin Trials. 2019;85:105819.
17. Schmeltz H, Rat C, Pogu C, Bianco G, Cowppli-Bony A, Gaultier A, Nguyen J-M. Effect of physician notification regarding nonadherence to colorectal cancer screening on early cancer detection. JAMA. 2020;323:2429–31.
18. Martin RM, Donovan JL, Turner EL, et al. Effect of a low-intensity PSA-based screening intervention on prostate cancer mortality: the CAP randomized clinical trial. JAMA. 2018;319:883–95.
19. Easter C, Thompson JA, Eldridge S, Taljaard M, Hemming K. Cluster randomized trials of individual-level interventions were at high risk of bias. J Clin Epidemiol. 2021;138:49–59.
20. Bolzern J, Mnyama N, Bosanquet K, Torgerson DJ. A review of cluster randomized trials found statistical evidence of selection bias. J Clin Epidemiol. 2018;99:106–12.
21. Li F, Tian Z, Bobb J, Papadogeorgou G, Li F. Clarifying selection bias in cluster randomized trials. Clin Trials. 2022;19:33–41.
22. Li F, Tian Z, Tian Z, Li F. A note on identification of causal effects in cluster randomized trials with post-randomization selection bias. Commun Stat - Theory Methods. 2024;53:1825–37.
23. Papadogeorgou G, Liu B, Li F, Li F. Addressing selection bias in cluster randomized experiments via weighting. 2024; https://doi.org/10.48550/arXiv.2309.07365.
24. Hemming K, Taljaard M, Moerbeek M, Forbes A. Contamination: how much can an individually randomized trial tolerate? Stat Med. 2021;40:3329–51.
25. Kenward MG, Roger JH. Small sample inference for fixed effects from restricted maximum likelihood. Biometrics. 1997;53:983–97.
26. Satterthwaite FE. An approximate distribution of estimates of variance components. Biom Bull. 1946;2:110–4.
27. Mohile SG, Epstein RM, Hurria A, et al. Communication with older patients with cancer using geriatric assessment: a cluster-randomized clinical trial from the National Cancer Institute Community oncology research program. JAMA Oncol. 2020;6:196–204.
28. Klabunde C, Blom J, Bulliard J-L, Garcia M, Hagoel L, Mai V, Patnick J, Rozjabek H, Senore C, Törnberg S. Participation rates for organized colorectal cancer screening programmes: an international comparison. J Med Screen. 2015;22:119–26.
29. Coronado GD, Vollmer WM, Petrik A, Taplin SH, Burdick TE, Meenan RT, Green BB. Strategies and opportunities to STOP colon cancer in priority populations: design of a cluster-randomized pragmatic trial. Contemp Clin Trials. 2014;38:344–9.
30. Cornfield J. Symposium on CHD prevention trials: design issues in testing life style intervention: randomization by group: a formal analysis. Am J Epidemiol. 1978;108:100–2.
31. Turner EL, Li F, Gallis JA, Prague M, Murray DM. Review of recent methodological developments in group-randomized trials: part 1—design. Am J Public Health. 2017;107:907–15.
32. Murray DM, Taljaard M, Turner EL, George SM. Essential ingredients and innovations in the design and analysis of group-randomized trials. Annu Rev Public Health. 2020;41:1–19.
33. Sample size estimation for modified Poisson analysis of cluster randomized trials with a binary outcome -Fan Li, Guangyu Tong. 2021. https://journals.sagepub.com/doi/full/10.1177/0962280221990415. Accessed 30 Sep 2024.
34. Donner A, Birkett N, Buck C. Randomization by cluster: sample size requirements and analysis. Am J Epidemiol. 1981;114:906–14.
35. Hemming K, Eldridge S, Forbes G, Weijer C, Taljaard M. How to design efficient cluster randomised trials. BMJ. 2017;358:j3064.
36. Shih WJ. Sample size and power calculations for periodontal and other studies with clustered samples using the method of generalized estimating equations. Biom J. 1997;39:899–908.
37. Rutterford C, Copas A, Eldridge S. Methods for sample size determination in cluster randomized trials. Int J Epidemiol. 2015;44:1051–67.
38. Wang X, Turner EL, Preisser JS, Li F. Power considerations for generalized estimating equations analyses of four-level cluster randomized trials. Biom J. 2022;64:663–80.
39. Eldridge SM, Ashby D, Kerry S. Sample size for cluster randomized trials: effect of coefficient of variation of cluster size and analysis method. Int J Epidemiol. 2006;35:1292–300.
40. Manatunga AK, Hudgens MG, Chen S. Sample size estimation in cluster randomized studies with varying cluster size. Biom J. 2001;43:75–86.
41. van Breukelen GJP, Candel MJJM, Berger MPF. Relative efficiency of unequal versus equal cluster sizes in cluster randomized and multicentre trials. Stat Med. 2007;26:2589–603.
42. Liu J, Colditz GA. Relative efficiency of unequal versus equal cluster sizes in cluster randomized trials using generalized estimating equation models. Biom J. 2018;60:616–38.
43. Li F, Lokhnygina Y, Murray DM, Heagerty PJ, DeLong ER. An evaluation of constrained randomization for the design and analysis of group-randomized trials. Stat Med. 2016;35:1565–79.
44. Kernan WN, Viscoli CM, Makuch RW, Brass LM, Horwitz RI. Stratified randomization for clinical trials. J Clin Epidemiol. 1999;52:19–26.
45. Donner A, Klar N. Pitfalls of and controversies in cluster randomization trials. Am J Public Health. 2004;94:416–22.
46. Chondros P, Ukoumunne OC, Gunn JM, Carlin JB. When should matching be used in the design of cluster randomized trials? Stat Med. 2021;40:5765–78.
47. Klar N, Donner A. The merits of matching in community intervention trials: a cautionary tale. Stat Med. 1997;16:1753–64.
48. Diehr P, Martin DC, Koepsell T, Cheadle A. Breaking the matches in a paired t-test for community interventions when the number of pairs is small. Stat Med. 1995;14:1491–504.
49. Moulton LH. Covariate-based constrained randomization of group-randomized trials. Clin Trials. 2004;1:297–305.
50. Li F, Turner EL, Heagerty PJ, Murray DM, Vollmer WM, DeLong ER. An evaluation of constrained randomization for the design and analysis of group-randomized trials with binary outcomes. Stat Med. 2017;36:3791–806.
51. Raab GM, Butcher I. Balance in cluster randomized trials. Stat Med. 2001;20:351–65.
52. de Hoop E, Teerenstra S, van Gaal BGI, Moerbeek M, Borm GF. The "best balance" allocation led to optimal balance in cluster-controlled trials. J Clin Epidemiol. 2012;65:132–7.
53. Zhou Y, Turner EL, Simmons RA, Li F. Constrained randomization and statistical inference for multi-arm parallel cluster randomized controlled trials. Stat Med. 2022;41:1862–83.
54. Chaussee EL, Dickinson LM, Fairclough DL. Evaluation of a covariate-constrained randomization procedure in stepped wedge cluster randomized trials. Contemp Clin Trials. 2021;105:106409.
55. Ciolino JD, Diebold A, Jensen JK, Rouleau GW, Koloms KK, Tandon D. Choosing an imbalance metric for covariate-constrained randomization in multiple-arm cluster-randomized trials. Trials. 2019;20:293.

56. Brown CA, Lilford RJ. The stepped wedge trial design: a systematic review. BMC Med Res Methodol. 2006;6:54.
57. Mdege ND, Man M-S, Taylor (nee Brown) CA, Torgerson DJ. Systematic review of stepped wedge cluster randomized trials shows that design is particularly used to evaluate interventions during routine implementation. J Clin Epidemiol. 2011;64:936–48.
58. Hemming K, Haines TP, Chilton PJ, Girling AJ, Lilford RJ. The stepped wedge cluster randomised trial: rationale, design, analysis, and reporting. BMJ. 2015;350:h391.
59. Nevins P, Ryan M, Davis-Plourde K, et al. Adherence to key recommendations for design and analysis of stepped-wedge cluster randomized trials: a review of trials published 2016–2022. Clin Trials. 2024;21:199–210.
60. Nevins P, Davis-Plourde K, Pereira Macedo JA, et al. A scoping review described diversity in methods of randomization and reporting of baseline balance in stepped-wedge cluster randomized trials. J Clin Epidemiol. 2023;157:134–45.
61. Hemming K, Taljaard M. Reflection on modern methods: when is a stepped-wedge cluster randomized trial a good study design choice? Int J Epidemiol. 2020;49:1043–52.
62. Copas AJ, Lewis JJ, Thompson JA, Davey C, Baio G, Hargreaves JR. Designing a stepped wedge trial: three main designs, carry-over effects and randomisation approaches. Trials. 2015;16:352.
63. Noordman BJ, Wijnhoven BPL, Lagarde SM, et al. Neoadjuvant chemoradiotherapy plus surgery versus active surveillance for oesophageal cancer: a stepped-wedge cluster randomised trial. BMC Cancer. 2018;18:142.
64. Ouyang Y, Li F, Preisser JS, Taljaard M. Sample size calculators for planning stepped-wedge cluster randomized trials: a review and comparison. Int J Epidemiol. 2022;51:2000–13.
65. Li F, Hughes JP, Hemming K, Taljaard M, Melnick ER, Heagerty PJ. Mixed-effects models for the design and analysis of stepped wedge cluster randomized trials: an overview. Stat Methods Med Res. 2021;30:612–39.
66. Hussey MA, Hughes JP. Design and analysis of stepped wedge cluster randomized trials. Contemp Clin Trials. 2007;28:182–91.
67. Rhoda DA, Murray DM, Andridge RR, Pennell ML, Hade EM. Studies with staggered starts: multiple baseline designs and group-randomized trials. Am J Public Health. 2011;101:2164–9.
68. Hemming K, Lilford R, Girling AJ. Stepped-wedge cluster randomised controlled trials: a generic framework including parallel and multiple-level designs. Stat Med. 2015;34:181–96.
69. Hemming K, Taljaard M. Sample size calculations for stepped wedge and cluster randomised trials: a unified approach. J Clin Epidemiol. 2016;69:137–46.
70. Ouyang Y, Hemming K, Li F, Taljaard M. Estimating intra-cluster correlation coefficients for planning longitudinal cluster randomized trials: a tutorial. Int J Epidemiol. 2023;52:1634–47.
71. Hooper R, Teerenstra S, de Hoop E, Eldridge S. Sample size calculation for stepped wedge and other longitudinal cluster randomised trials. Stat Med. 2016;35:4718–28.
72. Girling AJ, Hemming K. Statistical efficiency and optimal design for stepped cluster studies under linear mixed effects models. Stat Med. 2016;35:2149–66.
73. J Kasza, K Hemming, R Hooper, JNS Matthews, AB Forbes Impact of non-uniform correlation structure on sample size and power in multiple-period cluster randomised trials, 2019. https://journals.sagepub.com/doi/full/10.1177/0962280217734981. Accessed 10 Nov 2024.
74. Kasza J, Hooper R, Copas A, Forbes AB. Sample size and power calculations for open cohort longitudinal cluster randomized trials. Stat Med. 2020;39:1871–83.
75. Li F. Design and analysis considerations for cohort stepped wedge cluster randomized trials with a decay correlation structure. Stat Med. 2020;39:438–55.
76. Li F, Turner EL, Preisser JS. Sample size determination for GEE analyses of stepped wedge cluster randomized trials. Biometrics. 2018;74:1450–8.
77. Korevaar E, Kasza J, Taljaard M, Hemming K, Haines T, Turner EL, Thompson JA, Hughes JP, Forbes AB. Intra-cluster correlations from the CLustered OUtcome dataset bank to inform the design of longitudinal cluster trials. Clin Trials Lond Engl. 2021;18:529–40.
78. Hemming K, Kasza J, Hooper R, Forbes A, Taljaard M. A tutorial on sample size calculation for multiple-period cluster randomized parallel, cross-over and stepped-wedge trials using the shiny CRT calculator. Int J Epidemiol. 2020;49:979–95.
79. Chen J, Zhou X, Li F, Spiegelman D. Swdpwr: a SAS macro and an R package for power calculations in stepped wedge cluster randomized trials. Comput Methods Prog Biomed. 2022;213:106522.
80. Voldal EC, Hakhu NR, Xia F, Heagerty PJ, Hughes JP. swCRTdesign: an RPackage for stepped wedge trial design and analysis. Comput Methods Prog Biomed. 2020;196:105514.
81. Zhang Y, Preisser JS, Li F, Turner EL, Rathouz PJ. %CRTFASTGEEPWR: a SAS macro for power of the generalized estimating equations of multi-period cluster randomized trials with application to stepped wedge designs. 2022; https://doi.org/10.48550/arXiv.2205.14532.
82. Li F, Wang R. Stepped wedge cluster randomized trials: a methodological overview. World Neurosurg. 2022;161:323–30.
83. Kenny A, Voldal EC, Xia F, Heagerty PJ, Hughes JP. Analysis of stepped wedge cluster randomized trials in the presence of a time-varying treatment effect. Stat Med. 2022;41:4311–39.
84. Wang B, Wang X, Li F. How to achieve model-robust inference in stepped wedge trials with model-based methods? Biometrics. 2024;80:ujae123.
85. Taljaard M, Teerenstra S, Ivers NM, Fergusson DA. Substantial risks associated with few clusters in cluster randomized and stepped wedge designs. Clin Trials Lond Engl. 2016;13:459–63.
86. Tong G, Nevins P, Ryan M, et al. A review of current practice in the design and analysis of extremely small stepped wedge cluster randomized trials. Clin Trials. 2024:17407745241276137.
87. Lee KM, Cheung YB. The fixed-effects model for robust analysis of stepped-wedge cluster trials with a small number of clusters and continuous outcomes: a simulation study. Trials. 2024;25:718.
88. Odutayo A, Gryaznov D, Copsey B, et al. Design, analysis and reporting of multi-arm trials and strategies to address multiple testing. Int J Epidemiol. 2020;49:968–78.
89. Hemming K, Taljaard M, Grimshaw J. Introducing the new CONSORT extension for stepped-wedge cluster randomised trials. Trials. 2019;20:68.
90. Weijer C, Grimshaw JM, Eccles MP, McRae AD, White A, Brehaut JC, Taljaard M. The Ottawa statement on the ethical design and conduct of cluster randomized trials. PLoS Med. 2012;9:e1001346.

8 Systematic Reviews and Meta-Analysis

Andrew Sephien and Ambuj Kumar

Part 1: What Is a Systematic Review

A systematic review (SR) is a scientific method for searching, assembling, appraising, and quantifying results from similar studies to answer a specific question [1, 2]. The term "systematic review" was initially used by Archie Cochrane in 1989 in his compilation of research synthesis on pregnancy and childbirth, a concept that had been previously referred to as "research synthesis" by social scientists in the post-World War II period [3]. Systematic reviews may be accompanied by a meta-analysis (MA), which is a separate process of statistical or quantitative synthesis from all available similar studies for a specific outcome [3]. The term "meta-analysis" was first used by Gene V. Glass in 1976 to address the need for a quantitative synthesis of available evidence [3]. Synthesized research through systematic reviews and meta-analysis provides information on the totality of evidence and allows for informed decisions to be made on diagnosis, treatment, and healthcare management for both individual patients and populations.

As an example on the impact of a systematic review, a meta-analysis by Lau et al. assessing the effect of intravenous (IV) streptokinase as thrombolytic therapy for myocardial infarction was published in 1992 [4]. The food and drug administration approved IV streptokinase in the year 1987. However, the benefit of IV streptokinase was evident since 1973 through cumulative meta-analysis (cumulative Mantel-Haenszel method), long before its approval date [2, 4, 5]. One can make the assumption that had this meta-analysis been performed sooner, the approval and subsequent implementation of IV streptokinase would have had an earlier impact without need for further research and patients being unintentionally not receiving an ineffective intervention. Therefore, systematic review and meta-analysis findings is critical to informing patient care decisions.

Systematic Review Versus Narrative Review

It is important to understand the key differences between a systematic and a narrative review. The one broad difference between a narrative review and a systematic review is the presence or absence of a methodology for reproducibility. While a systematic review follows a specific methodology with clearly articulated steps, a narrative review is dependent on the skills of the author and, due to the lack of specific steps, is challenging to reproduce. The systematic review process is similar to a clinical trial except one exception which is the unit of analysis. In a clinical trial, the unit of analysis is the individual or the patient; in a systematic review, the unit of analysis is a study. The systematic review starts with a specific research question, and in a narrative review, the question is often broad. A systematic review requires the development of a protocol outlining the inclusion/exclusion criteria for studies, which are not required for a narrative review. A systematic review has a reproducible and robust search strategy (e.g., at least two databases), followed by clear criteria for inclusion of studies, which is not the case in a narrative review. In a systematic review, the selection of studies is followed by data abstraction from eligible studies on patient and intervention characteristics, methodological quality, and primary and secondary outcomes. Depending on the quality of the data, a meta-analysis (i.e., quantitative synthesis) could be performed as well. Narrative reviews do not have such a process for data abstraction or quantitative synthesis. In short, there are standards for conduct and reporting of systematic reviews. However, there are no such standards for the conduct and reporting of narrative reviews, and a narrative review lacks reproducibility, which is an essential element of the scientific process.

A. Sephien
Division of Cardiovascular Disease, University of Miami/Jackson Memorial Hospital, Miami, FL, USA

A. Kumar (✉)
Department of Internal Medicine, Research Methodology and Biostatistics Core, Office of Research, Morsani College of Medicine, University of South Florida, Tampa, FL, USA
e-mail: akumar6@usf.edu

J. Huang, H. S.L. Jim (eds.), *Cancer Research Guidance for Clinicians and Researchers*,
https://doi.org/10.1007/978-3-032-19175-5_8

Part 2: Conducting a Systematic Review

In this section we review the essential steps of performing a systematic review beginning with a specific question and ending with the reporting the findings in the form of a manuscript.

Step 1: Identifying the Specific Question and Matching the Study Design to the Research Question

As with any research study, a systematic review begins with a specific research question. One of the common formats/structures recommended for developing a specific research question is the use of the PICO framework, including the patient/population denoted by letter P, intervention or exposure or prognostic factor or a diagnostic test denoted by letter I, followed by comparison denoted by letter C, and the outcome denoted by letter O. After using PICO to formulate the research question, there are two additional elements needed to enhance the specificity of the PICO question, which is the type or domain of the question, denoted by letter T, and the study design that would be considered the most unbiased to provide reliable answers to the PICO question, denoted by letter S, resulting in PICOTS. The most common research question domain addressed in systematic reviews are treatments followed by prognosis, diagnostic accuracy, diagnostic utility, and/or harms, although these are by no means the only research questions that can be addressed by a systematic review. Accordingly, the next step is to determine what would be the optimal study design to address a specific type of question. As an example, if the PICO question for the systematic review is about diagnostic accuracy (T), a systematic review of cross-sectional analytic studies (S) would provide the most unbiased answer, whereas if the PICO question is about treatment (T), then a systematic review of randomized controlled trials (Table 8.1) would provide the most unbiased answer. Below is a clinical scenario and development of a specific question following the PICOTS model.

John is a 62-year-old male who was recently diagnosed with International Staging System (ISS) stage II, standard-risk cytogenetics, newly diagnosed multiple myeloma (NDMM). John has stage I hypertension, no cardiac disease, and ECOG performance status 1 and is an eligible candidate for autologous stem cell transplant (ASCT). The treating physician is conflicted between choosing a three- or four-drug regimen. Three-drug regimen with a proteasome inhibitor [PI], an immunomodulatory drug [IMiD], and dexamethasone has been the standard of care for patients with NDMM and is associated with improved progression-free survival (PFS) and overall survival (OS) [6]. Evidence from four-drug regimen with a PI, IMiD, dexamethasone, and anti-CD38 monoclonal antibody (mAb) also has been associated with improved PFS in patients with NDMM. For this clinical scenario, the PICOTS question will be as follows [7]:

P: Patients with NDMM
I: Four-drug regimen
C: Three-drug regimen
O: PFS, OS
T: Treatment
S: Randomized controlled trial

Since the above PICO question is a question regarding treatment, a systematic review and meta-analysis of all randomized controlled trials will be the most optimal strategy to provide the most conclusive answer to the efficacy question of four- versus three-drug regimen for the management of NDMM. As shown in Table 8.1, matching the study design to the question domain is a critical step to embarking on a systematic review. The *Cochrane Handbook for Systematic Reviews of Interventions*, which can be found online, provides additional details.

Step 2: Preparatory Work Before Embarking on a Systematic Review-Assess Feasibility

The conduct of a systematic review is dependent on the availability of existing studies for a specific question. Therefore, it is important to perform an informal literature search to assess how many potentially eligible studies exist to address the PICO question. There are no required number of studies for a systematic review, but a meta-analysis (quantitative synthesis) requires at least two studies.

In our example, now that our research question using the PICOTS has been formulated, a quick search of PubMed database for the feasibility assessment shows that there is more than one randomized controlled trial assessing the efficacy of four- versus three-drug regimens for the management of NDMM. The search also addresses the issue of futility. That is, if there is already a recent systematic review on a PICOTS, undertaking another systematic review would be considered a waste of resources and time unless there are valid reasons such as poorly or incorrectly performed systematic review, availability of newer RCTs since the publication of the most recent systematic review, etc. To further ensure that a systematic review is not currently being con-

Table 8.1 Optimal study design based on question domain

Diagnostic accuracy	Cross-sectional analytic study
Prognosis	Prospective cohort study
Treatment	Randomized controlled trial
Harms/side effects	Can vary

ducted with the PICOTS question of interest, a search of the PROSPERO register for systematic reviews (https://www.crd.york.ac.uk/prospero/) (a site where systematic review protocols are registered before conducting) should be performed to avoid duplicating efforts. Based on a positive feasibility assessment, one can proceed with performing a systematic review to address the PICOTS question.

Step 3: Developing a Protocol For a Systematic Review

The study protocol should follow a key rule of expected versus observed. All expectations and processes of the proposed research should be outlined a priori in a study protocol, and the results are considered observations resulting from that a priori process. Like the requirements in clinical research, articulating the specific questions, study eligibility criteria, search strategy to identify eligible studies, primary and secondary outcomes, methodology for study selection, data abstraction, data analysis plan, summary measures, etc. should be outlined in a study protocol. In summary, a study protocol should be developed before undertaking a systematic review. The systematic review protocol should follow the Preferred Reporting Items for Systematic reviews and Meta-Analyses (PRISMA) checklist up to the methods section. The protocol methods should be written in the future tense using the active voice and in simple language, avoiding technical jargon.

Study Protocol Registration

After the protocol is developed, it should be registered with a publicly accessible registry for several reasons. Prospective registration of a systematic review protocol ensures transparency and scientific integrity, prevents selective reporting of outcomes, allows for reproducibility, avoids research duplication, and is also required by many journals as a prerequisite for publication. Currently, there are three registries for registering systematic reviews, namely, PROSPERO, the Registry of Systematic Reviews/Meta-Analyses in Research Registry, and International Platform of Registered Systematic Review and Meta-Analysis (INPLASY).

Primary and Secondary Outcome Selection and Endpoint Multiplicity

The choice of outcomes should be based on their clinical importance and meaningfulness to relevant stakeholders (i.e., physicians, patients, scientists, and policymakers). A further issue is consideration of how many outcomes to include. To prevent information overload and inundating readers with too many outcomes, no more than seven outcomes are recommended. Another important consideration is to include a mix of patient- and disease-oriented outcomes when possible. As an example, for NDMM, overall survival is considered a hard/objective- or patient-oriented outcome, and response rate is considered a disease-oriented outcome. Another important tip is to include a mix of desirable/beneficial and undesirable/side-effect outcomes representing the benefits and risk profile of an intervention. Once the outcomes are decided for importance and relevance, one of these outcomes should be designated a priori as the primary outcome, and the rest as secondary outcomes.

Step 4: Literature Search and Study Selection

The next step would be to perform a systematic search to identify all potentially eligible studies. The search should be systematic and comprehensive to include all potentially eligible studies to minimize selection bias (which, as mentioned previously, is a significant concern in a narrative review). The Cochrane review recommends working with a librarian or information specialist to develop systematic search strategies specifically tailored to specific databases to identify potentially eligible studies [8, 9]. It is also important to document and save the specific search strategy, which is a key reporting requirement for reproducibility.

The search should include multiple databases (rather than relying exclusively on MEDLINE) and should not be limited by language or publication type (full text versus abstract) to maximize the likelihood of identification and nclusion of all eligible studies [8, 10–13]. To further emphasize the importance of using multiple databases, in a recent study by Ewald et al., they randomly selected 60 Cochrane reviews and found that using 2 or more databases decreased the risk of missing eligible studies [12]. The choice of databases is dependent on the context of the systematic review. For example, if the topic area is clinical oncology, searching Medline and EMBASE may be sufficient to identify all published studies. However, if the topic area relates to nonclinical medicine, the choice of database for searching will be different.

Should Only Peer-Reviewed Published Studies Be Included in the Systematic Review?

The goal of a systematic review is to assemble all eligible studies as per the PICOTS question, regardless of publication type (e.g., abstract, full text, etc.) and status (e.g., unpublished). The goal is to avoid publication bias as it is well documented that studies with statistically significant results are more likely to be published than those without significant results, and therefore, exclusion of unpublished studies may produce skewed results.

Step 5: Study Screening and Eligibility Assessment

Once the search results are collated, all resulting citations undergo an initial review of title and abstract to assess for eligibility independently by at least two reviewers. Review in duplicate avoids errors and enhances accuracy, reliability, and credibility. If, upon review of the title and abstract, a decision on inclusion could not be made, then the full text of the article is reviewed to determine eligibility. After the initial selection of potentially eligible studies, all the initially included studies should undergo an independent full-text review. If there is a disagreement among reviewers, there should be a prespecified plan as to how to deal with disagreements, such as reaching a consensus or discussing with a third reviewer who is independent of the initial selection process. Throughout the review process, the reasons for exclusion should be recorded, as this information will be used to generate a flow diagram. A flow diagram is essential to visualize the study selection process, enhance transparency, and support the reproducibility of the process. Resources for the selection process include Reference Manager (Mendeley) and QCRI (Rayyan).

Step 6: Data Abstraction—Collecting Necessary Information from Included Studies

Now that we have the denominator of included studies, we need to collect information from these included studies. The first consideration is what information/data to collect and how to collect. Depending on the context, the specific data items may vary. Broadly, data is collected for the following domains:

1. Study identification—Author names and year of publication. By convention, study identification is denoted by the first author's last name followed by the year of publication. For example, if the first author's name is John Doe and the year of publication is 2022, the study identification will be denoted as Doe, 2022.
2. Study and participant characteristics—Collect information on, but not limited to, study design (randomized controlled trial, prospective cohort, etc.); number of study arms; sample size in each arm; follow-up duration, if applicable; characteristics of patient population; intervention and comparison details; single versus multicenter; study setting; country of study; finding source (public versus industry); etc.
3. Primary and secondary outcomes—Details of primary and secondary outcomes, including the frequency of measurement, definitions, timepoints of outcome assessment, what tools or instruments were used to assess outcomes, etc.
4. Results for primary and secondary outcomes—Effect size (e.g., mean differences, risk ratio, odds ratio, rate of events in the intervention and comparison groups), confidence intervals, p-values, etc.
5. Risk of bias in individual studies—Choice of a validated tool for risk of bias assessment in individual studies is dependent on the study design of included studies. As an example, if the systematic review involves randomized controlled trials, the Cochrane risk of bias tool is a validated tool to assess for risk of bias. Similarly, there are specific checklists for various study designs. For observational studies, the use of the ROBINS-1 tool is recommended [14].

Included studies can have multiple publications and can have different pieces of information across these duplicate publications. Therefore, it is important to review these articles and assess each of them for the outcomes of interest. However, sometimes it can be difficult to ascertain if multiple articles are for the same study, given key characteristics may be excluded, such as different author order, abbreviated methodology reported, different characteristics and outcomes reported. Therefore, an investigation to assess similarity is essential, which may include checking protocol registration (i.e., clinicaltrials.gov) which may link publications, sponsors and sources of funding for the study, setting (i.e., study conducted in the same city/hospital), study duration, and similar authors (but different order of authors). Often, despite the above information, the data is not extractable due to poor quality of reporting. In such cases, reaching out directly to investigators (e.g., corresponding author) to request any unclear/missing information about any question results in getting the missing data.

Mode of Data Collection: Electronic Versus Paper Forms

Data for a systematic review can be extracted manually, where reviewers read the study and the information from the study is entered directly into a paper form or spreadsheet. While the use of a paper form or spreadsheet provides full control over the process, it is time-consuming and labor-intensive as it requires data reentry into analysis software and is prone to human error. It is also difficult to scale up for large systematic reviews with multiple people working across the globe on the same study. Given these challenges, in recent years, several tools or online platforms have come into existence to streamline data extraction and management. One common theme across these various platforms is that they allow for duplicate extraction, identify differences or disagreements in data extraction, and facilitate conflict resolution. However, use of these online or electronic platforms may be associated with significant costs, and there is a learning curve as well. In summary, electronic tools for data extraction may provide efficiency and accuracy, but manual oversight is critical to ensure quality and resolve discrepancies.

Understanding Quantitative Data Types for Data Extraction

The most common outcomes in clinical medicine are reported either as dichotomous, continuous, ordinal, counts and rates, or time-to-event data. All members of the systematic review should have a basic understanding of data types before commencing data extraction. All extraction should follow the intention-to-treat for desirable outcomes (i.e., benefits) and a per-protocol principle for undesirable outcomes (i.e., side effects).

Data Extraction for a Dichotomous Variable

Data can be extracted in the following forms for a dichotomous or categorical variable:

(a) Summary measures associated with pairwise comparison (e.g., odds ratio or risk ratio) along with 95% confidence intervals, and p-value
(b) Number of events, and total sample size in the intervention and the comparison groups, and p-value

Data Extraction for Continuous Variable

(a) Post-intervention means along with standard deviation and the total sample size for the intervention and the comparison groups
(b) Post-intervention medians along with interquartile range and the total sample size for the intervention and the comparison groups

Data Extraction for Time-to-Event Variable

(a) Summary measures associated with pairwise comparison (hazard ratio) along with 95% confidence intervals, and p-value
(b) Number of events, and total sample size in the intervention and the comparison groups and p-value

In cases where the abovementioned measures are not reported or different measures are reported across included studies, there are indirect methods to convert the various measures into a single measure for quantitative synthesis [8]. When using indirect methods for data extraction, quality assurance is important. The results computed using indirect methods should be matched against the original result in terms of effect size and direction. For example, if a study result favors an intervention, the indirect measurement should also show a benefit for the intervention. Regardless of the mode of data extraction, pilot testing the data extraction software and methodology is essential for avoiding any possible errors or issues down the road. Resources include the Cochrane Risk of Bias Tool, ROIBINS-I tool, Rayyan QCRI, and Systematic Review Data Repository, which are available online.

Step 7: Quantitative Synthesis—Meta-Analysis

Once data extraction is complete, the next step is quantitative synthesis, also called meta-analysis. A meta-analysis is a statistical method to combine the results from multiple studies on a specific PICOTS question. Meta-analysis is aimed at deriving a more accurate and precise estimate of the true effect associated with the intervention/prognostic factor/diagnostic test, etc. A meta-analysis is not a mega-trial, as study subjects from one study are not mixed with another study. A meta-analysis is performed in two steps, beginning with calculating the summary effect for each included study, followed by a weighted pooled estimate. Furthermore, it is important to realize that a systematic review can be conducted without a meta-analysis. However, a meta-analysis cannot be conducted without a systematic review. The exclusion of the "systematic review" is a methodological flaw and increases the risk of bias of a meta-analysis.

Selection of Fixed-Effect versus Random-Effects Models

The choice of model requires some assumption prior to analysis articulated a priori in the protocol. Under a fixed-effects model, the assumption is that all included studies estimate the same true effect size, and the inference is that studies are similar in PICOTS and any variation in results could be due to sampling error. Furthermore, larger studies receive more weight in pooling compared to smaller studies. On the other hand, under a random-effects model, the assumption is that each included study has a different but similar effect size. The weighting is more balanced across pooled studies and accounts for within and between study variances. In summary, the choice of random versus fixed model should be stated a priori and implemented accordingly.

Heterogeneity

Heterogeneity refers to the differences in results across included studies. Heterogeneity is commonly measured or quantified in two ways using either a Cochran's Q test or I^2 statistic. Cochran's Q test assesses whether the differences in pooled results are due to chance. A significant result indicates heterogeneity. An I^2 statistic provides a quantified percentage, between 0% and 100%, of variation across studies that could be attributed to heterogeneity rather than chance. Thresholds for interpretation of I^2 statistic could oversimplify inconsistency across pooled studies, which could be attributed to several factors. However, as per the Cochrane Handbook, an I^2 statistic of 0–40% could be interpreted as not important, 30–60% as moderate, 50–90% as substantial, and 75–100% as considerable heterogeneity. The choice of pooling model (random versus fixed) should not be dictated by the extent of heterogeneity. Additionally, it is critical to understand that heterogeneity without context is not informative. The presence of heterogeneity is not necessarily a bad thing. As an example, if the question is about the efficacy of watermelon versus oranges for lowering blood pressure, adding studies focused on other fruits would be considered inappropriate regardless of the level of heterogeneity. However, if the question is about the efficacy of fruits versus vegetables for lowering blood pressure, including studies with a variety of fruits versus vegetables would be considered appropriate regardless of the presence or absence of heterogeneity. While assessing heterogeneity is appropriate, without context, it may lead to erroneous conclusions.

Mixing study designs in a meta-analysis

Is it appropriate to mix study designs in the meta-analysis? The answer is no as mixing various study designs violates the key assumption of a meta-analysis, which is that similar studies with similar PICO question will produce similar results. Even in situations in which evidence is available from a randomized and non-randomized study, pooling from multiple study designs will lead to significant methodological and statistical heterogeneity, inaccurate risk of bias assessments, difficulty in interpreting the results, and questioning of the clinical validity with the use of different evidence hierarchies. Therefore, mixing study designs is not recommended. When including randomized and observational studies for a question, a feasible approach is to analyze the study designs separately or as subgroups. Online resources for conducting meta-analysis include RevMan software and OpenMeta.

Step 8: Assessing the Overall Certainty/Quality of Evidence

Before evaluating the overall certainty or quality of evidence, it is important to distinguish between risk of bias and overall certainty. While assessment of risk of bias is performed for each study and specific outcome included in the systematic review, the overall certainty of evidence or quality of evidence is assessed using the totality of the evidence (i.e., all studies included in the systematic review). The overall certainty of evidence or quality of evidence is assessed using the GRADE (Grading of Recommendations Assessment, Development and Evaluation) method. The aim is to assess the quality or certainty of evidence for a specific outcome and help to determine the confidence in the results of a systematic review or meta-analysis. GRADE assessment classifies evidence into four levels of high, moderate, low, and very low. The baseline rating starts with high for randomized controlled trials and low for observational studies. Based on specific qualifying factors, the evidence certainty or quality could be downgraded for randomized controlled trials or upgraded for observational studies. Qualifying factors that could result in a downgrade of certainty for randomized clinical trials include:

(a) Risk of bias—Refers to systematic errors affecting the validity of its results. The aim is to assess if issues in study design and execution impact our confidence in the summary effect.
(b) Inconsistency—Refers to systematic differences across the study results included in the systematic review. It applies only if there is more than one study in a systematic review. This could be explained by differences across included studies in PICO.
(c) Indirectness—Refers to issues related to applicability or generalizability of results from the systematic review. Indirectness could be determined by assessing how PICO of included studies aligns with PICO of interest in the systematic review.
(d) Imprecision—Refers to the confidence intervals associated with relative or absolute summary effects used to assess imprecision. Confidence intervals represent uncertainty around the summary effect. A predefined threshold for important effects should be used for specific outcomes and associated effect size to determine imprecision.
(e) Publication bias—Refers to the selective publication of studies based on the nature of results from a study. Publication bias could lead to skewed findings from systematic review and meta-analysis as exclusion of certain studies based on publication status goes against the goal of a systematic review to provide the totality of evidence.

Qualifying factors that could result in an upgrade of certainty for observational studies include:

(a) Large magnitude of effect—Refers to a very large effect size that could not be explained by factors such as risk of bias, inconsistency, indirectness, imprecision, and publication bias. The choice of large effect size threshold should be predetermined.
(b) Dose response—Refers to a consistent relationship between dose and response where a higher intensity of treatment results in superior outcomes compared to a lower intensity of treatment.
(c) Plausible residual and confounding—Refers to any specific factor that may potentially underestimate or overestimate the effect of an intervention.

Some GRADE factors may have an overlap, and the raters should be aware of this overlap to avoid double-counting. For example, factors of inconsistency and imprecision may overlap, and accordingly, discretion should be applied, and a detailed explanation should be provided to back the judgments. Like the conduct of a systematic review, dual and independent assessment is recommended for GRADE assessment, followed by a consensus meeting. Decisions to upgrade or downgrade each factor are based on judgment, and detailed reasoning for the assessment of each factor is helpful for the reconciliation discussions.

Step 9: Reporting the Findings of Systematic Review

Reporting of systematic reviews or any scientific reporting requires specificity. The reporting of systematic review should follow the PRISMA checklist. The latest version of the PRISMA checklist was published in the year 2020. The PRISMA checklist has 27 items covering all major sections of a manuscript including title, abstract, introduction/background, methods, results, discussion, and other information covering protocol registration; funding sources, if applicable; competing interests; and availability of data, data code, data collection forms, etc. The detailed instructions for each item in the PRISMA checklist are reported extensively in several publications [15]. When reporting, it is helpful to start with relatively easier tasks before proceeding to difficult tasks. Because the protocol is written in future tense, using the protocol content to complete the manuscript up to the methods section is a relatively easy task.

Results: Study Selection

The results section should start with the results of the search and selection process with a specific count of references identified in the initial search, the number of citations that passed the initial screening, and the number of citations included in the final screening, with reasons for exclusion at each step. The PRISMA checklist also recommends summarizing the study search and selection process using a flow diagram (Fig. 8.1).

Results: Study Characteristics

Reporting the results of search and selection should be followed by a section on reporting the characteristics of included studies. The recommendation is to provide details of partici-

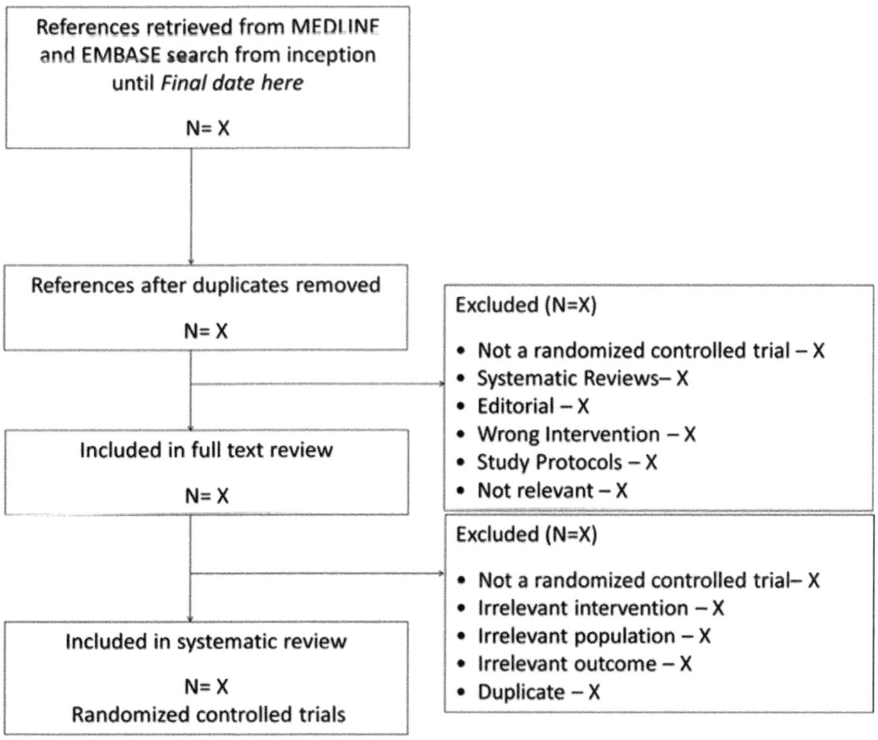

Fig. 8.1 A sample of how study selection can be summarized in a figure for a systematic review

pants, including number, intervention and comparison regimen, primary and secondary outcomes, setting, funding, etc.

Results: Risk of Bias in Included Studies

This section summarizes the results from assessments of risk of bias for each included study. Present quantitatively, of all the included studies how many satisfied the specific risk of bias item. Using the Cochrane Risk of Bias tool, generating a summary risk of bias assessment figure is recommended for reporting.

Results: Results of Individual Studies and Quantitative Synthesis (i.e., Meta-Analysis)

The results from individual studies, including a summary estimate for each included outcome with precision estimates (i.e., confidence intervals), should be reported in a standardized format. Reporting results from individual studies should be followed by reporting of pooled summary estimates along with confidence intervals, measures of statistical heterogeneity, and clearly articulating the direction of the findings (e.g., favors intervention or comparison group) for each outcome. After reporting the main results, report on the results of possible causes of heterogeneity (e.g., any subgroup or sensitivity analyses) followed by all sensitivity analyses performed to assess the robustness of the overall results. For each outcome, provide the overall certainty of evidence assessment (e.g., high, moderate, low, or very low). However, do not interpret the results in the results section. Report the results without any connotation and present the facts without any qualitative judgments or adjectives.

Organizing the Discussion

The discussion can be organized in five sections: (1) summary of key findings, (2) comparison of results to current literature, (3) limitations, (4) implications for research and practice, and (5) conclusion. The first paragraph of the discussion section should summarize the key findings using adjectives (rather than numerical) descriptives, such as significantly lower and higher. Depending on the context, authors should then provide an interpretation of the results which could include a balance of benefits and risks, applicability, overall certainty of evidence, recommendations for practice, etc. The summary results section should be followed by a discussion on how the results from the systematic review compares with other similar studies on the same topic. It is important to provide reasoning on why the results may be similar or different. Possible reasons could include differences in PICO, setting, risk of bias, etc. The next paragraph should focus on limitations of the current systematic review, and with each limitation, provide a counter focusing on how the limitation was minimized with a specific strategy used in the review process. The limitation section is followed by a conclusion with a broad focus on implications for research and practice and, specifically, recommendations regarding what remains answered or what was poorly addressed and should be addressed in future studies. For practice, provide specific recommendations on what should or should not change. Lastly, the conclusion should summarize the takeaway points from the systematic review.

Part 3: Common Myths About Systematic Reviews

There Are Not Enough Trials to Conduct a Systematic Review

It is often stated that there are not enough trials to conduct a systematic review and meta-analysis. The purpose of a systematic review is to summarize all available evidence on a specific PICO question. If there is more than one trial, a systematic review and meta-analysis is feasible. The summary estimate that is produced aids in determining if the results are precise and if further trials need to be conducted, or if the results are imprecise or inconsistent with the need for further trials for clarification.

We Already Know the Answer; No Need to Conduct a Systematic Review

Occasionally, there may be an incorrect assumption that the result of a PICO question is known, and there is no need to pool the results from all studies. However, summarizing results allows for quantitative synthesis, and, most importantly, allows for assessing the robustness of the results through risk of bias assessments and certainty assessments to increase or decrease the confidence in the estimates. Additionally, through assessment of the totality of evidence, recommendations can be made for future studies and practice. Bottomline, without a systematic approach the claims or lack there of is simply and assumption and remains unknown.

Most Studies Are of Low-Quality Studies So No Point in Synthesis: "Garbage In, Garbage Out"

This contradicts the purpose of a systematic review. The goal is to synthesize all available evidence and establish the quality (i.e., risk of bias) regardless of publication status. Furthermore, publication status, journal impact factor, reputation of the author or institution or any other factor is not an assurance of quality. There is no assumption. Unless the systematic review is completed, claims about the quality of studies are premature.

I Can Do It All Alone, No Need for a Team

We hope that what is provided above highlights the need for a team, given the unique skill sets and potentially overwhelming tasks that may come while conducting a systematic review. Ideally, a team should have people with methodological and content knowledge and skills.

References

1. Lasserson TJ, Thomas J, Higgins JP. Starting a review. In: Cochrane handbook for systematic reviews of interventions; 2019. p. 1–12.
2. Mulrow CD. Rationale for systematic reviews. BMJ. 1994;309(6954):597–9.
3. Chalmers I, Hedges LV, Cooper H. A brief history of research synthesis. Eval Health Prof. 2002;25(1):12–37.
4. Lau J, Antman EM, Jimenez-Silva J, Kupelnick B, Mosteller F, Chalmers TC. Cumulative meta-analysis of therapeutic trials for myocardial infarction. N Engl J Med. 1992;327(4):248–54.
5. Adivitiya KYP. The evolution of recombinant thrombolytics: current status and future directions. Bioengineered. 2017;8(4):331–58.
6. Moreau P , Hulin C , Perrot A , et al. Maintenance with daratumumab or observation following treatment with bortezomib, thalidomide, and dexamethasone with or without daratumumab and autologous stem-cell transplant in patients with newly diagnosed multiple myeloma (CASSIOPEIA): an open-label, randomised, phase 3 trial . Lancet Oncol . 2021 ;22 (10):1378 -1390 .
7. Sephien A, Dayto DC, Reljic T, et al. Efficacy of intravenous iron in patients with heart failure with reduced ejection fraction and iron deficiency: a systematic review and meta-analysis of randomized control trials. Am J Cardiovasc Drugs. 2024;24(2):285–302.
8. Higgins J, Thomas J, Chandler J, et al. Cochrane handbook for systematic reviews of interventions, version 6.4 (updated august 2023); Cochrane: London, UK, 2023.
9. Aamodt M, Huurdeman H, Stromme H. Librarian co-authored systematic reviews are associated with lower risk of bias compared to systematic reviews with acknowledgement of librarians or no participation by librarians. Evid Based Libr Inf Pract. 2019;14(4):103–27.
10. Bai Y, Gao J, Zou D, Li Z. Is MEDLINE alone enough for a meta-analysis? Aliment Pharmacol Ther. 2007;26(1):125–126; author reply 126.
11. Aali G, Shokraneh F. No limitations to language, date, publication type, and publication status in search step of systematic reviews. J Clin Epidemiol. 2021;133:165–7.
12. Ewald H, Klerings I, Wagner G, et al. Searching two or more databases decreased the risk of missing relevant studies: a metaresearch study. J Clin Epidemiol. 2022;149:154–64.
13. Booth A. Over 85% of included studies in systematic reviews are on MEDLINE. J Clin Epidemiol. 2016;79:165–6.
14. Sterne JA, Hernan MA, Reeves BC, et al. ROBINS-I: a tool for assessing risk of bias in non-randomised studies of interventions. BMJ. 2016;355:i4919.
15. Page MJ, McKenzie JE, Bossuyt PM, et al. The PRISMA 2020 statement: an updated guideline for reporting systematic reviews. BMJ. 2021;372:n71.

Part II

Data Analysis in Cancer Research

A Basic Overview of Statistics in Cancer Research

9

Julia N. Soulakova, Terrie Vasilopoulos, and Yajuan Si

Introduction

Any research study starts with the design stage. During this stage, the research questions are stated and "translated" into actionable, statistical language. For example, variables and parameters representing the study outcomes and measures, respectively, are identified, and corresponding statistical hypotheses are formulated. In addition, a study plan is developed, which includes several components such as power analysis (also known as sample size calculation) to determine the minimum required sample size, e.g., the required number of study participants. The power analysis should focus on the primary (and possibly secondary) endpoint(s) and reflect the statistical methods that will be used in the analytical stage. For studies involving primary data collection, the design stage is conducted prospectively, before the data collection stage. Post hoc power analysis, conducted after the primary data have been collected, raises a lot of issues and is generally not recommended [1]. Additional considerations for designing experimental studies, such as randomization and stratification, have been addressed in the context of oncology studies [2] and experimental studies, more generally [3].

In studies involving secondary data analysis, the researcher either has access to the data or possesses additional information that can inform the study design. For example, a questionnaire used to collect survey data could help refine the research questions to ensure they can be addressed using the data. Additionally, data exploration could be valuable for identifying data sources for linkage, assessing the adequacy of the data size, and comparing different data sources in terms of data completeness, among other aspects of study design [4]. Studies with secondary data should be designed with the same level of rigor as those involving primary data collection [4]. Additional considerations for designing observational studies have been addressed elsewhere [4, 5].

The stages of end-to-end statistical analysis following the design stage include the following: (1) data collection, preparation, and description; (2) data analysis; (3) interpretation of results; (4) validation of results; and (5) dissemination of study findings. In this chapter, we review key statistical concepts used in cancer research and discuss important considerations for several innovative statistical methods. The remainder of the chapter is organized as follows. Section "Risk assessment" provides a review of risk assessment, including key metrics such as the relative risk, number needed to treat, and odds ratio, with calculations demonstrated using a 2 × 2 contingency table. Section "Clinical diagnostic metrics" presents several clinical diagnostic metrics, including sensitivity and specificity, which are further discussed in section "Bayesian statistics" in the context of Bayesian inference, along with other considerations. Sections "Data imputation" and "Survey research methods in national surveys" provide concise reviews of data imputation methods and survey research methods, respectively. Section "Propensity score matching for causal inference" outlines causal inference methods based on propensity score matching. Section "Data integration" reviews the concept of data integration, i.e., the use of multiple data sources within the same study. Section "Statistical considerations in open science" outlines the key statistical considerations in open science. The chapter concludes with a summary provided in section "Summary".

J. N. Soulakova (✉)
Department of Population Health Sciences, College of Medicine, University of Central Florida, Orlando, FL, USA
e-mail: julia.soulakova@ucf.edu

T. Vasilopoulos
Department of Anesthesiology, Chief of Division of Education Research and Scholarship, Department of Orthopaedic Surgery and Sports Medicine, College of Medicine, University of Florida, Gainesville, FL, USA
e-mail: TVasilopoulos@anest.ufl.edu

Y. Si
Survey Research Center, Institute for Social Research, University of Michigan, Ann Arbor, MI, USA
e-mail: yajuan@umich.edu

J. Huang, H. S.L. Jim (eds.), *Cancer Research Guidance for Clinicians and Researchers*,
https://doi.org/10.1007/978-3-032-19175-5_9

The chapter is intended for clinicians who are familiar with conventional statistical methods used in oncology [2, 6, 7]. Some calculations, such as the formulas described in sections "Risk assessment" and "Clinical diagnostic metrics", are relatively basic and typically covered in first-year medical school statistics courses. These fundamental concepts should be manageable for clinicians to apply in their research. The other content, such as topics addressed in sections "Bayesian statistics" through "Statistical considerations in open science", expands on foundational statistics knowledge. Applying these more advanced concepts may require collaboration with a statistics expert.

Overview of Statistical Methods in Oncology

Risk Assessment

For clinicians and patients, it is important to understand the risk or likelihood of developing cancer or of going into remission given particularly predisposing factors. For prospective studies, including cohort studies and clinical trials, the relative risk (RR) can be calculated as the ratio of the probability of an event occurring in the treatment group to the probability in the control group. For the 2 × 2 contingency table shown in Fig. 9.1, the RR is calculated as the ratio of the event rate in the exposed (treatment) group to the event rate in the control group [8]. The experimental event rate (EER) represents the proportion of patients in the exposed group who experience the event, while the control event rate (CER) represents the proportion of patients in the control group who experience the event [8]. Figure 9.2 illustrates the calculation of the EER, CER, and RR for cancer in patients who smoke cigarettes compared to those who do not.

Since the RR is a ratio, a value of 1 is interpreted as indicating no association or effect (i.e., the null hypothesis) [8]. Typically, an RR greater than 1 indicates an increased risk of the event occurring in the exposed group compared to the control group, while an RR less than 1 indicates a decreased risk. It is important to calculate 95% confidence intervals (CIs) for RRs to assess their significance. A CI that does not include the value of 1 supports an association between a risk factor and the occurrence of an event. Relative risk reduction refers to the proportion by which the risk is decreased in the treatment group compared to the control group [9].

In addition to RR, understanding the differences in absolute risk of an event between the control and exposed groups is also important. These differences can be measured by absolute risk reduction (ARR) and absolute risk increase (ARI) [9], calculated using the formulas:

$$ARR = CER - EER \text{ and } ARI = EER - CER.$$

Exposure	Event	
	Yes (Event)	No (No Event)
Yes	*a*	*b*
No	*c*	*d*

$$EER = \frac{a}{a+b}, CER = \frac{c}{c+d}, RR = \frac{EER}{CER}, \text{ and } OR = \frac{\frac{a}{b}}{\frac{c}{d}} = \frac{a \cdot d}{b \cdot c},$$

where $a, b, c,$ and d denote the number of patients in the corresponding cross − group. For example, a is the number of patients who experienced the event in the exposed group.

Fig. 9.1 Formulas for calculating event rates in the exposed (EER) and control (CER) groups, relative risk (RR), and odds ratio (OR) of an event

Cigarette Use	Lung Cancer	
	Present	Absent
Yes	*75*	*25*
No	*25*	*75*

$$EER = \frac{a}{a+b} = \frac{75}{75+25} = 0.75, CER = \frac{c}{c+d} = \frac{25}{25+75} = 0.25,$$

$$RR = \frac{EER}{CER} = \frac{0.75}{0.25} = 3, \text{ and } OR = \frac{\frac{a}{b}}{\frac{c}{d}} = \frac{\frac{75}{25}}{\frac{25}{75}} = 9.$$

Fig. 9.2 Rates of lung cancer among patients who smoke (EER) and do not smoke (CER) cigarettes, relative risk (RR), and odds ratio (OR) of lung cancer for adults who smoke cigarettes versus those who do not

The most important and interpretable applications of ARR and ARI are the calculations of the number needed to treat (NNT) and the number needed to harm (NNH). These metrics indicate how many patients need to be treated to prevent one adverse event or cause one adverse event, respectively [9]. Specifically,

$$NNT = \frac{1}{ARR} \text{ and } NNH = \frac{1}{ARI}.$$

To standardize the interpretation, dividing 100 by NNT results in the number of additional patients prevented from having an adverse event (for every 100 patients treated) due to a given treatment or exposure [10]. For example, in a study comparing nivolumab in combination with chemotherapy to chemotherapy alone as treatment for advanced gastric cancer, gastroesophageal junction cancer, and esophageal adenocarcinoma, the calculated NNT for overall 1-year survival was 14. This means that seven additional patients are expected to survive due to receiving nivolumab in combination with chemotherapy rather than receiving chemotherapy alone [10]. Indeed,

$$\frac{100}{NNT} = \frac{100}{14} \approx 7.$$

In retrospective studies, such as case-control studies, risk cannot be directly determined; however, we can still assess the likelihood of an event given various factors. In these studies, we calculate the odds ratio (OR), which is defined as the odds of an event occurring in the treatment group divided by the odds of an event occurring in the control group [8]. The OR can be calculated from a contingency table, as illustrated in Figs. 9.1 and 9.2, or derived from regression coefficients in a logistic regression analysis. Similar to RR, the null value for ORs is 1, indicating that there is no association between the exposure and the event [8]. An OR greater than 1 indicates an increased likelihood of the occurrence of an event in the treatment group compared to the control group, while an OR less than 1 indicates a decreased likelihood. As with RRs, it is important to calculate 95% CIs to assess the significance of ORs. A word of caution, both RR and OR can be calculated from the same contingency tables in prospective studies; however, they yield different values and are not interchangeable. Figure 9.2 illustrates this discrepancy. The choice between RR and OR calculations depends on the study design and the research question [8].

Clinical Diagnostic Metrics

In oncology research, clinical diagnostic tests are crucial for early detection, accurate diagnosis, and monitoring of cancer. Sensitivity and specificity are vital for assessing the probability of true positive and true negative cases, respectively, ensuring that cancers are detected early and accurately. Sensitivity is calculated as the proportion of true positives, i.e., the proportion of positive cases among patients who have the disease, and specificity is the proportion of true negatives, i.e., the proportion of negative cases among those who do not have the disease. Both sensitivity and specificity range from 0 to 1 [11]. Figure 9.3 illustrates the formulas for computing sensitivity and specificity for a 2x2 contingency table. A highly sensitive test has a low false negative rate, meaning that if a test with high sensitivity gives a negative result, there is a greater likelihood that the patient does not have the disease. Highly sensitive tests are important for use in patient screening. An example of a highly sensitive test is the measurement of prostate-specific antigen (PSA) for prostate cancer screening. A sensitivity of the PSA test, PSA ≥ 4 ng/mL, is 0.93 [12], indicating that patients testing negative are unlikely to have prostate cancer. This high sensitivity makes the PSA test an excellent screening tool for prostate cancer. A highly specific test, on the other hand, has a low false positive rate, meaning that if a test with high specificity gives a positive result, there is a greater likelihood that the patient has the disease. Thus, highly specific tests are most useful for confirmatory, diagnostic testing. An example of a highly specific test is the Pap smear for the detection of cervical cancer. Numerous studies have demonstrated specificity values ranging from 0.86 to 1.00 for Pap smears, indicating that patients testing positive are likely to have cervical cancer [13].

Test Result	Actual Disease Status	
	Present	Absent
Positive	*a* (True Positive)	*b* (False Positive)
Negative	*c* (False Negative)	*d* (True Negative)

$$Sensitivity = \frac{a}{a+c},\quad Specificity = \frac{d}{b+d},\quad PPV = \frac{a}{a+b},\quad NPV = \frac{d}{c+d}$$

Fig. 9.3 Calculating the clinical diagnostic metrics

One aspect to consider regarding sensitivity and specificity is that they do not change with prevalence of a disease. Positive predictive value (PPV) and negative predictive value (NPV) account for disease prevalence and help determine the likelihood that a positive or negative test result is accurate. PPV is calculated as the proportion of true positives among all positive test results, and NPV is the proportion of true negatives among all negative test results. Like sensitivity and specificity, PPV and NPV range from 0 to 1 [11]. Figure 9.3 illustrates how PPV and NPV can be computed for a 2 × 2 table. High PPV indicates a high likelihood that a patient testing positive has the disease, while high NPV indicates a high likelihood that a patient testing negative does not have the disease. In terms of disease prevalence, higher prevalence increases PPV and decreases NPV, while lower prevalence decreases PPV and increases NPV [11]. To compare sensitivity and specificity to PPV and NPV, sensitivity and specificity are indicators of concordance between a test result and disease state, while PPV and NPV are indicators of likelihood that a given test will successfully identify someone's disease state based on test results.

Other useful metrics are the positive likelihood ratio (LR+) and negative likelihood ratio (LR-), which combine sensitivity and specificity into a single measure and are used to assess how much a test result will change the probability of having cancer, aiding in risk stratification [11]. These ratios are calculated as

$$LR+ = \frac{\text{Sensitivity}}{1-\text{Specificity}} \text{ and } LR- = \frac{1-\text{Sensitivity}}{\text{Specificity}}.$$

These ratios can be interpreted similarly to ORs. Specifically, an LR+ greater than 1 indicates that a positive test result is more likely to occur in patients with the disease. For example, an LR+ of 10 means that a positive test result is 10 times more likely to be found in patients with the disease than in those without the disease. Conversely, an LR- less than 1 indicates that a negative test result is more likely to occur in patients without the disease. For example, an LR- of 0.1 means that a negative test result is 10 times more likely to be found in patients without the disease than in those with it.

Receiver operating characteristic (ROC) curves and the area under the curve (AUC) are used to evaluate the overall performance of diagnostic tests. ROC curve analysis involves plotting the true positive rate (sensitivity) against the false positive rate (1 − specificity) at various threshold settings [14]. The AUC is an indication of the diagnostic accuracy of a given test or risk factor, with high AUC values signifying better diagnostic performance [15]. AUC can also be used to compare ROC curves of different tests or risk factors. An AUC of 0.5 suggests no discrimination (equivalent to random chance), while an AUC of 1 indicates perfect discrimination [14, 15]. When calculating AUC, it is important to also estimate the 95% CI to determine whether it includes 0.5. From the aforementioned review of the PSA test [12], the test had AUC = 0.72 with 95%CI = 0.68,0.76. First, the CI does not include 0.50, indicating support that the PSA test has discriminatory ability for prostate cancer. The AUC value of 0.72 can be interpreted as follows: if 100 patients are tested with the PSA test, 72 will be diagnosed correctly (for either having or not having prostate cancer). Thus, the test can reasonably differentiate between patients with prostate cancer and those without it. Additionally, ROC curve analysis can be used to determine cut points in continuous or ordinal biomarkers by estimating values that optimize sensitivity and specificity [12].

Bayesian Statistics

The field of statistics has two main perspectives: frequentist and Bayesian. Frequentist statistics assumes data are randomly selected and treats statistical model parameters as fixed quantities. In contrast, Bayesian statistics considers model parameters as random variables given collected data and thus allows for a probability statement for the estimand of interest, reallocating credibility across possibilities. Bayesian inference has become increasingly popular in clinical research, with broad applications from study design to analysis [16]. Bayesian statistics offers an intuitive view of statistical analysis and interpretation, incorporating prior knowledge and maintaining flexibility in handling complex data structures, which is particularly valuable given the unprecedented data sources available for clinical research.

Bayes' theorem combines the data and the prior information to generate the posterior distribution of the estimate. In diagnostic testing, discussed in section "Clinical diagnostic metrics", researchers are interested in estimating cancer incidence, and Bayesian analysis treats the probability of a new disease case as the unknown quantity of interest. Historical incidence (i.e., the incidence of a disease in a given population) can be included as prior knowledge, say $p_0 = 5\%$. If a new screening test result is positive, and the test has a sensitivity of 70% and a specificity of 90%, Bayesian inference yields the posterior probability of the diagnosed disease as

$$p = \frac{Sensitivity * p_0}{Sensitivity * p_0 + (1 - Specificity) * (1 - p_0)} = \frac{0.7 * 0.05}{0.7 * 0.05 + (1 - 0.9) * (1 - 0.05)} \approx 0.269\ (or 26.9\%)\ (26.9\%\$\$\ 26.9\backslash\%\ \$\$)$$

Hence, the posterior estimate is a weighted summary of the prior knowledge ($p_0 = 5\%$) and the data (a positive test result, with 70% sensitivity and 90% specificity).

The allocation weight assigned to the data depends on the sample size and variability. For a small trial with high variability, the posterior inference with the trial data may be dominated by the strong prior information. With large-scale studies, the data may dominate the posterior estimation. The prior can be informative or noninformative. With noninformative prior specifications, the Bayesian inference will be similar to that with the frequentist approaches. Informative prior specifications bring in the "effective prior sample data" and affect the posterior estimation. In practice, prior information can be solicited based on subjective knowledge, historical studies, and pilot or similar investigations. The power prior is a type of informative prior that is constructed from historical data and has applications in clinical trials [17]. Informative prior solicitation can be challenging as it requires quantifying and formulating external information into suitable probability distributions. Weakly informative prior distributions are often recommended to improve the posterior estimation [18]. The key steps of a Bayesian workflow include:

1. Identify the study design and data relevant to the research question.
2. Build a model for the relevant data, specifying the probability distributions and parameters.
3. Introduce a prior distribution for the parameters based on subjective knowledge, historical data, or other relevant sources.
4. Estimate the posterior distributions, reallocating credibility across parameter values, and interpret the results in terms of their substantive meanings.

The posterior computation can be analytic or approximated by Monte Carlo simulations. With specific prior and data distributions, such as conjugate prior specifications, the posterior distribution is analytically solvable. However, in practice, Monte Carlo approximations are typically used for Bayesian inference when dealing with complex data structures, with various Markov chain Monte Carlo (MCMC) algorithms (Chaps. 11 and 12 in [19]). The MCMC computation may require a large number of sampling iterations (e.g., tens of thousands, depending on the specific algorithm) and a long time to achieve convergence, which is a main reason why Bayesian inference is computationally intensive and has become popular due to recent advancements in computational resources.

Bayesian inference obtains the point estimates, standard error, and credible intervals based on the posterior samples for the quantities of interest or their functions. The interpretation is based on the parameters' probability distributions; for example, the 95% credible interval means that there is a 95% probability that the true (unknown) estimate would lie within the interval, given the evidence provided by the observed data and the prior information. [It's important to note that a 95% confidence interval in frequentist statistics does not represent the probability of the parameter being within the interval, which is a common misunderstanding.] The posterior samples allow for predictions of future events by generating the posterior predictive samples that propagate all sources of uncertainty estimating model parameters. Therefore, Bayesian inference is often more attractive than the frequentist approach that requires repeated sampling randomization, large-sample asymptotic approximations, and analytic forms.

Bayesian statistics has been applied to clinical trial designs (including adaptive randomization), trial monitoring, meta-analyses, and decision-making [20]. Because of their natural ability to incorporate prior information, Bayesian methods can flexibly model complex data structures through hierarchical models. The use of hierarchical models with group-level random effects can be treated as a Bayesian approach, where different groups share a common mean but present heterogeneity. Hierarchical Bayesian models can explicitly capture the data structure through multiple model levels, facilitate information sharing, and stabilize estimates for small groups. Cancer registry data are often collected across multiple centers, incorporating individual records and aggregated summaries from different time frames, necessitating the integration of multiple data sources. A Bayesian framework analyzing the heterogeneous cancer registry data accounts for the uncertainty associated with all data sources, facilitates information sharing across groups, and generates probability statements for inferences and predictions.

Data Imputation

Missing data is a frequent issue in national cancer datasets and registries [21]. Ignoring missing data in the analysis is only appropriate if the data are missing completely at random, which is often an unreasonable assumption and can lead to biased results. For example, a study examining missing data in the National Cancer Database found that cancer patients with complete data differed from those with missing data in terms of demographic characteristics, cancer stages, and treatments received [21]. Moreover, among patients with metastatic disease, those with missing data had worse overall survival [21]. Thus, excluding patients with missing values from the analysis may result in a more optimistic prognosis of overall survival among patients with metastatic disease [21].

Many data imputation methods have been proposed for studies in which missing is assumed to occur at random, and multiple imputation is probably the most commonly used approach [22]. In practice, multiple imputation creates several complete datasets that are analyzed separately, and then the results are combined. Sequential regression multiple imputation (also known as multiple imputation by chain equations) generates a complete dataset using an iterative process where each variable is imputed one at a time, conditional on the other variables [23]. The approach was used in a study examining the role of cannabis use in racial and ethnic disparities in testicular cancer incidence in the United States using data from the Surveillance, Epidemiology, and End Results (SEER) Program, the National Survey of Drug Use and Health, and several other sources [24]. Specifically, because SEER data are suppressed for small cell counts (fewer than 15) to protect patient confidentiality and ensure data reliability, missing data were highly prevalent, particularly for groups of color. To address this challenge, researchers performed 256 imputations, each with 20 iterations. This approach significantly reduced the extent of missing data; for example, in simple linear regression models for testicular cancer rates, the percentage of missing data decreased to 2.6% [24].

Survey Research Methods in National Surveys

Studies using secondary data from national surveys are common in cancer prevention and epidemiology. For example, national datasets such as the Tobacco Use Supplement to the Current Population Survey are used to estimate the prevalence of smoking and smoking cessation behaviors among various populations in the United States [25–27], which helps inform cancer prevention efforts. National surveys usually implement complex sampling (i.e., multistage sampling, such as stratified cluster sampling), resulting in a probability sample that is representative of the target population. In such samples, each respondent is assigned a primary sampling weight and possibly additional weights [28]. These weights should be incorporated into statistical analyses to ensure that the computed estimates of health characteristics, such as the incidence rate of breast cancer in the United States [29], actually reflect the target population (e.g., women in the United States).

Ignoring survey weights could lead to biased estimates. For example, discrepancies in estimates derived from correct and incorrect statistical methods were demonstrated in the context of smoking status and attitudes toward smoking bans among adult single parents in the United States [30]. Specifically, the estimated total number of single parents who have never smoked differed by 323,621 when comparing a method that incorrectly ignored survey weights to one that correctly incorporated them [30]. Moreover, discrepancies in the confidence intervals for proportions and totals between these methods were also highlighted [30]. Thus, researchers should apply appropriate survey statistical methods and adhere to the analysis guidelines provided with national surveys [30, 31]. Such methods should also be employed when handling missing data (e.g., fractional imputation) [32–34]. These key considerations form the foundation for understanding survey sampling techniques and their application in estimation and prediction [35].

Propensity Score Matching for Causal Inference

Propensity score matching (PSM) is a causal inference method used in observational studies with large datasets. It helps address the effects of confounding factors and thereby reduces bias associated with confounding (Part 2 in [5], [36, 37]). PSM enables the use of observational data to create matched groups that resemble treated and untreated groups in an experimental study, ensuring they are similar in terms of all observed baseline characteristics related to the study outcome. PSM is performed in three key steps (Part 2 in [5, 36, 37]). First, a logistic regression model (or another model suitable for a dichotomous outcome) is used to estimate propensity score, which represents the (conditional) probability of receiving the treatment given the observed covariates. The dependent variable is an indicator of receiving the treatment (versus no treatment). The covariates are all observed (baseline) characteristics relevant to the study outcome but not influenced by the treatment. For example, patient baseline demographic characteristics are commonly included, along with other relevant covariates [38]. Second, treated patients are matched with untreated patients so that both groups have similar observed characteristics (covariates) and propensity scores. Ideally, this matching results in two groups—treated and untreated—that are balanced in terms of all considered observed characteristics. Several methods, such as optimal pair matching, could be used to perform this matching (Chap. 8 in [5]). Third, the matched data are analyzed using traditional statistical methods for paired data, while unmatched patients are excluded from the analysis.

Rosenbaum provided an example of PSM applied to an oncology study, comparing medical oncologists and gynecologic oncologists in terms of the intensity of chemotherapy provided (measured by the number of weeks) and survival time among women older than 65 years with ovarian cancer (Chap. 8 in [5]). Patients treated by medical oncologists ("treated group") were matched to patients treated by gynecologic oncologists ("untreated group"). The observed baseline characteristics included the patient's age, cancer stage, tumor grade, and year of diagnosis, among several other factors. The two groups were well balanced. The analysis used Wilcoxon's signed-rank test to compare chemotherapy intensity and the Prentice-Wilcoxon test to compare survival times. The study indicated that medical oncologists appeared to administer chemotherapy more intensively compared to gynecologic oncologists, but there was no difference in survival time (Chap. 8 in [5]).

The PSM has been generalized for studies with multiple treatment groups [39, 40], continuous treatments [41], complex survey data [42, 43], and spatially indexed data [44], among others. Here we highlight one extension of PSM, the inverse probability of treatment weighting (IPTW) method. IPTW computes weights based on the propensity scores for all patients in the dataset and applies these weights to the data to create a weighted sample, which is then used in the analysis. Both PSM and IPTW methods were used in a recent study comparing two treatments for muscle-invasive bladder cancer, radical cystectomy, and trimodality therapy [38]. The primary study outcome was metastasis-free survival. Matching was used to create two groups that were similar in terms of age, biological sex, cT2 stage (i.e., percentage of patients with cT2 stage), presence of hydronephrosis, and receipt of neoadjuvant or adjuvant chemotherapy. The results of both methods were consistent—a finding that is not always guaranteed: radical cystectomy and trimodality therapy led to similar metastasis-free survival and other oncological outcomes. The authors concluded that trimodality therapy should be recommended to all eligible patients with muscle-invasive bladder cancer as part of a collaborative decision-making process, rather than being limited only to those patients who cannot undergo surgery [38].

Data Integration

Clinical research has long relied on data integration, combining multiple data sources including histology, genomics, radiology, and electronic health records. A single data source often cannot meet the growing demand to comprehensively capture the spectrum. Combining information from multiple sources has been widely implemented to generate high-quality statistical products, and it is crucial to understand the purpose and quality of each data source in a given analysis. Sample surveys, such as the national surveys discussed in section "Survey research methods in national surveys", often have a well-controlled sampling design and recruitment process to represent the target population. However, the sample sizes may be limited (e.g., for groups of color) due to high costs and nonresponse rates in data collection [45]. Electronic health records contain patient medical history, laboratory measures, and diagnostics; however, they often have significant missing information due to the reliance on patient engagement with the health system. Commercial claims, Medicare and Medicaid records, and registry data provide rich information on health utilization but linking across multiple databases may be incomplete due to nonconsent and inconsistent inputs. The scenarios for combining data include combining summary statistics, microdata, and aggregate and individual data. Below we discuss two examples of data integration to yield population-based research findings, combining probability and nonprobability surveys and combining clinical trials with real-world evidence.

Probability surveys start with a sampling frame representative of the population, select units with a known and nonzero probability, and allow for precision estimation. Probability sampling has been the ground for survey data collection intended for population inference, where the random sampling theory generalizes sample inference to the target population. Most national cancer epidemiology surveys, such as the National Health Interview Survey, have employed probability sampling, as was outlined in section "Survey research methods in national surveys". However, declining response rates have become a concern and could cause deviations from random sampling and make the design-based analysis assumptions invalid. Nonprobability surveys invite participants without known selection probabilities or in a deterministic inclusion fashion, for which response rates or sampling errors are inestimable. Nonprobability samples rely on statistical modeling to correct for nonrandom aspects of data collection [46]. Inferences of both kinds of samples require strong assumptions about how nonrandom features of the data collection process affect survey estimates. The modeling assumptions are similar to those in the missing data literature and aim to achieve ignorability [47], meaning that the selection mechanism is ignorable for the outcome variable of interest given the observed characteristics. In summary, strong assumptions are necessary to make population-based inference with a sample. Specifically, the sampled units must be conditionally exchangeable with nonsampled units that share common characteristics, and proper adjustments to the sampled units should ensure they represent the target population.

There is rich literature of methods adjusting for selection bias [48]. Design-based approaches focus on the selection mechanism and construct weights to accommodate unequal probabilities of selection, nonresponse, and coverage error. Model-based approaches focus on survey outcomes and fit models to predict nonsampled units. Doubly robust approaches combine weighting with predictions and offer protection against model misspecification under either weighting or prediction. One specific method, multilevel regression and poststratification (also known as MRP), fits a multilevel model to stabilize small group estimates and applies poststratification to adjust for selection bias [49]. To yield valid inference, the adjustment approaches must include all predictive auxiliary variables that are related to both the inclusion mechanism and survey variables. The practical constraint on the range of available auxiliary variables increases the challenge when the important factor related to the selection and outcome is not measured in any existing datasets. Often the relevant auxiliary information is partially collected and requires modeling to generate the synthetic population distribution [50].

Randomized trials have been the gold standard for assessing causal effects to achieve internal validity. Methods for causal inference with observational data, such as those discussed in section "Propensity score matching for causal inference", rely on strong but hard-to-verify assumptions, including ignorability, positivity, and the stable treatment value assumption. When the treatment effects are different across subgroups and the subgroup decomposition in the trial sample is different from that in the target population, the estimated causal effects cannot generalize to the population; i.e., the causal effects do not have external validity [51]. Evidence-based research combines data from controlled clinical trials with real-world evidence from electronic health records, ecological momentary assessments, environmental measures, administrative claims, cancer registries, and other medical data sources across multiple health systems. The adjustment methods include weighting, prediction, and doubly robust methods to achieve external and internal validity [52–54]. Careful consideration of each data type for data integration is necessary. The criteria assessing the integrated data quality include relevance, timeliness and punctuality, accessibility and clarity, coherence and comparability, and granularity [55].

Statistical Considerations in Open Science

Open science plays a pivotal role in advancing oncology research by promoting increased accessibility and collaboration among researchers worldwide. This collaborative approach is essential in oncology, where efforts across multiple clinical sites and researchers can lead to more comprehensive studies and faster advancements. Open-access articles often receive higher citation rates, enhancing the visibility and dissemination of crucial findings [56]. Additionally, open science encourages the sharing of vital datasets, such as genomics and proteomics data, which are fundamental for robust and reproducible cancer research; many institutions or researchers might not have access to this type of data otherwise [56, 57]. Moreover, merging data from multiple datasets or creating new datasets via data integration can be very time-consuming. Sharing these study datasets could not only facilitate replicability but also enhance the efficiency of research for other scientists. For example, data merged from two Current Population Survey Supplements were used in a study of smoking behaviors in the United States and shared via Harvard Dataverse to promote further tobacco research using this dataset [25]. Similarly, the merged dataset used in the study of testicular cancer incidence discussed in section "Data imputation" has been deposited in Mendeley Data [24]. However, it is important to be aware that not all study data may be sharable, even if the study utilizes publicly available data sources.

The National Institutes of Health (NIH), the National Cancer Institute (NCI) specifically, and many oncology journals, such as the *Journal of Clinical Oncology*, have enacted data sharing policies to support open science. The NIH (https://sharing.nih.gov/) and NCI (https://datascience.cancer.gov/data-sharing/policy-guidance) websites provide easily accessible details of their data sharing policies and what type of studies require data sharing plans. Researchers generating genomic data should pay special attention to specific policies for sharing this type of data. One key aspect of these policies is creating a data management and sharing plan to make data produced from funded studies publicly available, which often occurs via submission to a data repository. Data repositories range from general repositories to specialty or data-type specific repositories. Researchers can search and identify repositories via the NIH data sharing site (https://sharing.nih.gov) and the Data Citation Index (https://webofscience.help.clarivate.com/en-us/Content/data-citation-index/data-citation-index.htm). By making research more transparent and accessible, open science improves the quality and reliability of findings [56, 57]. Furthermore, it accelerates the translation of research into clinical practice, ultimately benefiting patients through the development of personalized medicine approaches and more efficacious treatments [57]. Oncology research will increasingly benefit from the continued support and implementation of open science practices.

Summary

In this chapter, we focused on several traditional and innovative statistical strategies, addressing only some of the methods commonly used in cancer research. Other important methods, such as survival analysis, multiple comparisons adjustments, and sensitivity analysis, as well as common statistical pitfalls, have been discussed elsewhere [2, 6, 7]. Likewise, the chapter did not address the use of artificial intelligence methods, such as machine learning, which are becoming increasingly popular in oncology studies involving high-dimensional data [58–60]. The development and application of these methods require expertise in bioinformatics and are thus outside of the scope of this chapter.

As mentioned in section "Introduction", applying some of the methods discussed in this chapter in practice may require collaboration with a biostatistician. This collaboration is vital for ensuring that the study aims are accurately translated into statistical hypotheses, that the study design and analyses are appropriate for the aims, and that the results and limitations are interpreted correctly. Moreover, in the context of open science, such collaboration promotes effective data sharing, facilitating the replicability of the findings, and, hence, improves the quality of cancer research.

Acknowledgements The initial draft of the chapter was prepared with the assistance of ChatGPT, an AI language model developed by OpenAI, for editing purposes. The authors would like to thank Bryan Penberthy for his assistance in editing the final draft of the chapter.

References

1. Dziak JJ, Dierker LC, Abar B. The interpretation of statistical power after the data have been gathered. Curr Psychol. 2020;39:870–7. https://doi.org/10.1007/S12144-018-0018-1/METRICS.
2. Xu W, Huang SH, Su J, et al. Statistical fundamentals on cancer research for clinicians: working with your statisticians. Clin

Transl Radiat Oncol. 2021;27:75–84. https://doi.org/10.1016/J.CTRO.2021.01.006.
3. Aberson CL. Statistical power analysis. In: Scott R, Kosslyn S, editors. Emerging trends in the social and behavioral sciences. Wiley; 2015.
4. Sarensen HT, Sabroe S, Olsen J. A framework for evaluation of secondary data sources for epidemiological research. Int J Epidemiol. 1996;25:435–42.
5. Rosenbaum PR. Design of Observational Studies. 2nd ed. Cham: Springer; 2020.
6. Katz MH. Multivariable analysis: a practical guide for clinicians and public health researchers. 3rd ed. Cambridge University Press; 2011.
7. Katz M. Study design and statistical analysis: a practical guide for clinicians. Cambridge University Press; 2004.
8. Khan S, Memon MA. Measuring association between two categorical variables: revisiting risk ratio and odds ratio. Int J Stat Sci. 2020;20:153–70.
9. D'Arrigo G, Gori M, Pitino A, et al. Measures of frequency and effect in clinical research. Int Urol Nephrol. 2023;55:3147–52. https://doi.org/10.1007/S11255-023-03626-W/TABLES/3.
10. Janjigian YY, Shitara K, Moehler M, et al. First-line nivolumab plus chemotherapy versus chemotherapy as first-line treatment for advanced gastric cancer/gastroesophageal junction cancer/oesophageal adenocarcinoma (CheckMate 649): a multicentre, randomised, open-label, phase 3 trial. Lancet. 2021;398:27–40. https://doi.org/10.1016/S0140-6736(21)00797-2.
11. Monaghan TF, Rahman SN, Agudelo CW, et al. Foundational statistical principles in medical research: sensitivity, specificity, positive predictive value, and negative predictive value. Medicina (B Aires). 2021;57:503. https://doi.org/10.3390/MEDICINA57050503.
12. Merriel SWD, Pocock L, Gilbert E, et al. Systematic review and meta-analysis of the diagnostic accuracy of prostate-specific antigen (PSA) for the detection of prostate cancer in symptomatic patients. BMC Med. 2022;20:1–11. https://doi.org/10.1186/S12916-021-02230-Y/FIGURES/4.
13. Nanda K, McCrory DC, Myers ER, et al. Accuracy of the Papanicolaou test in screening for and follow-up of cervical cytologic abnormalities: a systematic review. Ann Intern Med. 2000;132:810–9. https://doi.org/10.7326/0003-4819-132-10-200005160-00009.
14. Carter JV, Pan J, Rai SN, Galandiuk S. ROC-ing along: evaluation and interpretation of receiver operating characteristic curves. Surgery. 2016;159:1638–45. https://doi.org/10.1016/J.SURG.2015.12.029.
15. Mandrekar JN. Receiver operating characteristic curve in diagnostic test assessment. J Thorac Oncol. 2010;5:1315–6. https://doi.org/10.1097/JTO.0b013e3181ec173d.
16. Adamina M, Tomlinson G, Guller U. Bayesian statistics in oncology: a guide for the clinical investigator. Cancer. 2009;115:5371–81. https://doi.org/10.1002/CNCR.24628.
17. Ibrahim JG, Chen MH, Gwon Y, Chen F. The power prior: theory and applications. Stat Med. 2015;34:3724–49. https://doi.org/10.1002/SIM.6728.
18. Gelman A, Jakulin A, Pittau MG, Su YS. A weakly informative default prior distribution for logistic and other regression models. Ann Appl Stat. 2008;2:1360–83. https://doi.org/10.1214/08-AOAS191.
19. Gelman A, Carlin JB, Stern HS, et al. Bayesian Data Analysis. 3rd ed. London: CRC Press; 2013.
20. Lee SY. Using Bayesian statistics in confirmatory clinical trials in the regulatory setting: a tutorial review. BMC Med Res Methodol. 2024;24:110. https://doi.org/10.1186/S12874-024-02235-0.
21. Yang DX, Khera R, Miccio JA, et al. Prevalence of missing data in the National Cancer Database and association with overall survival. JAMA Netw Open. 2021;4:e211793–e211793. https://doi.org/10.1001/JAMANETWORKOPEN.2021.1793.
22. Little RJA, Rubin DB. The analysis of social science data with missing values. Sociol Methods Res. 1989;18:292–326. https://doi.org/10.1177/0049124189018002004.
23. Raghunathan TE, Lepkowski JM, Van Hoewyk J, Solenberger P. A multivariate technique for multiply imputing missing values using a sequence of regression models. Surv Methodol. 2001;27:85–95.
24. Reece AS, Hulse GK. Causal inference multiple imputation investigation of the impact of cannabinoids and other substances on ethnic differentials in US testicular cancer incidence. BMC Pharmacol Toxicol. 2021;22:1–32. https://doi.org/10.1186/S40360-021-00505-X/FIGURES/20.
25. Soulakova JN, Crockett LJ. Current use of cigarettes in the United States: the joint role of race/ethnicity and health insurance coverage. Healthcare. 2023;11:3014. https://doi.org/10.3390/healthcare11233014.
26. Soulakova JN, Crockett LJ. Level of cigarette consumption and duration of smoking abstinence during failed quit attempts among long-term daily smokers: the role of race/ethnicity and cessation aids. J Racial Ethn Heal Disparities. 2018;5:293–303. https://doi.org/10.1007/s40615-017-0370-0.
27. Mai Y, Soulakova JN. Retrospective reports of former smokers: receiving doctor's advice to quit smoking and using behavioral interventions for smoking cessation in the United States. Prev Med Reports. 2018;11:290–6. https://doi.org/10.1016/j.pmedr.2018.07.012.
28. Si Y, Lee S, Heeringa SG. Population weighting in statistical analysis. JAMA Intern Med. 2024;184:98–9. https://doi.org/10.1001/JAMAINTERNMED.2023.6300.
29. Siegel RL, Giaquinto AN, Jemal A. Cancer statistics, 2024. CA Cancer J Clin. 2024;74:12–49. https://doi.org/10.3322/caac.21820.
30. Ha T, Soulakova JN. Importance of adjusting for multi-stage design when analyzing data from complex surveys. In: Zhao Y, Chen D-G, editors. New Frontiers of biostatistics and bioinformatics. Springer; 2018. p. 257–68.
31. Gomez C, Goponenko AV, Soulakova JN. Constructing UpSet plot for survey data with weights using SAS and R software. Commun Stat – Simul Comput. 2021;52:2320–6. https://doi.org/10.1080/03610918.2021.1904142.
32. Kim JK, Fuller W. Fractional hot deck imputation. Biometrika. 2004;91:559–78. https://doi.org/10.1093/biomet/91.3.559.
33. Rubin DB. Multiple imputation for nonresponse in surveys. New York: John Wiley & Sons; 1987.
34. Yang S, Kim JK. Fractional imputation in survey sampling: a comparative review. Stat Sci. 2016;31:415–32. https://doi.org/10.1214/16-STS569.
35. Lohr SL. Sampling: design and analysis. 3rd ed. Chapman and Hall/CRC; 2021.
36. Rosenbaum PR, Rubin DB. The central role of the propensity score in observational studies for causal effects. Biometrika. 1983;70:41–55. https://doi.org/10.1093/BIOMET/70.1.41.
37. Umberto B, Head SJ, Angelini GD, Blackstone EH. Statistical primer: propensity score matching and its alternatives. Eur J Cardio-Thorac Surg. 2018;53:1112–7. https://doi.org/10.1093/ejcts/ezy167.
38. Zlotta AR, Ballas LK, Niemierko A, et al. Radical cystectomy versus trimodality therapy for muscle-invasive bladder cancer: a multi-institutional propensity score matched and weighted analysis. Lancet Oncol. 2023;24:669–81. https://doi.org/10.1016/S1470-2045(23)00170-5.
39. Imai K, Van Dyk DA. Causal inference with general treatment regimes. J Am Stat Assoc. 2004;99:854–66. https://doi.org/10.1198/016214504000001187.

40. Tchernis R, Horvitz-Lennon M, Normand SLT. On the use of discrete choice models for causal inference. Stat Med. 2005;24:2197–212. https://doi.org/10.1002/SIM.2095.
41. Zhu Y, Coffman DL, Ghosh D. A boosting algorithm for estimating generalized propensity scores with continuous treatments. J Causal Inference. 2015;3:25–40. https://doi.org/10.1515/JCI-2014-0022.
42. Dong N, Stuart EA, Lenis D, Quynh Nguyen T. Using propensity score analysis of survey data to estimate population average treatment effects: a case study comparing different methods. Eval Rev. 2020;44:84–108. https://doi.org/10.1177/0193841X20938497.
43. Austin PC, Jembere N, Chiu M. Propensity score matching and complex surveys. Stat Methods Med Res. 2018;27:1240–57. https://doi.org/10.1177/0962280216658920/ASSET/IMAGES/LARGE/10.1177_0962280216658920-FIG10.JPEG.
44. Giffin A, Reich BJ, Yang S, Rappold AG. Generalized propensity score approach to causal inference with spatial interference. Biometrics. 2023;79:2220–31. https://doi.org/10.1111/BIOM.13745.
45. Si Y, Little R, Mo Y, Sedransk N. Nonresponse bias analysis in longitudinal studies: a comparative review with an application to the early childhood longitudinal study. Int Stat Rev. 2024;92:383–405. https://doi.org/10.1111/insr.12566.
46. Elliott MR, Valliant R. Inference for nonprobability samples. Stat Sci. 2017;32:249–64. https://doi.org/10.1214/16-STS598.
47. Rubin DB. Inference and missing data. Biometrika. 1976;63:581–92. https://doi.org/10.1093/BIOMET/63.3.581.
48. Wu C. Statistical inference with non-probability survey samples. Surv Methodol. 2022;48:283–311.
49. Si Y. On the use of auxiliary variables in multilevel regression and Poststratification. ar XivPrepr. 2022:arXiv201100360.
50. Li K, Si Y. Embedded multilevel regression and poststratification: model-based inference with incomplete auxiliary information. Stat Med. 2024;43:256–78. https://doi.org/10.1002/SIM.9956.
51. Cole SR, Stuart EA. Generalizing evidence from randomized clinical trials to target populations: the ACTG 320 trial. Am J Epidemiol. 2010;172:107–15. https://doi.org/10.1093/AJE/KWQ084.
52. Degtiar I, Rose S. A review of generalizability and transportability. Annu Rev Stat Its Appl. 2023;10:501–24. https://doi.org/10.1146/ANNUREV-STATISTICS-042522-103837/CITE/REFWORKS.
53. Paddock SM, Franco C, Breidt FJ, Betancourt B. Statistical data integration for health policy evidence-building. Annu Rev Stat Its Appl. 2024;12 https://doi.org/10.1146/ANNUREV-STATISTICS-112723-034507.
54. Elliott MR, Carroll O, Grieve R, Carpenter J. Improving transportability of randomized controlled trial inference using robust prediction methods. Stat Methods Med Res. 2023;32:2365–85. https://doi.org/10.1177/09622802231210944.
55. Smeeding T, Johnson D, Citro C. Creating an integrated system of data and statistics on household income, consumption, and wealth: time to build. National Academies Press; 2024.
56. Rius C, Liu Y, Sixto-Costoya A, et al. State of open science in cancer research. Clin Transl Oncol. 2024;26:2457–65. https://doi.org/10.1007/S12094-024-03468-7.
57. Nilbert M. Turning the page on 2024—embracing Open Science. Acta Oncol (Madr). 2024;63:25815. https://doi.org/10.2340/1651-226X.2024.25815.
58. Bhinder B, Gilvary C, Madhukar NS, Elemento O. Artificial intelligence in cancer research and precision medicine. Cancer Discov. 2021;11:900–15. https://doi.org/10.1158/2159-8290.CD-21-0090.
59. Boehm KM, Khosravi P, Vanguri R, et al. Harnessing multimodal data integration to advance precision oncology. Nat Rev Cancer. 2021;22:114–26. https://doi.org/10.1038/s41568-021-00408-3.
60. Zhang B, Shi H, Wang H. Machine learning and AI in cancer prognosis, prediction, and treatment selection: a critical approach. J Multidiscip Healthc. 2023;16:1779–91. https://doi.org/10.2147/JMDH.S410301.

Statistical Methods in Epidemiology

10

Christian A. Maino Vieytes

Introduction

Epidemiology as a Population Science

As a broad discipline, epidemiology sits at the crossroads of several fields, including the biomedical and biological sciences, bioinformatics, sociology, economics, demography, geography, biostatistics, and countless others. Nevertheless, *epidemiology* is unique in its stated intent, which is that it strives to understand the distribution and determinants of health-related events or outcomes in populations [1, 2]. Epidemiological practice has deep implications for understanding and promoting population health. It also plays an important role in shaping public health decisions at all levels of public administration. Within the field of cancer research, epidemiology is central to understanding the distributions of certain cancers and disproportionate burdens of cancer experienced by certain populations; identifying risk factors for cancer; and assessing the efficacy of novel interventions, treatments, and policies for their potential to curb cancer incidence, mortality, and other cancer-related outcomes.

Two major dimensions of epidemiological research include *descriptive epidemiology*, which is tasked with describing the distribution or burden of disease or health-related event (i.e., answering questions such as: "Who is affected by disease?" "When were they affected by disease?" "Where were they affected by disease?"), and *analytical epidemiology*, which is concerned with identifying causes and risk factors of a disease or health-related event (e.g., does factor X cause disease Y?) [3]. Often, a repertoire of statistical tools and expertise in their use is required to gauge research questions in either of these pillars of epidemiology. Indeed, being able to conduct *statistical analysis* and interpret results and findings encompasses two central responsibilities of an epidemiologist, which add to their subject-matter expertise and engagement in other activities such as planning and implementing study designs, engaging in data management and surveillance, developing and implementing interventions and programs, liaising with policymakers and the public through varied mediums of communication, among others [4].

A Cautionary Note on Causality

As noted, a cornerstone of epidemiology is the delineation of determinants, or causes, of health-related events. Regression and other statistical techniques are regularly adopted by epidemiologists to this end, although sometimes irresponsibly. The models routinely employed by epidemiologists to address research questions are *probabilistic*, while the models required to make claims with absolute certainty would be *deterministic*. All estimated model parameters bear a certain degree of uncertainty. Indeed, quantifying uncertainty is a critical objective in statistics. To make authoritative claims about causes, several assumptions must be adjudicated. Chiefly among these are the assumptions that there is no measurement error in the dependent or independent variables, that there is no unmeasured *confounding* of the relationship between *X* and *Y*, and that all relevant variables are included and their causal progression known (i.e., *correct model specification*) [5–7]. A field dedicated to exploring causal relationships using probabilistic models (i.e., the field of *causal inference*) has grown over the preceding decades but will not be covered in this chapter [5, 7, 8]. Despite the clear advances in model-based approaches for delineating causal effects, it is noteworthy that these methods will be valid to the extent that the data they harness are free from bias introduced during the collection process. Therefore, it becomes prudent and customarily necessary to exercise caution in making causal statements from relationships or associations borne of the data. Nevertheless, certain criteria, such as the Bradford-Hill framework, may help guide judging the

C. A. M. Vieytes (✉)
DC Health, Washington, DC, USA

J. Huang, H. S.L. Jim (eds.), *Cancer Research Guidance for Clinicians and Researchers*,
https://doi.org/10.1007/978-3-032-19175-5_10

causal extent of a posited epidemiological relationship [9]. Generally, the consistency of an association (i.e., the reproducibility and replication of an observed result) across different studies, samples, and time is an appropriate barometer for broaching the subject of causality [10].

Statistical Software

Epidemiologists and statisticians rely on statistical software to perform data management, analysis, and related computations. The need for modern and flexible software that remains caught up to the rapid advances in statistical theory and practice, particularly in the era of big data and machine learning, is patent. Commercial software such as SAS, SPSS, and Stata are popular options and require annual and renewable licenses for operation. R is a free open-source programming language and statistical software that provides a vast ecosystem of collaborative and user-developed packages and libraries and an enthusiastic community of users that facilitate the implementation of complex statistical techniques and models [11]. R is typically interfaced through RStudio, an *integrated development environment* (IDE), which yields a user-friendly interface and that provides a bounty of auxiliary tools such as R Shiny, for web application/dashboard development; R Markdown, for creating dynamic documents that combine R code with narrative text; and several others [11]. Furthermore, it provides a user-friendly interface to version-control systems such as Git and GitHub, which are becoming exceedingly common and indispensable in the face of increasing efforts to bolster reproducibility in science and epidemiology [12–14]. This chapter will provide reproducible examples using R to motivate study and practice and to highlight theoretical concepts.

Linear Regression

Statistics in Epidemiology and Basic Terminology

Implementing modern statistical theory within epidemiological practice is central to the stated goals of epidemiology, which focus on uncovering and making inferences about population-level phenomena. The essential framework of harnessing *samples* and conducting inference on those samples to draw conclusions about *populations*, a concept fundamental to the field of statistics, is ubiquitous in epidemiology. It is impractical, and not to mention nearly impossible, to collect data on every individual in a population for surveillance and analysis. Hence, we rely on practical and representative samples (e.g., patients, study participants, drug recipients, etc.) to conduct our inference. As epidemiologists, we seek to quantify or deduce patterns in population *parameters* (i.e., quantifiable population characteristics that are unknown) using data collected from samples, which are then used to generate *estimates* of those parameters using the sample data. The discernible patterns alluded to are often referred to as *associations*.[1]

Simple Linear Regression

We harness the rudimentary, yet powerful, example of *simple linear regression* (SLR) to highlight key statistical terminology and notation frequently encountered in this chapter:

$$E(Y|X) = \beta_0 + \beta_1 X + \epsilon \quad where \quad \epsilon \sim NIID\left(0, \sigma^2\right) \quad (10.1)$$

Equation 10.1 is the SLR model widely implemented across disciplines for examining the bivariate relationship between an *independent variable*, *X*, and a *dependent variable*, *Y*. Epidemiologists may opt for alternative vocabulary to refer to these terms. For instance, *exposure*, *treatment*, or *predictor* may be used to describe *X*, and *outcome* or *response* may be used to describe *Y*. Moreover, *X* and *Y* are assumed to be *continuous*, i.e., numeric variables that are not constrained and lie on the real number line. The left-hand side of the equation, $E(Y|X)$, denotes the conditional expectation, or mean, of the response, *Y*, given *X*, which is a function of the sum of a fixed population parameter; β_0, colloquially referred to as "the intercept," another fixed population parameter; and β_1, colloquially referred to as "the slope," multiplied by the value of *X*. ϵ is an error term that allows random error to be introduced (i.e., it suggests the relationship between *X* and *Y* is not perfectly described by β_0 and β_1 alone). ϵ is assumed to be *normally*, *identically*, and *independently distributed* (NIID) with mean 0 and variance, σ^2, another population parameter of interest. By normally, identically, and independently distributed, we mean that the random error values, ϵ, are all independent draws from the same probability distribution, assumed to be a normal distribution with mean 0 and a variance that will be estimated from the data. Note that, by convention, Greek letters are used to symbolize parameters while English alphabet letters are used to symbolize variables. The error term, ϵ, can also be understood as the variation in the response, *Y*, which is not captured by *the model* (i.e., the parts of Equation 10.1 we estimate: β_0 and β_1), as is conveyed by Equation 10.2):

$$\epsilon = E(Y|X) - (\beta_0 + \beta_1 X) \quad (10.2)$$

[1]This chapter will not cover techniques or principles of sampling, increasingly germane topics which are integral to study design and to the collection of data that leads to unbiased estimates of epidemiological *measures of association*. For further reading, we refer the reader to the work by Thompson [15] and others.

The SLR model in Equation 10.1 is only theoretical, given that epidemiologists work with data collected from samples derived from populations. Consequently, the parameters β_0, β_1, and σ^2 must be estimated, and we can apply an SLR to the data on hand, as expressed in Equation 10.3:

$$\hat{y}_i = \hat{\beta}_0 + \hat{\beta}_1 x_i + \hat{\epsilon_i}, \quad where \quad \hat{\epsilon_i} \sim NIID\left(0, \hat{\sigma}^2\right) \quad (10.3)$$

In this notation, we also introduce the subscript i, which represents an observation, participant, or unit of analysis in the population under study. If we were to consider the example of a clinical trial for a novel cancer therapeutic, i could refer to, for instance, a study participant. Note that the "hat" symbol, ^, indicates estimates of parameters and variables. Therefore, the coefficients $\hat{\beta}_0$ and $\hat{\beta}_1$ are sample-based estimates of the regression parameters, and x_i represents the realized, or observed, value of the random variable X for the ith observation. $\hat{y}_i$ is the regression estimate of the random variable Y for the ith observation, and $\hat{\epsilon_i}$ is an estimate of the error term, again specific to the ith observation, which accounts for random variation. We generally use capital letters to represent random variables and lowercase letters to represent their realizations in data.

The coefficient, β_1, is an epidemiological measure of association that describes the relationship between X and Y. Its interpretation follows that β_1 is the expected change in Y when considering a one-unit increase in X (Equation 10.4):

$$\beta_1 = Y_{X=1} - Y_{X=0} \quad (10.4)$$

Assuming that X is continuous, $Y_{X=1}$ is the value of Y when $X = 1$ and $Y_{X=0}$ is the value of Y when $X = 0$. The difference, therefore, is the expected rate of change in Y when X increases by 1.

Multiple Linear Regression

"Adjusted" estimates of the coefficients that account for *confounding variables* are estimated with the multiple regression model (MLR), which introduces additional coefficient-variable pairs to the SLR model in an additive fashion (Equation 10.5):

$$\hat{y}_i = \hat{\beta}_0 + \hat{\beta}_1 x_{1i} + \hat{\beta}_2 x_{2i} + \ldots + \hat{\beta}_p x_{pi} + \hat{\sigma_i},$$
$$where \quad \hat{\sigma_i} \sim NIID\left(0, \hat{\sigma}^2\right) \quad (10.5)$$

This notation introduces an additional subscript that denotes the variable index (i.e., 1, 2,…, p), which is essential when we have multiple variables we want to include in the model. If we assign x_1 as the independent variable of analytic interest and the remaining $p - 1$ variables as the "confounders"—or additional *covariates* we are adjusting for, then $\hat{\beta}_1$ is the adjusted regression coefficient, or epidemiological measure of association of interest between X_1 and Y. Any substantial change in the value of $\hat{\beta}_1$ from the SLR to the MLR is suggestive of possible confounding by any of the other variables included in the MLR that were not in the SLR [16]. The fundamental principles and concepts in linear regression that we introduced herein will reappear as we introduce logistic and Poisson regression in subsequent sections.

Estimation

Model specification refers to the declaration of a model that is apt for invoking the epidemiological research question. It involves assigning and indicating the response and exposure variables, covariates, and the parameters to be estimated. The process of estimating the values of the model parameters (e.g., $\hat{\beta}_0$ and $\hat{\beta}_1$) is termed *estimation* and typically requires numerical algorithms that are beyond the scope of what this chapter is meant to cover [17]. *Maximum likelihood estimation* (MLE) is a method of estimation implemented frequently in regression contexts. The likelihood is defined as how probable the observed data are given the values of the parameters in the model [5]. When we assume a particular probability distribution (e.g., that the response follows a normal distribution) in a regression model, we use the function of that probability distribution to derive the *likelihood function*. Because there is no closed-form solution (i.e., an exact equation) to this mathematical problem, we rely on calculus and algebraic methods to find the values of the parameters that maximize the likelihood function. All these computations are carried out by statistical software, and nothing more than a conceptual understanding of MLE is required to fit statistical models with it.

Expressing Uncertainty

The *confidence interval* is a tool for capturing the uncertainty associated with a parameter estimate or measure of association. Conventionally, the 95% confidence interval is used to express this uncertainty. In the setting of SLR, 95% confidence intervals are computed for the estimated parameters (β_0 and β_1). Consider a 95% confidence interval for β_1 with lower bound z_l and upper bound z_u. From this, the researcher concludes with 95% confidence that the true population value of β_1 lies within the interval $[z_l, z_u]$, in the sense that with repeated sampling, they would expect 95% of confidence intervals to include the true β_1. Equations for 95% confidence intervals abound, and we refrain from providing exact equations. Depending on the method of estimation used (e.g., the method of least squares or MLE for SLR), we employ alternate closed forms of the 95% confidence intervals (e.g., the Wald confidence interval). In a practical setting, we employ statistical software to compute these intervals.

Discrete Data Models

Introduction

Discrete, or countably finite, data types abound in the biomedical sciences and epidemiology. In the setting of cancer research, such data may manifest as variables measuring whether or not a study participant received a candidate drug or the placebo in a clinical trial, for which we would say that variable is *binary* or *dichotomous* (i.e., consisting of only two levels), or the integer frequency of individuals in a census block diagnosed with lung cancer over a specified time interval, for which we would say that variable is a count variable. Other forms of discrete data include *nominal* variables, which are categorical variables that do not have an inherent order or ranking, and *ordinal* variables, categorical variables that, in contrast, do have an intrinsic order. This section will focus on modeling approaches for binary and count data, which are data types repeatedly encountered by epidemiologists in practice.

Binary Data and Binary Probability Models

We begin by evaluating the case of a binary random variable that assumes one of two possible values (i.e., "Yes"/"No" or 1/0). In our example, we will use data from the Ohsaki National Health Insurance (NHI) study analysis by Li et al. that examined the relationship between green tea consumption and lung cancer risk [18]. The NHI was a prospective longitudinal cohort study of over 52,000 beneficiaries aged 40–79 from the Miyagi Prefecture of Japan, which collected robust lifestyle and medical history data [19]. The goal of epidemiological analysis in this scenario, and in many scenarios involving binary data, was to generate probability estimates of the response, in this case lung cancer, and to understand whether that probability is modified by the exposure, daily green tea consumption. Again, we underscore the fact that the models we work with are probabilistic, as the risk of any individual from the target population developing lung cancer cannot be determined with absolute certainty. The crude incidence data (taken from the manuscript we cite here [18]) are presented in the two-by-two table below.

Cancer status			
Daily green tea consumption	Lung cancer	No lung cancer	Total
0–2 cups	127	19,806	19,933
≥ 3 cups	175	21,332	21,507
Total	302	41,138	41,440

These data summarize the cumulative incidence of lung cancer within the study sample between the study's initiation in 1994 through the end of the follow-up period in 2001. There are several *binary probability models* or epidemiological measures of association that we could compute with these data. We begin with the *relative risk* (RR), which can be defined as the ratio of risk (i.e., the probability of having the outcome of interest, e.g., lung cancer) in the exposed group to the risk in the nonexposed group. For this example, we arbitrarily assign the ≥ 3 cups of green tea group as the "exposed" group, although it is inconsequential and only pertains to the assignment of numerators and denominators in our model construction. In subsequent equations, the risk, or probability, of the response, incident lung cancer, is denoted by π:

$$RR = \frac{\pi_{exposed}}{\pi_{non-exposed}} = \frac{\pi_{\geq 3 Cups}}{\pi_{0-2 Cups}} = \frac{\frac{175}{175+21332}}{\frac{127}{127+19806}} = 1.277$$

The interpretation that follows is that the risk, or probability, of lung cancer in those consuming ≥ 3 cups of green tea daily is 1.277 times greater than that of individuals consuming 0–2 cups daily. Had this measure of association been equal to 1, we would have concluded that there is no relationship between green tea consumption and lung cancer, and had it been less than 1, we would have concluded that those drinking more green tea have a lower risk of lung cancer compared to those drinking less of it. An alternative conceptualization of event risk is the *odds*, the ratio of the probability of an event occurring to the probability of it not occurring (Equation 10.6), which we denote Ω [20]:

$$\Omega = \frac{\pi}{1-\pi} \tag{10.6}$$

We would find the odds of lung cancer in those drinking ≥ 3 cups of green tea daily is

$$\Omega_{\geq 3 Cups} = \frac{\frac{175}{175+21332}}{\frac{21332}{175+21332}} = \frac{175}{21332} = 0.0082$$

One interpretation of this estimate could be that, among individuals in the target population drinking ≥ 3 cups of green tea daily, we expect there to be 175 individuals diagnosed with lung cancer for every 21,332 individuals in this group that are lung cancer-free. Therefore, the odds of at-risk individuals (i.e., those individuals in the ≥ 3 cups exposure category) being affected by lung cancer could be considered small. Despite the small absolute odds of lung cancer in this group, the measure of association that is of greater interest to epidemiologists is the odds ratio (OR), which is the ratio of the odds of an event within an exposure category to the odds in another level of the exposure. In our example, we would compute the following odds ratio:

$$OR = \frac{\Omega_{exposed}}{\Omega_{non-exposed}} = \frac{\Omega_{\geq 3Cups}}{\Omega_{0-2Cups}} = \frac{\left(\dfrac{\frac{175}{175+21332}}{\frac{21332}{175+21332}}\right)}{\left(\dfrac{\frac{127}{127+19806}}{\frac{19806}{127+19806}}\right)} = \frac{\frac{175}{21332}}{\frac{127}{19806}}$$

$$= 1.279$$

We conclude that the odds of incident lung cancer in those consuming ≥ 3 cups of green tea daily are 1.279 times greater than those of individuals consuming 0–2 cups daily. It is noteworthy that the computed OR approximated the RR in this example. However, this is a common phenomenon that tends to occur when the absolute risk of the event in question is exceedingly small, but it will not hold in all cases [5].

Introducing Binary Logistic Regression

The odds ratio introduced previously is regarded as the *crude* or *unadjusted* odds ratio because it does not account for extraneous sources of variation (i.e., other variables) that may have distorted or *confounded* the relationship between the exposure and the response. For a more nuanced analysis, we look at the tools afforded by regression. Adjusted odds ratios can be estimated with *logistic regression* models. In these models, the binary response variable will be coded using "1" or "0." For instance, study participants with lung cancer, from our example, would have a 1 for their value of the response variable, while the subjects without lung cancer would be coded as 0.

Generalized Linear Models

The linear regression model in Equation 10.1 belongs to a larger family of *generalized linear models* (GLMs) that extend the linear regression model to cases where the response variable is not necessarily continuous or does not follow a normal distribution. In the setting of a binary response, it would be inappropriate to use a normal distribution to model a response that takes only the values 1 or 0. Instead, our goal is to model the probability, π, of the outcome, Y, given the exposure, X (Equation 10.7):

$$\mu = \pi = \Pr\left(Y = 1 | X = x\right) \qquad (10.7)$$

Thus, an alternative distribution must be specified. A GLM takes the following broad form (Equation 10.8):

$$g\left(\mu\right) = \beta_0 + \beta_1 X_1 + \beta_2 X_2 + \ldots + \beta_p X_p \qquad (10.8)$$

$$where\ \mu = E\left[Y | X\right] and\ p = total\ no.of\ variables$$

g is what we term the *link function*, which essentially allows the expected value of the response given the exposure, $E[Y | X]$, to be "linked" to a linear model expressed on the right-hand side of the equation, which is like what we encountered in linear regression. Assuming X_1 is the independent variable of analytic interest, we can "control" for other confounding variables by including them in the linear model (i.e., these are the variables X_2 to X_p). Generally, there are two important preemptive steps for implementing a GLM:

1. *Select a distribution*[2] *to model the response*—This is used to formulate the likelihood function for estimating the model parameters.
2. *Select a link function*—Note that in the special case of linear regression, the distribution we choose is the normal distribution, and the link function is the identity function, where $g(E[Y \mid X]) = E[Y \mid X]$.

Logistic Regression as a GLM

For modeling a binary response variable, we could specify a *Bernoulli distribution* (a special case of the binomial distribution) and the *logit* link function (depicted generally in Equation 10.9 and specific to logistic regression in Equation 10.10):

$$logit\left(x\right) = \log\left(\frac{x}{1-x}\right) \qquad (10.9)$$

$$logit\left(\pi\right) = \log\left(\frac{\pi}{1-\pi}\right), \quad where\ \pi = \Pr\left(Y = 1 | X = x\right) \qquad (10.10)$$

[2] The family of distributions at our disposal for use in GLMs is the *exponential family*. For further reading, see Dobson and Barnett [17].

If π is the probability of the outcome given some value of the exposure, then the rational expression, $\frac{\pi}{1-\pi}$ should appear familiar since it is the equation for the odds, which we introduced in Equation 10.6. Note that if π = 1, then $logit(\pi) \rightarrow \infty$ and if π = 0, then $logit(\pi) \rightarrow -\infty$, which highlights how the link function abrogates the dilemma of modeling a response that is naturally bounded above at 1 and below at 0. Putting it all together, we present the logistic regression model in Equation [11]:

$$logit(\pi) = \log\left(\frac{\pi}{1-\pi}\right) = \beta_0 + \beta_1 X_1 + \beta_2 X_2 + \ldots + \beta_1 X_p \tag{10.11}$$

With this model of the log odds, computing a study participant's estimated probability of the response ($\hat{\neq}_i$), e.g., their probability of having lung cancer given the values of their covariates becomes easily attainable. We could also use it to predict this probability, with caution, for an individual outside the study sample, but within the same population. After performing some algebraic rearrangement[3] to Equation 10.11 and substituting parameter estimates for parameters, we have:

$$\hat{\pi}_i = \frac{\exp\left(\hat{\beta}_0 + \hat{\beta}_1 x_1 + \hat{\beta}_2 x_2 + \ldots + \hat{\beta}_p x_p\right)}{1 + \exp\left(\hat{\beta}_0 + \hat{\beta}_1 x_1 + \hat{\beta}_2 x_2 + \ldots + \hat{\beta}_p x_p\right)}$$

Interpretation of β as an Odds Ratio in the Logistic Regression Model

Beyond predicting a subject's probability of a binary outcome, the logistic regression model also provides information, encoded in the model's parameters, about the relationship between the exposure, *X*, and the outcome, *Y*, in the population under study. If we were to fit a logistic regression model with X_1 as the only predictor on the right-hand side of the equation, we would essentially compute the unadjusted odds ratio we defined earlier (based on the method we describe below). In contrast, fitting a logistic regression model that adjusts for multiple confounding variables allows us to estimate the *adjusted odds ratio*. The question of how we obtain the odds ratio from the logistic model is deduced from some algebraic rearranging of Equation 10.12.

Assume we are interested in computing an unadjusted odds ratio and are interested in assessing the relationship of a continuous variable, X_1, to some binary disease outcome (i.e., disease present/disease not present). To do so, we could fit the following simple logistic regression model:

[3]Note: exp *x* = *ex*, where *e* is Euler's number: 2.71828…

$$\log\left(\frac{\pi}{1-\pi}\right) = \beta_0 + \beta_1 X_1 \tag{10.12}$$

Recall that in linear regression, β_1 would be interpreted as the change in *Y* that would be expected for a unit increase in X_1. However, in this new scenario, the interpretation of β_1 would change to that of the expected change in the log odds for a unit increase in X_1. This interpretation can be expressed as follows:

$$\beta_1 = \log\left(\frac{\pi}{1-\pi}\right)_{X_1=1} - \log\left(\frac{\pi}{1-\pi}\right)_{X_1=0}$$

However, interpreting the log odds is not practical, and the interpretation is muddled. Thus, we exponentiate the previous expression:

$$\exp(\beta_1) = \exp\left(\log\left(\frac{\pi}{1-\pi}\right)_{X_1=1} - \log\left(\frac{\pi}{1-\pi}\right)_{X_1=0}\right)$$
$$= \frac{\left(\frac{\pi}{1-\pi}\right)_{X_1=1}}{\left(\frac{\pi}{1-\pi}\right)_{X_1=0}} = \frac{\Omega_{X_1=1}}{\Omega_{X_1=0}}$$

Therefore, we find that the exponent of the coefficient, β_1, is interpreted as the odds ratio associated with a one-unit increase in the independent variable, X_1, when X_1 is a continuous variable. However, if X_1 is a categorical variable, then the exponent of the coefficient β_1 is the ratio of the odds ratio for some level of X_1 to the odds ratio for the level of X_1 that is set as the *referent*:

$$\exp(\beta_1) = \exp\left(\log\left(\frac{\pi}{1-\pi}\right)_{X_{1_k}} - \log\left(\frac{\pi}{1-\pi}\right)_{X_{1_{ref}}}\right)$$
$$= \frac{\left(\frac{\pi}{1-\pi}\right)_{X_{1_k}}}{\left(\frac{\pi}{1-\pi}\right)_{X_{1_{ref}}}} = \frac{\Omega_{X_{1_k}}}{\Omega_{X_{1_{ref}}}} \tag{10.13}$$

In Equation 10.13, X_{1_k} is some level of X_1, which we can say has *K* levels and *k* represents one of those levels. $X_{1_{ref}}$ is the level of X_1 that is arbitrarily set as the referent.

Count Data

Another, often-encountered, data type in epidemiological practice is the count variable. At the individual level, count variables can include the whole number of visits a cancer patient had during a specified period, the whole number of drugs a patient is currently taking, or the number of claims filed for a specific procedure at a clinic. However, count data are especially common when dealing with *data aggregation*, whereby micro-level, e.g., individual-level, data are aggregated, or combined (i.e., through some real number operation such as the sum, mean, or median), to a higher, macro-level unit of analysis. For instance, the self-identified race of an individual can be aggregated to their neighborhood of residence, whereby race becomes an aggregate count (i.e., a sum) of individuals in that neighborhood belonging to each of the race classifications. Often, we aggregate variables to spatial units (e.g., neighborhood, census blocks or tracts, counties, or states, etc.), time periods (e.g., 2024 or March 2023, etc.), or events (e.g., pre-COVID-19/post-COVID-19). These data types may be encountered, for instance, by exposure epidemiologists investigating environmental exposures and their relationships to cancer incidence and other outcomes.

We employ the *Poisson distribution*, which can also be derived from the binomial distribution, to model count data [21]. A Poisson random variable, Y, can be defined as one that counts the number of occurrences of a phenomenon during a specific period of study or time and is contained in the set of natural numbers (i.e., $N \in 0, 1, 2, \ldots$). Poisson regression is, therefore, a method for assessing the relationships between a set of covariates, $x_1, x_2, \ldots, x_p$, to the Poisson random variable, Y. Like logistic regression, it belongs to the family of GLMs. The Poisson regression model is expressed as follows in Equation 10.14:

$$E[Y|X] = \exp\left(\beta_0 + \beta_1 X_1 + \beta_2 X_2 + \ldots + \beta_p X_p\right) \quad (10.14)$$

To change Equation 10.14 to the more familiar regression form in Equation 10.8, we take the logarithm of both sides:

$$\log\left(E[Y|X]\right) = \beta_0 + \beta_1 X_1 + \beta_2 X_2 + \ldots + \beta_p X_p \quad (10.15)$$

Thus, it is easier to identify that the link function is the logarithmic function (which is also why you may see this model referred to as the *log-linear model* in other texts), and the distribution is the Poisson distribution, which has a single parameter, λ, which is defined as the average number of occurrences. Notably, this λ can be substituted into Equations 10.14 and 10.15:

$$let\ E[Y|X] = \lambda$$

$$\log(\lambda) = \beta_0 + \beta_1 X_1 + \beta_2 X_2 + \ldots + \beta_p X_p$$

Therefore, the interpretation of β_1 is expressed as the change in $log(\lambda)$ associated with a one-unit increase in the independent variable, X_1. Similar to the issues arising from interpreting the log-odds in logistic regression, the log of λ is not particularly meaningful to the epidemiologist. Consequently, we exponentiate it to provide an intelligible conclusion:

$$\beta_1 = \log(\lambda)_{X_1=1} - \log(\lambda)_{X_1=0}$$

$$\exp(\beta_1) = \frac{\lambda_{X_1=1}}{\lambda_{X_1=0}}$$

Likewise, in the case of categorical independent variables, we can get the ratio of λ for a level of a categorical independent variable relative to some referent category:

$$\exp(\beta_1) = \frac{\lambda_{X_{1_k}}}{\lambda_{X_{1_{ref}}}}$$

The Issue of Overdispersion

In practice, we often experience an issue with the Poisson regression model. That is, the outcome variable is *overdispersed*, or the variance in the response variable is greater than what is expected. One of the key assumptions of the Poisson regression model is that the mean of the random variable Y is also equal to the variance of Y. The negative binomial distribution provides a solution to this issue by introducing an additional parameter that accounts for the overdispersion. We refer the readers to other texts for greater detail on the negative binomial distribution [21]. Nevertheless, the use of the negative binomial regression model and the interpretation of its parameters proceed similarly to that of the Poisson regression model.

Mortality Metrics

Another motivating objective in epidemiology is to understand patterns of mortality, and methods for estimating the extent of mortality are therefore of interest to epidemiologists for guiding policy recommendations, allocation of resources, and to identify areas where treatment advances are urgently needed. We will introduce two metrics of mortality in this section to showcase how Poisson regression is used to model them in a regression context, where we may have datasets with many rows (i.e., observations) and many columns (i.e., variables). The first metric we introduce is the *crude mortality rate* (CMR), which is expressed in Equation 10.16 and reflects the number of deaths, among all causes or for a given cause, among individuals in a population:

$$CMR = 10^r \frac{No. Deaths\ in\ Population\ During\ Some\ Time\ Interval}{Midinterval\ Population} \quad (10.16)$$

The CMR is often expressed in terms of 1,000, 10,000, or 100,000 persons. For instance, if disease Z caused 643 deaths in 2024 among the population of county U (with a midyear population size of 987,541 persons), then we could express the CMR (per 10,000 persons—i.e., $r = 4$) as follows:

$$CMR_Z = 10^4 \frac{643}{987,541} = 6.51\, deaths\ per\ 10,000\ persons$$

Another commonly referenced mortality metric is the standardized mortality ratio (SMR), which, unlike the CMR, does not provide information about the rate of mortality but, rather, the ratio of deaths to the number of deaths that would be otherwise expected based on some reference population:

$$SMR = 10^r \frac{\begin{array}{c}No.Deaths\ in\ Population\\ During\ Some\ Time\ Interval\end{array}}{\begin{array}{c}No.Deaths\ Expected\ in\ that\ Population\\ During\ the\ Same\ Time\ Interval\end{array}}$$

Therefore, the SMR can be interpreted by its value relative to 1. If the SMR > 1, then the number of deaths in that population exceeded what was expected. Accordingly, if the SMR < 1, the number of deaths was less than what was expected, and if the SMR = 1, then the number of deaths was exactly what was expected. Biting off the same example we painted for the CMR, we could add that we know that the national crude mortality rate of disease Z is 7.86 deaths per 10,000 persons. Using this datum, we can compute the expected deaths and SMR of disease Z for county U:

$$\mathrm{Exp}.\ Deaths = \left(\frac{7.86\, deaths}{10,000\, persons}\right)(987,541) = 776.2\, deaths$$

$$SMR = \frac{643\, deaths}{776.2\, expected\ deaths} = 0.83$$

Consequently, we conclude that the deaths due to disease Z in county U are 17% lower than what would be expected based on the national figure.

Modeling Mortality with Poisson Regression and the Offset Term

The mortality metrics we introduced above can be modeled with Poisson or negative binomial regression. To do so, the *offset term* is introduced, which is represented by $log(c)$ in the following form:

$$\log(\lambda) = \beta_0 + \beta_1 X_1 + \log(c) \qquad (10.17)$$

From this representation, it is intuitive that there is no parameter to be estimated for the offset term; it modifies the likelihood function (not shown here) used to arrive at estimates of the model parameters. Let us assume the response variable is the number of cancer deaths in a county. Therefore, λ represents the average number of cancer deaths in a county. In this case, c would be another variable with the same units as λ. To model the mortality rate (see Equation 10.16 above) as an outcome, we could specify c as the county population. Rearranging Equation 10.17 using some algebra, we can derive the mortality rate:

$$\log(\lambda) - \log(c) = \beta_0 + \beta_1 X_1$$

$$\log\left(\frac{\lambda}{c}\right) = \beta_0 + \beta_1 X_1$$

$$\frac{\lambda}{c} = \exp(\beta_0 + \beta_1 X_1) \qquad (10.18)$$

In Equation 10.18, $\frac{\lambda}{c}$ is the mortality rate, which is expressed as a function of the right-hand side of the equation. In this case, $exp(\beta_1)$ is interpreted as the change in the mortality rate $\frac{\lambda}{c}$ that coincides with a one-unit increase in X_1. If the desire, in contrast, was to model the SMR, we could specify c as the expected cancer death count, which could be computed for each county using the cancer mortality rate of a reference population.

Examples

A GitHub repository of R code with examples can be found at https://github.com/cmainov/epistats-examples (accessed 2026-02-16). Examples involving real-world data are provided.

References

1. A dictionary of epidemiology. Oxford University Press; 2008. https://doi.org/10.1093/acref/9780195314496.001.0001.
2. Gordis L. Epidemiology. 4th ed, [Nachdr.]. Saunders: Elsevier; 2009.
3. Mitra AK, ed. Statistical approaches for epidemiology: from concept to application. 1st ed. 2024. Springer. doi:https://doi.org/10.1007/978-3-031-41784-9
4. Samet JM, Woodward A. On Being an Epidemiologist. Am J Epidemiol. 2019;188(5):818–24. https://doi.org/10.1093/aje/kwy279.
5. Clayton D, Hills M. Statistical models in epidemiology. Oxford University Press; 2013.
6. Freedman D. From association to causation via regression. Adv Appl Math. 1997;18(1):59–110. https://doi.org/10.1006/aama.1996.0501.
7. Hernán M, Robins JM. Causal inference: what if. 1st edition. Taylor; Francis; 2023.
8. Robins JM, Hernán MA, Brumback B. Marginal structural models and causal inference in epidemiology. Epidemiology. 2000;11(5):550–60. https://doi.org/10.1097/00001648-200009000-00011.

9. Hill AB. The environment and disease: association or causation? J R Soc Med. 2015;108(1):32–7. https://doi.org/10.1177/0141076814562718.
10. Lash TL, Collin LJ, Van Dyke ME. The replication crisis in epidemiology: snowball, snow job, or winter solstice? Curr Epidemiol Rep. 2018;5(2):175–83. https://doi.org/10.1007/s40471-018-0148-x.
11. Gandrud C. Reproducible research with R and RStudio. 2nd ed. Chapman; Hall/CRC; 2018. doi:https://doi.org/10.1201/9781315382548.
12. Mathur MB, Fox MP. Toward open and reproducible epidemiology. Am J Epidemiol. 2023;192(4):658–64. https://doi.org/10.1093/aje/kwad007.
13. Wilson G, Aruliah DA, Brown CT, et al. Best Practices for Scientific Computing. Eisen JA, ed. PLoS Biol. 2014;12(1):e1001745. https://doi.org/10.1371/journal.pbio.1001745.
14. Hicks DJ. Open science, the replication crisis, and environmental public health. Account Res. 2023;30(1):34–62. https://doi.org/10.1080/08989621.2021.1962713.
15. Thompson SK. Sampling. 3rd ed. Wiley; 2012. https://doi.org/10.1002/9781118162934.
16. Kestenbaum B. Epidemiology and biostatistics: an introduction to clinical research. New York: Springer; 2009. https://doi.org/10.1007/978-0-387-88433-2.
17. Dobson AJ, Barnett AG. An introduction to generalized linear models. 4th ed. Chapman: Hall/CRC; 2018.
18. Li Q, Kakizaki M, Kuriyama S, et al. Green tea consumption and lung cancer risk: the Ohsaki study. Br J Cancer. 2008;99(7):1179–84. https://doi.org/10.1038/sj.bjc.6604645.
19. Tsuji I, Nishino Y, Ohkubo T, et al. A prospective cohort study on National Health Insurance beneficiaries in Ohsaki, Miyagi prefecture, Japan: study design, profiles of the subjects and medical cost during the first year. J Epidemiol. 1998;8(5):258–63. https://doi.org/10.2188/jea.8.258.
20. Katz KA. The (relative) risks of using odds ratios. Arch Dermatol. 2006;142(6):761–4. https://doi.org/10.1001/archderm.142.6.761.
21. Hilbe JM. Negative Binomial Regression. 2nd ed. Cambridge University Press; 2011.

Statistics of Randomized Clinical Trials

11

Tho Nguyen, Chang Liu, Liqiang Ni, and Rui Xie

Introduction

Randomized clinical trials (RCTs) are universally recognized as the preeminent methodology for evaluating the clinical efficacy of novel oncological interventions [1, 2]. The cornerstone of their methodological rigor lies in prospective randomization, where individuals are randomly assigned to different treatment groups (arms). This fundamental design principle prevents selection bias and ensures baseline comparability between groups, effectively controlling for both observed and unobserved prognostic factors. As a result, differences observed in outcomes can be robustly attributed to the tested interventions rather than to preexisting group differences [3]. By mitigating systematic bias and confounding variables, RCTs enable robust causal inference regarding treatment-specific effects, establishing them as the linchpin of evidence-based oncology. Moreover, the link between randomization and causal inference has been further strengthened through advanced statistical methodologies that address trial complexities, ensuring that RCT conclusions remain both internally valid and clinically relevant [3]. Consequently, findings from and well-designed RCTs are central to oncology: Regulatory approvals for new cancer treatments, the formulation of clinical practice guidelines, and the definition of standard-of-care protocols are all predominantly informed by the results of rigorously conducted RCTs [4]. The modern landscape of oncology continues to rely on this evidence hierarchy, with RCT results shaping decisions from drug approvals to patient care pathways and healthcare policy.

In oncological research, RCTs face distinct challenges that are not uniformly encountered in other clinical disciplines. A notable challenge pertains to the widespread utilization of time-to-event endpoints, such as overall survival (OS, the time from randomization until death from any cause), progression-free survival (PFS, the time from randomization until disease progression or death), disease-free survival (DFS, the time until recurrence of disease or death), and objective response rate (ORR, the proportion of patients with a predefined reduction in tumor burden), which differ fundamentally from the simpler endpoints often assessed in non-oncology trials [5]. OS is widely regarded as the most robust and clinically relevant outcome measure; however, it may require extensive follow-up durations due to time to cancer progression and mortality. Extended follow-up can exacerbate trial adherence challenges, increase trial costs, and delay the availability of crucial efficacy and safety information, hindering timely decisions on the approval and clinical use of new treatments [6]. Consequently, surrogate endpoints, including PFS, DFS, and ORR, are frequently utilized as earlier indicators of therapeutic benefit. Rigorous statistical validation of these surrogate endpoints continues to be an area of active research, given that their predictive validity may exhibit heterogeneity across distinct oncological subtypes and clinical contexts. The US Food and Drug Administration (FDA) and the European Medicines Agency (EMA) have issued guidelines to govern the application of surrogate endpoints within oncological RCTs, thereby aiming to find a balance the imperative for expediting patient access to promising therapies against the necessity of establishing clear, clinically relevant benefits to patient survival and quality of life [7, 8]. These rules try to find a balance between the need to get promising treatments to patients

Authors 'Tho Nguyen' and 'Chang Liu' have been equally contributed to this work.

T. Nguyen · R. Xie (✉)
School of Data, Mathematical, and Statistical Sciences, College of Sciences, University of Central Florida, Orlando, FL, USA

College of Nursing, University of Central Florida, Orlando, FL, USA
e-mail: tho.nguyen@ucf.edu; rui.xie@ucf.edu

C. Liu · L. Ni
School of Data, Mathematical, and Statistical Sciences, College of Sciences, University of Central Florida, Orlando, FL, USA
e-mail: ch786084@ucf.edu; liqiang.ni@ucf.edu

J. Huang, H. S.L. Jim (eds.), *Cancer Research Guidance for Clinicians and Researchers*,
https://doi.org/10.1007/978-3-032-19175-5_11

quickly and the need to show clear, clinically relevant benefits to patients' disease and survival outcomes.

Another methodological complexity in oncology RCTs arises from intercurrent events, which occur after treatment initiation and can complicate the interpretation of treatment effects. Common examples include treatment switching, dose modifications, early discontinuation due to toxicity, or the initiation of subsequent lines of therapy, all of which disrupt the pure comparison between randomized treatment arms and may obscure the true effect of the assigned intervention [9]. These intercurrent events pose substantial challenges, particularly for survival outcomes and other time-to-event endpoints, by affecting both the measurement and existence of outcome data. For instance, treatment switching can dilute the contrast between study arms, dose changes might alter post-randomization exposures, and discontinuations can lead to missing or censored data, all complicating straightforward causal interpretation. To address these challenges, the ICH E9(R1) Addendum [10, 11] provides a formal and structured framework that aligns the trial's objectives, design, and analytical strategies with the clinical questions of interest while explicitly accounting for intercurrent events. The estimand framework encourages careful prospective specification of how such events will be handled when defining the treatment effect, facilitating clarity and consistency in interpretation [11]. For example, in oncology trials, it may be critical to define whether the treatment effect estimation should consider outcomes only while on assigned therapy (a "while on treatment" strategy) or regardless of subsequent treatments received by patients (a "treatment policy" strategy). This distinction has direct implications for regulatory decisions, clinical guidelines, and personalized care, as it determines what precisely is being measured and influences how results apply to real-world clinical scenarios. Modern oncology RCTs are increasingly influenced by the evolving therapeutic landscapes, with innovations in immuno-oncology and targeted therapies often resulting in nonproportional hazards in survival outcomes. This shift challenges the applicability of traditional Cox proportional hazards model and has catalyzed the adoption of alternative statistical approaches, including restricted mean survival time (RMST) [12], weighted log-rank tests, and milestone survival analyses [13, 14], which offer more practical and interpretable summaries of treatment effects in settings where hazards are not constant over time. In parallel, there is continuous emphasis on rigorous reporting and transparency, reflecting the profound impact of oncology RCTs on clinical recommendations and patient care. The CONSORT 2025 update [15] strengthens reporting standards by promoting the explicit pre-specification of estimands, systematic handling of intercurrent events, and the prioritization of patient-centered outcomes. Coupled with established SPIRIT protocol guidelines [16], these advances foster reproducibility, facilitate critical appraisal, and ensure that research findings can be translated reliably into practice.

This chapter focuses specifically on the statistical principles and practices of RCTs in oncology. We review the foundations of randomization (Section "Randomization in Oncology Randomized Clinical Trials") and key oncology endpoints (Section "Endpoints in Oncology RCTs"), followed by a discussion of sample size planning for superiority, non-inferiority, and equivalence objectives (Section "Trial Designs in Cancer Randomized Clinical Trials"). The chapter further provides methodological guidance for the analysis of different types of endpoints and time-to-event outcomes (Section "Statistical Analysis of Oncology RCTs"), as well as discussing strategies for handling missing data and intercurrent events, and navigating multiplicity and subgroup analyses. In section "Interpreting and Critically Appraising RCT Results", we highlight current best practices in statistical reporting to ensure transparency, reproducibility, and relevance to clinical audiences. Throughout, real-world examples from landmark oncology RCTs are presented to illustrate these principles and demonstrate their significance in advancing cancer treatment and care. By navigating the interface of advanced statistical methods and oncological realities, this chapter equips researchers and clinicians with the tools and understanding necessary to design, analyze, and interpret RCTs that not only meet methodological standards but also meaningfully inform patient-centered oncology practice.

Randomization in Oncology Randomized Clinical Trials

Randomization is the defining feature of RCTs and is essential for ensuring the internal validity of oncology trials [17]. For clinicians and public health professionals, randomization provides a clear mechanism for preventing systematic differences between treatment groups [17, 18]. Randomization ensures that any observed differences in survival, progression, quality of life, or other outcomes can be attributed to the treatments themselves rather than preexisting differences among patients [19]. For statisticians, randomization is also a methodological tool that creates the conditions for unbiased estimation and valid causal inference by balancing both known and unknown prognostic factors across study arms [20].

In oncology, the role of randomization is particularly important, because patient populations are highly heterogeneous, with variation in tumor biology, stage at diagnosis, and prior treatment history. Without careful design and concealment of treatment allocation, these differences could bias the trial results and reduce confidence in new therapies. This section examines both the rational and the practical implementation of randomization in cancer trials. We begin by outlining the purpose of randomization and the importance of allocation concealment and then review major randomization methods commonly used in oncology research. We highlight why stratification is often essential for achieving balance on key prognostic factors,

and finally, we discuss approaches to maintain validity and comparability in large, heterogeneous, and multicenter oncology populations.

Purpose of Randomization and Allocation Concealment

The main reason to randomize patients in clinical trials is to protect the study from selection bias. Selection bias happens when the way patients are assigned to treatment groups is influenced by their health status or other prognostic factors, either intentionally or unintentionally [21, 22]. If researchers can predict who will be assigned next, they might put patients with better outlooks in the experimental group, or sicker patients in the control group, which would distort the results. Randomization prevents this bias by leaving the assignment entirely to chance.

Without randomization, both researchers and patients might make enrollment decisions based on assumptions about which group a patient will enter [23]. For instance, in an oncology trial, a doctor might try to place a patient with advanced disease into the experimental arm in the hope of access to a new therapy. If they expect the patient to be assigned to the control arm instead, they may even avoid enrolling that patient at all. These seemingly small decisions, when repeated across many patients, can create systematic differences between groups that compromise the validity of the trial.

By making allocation unpredictable, randomization prevents such manipulation and keeps the treatment groups comparable at the start [24]. This unpredictability is not only a convenience but also a fundamental part of rigorous trial design. It ensures that differences in outcomes are the result of the treatment itself, not differences in who was assigned to which group. Studies have shown that trials without proper randomization or concealment often overestimate treatment benefits, highlighting how crucial this step is [25].

From a statistical perspective, randomization balances both measured and unmeasured prognostic factors between groups [26, 27]. Known or measured variables like tumor stage, age, or performance status can be adjusted for in the analysis, but unknown or unmeasured factors cannot [28]. Randomization distributes these factors evenly across groups in expectation, allowing researchers to draw conclusions about treatment effects without bias from confounding. This balance is the foundation for valid causal inference [29, 30]. Randomization makes the groups exchangeable, which means that outcome differences can be interpreted as treatment effects rather than background differences [31]. Without randomization, causal conclusions would rely heavily on assumptions and complex modeling. With randomization, the interpretation is much clearer, giving clinicians, statisticians, and policy-makers confidence in the results of oncology trials [17, 31].

In oncology, the importance of this principle is amplified by the high degree of heterogeneity among patients. Tumor biology, disease stage, molecular characteristics, and prior treatment history all strongly influence outcomes [32]. If these factors are unevenly distributed, the apparent treatment effect could be confounded. Randomization helps equalize these characteristics across groups, thereby strengthening the internal validity of the trial and providing a reliable foundation for drawing clinical and scientific conclusions [31]. However, this benefit can only be preserved if the randomization sequence is properly concealed at the time of enrollment.

Allocation concealment complements randomization by preventing foreknowledge of upcoming assignments [33]. Without concealment, investigators may consciously or unconsciously influence enrollment, undermining the integrity of the trial [34]. This problem can be especially acute in high-stakes oncology settings where treatment options are limited and where clinicians may have strong preferences about giving patients access to novel therapies [35, 36]. Techniques such as central randomization via web-based or telephone systems, or sequentially numbered, opaque, sealed envelopes (SNOSE), are commonly used to ensure concealment in oncology RCTs [23, 37, 38]. When properly implemented, allocation concealment preserves the integrity of the randomization process and maintains the credibility of trial findings [33].

Randomization Methods

Randomization is the defining feature of randomized clinical trials [31], and multiple methods have been developed to implement it in practice. Each method carries strengths and limitations, and the choice depends on sample size, complexity of the trial, and the importance of covariate balance in the disease setting. In oncology, where patient heterogeneity is often pronounced and trial outcomes are high stakes, the selection of a randomization strategy can directly affect the credibility of trial conclusions [35].

Simple Randomization

Simple randomization is the most elementary method of treatment allocation, in which each patient is randomly and independently assigned to a study arm with equal probability

[31]. It can be thought of as flipping a coin or using a random number generator, and its strength lies in both simplicity and methodological rigor [17]. Over the long run, this approach guarantees an unbiased distribution of patients, making it an attractive option for large oncology trials where thousands of participants are enrolled. In such settings, the law of large numbers ensures that treatment arms are well-balanced [17].

In smaller trials, however, which are common in early-phase oncology studies or in rare cancers, chance imbalances may become problematic. For instance, in a phase II study with only 80 patients, simple randomization could by chance assign more patients with advanced-stage disease to one arm, leading to an apparent difference in outcomes that is unrelated to treatment [39, 40]. These imbalances can reduce statistical power, complicate the analysis, and undermine the credibility of findings. While post hoc adjustments with regression models can partially address the issue, it is often preferable to mitigate the risk at the design stage by using more structured randomization methods [31].

Block Randomization

Block randomization was developed to maintain balance throughout the course of enrollment, not just at the end of the trial. Patients are randomized in blocks of predetermined size, ensuring that each block contains equal numbers of participants in each treatment arm [41]. This approach is especially valuable in multicenter oncology RCTs, where enrollment is staggered across hospitals and countries [42]. For example, in a large breast cancer trial conducted by cooperative oncology groups, block randomization ensures that each center contributes a balanced number of patients to each treatment arm [42]. Without this mechanism, sites with slower accrual might distort allocation patterns, complicating interim analyses or delaying regulatory review.

One limitation of block randomization is predictability when block sizes are fixed and known to investigators [42]. If researchers suspect a pattern, they may anticipate upcoming assignments and potentially influence enrollment. To mitigate this risk, modern trials often use random block sizes, which preserve unpredictability while maintaining balance [43].

Stratified Randomization

Stratified randomization builds on block randomization by incorporating clinically important prognostic factors into the allocation process [44]. Patients are first categorized into strata based on variables that are strongly associated with outcomes and then randomized within each stratum. In oncology, these variables typically include tumor stage, biomarker status, prior treatment, or performance measures such as the ECOG score [45].

This method is particularly effective in preventing confounding by key covariates [46]. For example, in the pivotal KEYNOTE-189 trial of immunotherapy for non-small cell lung cancer, patients were stratified by PD-L1 expression because of its known predictive value for response [46, 47]. Similarly, breast cancer trials are frequently stratified by hormone receptor and HER2 status to ensure that the distribution of molecular subtypes is balanced across groups [48]. By improving comparability between treatment arms, stratified randomization increases both the credibility of causal inference and the interpretability of subgroup analyses [29, 44].

Despite its advantages, stratified randomization becomes unwieldy when many stratification factors are included. As the number of strata increases, the number of patients in each stratum may be too small for effective randomization to occur. Consequently, researchers must carefully prioritize which prognostic factors are most essential to include [44, 49].

Minimization

Minimization is an adaptive allocation technique that dynamically assigns each new patient to the treatment arm that minimizes overall imbalance across several covariates [50, 51]. Unlike stratified randomization, which requires prespecified strata, minimization evaluates the current state of balance across all relevant variables and makes the allocation accordingly [50].

This approach is particularly valuable in oncology trials where multiple covariates simultaneously affect prognosis, such as genomic subtypes, tumor burden, and prior lines of therapy [51]. In such cases, conventional stratified randomization might be impractical due to the large number of strata, whereas minimization provides a flexible solution.

For example, in trials of targeted therapies for hematologic malignancies, where outcomes may be influenced by age, cytogenetic abnormalities, and treatment history, minimization ensures that no treatment arm is disproportionately populated by high-risk patients [52]. Although it requires a more complex implementation, often involving centralized software, minimization is well-suited to modern precision oncology trials, where balancing many small but important subgroups is crucial for valid inference [51].

Importance of Stratification in Oncology

Stratification is of particular importance in oncology RCTs, because cancer is not a single disease but a collection of biologically and clinically diverse conditions. Prognosis is shaped by multiple factors, including tumor biology, disease stage, molecular subtype, and patient comorbidities [53, 54].

For example, outcomes for patients with early-stage, surgically resectable disease differ dramatically from those with advanced metastatic cancer [55]. Likewise, within breast cancer, triple-negative tumors have a markedly poorer prognosis compared with hormone receptor-positive or HER2-positive subtypes [56].

Without stratification, randomization may produce treatment groups that differ substantially with respect to these critical prognostic variables [44]. Such imbalances can confound the treatment effect, making it unclear whether differences in outcomes are due to the therapy or to baseline differences between groups [57]. Stratification reduces this risk by ensuring that each treatment arm includes a representative mix of patients across key variables [44].

The practical impact of stratification is well illustrated by landmark oncology trials. In the KEYNOTE-189 trial of immunotherapy in non-small cell lung cancer, stratification by PD-L1 status was essential to produce valid comparisons between groups [58]. Similarly, colorectal cancer trials often stratify by tumor sidedness, given its strong association with prognosis and treatment response [59]. By controlling for heterogeneity at the design stage, stratification strengthens internal validity, improves statistical efficiency, and enhances the interpretability of subgroup analyses [44].

Balancing Prognostic Factors in Heterogeneous Populations

Oncology RCTs often recruit patients across multiple centers, regions, and healthcare systems, introducing additional variability into the study population. Patients may differ not only in biological characteristics but also in access to care, supportive treatments, and background therapies [60]. This diversity makes oncology trials particularly vulnerable to imbalances between treatment groups, which in turn can obscure or exaggerate treatment effects [61].

Randomization provides the primary safeguard against such imbalances, ensuring that treatment groups are comparable in expectation [17]. Even when a perfect balance is not achieved in small subgroups, randomization guarantees unbiased estimation under the intention-to-treat principle [62]. However, additional methods such as stratification and minimization can further improve balance, particularly in trials where prognostic heterogeneity is extreme [60].

Balancing prognostic factors is especially important in the era of precision oncology. Modern therapies often target specific molecular alterations, meaning that trial populations may be small and highly heterogeneous [63]. In these settings, even modest imbalances in biomarker distribution can lead to misleading conclusions about treatment benefit [64]. For instance, if one arm includes a disproportionate number of patients with a favorable mutation, the treatment effect may appear larger than it actually is [65, 66]. By carefully designing randomization strategies to control for such factors, researchers ensure that oncology trials yield reliable, interpretable, and generalizable results [67].

Trial Designs in Cancer Randomized Clinical Trials

Randomized clinical trials (RCTs) not only establish whether a new therapy works but also guide regulatory approvals, reimbursement decisions, and treatment guidelines [68, 69]. Designing RCTs in cancer is particularly challenging, because the disease is heterogeneous, patient populations can be small, and endpoints such as overall survival require long follow-up. At the same time, the urgency of delivering effective therapies to patients has pushed the field to adopt more innovative designs [70]. This section reviews the spectrum of trial designs in oncology, from traditional approaches to the cutting edge of precision medicine.

Statistical Aims in Phases of Clinical Trials

The development of new cancer therapies proceeds through a series of clinical trial phases, each with distinct goals. Phase I trials are primarily concerned with safety. Unlike in most other disciplines, these studies rarely involve healthy volunteers, because anticancer agents are often too toxic to administer to individuals without disease [71]. Instead, patients with advanced cancers are recruited, usually those who have exhausted standard options. The statistical focus is to determine the maximum tolerated dose or the recommended dose for subsequent trials [72]. Historically, this was done using simple rule-based dose-escalation methods, where small groups of patients were treated at increasing dose levels until unacceptable toxicity occurred [73]. In recent decades, more sophisticated model-based approaches such as the continual reassessment method and Bayesian optimal interval designs have been introduced. These methods make more efficient use of toxicity data and allow faster identification of safe and active doses, exposing fewer patients to harmful or ineffective regimens [74].

Phase II trials move beyond safety to examine preliminary efficacy. The key question in phase II is whether a therapy shows enough promise to justify a larger, definitive trial [75]. Designs often incorporate mechanisms to stop early if a therapy appears ineffective, thereby protecting patients and conserving resources. Simon's two-stage design [76], for example, allows investigators to assess early results and terminate the study before full accrual if the likelihood of success is low. Increasingly, randomized phase II trials are used, since they provide stronger comparative evidence than single-arm studies. A positive phase II result does not guarantee ultimate success, but it serves as an important gatekeeper before the significant investment of a phase III study [77].

Phase III trials are large randomized studies that provide definitive evidence about efficacy and safety. They are designed to detect superiority, non-inferiority, or equivalence of a new intervention compared to the standard of care [78]. Sample size calculations are based on assumptions about expected effect sizes, event rates, and acceptable levels of type I and type II error [79], where type I error refers to the probability of incorrect rejection of the null hypothesis (a false positive) and type II error refers to the probability of failing to detect a true effect (a false negative). A well-conducted phase III trial can directly change clinical practice and inform international treatment guidelines. A clear example is the KEYNOTE-024 trial, which demonstrated that pembrolizumab significantly improved survival outcome compared with chemotherapy in patients with advanced non-small cell lung cancer expressing PD-L1 [80].

Phase IV trials occur after regulatory approval and extend evaluation into real-world practice. Their goals include monitoring for rare or late adverse events, assessing effectiveness in broader populations, and understanding long-term quality of life [81]. These studies often adopt pragmatic designs that reflect routine care and may draw on data from cancer registries, electronic patient records, or insurance claims. Phase IV studies are increasingly important in oncology, where treatments are used for many years and in populations that were underrepresented or excluded in earlier trials. For example, a recent review of trial registries found that phase IV oncology trials often focus on long-term safety, effectiveness in broader real-world patient groups, and detection of late or rare adverse events not evident during preapproval phases [82]. Furthermore, phase IV trials allow researchers to assess how therapies perform under usual clinical conditions outside of the controlled settings of early trials, making them essential for refining treatment recommendations and improving patient care [83].

Parallel-Group Superiority Trials

The parallel-group superiority trial is the most familiar and widely used design in cancer research [84]. In its simplest form, patients are randomly allocated to one of two groups: One group receives the experimental treatment, while the other receives either the standard therapy or, when no established treatment is available, a placebo [31]. The groups are then followed over time, and outcomes such as overall survival or symptom control are compared. Because randomization balances both known and unknown characteristics between groups, the design allows researchers to conclude with confidence that any differences observed are due to the treatment itself rather than to patient differences [84].

This design is chosen, because it provides the clearest and most direct answer to the question patients and clinicians care about most: Does the new treatment work better than the comparator [85]? It is also highly accepted by regulators and guideline committees, because the results are straightforward to interpret. The results of superiority trials often become the evidence that shapes everyday practice, since these trials form the backbone of clinical guidelines [86].

The CALGB 9741 trial in breast cancer provides a good example. In this study, patients were randomized to receive standard chemotherapy every 3 weeks or the same drugs given every 2 weeks, a strategy known as "dose-dense" scheduling [87]. The trial demonstrated that the more frequent schedule significantly improved survival. This finding immediately changed how oncologists prescribed chemotherapy and affected nursing care as well [88]. Nurses had to provide patient education more frequently, monitor for toxicities at shorter intervals, and coordinate supportive treatments such as growth factor injections more carefully [87, 88]. This illustrates how the results of superiority trials not only shape drug approvals but also directly affect how care teams deliver treatment.

Another landmark superiority trial was KEYNOTE-024 [89], which tested the immunotherapy pembrolizumab against chemotherapy in patients with advanced non-small cell lung cancer who expressed the PD-L1 biomarker. The study found a significant improvement in survival with pembrolizumab, leading to its rapid adoption as the standard of care [90]. For clinicians, this trial changed the way treatment decisions were made, introducing routine biomarker testing into practice [89]. For nurses, it meant educating patients about the different side effect profile of immunotherapy compared with chemotherapy, such as immune-related toxicities that require monitoring and prompt intervention [89].

Parallel-group superiority trials typically use survival analysis statistical methods to compare outcomes, since many cancer endpoints involve time until progression or death [84]. From a clinical perspective, this means these trials often run for several years to ensure that enough events occur to detect a meaningful difference. The long timelines require sustained patient follow-up, careful data collection, and consistent nursing engagement to monitor symptoms and adherence [20].

Understanding superiority trials is important for healthcare providers, because they are the clearest indicator of when a new therapy is ready to replace an older one [84]. They provide the evidence base for clinical guidelines, shape the standard of care, and influence the daily work of nurses and physicians alike [20, 84]. In oncology, where the ultimate aim is to improve survival and quality of life, superiority trials are the most direct way to demonstrate progress [20].

Non-inferiority and Equivalence Trials

In many cases, the question is not whether a new therapy is superior, but whether it is close enough in efficacy to the standard while offering other meaningful benefits. Non-inferiority trials are designed to prove that a new intervention is not unacceptably worse than the control by more than a prespecified margin [91]. In oncology, these designs are particularly valuable in treatment de-escalation, supportive care, or when evaluating therapies that may reduce toxicity or cost [92]. Equivalence trials, in contrast, aim to show that two therapies have outcomes so similar that any differences fall within a narrow, predefined range [92]. This design is often used in the development of biosimilars, which are highly similar versions of complex biologic drugs [93]. Because biologics like trastuzumab or rituximab are expensive, biosimilars must prove that they have the same effectiveness and safety as the original drugs before being approved for use [94].

The process of conducting these trials requires careful thought about the margin of difference allowed [91]. If the margin is too wide, an inferior treatment could be mistakenly accepted. If it is too narrow, the study may need to be so large that it becomes impossible to conduct [95]. This is why both clinicians and statisticians must work together to define a margin that is both clinically meaningful and practically feasible [91].

A good example of a non-inferiority trial is the START series of studies in breast cancer. These trials compared shorter courses of radiotherapy with the traditional longer schedule [96]. The findings indicated that the shorter schedule was not inferior to the longer one in terms of cancer control. This was a major shift for patients and healthcare providers alike [96]. For patients, it meant fewer trips to the hospital and less disruption to daily life. For nurses and radiation therapists, it changed treatment planning, follow-up care, and the way side effects were monitored, since the shorter schedule delivered higher daily doses but over fewer sessions [96].

Equivalence trials have been especially important in the field of supportive oncology [91]. For example, biosimilar versions of trastuzumab and rituximab were tested in equivalence designs that compared their effectiveness and safety directly to the original biologics [97]. The results confirmed that the biosimilars performed the same as the reference drugs. This has allowed healthcare systems to adopt lower-cost alternatives without compromising patient outcomes, freeing resources that can be redirected to other aspects of patient care. Nurses, pharmacists, and physicians have all had to adapt by learning how to explain biosimilars to patients, manage any concerns about switching from the original drug, and monitor for side effects with the same vigilance as before [93].

Factorial Designs

A factorial design allows researchers to test more than one intervention at the same time within a single study [98]. Instead of studying just one new treatment against the standard, a factorial trial can evaluate two or more treatments simultaneously, either alone or in combination. This is especially relevant in oncology, where patients often receive multiple therapies together such as chemotherapy, hormone therapy, radiation, immunotherapy, or targeted drugs rather than a single treatment [99].

The main reason to use a factorial design is efficiency. It enables investigators to answer several research questions in a single trial rather than running multiple separate studies [100]. For instance, a 2×2 factorial design might randomize patients to chemotherapy with or without an immune checkpoint inhibitor while at the same time randomizing them to either a standard or higher dose of radiation. In this way, researchers can determine not only whether immunotherapy helps, and whether a higher radiation dose helps, but also whether the combination of treatments has an added or unexpected effect [101].

The way a factorial trial works is straightforward in concept but requires careful planning [101]. Patients are randomized into groups that represent all possible combinations of the treatments being studied. For a 2×2 factorial design, there are four groups: One gets chemotherapy alone with standard radiation, another gets chemotherapy plus immunotherapy with standard radiation, a third gets chemotherapy with higher-dose radiation, and the fourth gets chemotherapy plus immunotherapy with higher-dose radiation. After follow-up, researchers compare results across groups, looking for both the independent effects of each treatment and any interaction between them [100, 101].

The attraction of factorial trials lies in their ability to maximize what is learned from a single group of patients [100]. However, this efficiency comes with challenges. If the treatments interact strongly, meaning that the effect of one treatment depends on whether the other is given, the results can be harder to interpret. Additionally, because multiple comparisons are being made, the number of patients required can be quite large to ensure that the results are reliable [100, 102].

Despite these difficulties, factorial designs have played an important role in oncology. In prostate cancer, for example, researchers have used factorial trials to study both the duration of androgen deprivation therapy and the use of radiation therapy within the same trial [103]. This design allowed investigators to answer questions about hormonal treatment and local therapy simultaneously, providing comprehensive evidence that shaped treatment guidelines [100]. In breast cancer, factorial trials have been used to evaluate the combined effects of chemotherapy and hormonal therapy, demonstrating how the integration of multiple treatments improved patient outcomes [104].

For healthcare providers, understanding factorial designs is valuable, because they often underpin decisions about multimodal therapy, such as the kinds of complex regimens that nurses and physicians manage daily [105]. When two or more interventions are shown to work well together in a factorial trial, the result directly influences how treatment plans are structured, how supportive care is scheduled, and how patients are counseled about what to expect. These trials reflect the real-world reality of oncology care, where treatment success usually depends not on a single drug but on the thoughtful combination of several therapies [105].

Crossover Trials

In crossover trials, each patient receives more than one treatment in sequence [106]. For example, a participant may receive one treatment first, then after a washout period, switch to the other treatment. Because every patient tries both treatments, each individual essentially acts as their own control. This reduces the impact of differences between patients, making it easier to detect differences between treatments using a smaller sample size [107].

In oncology, however, crossover trials are not commonly used. The main reason is that most cancer treatments, such as chemotherapy, radiation, or targeted therapies, have long-lasting biological effects [108]. Once a patient receives one of these treatments, its impact on the body and on the cancer often continues well into the future [109]. As a result, it is difficult to clearly distinguish the effect of the first treatment from the second. In addition, cancer is a progressive disease. If a patient's cancer worsens during the first treatment period, this can complicate or even prevent the second treatment period, making the results hard to interpret. For these reasons, crossover designs are generally unsuitable for studies focused on survival outcomes or curative treatments [110].

Despite these limitations, crossover trials are valuable in supportive care, where treatments tend to act quickly and their effects wear off within a short time [111]. When testing interventions for cancer-related symptoms such as nausea, vomiting, pain, fatigue, or sleep disturbances [108], these trials are particularly useful. For instance, in studies of antiemetic drugs for chemotherapy-induced nausea and vomiting, patients may receive one drug during their first cycle of chemotherapy and then switch to another drug during the next cycle. A washout period is built in to minimize carryover effects [109]. This design allows researchers to directly compare how well each drug works in the same patient, removing variability between different patients.

The efficiency of this design means that crossover trials often require fewer participants to reach meaningful conclusions. This is especially valuable in supportive oncology, where resources may be limited and where rapid answers are needed to improve patient comfort [108]. Results from such studies have had a direct impact on practice. For example, crossover trials comparing ondansetron with older antiemetics in the 1990s helped establish ondansetron as the preferred agent for preventing chemotherapy-induced nausea, changing the standard of care [112].

Multicenter and Global Trials

Multicenter and global trials are studies that take place across multiple hospitals, often spanning different regions or countries [113]. In modern oncology, most large clinical trials use this approach, because no single hospital or even one country alone can recruit enough patients quickly enough to answer important questions [114]. By combining sites, researchers can reach the necessary number of participants more efficiently. This not only speeds up the trial but also increases the statistical strength of the findings. Just as importantly, it ensures that results are generalizable, meaning they are more likely to apply to patients in everyday practice because the study population is more diverse [113]. The main reason these trials are used in oncology is that cancers are increasingly divided into smaller and smaller subgroups [114]. For example, treatments may target a specific gene mutation that is only present in a small percentage of patients. To study such groups, researchers must pool patients from many centers and sometimes from multiple countries [115]. Global trials also make it possible to perform subgroup analyses, looking at whether treatment effects differ based on geography, ethnicity, or healthcare system differences [116]. This helps ensure that the therapy is effective not just in one setting but across many different real-world contexts.

Conducting trials across multiple centers, however, is complex. Each site may have different diagnostic standards, healthcare infrastructure, and patient populations. Regulatory requirements also differ by country, which can slow approvals and complicate trial conduct [117]. To reduce these risks, trials often use strategies such as stratified randomization by site, centralized pathology or imaging review, and oversight by independent data and safety monitoring committees [118]. These measures help ensure consistency and reliability across sites, so that results can be trusted.

The MONALEESA program of trials for CDK4/6 inhibitors in breast cancer illustrates the value of multicenter and global designs [119, 120]. These studies enrolled thousands of women from dozens of countries around the world [119]. The inclusion of diverse populations made the results more compelling and applicable across different health systems. The findings were robust enough to change international guidelines, firmly establishing CDK4/6 inhibitors as part of the standard treatment for hormone receptor-positive breast cancer [120].

Treatments that emerge from such trials are more likely to be broadly effective, because they have been tested in patients from different backgrounds and healthcare settings. Providers in local clinics can be confident that the evidence supporting a new therapy does not only apply to patients from one specialized center but is relevant to the diverse populations they see in practice [118]. Nurses often play a critical role in these trials by ensuring protocol adherence across sites, supporting patients through complex treatment regimens, and contributing to the collection of high-quality, consistent data [81]. In this way, multicenter and global trials not only drive progress in oncology but also highlight the essential role of healthcare teams in making research meaningful and reliable.

Adaptive Designs

Adaptive designs are an innovative type of clinical trial that allow certain modifications to be made as the study progresses while still maintaining statistical validity [121]. Unlike traditional trials, which are fixed from the start and cannot change without compromising reliability, adaptive trials are planned with built-in flexibility. This means that researchers can respond to the data as it emerges rather than waiting until the trial is completely finished [122]. In oncology, where time is critical and patients often have limited treatment options, this approach has become increasingly attractive.

The main reason adaptive designs are used in cancer research is efficiency. They can shorten the timeline for finding answers, minimize the number of patients receiving ineffective treatments, and sometimes allow promising therapies to reach patients sooner [122]. From an ethical standpoint, they can also be appealing, because patients are more likely to receive treatments that show early signs of benefit as the trial continues.

Adaptive designs are important, because they can accelerate the development of treatments that may soon enter standard practice [121]. For instance, the number of patients recruited may increase, or the distribution of patients between arms may shift. This requires flexibility in trial management, close communication with patients, and careful attention to informed consent, since participants need to understand that the trial design is dynamic [123].

Although adaptive trials hold great promise, they also require careful planning and strict oversight. Complex statistical modeling is needed to ensure results remain valid, and regulatory agencies expect strong justification for the adaptive methods chosen. Still, in oncology, where patient lives and time are so precious, adaptive designs represent a powerful tool to make research more efficient, ethical, and responsive to patient needs [124]. There are several ways adaptive trials may work in practice.

Group-Sequential Designs

A group-sequential design is an adaptive approach that allows researchers to analyze the data at several points during the trial rather than only at the end. At these interim analyses, the study can be stopped early if results are already compelling [125]. For example, if a treatment is clearly superior, it is more ethical to stop the trial, so that more patients outside the study can access the effective therapy. Conversely, if the treatment is clearly not working, the trial can also be stopped early to prevent further patient exposure to an ineffective option.

In oncology, this type of design is particularly appealing, because waiting years for final results may delay the introduction of effective therapies for patients with life-threatening disease [126]. An example is seen in some large breast cancer trials, where interim analyses allowed early recognition of survival benefits and sped up changes in treatment guidelines. For healthcare providers, group-sequential designs mean that practice may change sooner and nurses may need to adjust patient education and supportive care as new therapies are adopted earlier than expected [127].

Another form of adaptive design is sample size reestimation. In traditional trials, the number of patients is fixed from the start, based on assumptions about how large the treatment effect will be and how much variability there will be in the data [121]. If these assumptions are wrong, the study may lack sufficient power to identify real differences. Sample size reestimation addresses this problem by allowing researchers to adjust the number of participants, while the trial is ongoing. In practice, if early results suggest that the effect size is smaller than expected, more patients can be added to ensure the trial still has enough power [125]. On the other hand, if results show less variability than expected, the study size may be reduced, saving time and resources. In oncology, where patient populations may be small and treatments expensive, this flexibility is especially valuable. For clinicians and nurses, sample size reestimation means that recruitment periods may be extended and care teams need to remain prepared for changes in how many patients are enrolled at their site [127].

Adaptive Randomization

Adaptive randomization is a design in which the probability of assigning patients to different treatment arms is adjusted as the trial progresses [127]. As more data accumulate, the likelihood of patients assigned to more effective treatment also increases [17]. This design is appealing in oncology, because it addresses an important ethical concern: Rather than continuing to assign half the patients to a treatment that is likely less effective, more patients receive the option that shows early signs of benefit [17]. A clear example of adaptive randomization is the BATTLE trial in non-small cell lung cancer [128]. In that study, patients were adaptively assigned to therapies based on both their biomarker profiles and the emerging results of the trial, meaning that as data suggested certain subgroups benefited more from specific drugs, more patients with those profiles were assigned to those therapies [117]. For healthcare providers, adaptive randomization highlights the growing role of precision medicine. Nurses and physicians caring for trial participants must be able to explain to patients why their chance of receiving one treatment may differ from another patient, and they must be vigilant in monitoring for treatment-specific side effects as assignments change over time [124].

Adaptive designs are important, because they can accelerate the development of treatments that may soon enter standard practice [122]. For example, the number of patients recruited may increase or the distribution of patients between arms may shift. This requires flexibility in trial management, close communication with patients, and careful attention to informed consent, since participants need to understand that the trial design is dynamic [129].

Master Protocols in Oncology

The rise of precision oncology has transformed how cancer trials are designed [117]. Instead of testing one therapy in one type of cancer at a time, researchers increasingly use what are called master protocols [130]. A master protocol is an overarching trial framework that can evaluate multiple treatments or hypotheses simultaneously. This structure is especially important in the genomic era, where cancers are defined not only by their tissue of origin but also by their molecular features [117]. Many genetic subgroups are rare, and studying them separately would be inefficient. Master protocols solve this problem by testing therapies in a way that is both more flexible and more efficient. The three main types of master protocol designs used in oncology today are umbrella trials, basket trials, and platform trials [130].

Umbrella Trials

An umbrella trial focuses on a single cancer type but tests multiple therapies, with patients assigned to specific treatment arms according to the molecular characteristics of their tumor [130]. This design is useful, because many cancers, such as lung cancer, are not one disease but a collection of subtypes driven by different genetic mutations. By bringing these subgroups together under one protocol, researchers can more efficiently study several targeted therapies at once without setting up separate trials for each mutation [131].

The Lung-MAP trial in non-small cell lung cancer is a prime example. Patients are screened for a panel of biomarkers, and they are directed to the treatment arm most relevant to their tumor's genetic profile based on their results [132]. For nurses and physicians, umbrella trials change how care is delivered: Patients must undergo biomarker testing as part of routine care, and clinicians must be prepared to explain to patients why their treatment pathway may differ from others with the same type of lung cancer [130].

Basket Trials

Basket trials take the opposite approach. Instead of focusing on one cancer type, they evaluate a single therapy across many different cancers that share a common molecular alteration [131, 133]. The logic here is that if a drug targets a specific mutation, it might work in any tumor that carries that mutation, regardless of where in the body the cancer started [133].

The molecular analysis for therapy choice (NCI-MATCH) trial is one of the best-known examples of a basket trial [134]. In this trial, patients with many different cancers were tested for genetic changes, and those with certain mutations were assigned to therapies designed to target those changes [134]. This approach is particularly helpful for rare mutations that occur in only a small percentage of patients within each cancer type but add up across multiple cancers. For providers, basket trials highlight the importance of genomic testing and require coordination between oncologists, pathologists, and nurses to ensure patients are screened and matched to the right treatment arm [133].

Platform Trials

Platform trials are the most flexible form of master protocol. They are designed to continuously evaluate multiple therapies against a shared control group [135]. Treatments that prove ineffective can be dropped, while new treatments can be added as they become available, all under the same protocol. This allows the trial to adapt to new scientific discoveries and drug developments without having to start from scratch each time [135].

The I-SPY 2 trial in breast cancer is a leading example. It uses a common control arm and adaptively randomizes patients to experimental therapies based on early results. Promising drugs move forward more quickly, while ineffective ones are discontinued [136]. This trial has accelerated the pace of breast cancer drug development and created a model that is now being applied to other cancers. Platform trials demand flexibility, as the therapies under study may change during the course of the trial. Patient education also becomes critical, since patients need to understand that they are part of a dynamic trial where new arms may be introduced and others may close [135, 136].

Endpoints in Oncology RCTs

The choice of endpoints in oncology randomized clinical trials (RCTs) is central to trial design, interpretation, and regulatory approval. Endpoints are used in trials to measure the validity, generalizability, and clinical impact of the study, and the evidence they generate guides both clinicians and patients in decision-making. Endpoints should be easy to measure either objectively or subjectively by a clinician, observer, or patient themselves [137]. High-quality endpoints must reflect clinically meaningful benefits, be measurable within feasible timeframes, and align closely with the scientific and therapeutic objectives of the trials [137, 138]. Most importantly, a primary clinical endpoint should demonstrate clear patient relevance and directly measure their survival, functional ability, or quality of life. In many cases, using multiple endpoints to assess changes in clinical course provide a more comprehensive view of how an intervention influences the course of disease [137–139].

Oncology trials present unique challenges; for example, survival outcomes often require long follow-up, while intermediate and surrogate endpoints such as progression-free survival or biomarker-based measures can provide earlier signals of efficacy [137, 140]. The balance between clinical relevance, timeliness of assessment, and regulatory acceptability makes endpoint choice particularly complex in oncology research.

Primary Endpoints

Overall Survival (OS)

Overall survival (OS) is recognized as the gold standard endpoint in oncology, which records the length of time from a patient's randomization until death from any cause [140]. OS is objective, clinically meaningful, and unambiguous. However, it often requires long follow-up and large sample sizes, particularly in cancers with prolonged survival (e.g., early stage cancers), and may be confounded by therapies after disease progression [141, 142]. Regulatory bodies such as the FDA have regarded OS as the preferred primary endpoint and definitive measure of direct benefit especially in phase III clinical trials [140].

Similar to OS, cancer-specific survival is another commonly used primary endpoint which measures the time from randomization to death related to the index cancer or secondary tumor of the same type [137, 143]. Deaths due to other causes, lost to follow-up, and patients alive at the end of study are excluded from this measure. The primary challenge in using this type of survival lies in accurately determining the cause of death, which is often subject to misclassification. In addition, because it integrates multiple considerations, this endpoint is inherently composite and therefore somewhat difficult to define with precision.

Progression-Free Survival (PFS)

When OS is impractical due to extended survival or post-progression crossover, PFS is widely used as a primary endpoint. PFS is defined as the length of time from randomization or initiation of treatment until disease progression or death. PFS offers earlier readouts and requires fewer patients than OS, but its clinical relevance can vary by disease type and may be influenced by assessment frequency and progression criteria such as RECIST [144]. Therefore, PFS is prone to assessment bias and may not always correlate with survival [140, 145].

Disease-Free Survival (DFS)

Commonly used in the adjuvant setting following definitive surgery or radiotherapy, DFS captures the time from randomization to recurrence of disease or death from any cause. Unlike PFS which accounts for both the initial progression of measurable disease and recurrence, DFS is specifically concerned with the duration a patient remains free of detectable disease following curative treatment, thus excluding the progression of non-eradicated, preexisting tumors. DFS is particularly relevant in early-stage cancers where curative intent is plausible, as it captures the interval during which a patient remains free of detectable disease after primary therapy [137]. Similar to PFS, DFS allows for earlier outcome assessment but requires careful specification of recurrence events and standardized follow-up schedules [146, 147]. Challenges include variability in the interpretation of recurrence events and the potential for misclassification, for example, distinguishing between a true recurrence and a new primary tumor. Despite these complexities, DFS has served as a basis for traditional regulatory approval in several malignancies, including breast cancer, colorectal cancer, melanoma, and renal cell carcinoma [140].

Secondary Endpoints

Objective Response Rate (ORR)

ORR refers to the proportion of patients who achieve tumor shrinkage that meets predefined criteria for a specified minimum duration after treatment, which typically encompasses complete or partial response, as defined by standardized criteria such as RECIST [144]. The FDA defines ORR as the sum of complete and partial response rates, making it a direct measure of a drug's antitumor activity, commonly evaluated in single-arm studies [140]. Moreover, ORR is frequently used as a secondary endpoint in phase II and III trials and serves as a rapid measure of drug activity, though it may not always correlate with long-term outcomes [148]. To ensure consistency and reliability, response criteria should be standardized and predefined in the clinical trial protocol, where RECIST guidelines are often considered appropriate. The importance of ORR is determined by both the magnitude and duration of the responses and by the percentage of complete responders.

Duration of Response (DoR)

DoR measures the length of time from first response (either complete or partial response) until the progression of disease or death. It complements ORR by quantifying the sustainability of tumor control, providing insights into treatment durability [149]. DoR has emerged as a clinically meaningful endpoint for assessing treatments that provide both rapid and lasting effects, especially in single-arm studies where PFS or OS data are not yet mature [140, 150].

Time to Treatment Failure (TTF)

TTF measures the duration from randomization to treatment discontinuation for any reason, including progression, toxicity, or death [140]. This endpoint is often used for treatments that are administered continuously until disease progression, such as immune checkpoint inhibitors, targeted therapies, and other maintenance treatments. In contrast to time-limited treatment modalities like chemotherapy or radiation therapy, where treatment duration is predetermined, continuous therapies require endpoints that capture the full treatment experience until discontinuation becomes necessary. While less commonly used as a primary endpoint, especially in new molecular entity drug approval [140], TTF provides a pragmatic measure of overall treatment effectiveness, making it valuable for understanding both efficacy and tolerability in oncology.

Patient-Reported Outcomes (PROs)

Quality of life, symptom burden, and functional status are increasingly recognized as key secondary endpoints. PROs provide direct patient perspectives on treatment benefit and toxicity rather than from a clinician or observer, complementing survival outcomes. PROs are assessed through patient-reported outcome measures (PROMs), which are standardized, validated questionnaires or survey tools administered during illness, throughout treatment, or after interventions to monitor changes in health status over time [151, 152]. Regulatory bodies, including the FDA and EMA, emphasize the importance of PROs in evaluating clinical benefit [140].

Quality of Life (QoL)

QoL serves as a crucial endpoint in oncology, complementing traditional outcomes by incorporating the patient's subjective experience of their cancer and treatment. Measured through PROs, QoL assessments evaluate the physical, mental, and emotional impact of both the disease and therapy, providing a more complete picture of treatment benefit beyond survival or disease progression [153]. This patient-centered approach can help to educate patients and families about what to expect on treatment, inform clinical decisions, and enhance overall patient care.

Surrogate Endpoints: Regulatory Use and Validation

Surrogate endpoints such as PFS and ORR are often used for accelerated approval of oncology drugs, because they permit earlier evaluation of treatment effects and often enable smaller, less resource-intensive trials [154]. However, the reliability and acceptance of surrogate endpoints hinge on robust evidence linking improvements in these measures to meaningful benefits such as extended OS or enhanced QoL. Validation of surrogates requires rigorous meta-analytic assessment across multiple trials and cancer types to confirm that benefits on the surrogate translate into real-world patient gains [155]. While surrogate endpoints can speed up drug development, reduce required sample sizes, and facilitate earlier regulatory decisions, overreliance on weak or inadequately validated surrogates introduces significant uncertainty for patients, clinicians, and regulatory agencies. If drugs are approved on the basis of surrogate outcomes that are not associated with true clinical benefit, patients may be exposed to unnecessary risks including toxicities and costs, without a reasonable expectation of survival or QoL improvement [156]. Thus, the use of surrogate endpoints should be accompanied by rigorous scientific justification and strict post-marketing confirmation whenever used as a basis for regulatory approval [8, 154].

Minimal Residual Disease (MRD) as an Emerging Endpoint

Minimal residual disease (MRD), referring to the presence of subclinical cancer cells detected by sensitive molecular or immunologic assays, has become a powerful endpoint in hematologic malignancies [157]. Detecting MRD helps doctors assess a patient's response to treatment, predict the risk of relapse, and guide future treatment decisions. MRD negativity has been strongly associated with improved survival in leukemias and lymphomas, and regulatory agencies increasingly recognize MRD as an accelerated surrogate endpoint [8]. Ongoing research aims to refine and standardize MRD assessment methods and establishes its prognostic and predictive validity across malignancies [157].

Statistical Analysis of Oncology RCTs

Statistical analysis in oncology RCTs requires careful consideration of endpoint types, population heterogeneity, and disease-specific complexities. The goal is to provide reliable evidence on the efficacy and safety of novel cancer therapies, often under complex scenarios such as biomarker-driven subgroups or adaptive trial designs. The following subsections outline the main statistical principles and methods commonly applied in oncology RCTs.

Intention-to-Treat (ITT) vs. per-Protocol Analysis

In oncology RCTs, the intention-to-treat (ITT) principle is widely considered the gold standard as it preserves the prognostic balance achieved by randomization and reduces the risk of bias [158]. The principle utilizes all randomized participants regardless of their adherence, crossover, or protocol deviations. ITT analysis provides an unbiased estimate of treatment effect reflective of real-world clinical application, even when participants discontinue or switch therapy, such as in immuno-oncology studies [158]. In contrast, per-protocol (PP) analysis is only restricted to participants who adhered to the protocol, though offering additional context on efficacy under ideal conditions, it potentially introduces bias due to loss of randomization benefits [159]. As a result, PP analyses should utilize statistical approaches commonly used in nonrandomized studies to address potential patient differences and reduce confounding effects [159]. In cancer research, where treatment discontinuation, crossover, or deviations are frequent, reporting both ITT and PP analyses can yield complementary benefits by balancing rigorous assessment of effectiveness in the total randomized cohort with consideration of outcomes in fully adherent patients.

Analysis of Dichotomous Outcomes

Binary outcomes, such as objective response rate or complete remission rate in hematologic malignancies, are common in oncology research. The following statistical methods are used to analyze these dichotomous outcomes, providing intuitive interpretations and clear communication of treatment effects, and allowing appropriate adjustment of important covariates when necessary.

Proportions and Risk Ratios (RR)

Proportions summarize the rates of outcomes within groups, and risk ratios (RRs, also referred to as relative risks) quantify the probability of an event in one group relative to another, offering an interpretable measure of comparative likelihood. RR is often preferred for direct interpretability in RCTs and cohort studies of cancer outcomes, making them easier to communicate and interpret in clinical contexts. In addition to simple calculations, regression-based approaches such as log-binomial models or Poisson regression with robust variance estimation are commonly used to obtain direct estimates of RRs, particularly when adjusting for covariates or handling complex study designs. These methods extend the applicability of RR estimation beyond unadjusted comparisons, thereby providing a more nuanced understanding of treatment effects in cancer research.

Chi-Squared Test or Fisher's Exact Test

For comparing binary outcomes between two independent groups, the Chi-square test is the classical standard when the sample size is sufficient, and expected cell counts meet threshold criteria (generally, no more than 20% of expected counts below 5). The Fisher's exact test is recommended when expected counts are small, as it computes exact p-values without relying on large-sample approximations. Both tests assume independent observations. These methods are widely applied in oncology screening trials and treatment comparisons to test equality of proportions.

For paired binary (dichotomous) data, as in assessing two interventions or diagnostic tests in the same sample or matched cohorts, McNemar's test is appropriate. This test evaluates the differences of the treatments by focusing on discordant pairs, the pairs of responses in which there is a disagreement between the two measurements.

Logistic Regression and Odds Ratio (OR)

Logistic regression plays a fundamental role when it is necessary to adjust for covariates (or stratification factors), such as disease stage or biomarker status, which may confound the effect of treatment on dichotomous results. By modeling the logodds of the binary response (presence or absence of cancer, treatment success) as a function of covariates, logistic regression facilitates hypothesis testing and estimation of the (adjusted) odds ratios (ORs, or relative odds) while controlling for common stratification factors in RCTs. This adjustment is particularly important to isolate the effect of experimental interventions when prognostic factors or baseline imbalances are present. Proper covariate adjustment generally leads to greater efficiency by reducing variability and enhancing statistical power, particularly when prognostic covariates are included in the model.

Analysis of Continuous Outcomes

Continuous endpoints, such as PROs, QoL scores, or tumor burden (e.g., percentage reduction in lesion size), are frequently encountered in RCTs and observational studies. The analysis of these outcomes centers on quantifying group differences, assessing variability, and modeling intervention effects using established statistical methods.

Measures of Central Tendency and Measures of Dispersion

- Descriptive statistics are foundational in summarizing continuous outcomes.
- Measures of central tendency consist of the mean, median, and mode. The mean provides the arithmetic average, the median indicates the middle value in the order sample, and the mode identifies the most frequent observation.
- Measures of dispersion quantify variability, commonly using the standard deviation (SD), interquartile range (IQR), and range. These describe the spread of observations and aid in characterizing population heterogeneity.

Comparison of the Means

Statistical comparison of continuous outcomes across groups employs several inferential methods:

- Independent t-tests are used to compare the means of two unrelated groups to determine if a significant difference exists between them. In contrast, paired t-tests assess whether the means differ significantly within the same group measured at two different times or under two conditions by analyzing matched or paired observations. These tests require a normality assumption.
- Analysis of variance (ANOVA) extends the independent t-tests to more than two groups or factors, detecting overall differences in means. The core principle of ANOVA is to partition the total observed variability in the data into components attributable to between-group differences and within-group (error) variability. While ANOVA determines if any overall differences exist, it does not specify which groups contribute the difference. Post hoc tests such as Bonferroni, Tukey's HSD, or Scheffe's test are used following a significant ANOVA to identify specific group contrasts. Its flexibility and capacity to handle complex experimental designs make ANOVA widely used in clinical trials and biomedical research to assess treatment effects and interactions among factors.
- Nonparametric methods (such as Wilcoxon rank-sum, Kruskal-Wallis) are alternatives when assumptions of normality or equal variances are violated.

Linear Regression and Mixed-Effects Models

Linear regression models estimate the relationship between a continuous outcome and one or more predictors, yielding both effect size estimates and p-values. The model assumes a linear relationship between the predictor and the outcome variable. Linear regression is flexible for adjusting multiple covariates simultaneously and is widely used for cross-sectional or single-time-point data where observations are independent.

However, when data consist of repeated measurements over time or clustering (e.g., multiple observations per subject or patients nested within hospitals), the independence assumption of linear regression is violated. This is where mixed-effects models play a key role. Mixed-effects models incorporate both fixed effects, which estimate the average population-level relationship between predictors and outcome, and random effects that account for subject-specific or cluster-specific deviations. By modeling these random effects, mixed-effects models handle within-subject correlation, irregular and unequal numbers of repeated measurements, and missing data, producing more precise and valid estimates [160]. In longitudinal studies, mixed-effects models allow each subject's trajectory to vary while estimating overall treatment effects. They effectively use all available data without requiring complete data at every time point and can model nonlinear trends through extensions such as spline functions. This adaptability makes mixed-effects models widely favored in oncology research for analyzing longitudinal endpoints or other hierarchical data structures, providing predictions at both the population and individual levels.

Survival Analysis: The Backbone of Cancer Trial Statistics

Time-to-event outcomes are central in oncology RCTs, particularly for survival endpoints. Survival analysis methods enable researchers to appropriately account for varying follow-up times, censoring, and the timing of events, which are inherent in oncology studies.

Censoring: What It Means and Why It Is Necessary

Censoring occurs when a patient's event time (e.g., death, disease progression, or recurrence) is not fully observed. This is common in oncology trials due to loss to follow-up, withdrawal, or because the patients have not experienced the event of interest when the study ends. Two main types of censoring are particularly relevant in oncology:

- Right censoring: This is the most common type and happens when the event of interest has not occurred by the last time the patient is observed. For example, a patient is still alive without progression at the study cutoff date, or they are lost to follow-up/move out of the community before progression is documented. The actual event time is only known to occur after the censoring time (if at all). Right censoring is standard in oncology survival analysis and is directly handled by Kaplan-Meier curves and Cox models.

- Left censoring: This occurs when the patients had already had the event prior to entering the study, but the exact timing is unknown. For instance, if a patient's cancer recurrence is discovered at enrollment but the precise date of recurrence is not available, only their true event time is known to be before the observed entry time. Left censoring is less common in oncology trials but may arise in registry studies, retrospective cohorts, or when biomarkers are measured after the onset of disease. Specialized statistical approaches (e.g., parametric survival models or Turnbull's estimator) are needed to address left censoring.

Life Table

Life tables were one of the earliest statistical tools used to summarize survival experience in clinical and epidemiological studies [161]. The method divides the total follow-up period into discrete intervals (e.g., weeks, months, or years) and estimates the probability of surviving through each interval. At the start of each interval, the number of individuals at risk is recorded, and the number of events (e.g., deaths, disease recurrence) and censored observations are noted. From this information, interval-specific survival probabilities are calculated, and these can be combined to estimate the cumulative probability of survival over time. Life tables also provide descriptive statistics such as median survival time, interval-specific mortality rates, and remaining life expectancy. In oncology, although Kaplan-Meier curves have largely replaced life tables for estimating survival, life tables remain valuable in certain contexts, such as population level cancer registries or and health economic evaluations.

Kaplan-Meier Curves: Reading and Interpreting Survival Plots

Kaplan-Meier (KM) curves provide nonparametric estimates of the survival function, plotting the probability of surviving beyond each time point. These curves visually demonstrate differences in survival between treatment arms, highlight periods of rapid risk change, and identify censoring times. Drops in the curve represent events, while tick marks indicate censoring. Key features include median survival, fixed-time survival rates (e.g., 1- or 5-year), and visual separation between treatment arms. Crossing curves may signal nonproportional hazards, such as delayed immunotherapy effects. While offering an intuitive summary, KM curves lack covariate adjustment and are less precise at later time points. They are typically complemented by Cox models to provide adjusted estimates and hazard ratios [162].

Log-Rank Test: Comparing Survival Distributions

The log-rank test is a nonparametric hypothesis test and commonly used alongside KM plots to compare survival distributions of two or more groups. By weighting observed versus expected event counts over time, the test assesses whether survival curves differ significantly across treatment arms. The stratified log-rank test extends the standard version to adjust for the effects of stratification variables (such as age groups, gender, or risk categories). Within each stratum, observed and expected event counts are calculated, and the overall test statistic is constructed by summing across strata. This approach controls for potential confounding by balancing risk factors, thus providing a fairer comparison between treatment arms when baseline covariates differ. Weighted log-rank tests (such as Tarone-Ware, Peto-Prentice, or Fleming- Harrington) introduce weights that emphasize specific time intervals, allowing better sensitivity when the proportional hazards assumptions do not hold [162]. For instance, the Fleming-Harrington test can give more importance to early or late differences between survival curves. These methods are especially valuable if hazards are expected to cross, or if treatment effects are delayed or diminish over time [163].

Choosing the appropriate weighting scheme should be matched to the expected pattern of nonproportionality. A significant log-rank result indicates a statistically significant difference in the OS experience between groups but does not quantify effect size nor specify when or how curves differ. Therefore, hazard ratios from the Cox models are often reported alongside log-rank p-values to give an estimate of effect magnitude.

Hazard Ratio and the Cox Proportional Hazards Model

Hazard ratios (HRs), which are estimated from the Cox proportional hazards model, quantify the relative risk of events between treatment arms while adjusting for covariates such as age or biomarker status. This semi-parametric model is the workhorse of oncology trials, enabling multivariable adjustment and interpretation of treatment effects on OS and PFS [162]. In immuno-oncology and other areas, the proportional hazards assumption often fails due to delayed treatment effects or crossing survival curves [163]. This has led to alternative analytic strategies, such as weighted log-rank tests that emphasize specific time ranges, restricted mean survival time (RMST) analyses that summarize average survival up to a fixed time, and landmark or milestone survival rates (e.g., 12- or 24-month OS). These methods provide robust inference when conventional Cox model assumptions are violated, ensuring reliable and clinically meaningful interpretation of survival benefits [12].

Subgroup and Biomarker Analyses

Heterogeneity in cancer biology often necessitates subgroup and/or biomarker analyses to evaluate whether some patients benefit more from treatment than others. For example, programmed death-ligand 1 (PD-L1) expression or genomic alterations (e.g., EGFR, ALK mutations in lung cancer) often inform treatment benefit. Additionally, subgroup analyses may be conducted based on non-biomarker characteristics such as sex (men vs. women), age groups, performance status, disease stage, or people with a particular germline genetic variant (e.g., BRCA1/2 mutations in breast and ovarian cancers). Prespecified subgroup analyses are typically explored using interaction tests within regression frameworks. While a priori subgroup analyses can provide critical insights into precision oncology, caution is warranted regarding post hoc analyses due to multiplicity and the risk of false-positive findings [70]. When interpreting the study results in the total study population, it is crucial to consider the generalizability, appropriateness, and sufficiency of the complementary subgroup, particularly in light of the disease context.

Interpreting and Critically Appraising RCT Results

Accurate interpretation and transparent reporting of oncology RCTs are essential for interpreting statistical findings to support evidence-based treatment decisions that matter to patients [118]. Oncology trials pose unique challenges, as they frequently deal with time-to-event outcomes like OS or PFS, as well as complex composite endpoints, and adaptive designs that allow for midcourse adjustments [117]. In this section, we discuss the principles that guide the interpretation of results, the distinction between clinical and statistical significance, and the importance of following reporting standards, so that research can be trusted and applied in practice.

Assessing Study Validity: Internal and External Validity

When reading a trial report, the first question is whether the study results can be trusted. This is often described in terms of internal validity, which refers to whether the observed results truly reflect the effect of the intervention under study. Threats to internal validity arise from different types of bias [164]. As described above, selection bias occurs if participants entering the trial differ systematically between treatment groups [165, 166]. Performance bias may appear if one group receives more attention or supportive care than another [167]. Detection bias arises when outcomes are assessed differently between groups, perhaps because investigators know which treatment was given [168]. Attrition bias occurs when patients drop out of the study unequally across groups, leaving incomplete data that can distort results [169]. Understanding these biases helps the reader judge whether the results are reliable.

External validity, or generalizability, answers a different question: Will these results apply to patients outside the context of an RCT (e.g., in the "real world") [116]? A trial may show a benefit in a highly selected group of patients, but if those patients are younger, healthier, or from a different population than the patients seen in practice, the findings may not be directly transferable [170]. For instance, an oncology trial limited to patients under the age of 60 may not reflect outcomes for older adults who may be more vulnerable to treatment toxicity [171]. Researchers should always carefully consider how closely the study participants resemble patients to which study results will be generalized [172].

Understanding the Clinical Significance of Results

Many readers focus first on whether a result is statistically significant, usually reported through a p-value or a confidence interval [172]. While this tells us how likely it is that the observed effect could be due to chance, it does not necessarily mean that the result is important for patient care. In contrast, clinical significance is about whether the effect size is large enough and relevant enough to change treatment decisions [173].

In oncology, some randomized trials demonstrate statistically significant survival improvements of only a few weeks, raising debate about clinical significance [174, 175]. While such a difference may reach the conventional threshold of statistical significance, many clinicians and patients would question whether such a small gain justifies exposure to toxic therapies or high treatment costs [176]. On the other hand, a study might show a clinically meaningful benefit, such as improved quality of life or a large survival gain, but fail to reach statistical significance if the sample size is small (e.g., if the study was an early-phase trial) [177].

The key point is that interpretation of both statistical and clinical significance is necessary. A trial with a p-value below 0.05 but minimal improvement in patient outcomes may not be worth adopting widely [178]. Conversely, results that are promising but not statistically definitive may still support further research or careful clinical use in selected patients [115]. For example, adjuvant treatments in early-stage breast cancer often undergo initial studies where benefits appear encouraging but need confirmation in larger, adequately powered trials. Balancing both views helps clinicians make patient-centered decisions [179].

Reporting Guidelines: CONSORT 2025 and Oncology-Specific Extensions

High-quality reporting is the foundation of transparency. The Consolidated Standards of Reporting Trials 2025 (CONSORT 2025) Statement provides updated guidance for randomized clinical trials, emphasizing the need to prespecify endpoints, estimands, and analysis strategies before the trial begins [180]. This avoids selective reporting and ensures that readers understand what the investigators intended to measure.

Oncology trials require additional considerations. Many use time-to-event endpoints such as OS, PFS, or DFS [15]. Each of these must be clearly defined, because different definitions can change how results are interpreted. Surrogate endpoints, such as tumor response rate, should be reported with a discussion of how well they predict long-term outcomes. Subgroup analyses, especially those based on biomarkers, are increasingly important in precision oncology, but they must be carefully reported to avoid overinterpretation [15]. Adaptive and multi-arm designs, which allow treatments to be added or dropped as data accumulate, require detailed explanation, so readers can follow how the trial evolved. Adhering to CONSORT and its oncology extensions allows clinicians, regulators, and patients to interpret findings with confidence [129].

Transparent Reporting of Estimands, Endpoints, and Interim Analyses

In recent years, the ICH E9(R1) addendum has emphasized the concept of estimands [181]. An estimand clearly specifies the treatment effect of interest while accounting for relevant events that occur after treatment starts, such as treatment switching, dose reductions, or discontinuations [11, 182]. Without clarity, two trials that both report overall survival may actually be answering different questions [141]. For example, one trial may analyze survival regardless of what treatment patients receive after disease progression, while another may analyze survival only while patients remain on the assigned therapy. These differences may result in significantly different conclusions, even though the outcome is labeled the same [183].

Similarly, interim analyses should be reported transparently. Oncology trials often stop early for benefit, futility, or safety [184]. If the stopping rules and timing are not clearly described, readers may overestimate the reliability of early results [184]. By specifying estimands, endpoints, and interim analyses in detail, trialists help prevent misinterpretation and enable fair comparisons across studies. This transparency also facilitates systematic reviews and regulatory assessments [11].

Conclusion: Translating Trial Evidence into Practice

Randomized clinical trials (RCTs) are the cornerstone of evidence generation in oncology, offering the most reliable foundation for assessing the efficacy and safety of new cancer treatments. This chapter has highlighted the key statistical considerations essential for the trial design, analysis, and interpretation of oncology RCTs.

We began by emphasizing the importance of randomization and allocation concealment in balancing prognostic factors across heterogeneous cancer populations. Various randomization methods, including simple, block, stratified, and minimization, allow flexibility depending on trial size, stratification requirements, and ethical considerations.

We also reviewed the spectrum of trial designs in oncology, from parallel-group superiority trials to non-inferiority and equivalence studies, factorial designs for combination therapies, and limited-use crossover trials. The design of randomized clinical trials in oncology has evolved to meet the unique challenges of cancer research, including disease complexity, long follow-up times, and the need for increasingly personalized therapies [88]. Each trial design serves a specific purpose and brings its own advantages and limitations. Parallel-group superiority trials remain the cornerstone, providing clear evidence when a new treatment improves outcomes [84]. Non-inferiority and equivalence trials are valuable when the objective is to demonstrate that a treatment is nearly as effective as the standard but safer, less costly, or more convenient [95]. Factorial designs allow multiple questions to be addressed simultaneously [100], while crossover designs, though rare in oncology, are particularly useful in supportive care studies [111]. Moreover, multicenter and global trials highlight the importance of diversity and generalizability, ensuring that findings apply across healthcare systems and populations worldwide [113]. This section also introduced advanced adaptive designs and master protocols such as umbrella, basket, and platform trials, which are increasingly important in the era of precision oncology. Adaptive designs represent a new era of efficiency and ethics, allowing researchers to make midcourse changes that benefit patients and accelerate discovery [122]. Master protocols embody the spirit of precision oncology, testing therapies in flexible, biomarker-driven ways that better match treatments to patients [124].

We discussed sample size and power considerations, highlighting the role of effect size assumptions, event-driven designs, stratification, interim analyses, and multiplicity in multi-arm and platform trials. Careful planning ensures trials are sufficiently powered to detect clinically meaningful effects while maintaining ethical standards.

Endpoints in oncology RCTs range from traditional survival measures such as OS to intermediate markers of disease activity like PFS, and most recently, novel biomarkers including MRD. Although OS remains the gold standard primary endpoint, increasing attention is being paid to the complementary role of alternative endpoints, particularly in the evaluation of adjuvant and neoadjuvant therapies [137]. Selecting appropriate endpoints involves balancing scientific rigor, clinical relevance, and regulatory requirements to ensure that the trial effectively captures clinically meaningful benefits while remaining feasible. The rise of precision oncology and adaptive trial designs has further complicated this process, underscoring the need for flexible and nuanced approaches. In addition, as cancer treatment modalities evolve, especially with the advent of new immunotherapies and the extension of patient survival, qualitative measures of clinical benefit, such as QoL and functional outcomes, are becoming essential secondary endpoints. Overall, endpoint selection in oncology trials must continue to adapt to align with emerging therapies, patient-centered priorities, and regulatory guidance to optimize both scientific validity and clinical impact.

Analytical approaches range from classical ITT analyses to advanced methods addressing nonproportional hazards and biomarker-defined subgroups. We summarized methods for binary outcomes (chi-square tests, logistic regression), continuous outcomes (t-test, ANOVA, regression, mixed models), and time-to-event outcomes (Kaplan-Meier estimation, log-rank tests, Cox proportional hazards regression, and methods for nonproportional hazards). Statistical analysis of oncology RCTs requires methodological rigor tailored to the complexity of endpoints and patient heterogeneity. Many common inaccuracies can be avoided by adhering to established statistical principles and guidelines, thereby enhancing the quality of research. Ultimately, careful methodological considerations are essential to ensure reliable evidence that supports both regulatory approval and clinical practice in oncology. Subgroup and biomarker analyses were emphasized to account for patient heterogeneity and facilitate precision oncology.

Finally, the chapter addressed interpretation and reporting, highlighting the distinction between statistical and clinical significance, the importance of both relative and absolute effect measures, and adherence to contemporary guidelines such as CONSORT 2025 and ICH E9(R1) estimand frameworks. Interpreting results from oncology RCTs requires more than checking whether the p-values are significant. It requires integrating statistical findings with clinical judgment, understanding potential sources of bias, and considering whether the study population reflects real-world patients. Absolute and relative measures should both be reported, and the clinical meaning of results should be explicitly discussed. Adherence to contemporary reporting standards, including CONSORT 2025 and ICH E9(R1), ensures that results can be trusted and applied to practice. Ultimately, careful interpretation helps bridge the gap between statistical analysis and meaningful improvements in patient care. Transparent reporting of endpoints, estimands, and interim analyses ensures reproducibility and regulatory compliance.

In summary, rigorous statistical design and analysis in oncology RCTs, combined with transparent and clinically relevant reporting, are essential for advancing cancer treatment and enhancing patient outcomes. As oncology trials continue to evolve with adaptive designs, biomarker-driven strategies, and novel endpoints, statisticians play a central role in ensuring that evidence is robust, interpretable, and actionable.

References

1. Gale RP, Zhang M-J, Lazarus HM. The role of randomized controlled trials, registries, observational databases in evaluating new interventions. Best Pract. Res. Clin. Haematol. 2023;36(4):101523. https://doi.org/10.1016/j.beha.2023.101523.
2. Harbour R, Miller J. A new system for grading recommendations in evidence based guidelines. BMJ. 2001;323(7308):334–6. https://doi.org/10.1136/bmj.323.7308.334.
3. Del Paggio JC, et al. Evolution of the randomized clinical trial in the era of precision oncology. JAMA Oncol. 2021;7(5):728–34. https://doi.org/10.1001/jamaoncol.2021.0379.
4. Booth CM, et al. Evolution of the randomized controlled trial in oncology over three decades. J. Clin. Oncol. 2008;26(33):5458–64. https://doi.org/10.1200/JCO.2008.16.5456.
5. Sankar K, et al. Pragmaticism in cancer clinical trials. Am Soc Clin Oncol Educ Book. 2024;44:e100040. https://doi.org/10.1200/EDBK100040.
6. Enserro DM, Gunn HJ, Elsaid MI, Duan F, Pugh SL. Challenges to and considerations of designing cancer prevention trials. JNCI Monogr. 2025;2025(68):49–55. https://doi.org/10.1093/jncimonographs/lgae044.
7. European Medicines Agency. Guideline on the evaluation of anticancer medicinal products in man. https://www.ema.europa.eu, 2023.
8. U.S. Food and Drug Administration. Table of surrogate end- points that were the basi of drug approval ORL ICEN sure. https://www.fda.gov/drugs/development-resources/table-surrogate-endpoints--were-basis-drug-approval-or-licensure. Accessed 20 Sept 2025.
9. Rojas-Saunero LP, et al. Intercurrent events in clinical research: the norm, not the exception. J. Bras. Pneumol. 2022;48(4):e20220310. https://doi.org/10.36416/1806-3756/e20220310.
10. International Council for Harmonisation (ICH). Ich e9(r1) statistical principles for clinical trials: addendum on estimands and sensitivity analysis in clinical trials. https://database.ich.org/sites/default/files/E9-R1_Step4_ Guideline_2019_1203.pdf, 2019.
11. Kahan BC, Morris TP, Scott JM, et al. The estimands framework: a primer on the ich e9(r1) addendum. BMJ. 2024;384:e076316. https://doi.org/10.1136/bmj-2023-076316.
12. Royston P, Parmar MKB. Restricted mean survival time: an alternative to the hazard ratio for the design and analysis of randomized trials with a time- to-event outcome. BMC Med. Res. Methodol. 2013;13:152. https://doi.org/10.1186/1471-2288-13-152.

13. Chen TT. Milestone survival: a potential intermediate endpoint for immune checkpoint inhibitors. J. Natl. Cancer Inst. 2015;107(9):djv156. https://doi.org/10.1093/jnci/djv156.
14. Wang Z, Wu H, Xie L, et al. Correlation of milestone restricted mean survival time ratio with overall survival hazard ratio in randomized clinical trials of immune checkpoint inhibitors: a systematic review and meta-analysis. JAMA Netw. Open. 2019;2(5):e193433. https://doi.org/10.1001/jamanetworkopen.2019.3433.
15. Hopewell S, Welch V, Boutron I, et al. Consort 2025: updated guideline for reporting randomised trials. JAMA. 2025;334(3):e2832868. https://doi.org/10.1001/jama.2025.2832868.
16. Tunn R, Bartlett V, Chan A-W, et al. Methods used to develop the spirit 2024 and consort 2024 statements. J. Clin. Epidemiol. 2024;163:1–11. https://doi.org/10.1016/j.jclinepi.2024.06.006.
17. Rosenberger WF, Lachin JM. Randomization in clinical trials: theory and practice. 2nd ed. Hoboken: Wiley; 2015.
18. Victora G, Habicht JP, Bryce J. Evidence-based public health: moving beyond randomized trials. Am. J. Public Health. 2004;94(3):400–5. https://doi.org/10.2105/AJPH.94.3.400.
19. Lustberg MB, Kuderer NM, Desai A, Bergerot C, Lyman GH. Mitigating long-term and delayed adverse events associated with cancer treatment: implications for survivorship. Nat. Rev. Clin. Oncol. 2023b;20(8):527–42. https://doi.org/10.1038/s41571-023-00776-9.
20. Piantadosi S. Clinical trials: a methodologic perspective. 3rd ed. Hoboken: Wiley; 2024.
21. Altman DG, Bland JM. Treatment allocation in controlled trials: why randomise? BMJ. 1999;318(7192):1209. https://doi.org/10.1136/bmj.318.7192.1209.
22. Altman DG, Schulz KF, Moher D, Egger M, Davidoff F, Elbourne D, et al. The revised consort statement for reporting randomized trials: explanation and elaboration. Ann. Intern. Med. 2001;134(8):663–94. https://doi.org/10.7326/0003-4819-134-8-200104170-00012.
23. Doig GS, Simpson F. Randomization and allocation concealment: a practical guide for researchers. J. Crit. Care. 2005;20(2):187–91. https://doi.org/10.1016/j.jcrc.2005.04.005.
24. Holmberg MJ, Andersen LW. Adjustment for baseline characteristics in randomized clinical trials. JAMA. 2022;328(21):2155–6. https://doi.org/10.1001/jama.2022.21506.
25. Wood L, Egger M, Gluud LL, Schulz KF, Juni P, Altman DG, et al. Empirical evidence of bias in treatment effect estimates in controlled trials with different interventions and outcomes: meta-epidemiological study. BMJ. 2008;336(7644):601–5. https://doi.org/10.1136/bmj.39465.451748.AD.
26. Little RJ, Rubin DB. Causal effects in clinical and epidemiological studies via potential outcomes: concepts and analytical approaches. Annu. Rev. Public Health. 2000;21(1):121–45. https://doi.org/10.1146/annurev.publhealth.21.1.121.
27. Pocock SJ, Simon R. Sequential treatment assignment with balancing for prognostic factors in the controlled clinical trial. Biometrics. 1975;31(1):103–15. https://doi.org/10.2307/2529712.
28. Seve P, Sawyer M, Hanson J, Broussolle C, Dumontet C, Mackey JR. The influence of comorbidities, age, and performance status on the prognosis and treatment of patients with metastatic carcinomas of unknown primary site: a population-based study. Cancer. 2006;106(9):2058–66. https://doi.org/10.1002/cncr.21.833.
29. Colnet B, Mayer I, Chen G, Dieng A, Li R, Varoquaux G, Vert JP, Josse J, Yang S. Causal inference methods for combining randomized trials and observational studies: a review. Stat. Sci. 2024;39(1):165–91. https://doi.org/10.1214/23-STS889.
30. Greenland S. Randomization, statistics, and causal inference. Epidemiology. 1990;1(6):421–9. https://www.jstor.org/stable/25759845
31. Lachin JM. Statistical properties of randomization in clinical trials. Control. Clin. Trials. 1988;9(4):289–311. https://doi.org/10.1016/0197-2456(88)90045-1.
32. Bertram JS. The molecular biology of cancer. Mol. Asp. Med. 2000;21(6):167–223. https://doi.org/10.1016/S0098-2997(00)00007-8.
33. Schulz KF, Grimes DA. Allocation concealment in randomised trials: Defending against deciphering. Lancet. 2002a;359(9306):614–8. https://doi.org/10.1016/S0140-6736(02)07750-4.
34. Devine EG, Waters ME, Putnam M, Surprise C, O'Malley K, Richambault C, Ciraulo DA. Concealment and fabrication by experienced research subjects. Clinl Trials. 2013;10(6):935–48. https://doi.org/10.1177/1740774513492917.
35. Nathe JM, Krakow EF. The challenges of informed consent in high-stakes, randomized oncology trials: A systematic review. MDM Pol Pract. 2019;4(1):2381468319840322. https://doi.org/10.1177/2381468319840322.
36. Tate, Spencer KL. High-stakes treatment negotiations gone awry: the importance of interactions for understanding treatment advocacy and patient resistance. J. Health Soc. Behav. 2024;65(2):237–55. https://doi.org/10.1177/00221465231204354.
37. Clark L, Fairhurst C, Torgerson DJ. Allocation concealment in randomised controlled trials: Are we getting better? BMJ. 2016;355:i5663. https://doi.org/10.1136/bmj.i5663.
38. Clark L, Dean A, Mitchell A, Torgerson DJ. Envelope use and reporting in randomised controlled trials: a guide for researchers. Res Methods Med Health Sci. 2021;2(1):2–11. https://doi.org/10.1177/2632084320957204.
39. Fisher RI, Miller TP, O'Connor OA. Diffuse aggressive lymphoma. ASH Educ Program Book. 2004;2004(1):221–36. https://doi.org/10.1182/asheducation-2004.1.221.
40. Stathis, Moore MJ. Advanced pancreatic carcinoma: Current treatment and future challenges. Nat Rev Clin. Oncol. 2010;7(3):163–72. https://doi.org/10.1038/nrclinonc.2009.236.
41. McEntegart D. Chapter 11: Block randomization. In: Balakrishnan N, editor. Methods and applications of statistics in clinical trials: concepts, principles, trials, and design. Wiley; 2014. p. 125–38. https://doi.org/10.1002/9781118736863.
42. Matts JP, Lachin JM. Properties of permuted-block randomization in clinical trials. Control. Clin. Trials. 1988;9(4):327–44. https://doi.org/10.1016/0197-2456(88)90047-5.
43. Schulz KF, Grimes DA. Generation of allocation sequences in randomised trials: Chance, not choice. Lancet. 2002b;359(9305):515–9.
44. Kernan WN, Viscoli CM, Makuch RW, Brass LM, Horwitz RI. Stratified randomization for clinical trials. J. Clin. Epidemiol. 1999;52(1):19–26.
45. Broglio K. Randomization in clinical trials: permuted blocks and stratification. JAMA. 2018;319(21):2223–4.
46. Chen X, Jing Y, Zhu H, Wang L. Sequential monitoring of covariate adaptive randomized clinical trials with non-parametric approaches. Stat. Med. 2025;44(6):e70042.
47. Gadgeel S, Rodr'ıguez-Abreu D, Speranza G, Esteban E, Felip E, Do'mine M, Hui, Garassino MC. Updated analysis from keynote-189: Pembrolizumab or placebo plus pemetrexed and platinum for previously untreated metastatic nonsquamous non-small-cell lung cancer. J. Clin. Oncol. 2020;38(14):1505–17.
48. Russnes HG, Lingjarde OC, Borresen-Dale A, Caldas C. Breast cancer molecular stratification: From intrinsic subtypes to integrative clusters. Am. J. Pathol. 2017;187(10):2152–62.
49. Trusheim R, Burgess B, Hu SX, Long T, Averbuch SD, Flynn AA, Lieftucht, et al. Quantifying factors for the success of stratified medicine. Nat. Rev. Drug Discov. 2011;10(11):817–33.

50. Coart E, Bamps P, Quinaux E, Sturbois G, Saad ED, Burzykowski T, Buyse M. Minimization in randomized clinical trials. Stat. Med. 2023;42(28):5285–311.
51. Lin Y, Zhu M, Su Z. The pursuit of balance: an overview of covariate-adaptive randomization techniques in clinical trials. Contemp Clin Trials. 2015;45:21–5.
52. Rosenquist R, Bernard E, Erkers R, Scott AW, Itzykson R, Rousselot P, Smedby KE, et al. Novel precision medicine approaches and treatment strategies in hematological malignancies. J. Intern. Med. 2023;294(4):413–36.
53. Azuaje F. Artificial intelligence for precision oncology: Beyond patient stratification. NPJ Precis Oncol. 2019;3(1):6.
54. Halabi S, Owzar K. The importance of identifying and validating prognostic factors in oncology. Semin. Oncol. 2010;37(2):e9–e18.
55. Crino L, Weder W, Van Meerbeeck J, Felip E, ESMO Guidelines Working Group. Early stage and locally advanced (non-metastatic) non-small-cell lung cancer: Esmo clinical practice guidelines for diagnosis, treatment and follow-up. Ann. Oncol. 2010;21(Suppl 5):v103–15.
56. Bae SY, Kim S, Lee JH, Lee H, Lee SK, Kil WH, Kim SW, Lee JE, Nam SJ. Poor prognosis of single hormone receptor-positive breast cancer: similar outcome as triple-negative breast cancer. BMC Cancer. 2015;15(1):138.
57. Roberts C, Torgerson DJ. Baseline imbalance in randomised controlled trials. BMJ. 1999;319(7203):185.
58. Garassino MC, Gadgeel S, Esteban E, Felip E, Speranza G, Domine M, Rodr'guez-Abreu D, et al. Patient-reported outcomes following pembrolizumab or placebo plus pemetrexed and platinum in patients with previously untreated, metastatic, non-squamous non-small-cell lung cancer (keynote-189): a multicentre, double-blind, randomised, placebo-controlled, phase 3 trial. Lancet Oncol. 2020;21(3):387–97.
59. Schrag D, Weng S, Brooks G, Meyerhardt JA, Venook AP. The relationship between primary tumor sidedness and prognosis in colorectal cancer. JAMA Oncol. 2016;2(12):1557–9.
60. Stout RL, Wirtz PW, Carbonari JP, Del Boca FK. Ensuring balanced distribution of prognostic factors in treatment outcome research. J. Stud. Alcohol Suppl. 1994;12:70–5.
61. Gross AS, Harry AC, Clifton CS, Della Pasqua O. Clinical trial diversity: an opportunity for improved insight into the determinants of variability in drug response. Br. J. Clin. Pharmacol. 2022;88(6):2700–17.
62. Lachin JM. Statistical considerations in the intent-to-treat principle. Control Clin Trials. 2000;21(3):167–89. https://doi.org/10.1016/S0197-2456(00)00046-5. ISSN 0197–2456. https://www.sciencedirect.com/science/article/pii/S0197245600000465
63. Fisher R, Pusztai L, Swanton C. Cancer heterogeneity: Implications for targeted therapeutics. Br. J. Cancer. 2013;108(3):479–85.
64. Polley MC, Freidlin B, Korn EL, Conley BA, Abrams JS, McShane LM. Statistical and practical considerations for clinical evaluation of predictive biomarkers. J. Natl. Cancer Inst. 2013;105(22):1677–83.
65. Sabapathy K, Lane DP. Therapeutic targeting of p53: all mutants are equal, but some mutants are more equal than others. Nat. Rev. Clin. Oncol. 2018;15(1):13–30.
66. Schmitt MW, Loeb LA, Salk JJ. The influence of subclonal resistance mutations on targeted cancer therapy. Nat. Rev. Clin. Oncol. 2016;13(6):335–47.
67. Msaouel P, Lee J, Thall PF. Interpreting randomized controlled trials. Cancers. 2023;15(19):4674.
68. Rosemann A. Alter-standardizing clinical trials: the gold standard in the crossfire. Sci. Cult. 2019;28(2):125–48.
69. Tannock IF, Amir E, Booth CM, Niraula S, Ocana A, Seruga B, Vera- Badillo F, et al. Relevance of randomised controlled trials in oncology. Lancet Oncol. 2016;17(12):e560–7.
70. Hu C, Dignam JJ. Biomarker-driven oncology clinical trials: key design elements, types, features, and practical considerations. JCO Precision Oncol. 2019;1:1–12.
71. Freidlin B, McShane LM, Korn EL. Randomized clinical trials with biomarkers: design issues. J. Natl. Cancer Inst. 2010;102(3):152–60.
72. Iasonos A, O'Quigley J. Adaptive dose-finding studies: a review of model- guided phase I clinical trials. J. Clin. Oncol. 2014;32(23):2505–11.
73. Le Tourneau C, Lee JJ, Siu LL. Dose escalation methods in phase I cancer clinical trials. JNCI J. Natl. Cancer Inst. 2009;101(10):708–20.
74. Yin G, Yuan Y. Bayesian model averaging continual reassessment method in phase I clinical trials. J. Am. Stat. Assoc. 2009;104(487):954–68.
75. Rubinstein LV, Korn EL, Freidlin B, Hunsberger S, Ivy SP, Smith MA. Design issues of randomized phase II trials and a proposal for phase II screening trials. J. Clin. Oncol. 2005;23(28):7199–206.
76. Simon R. Optimal two-stage designs for phase ii clinical trials. Control. Clin. Trials. 1989;10(1):1–10.
77. Sharma MR, Stadler WM, Ratain MJ. Randomized phase II trials: a long-term investment with promising returns. J. Natl. Cancer Inst. 2011;103(14):1093–100.
78. Strober E, Crowley JJ, Yamauchi PS, Olds M, Williams DA. Efficacy and safety results from a phase III, randomized controlled trial comparing the safety and efficacy of briakinumab with etanercept and placebo in patients with moderate to severe chronic plaque psoriasis. Br. J. Dermatol. 2011;165(3):661–8.
79. Noordzij M, Tripepi G, Dekker FW, Zoccali C, Tanck MW, Jager KJ. Sample size calculations: basic principles and common pitfalls. Nephrol. Dial. Transplant. 2010;25(5):1388–93.
80. Mok SK, Wu Y, Kudaba I, Kowalski DM, Cho BC, Turna HZ, Castro G, Srimuninnimit KK, Laktionov I, Bondarenko K, Kubota GM, Lubiniecki Z, Kush D, Lopes G. Pembrolizumab versus chemotherapy for previously untreated, pd-l1-expressing, locally advanced or metastatic non-small- cell lung cancer (keynote-042): a randomised, open-label, controlled, phase 3 trial. Lancet. 2019;393(10183):1819–30.
81. Lustberg MB, Kuderer NM, Desai A, Bergerot C, Lyman GH. Mitigating long-term and delayed adverse events associated with cancer treatment: Implications for survivorship. Nat. Rev. Clin. Oncol. 2023a;20(8):527–42.
82. Henry BM, Lippi G, Nasser A, Ostrowski P. Characteristics of phase IV clinical trials in oncology: an analysis using the clinicaltrials.gov registry data. Curr. Oncol. 2023;30(6):5932–45.
83. Hill TP. Conducting phase IV clinical studies: a moral imperative? ecancermedicalscience. 2012;6:276.
84. Richens A. Proof of efficacy trials: Cross-over versus parallel-group. Epilepsy Res. 2001;45(1–3):43–7.
85. Moher D, Hopewell S, Schulz KF, Montori V, Gøtzsche PC, Devereaux PJ, Elbourne D, Egger M, Altman DG. Consort 2010 explanation and elaboration: updated guidelines for reporting parallel group randomised trials. BMJ. 2010;340
86. Mentz RJ, Hernandez AF, Berdan LG, Rorick T, O'Brien EC, Ibarra JC, Curtis LH, Peterson ED. Good clinical practice guidance and pragmatic clinical trials: balancing the best of both worlds. Circulation. 2016;133(9):872–80.
87. Ligibel JA, Cirrincione CT, Liu M, Citron M, Ingle JN, Gradishar W, Martino S, Sikov W, Michaelson R, Mardis E, et al. Body mass index, pam50 subtype, and outcomes in node-positive breast cancer: Calgb 9741 (alliance). J. Natl. Cancer Inst. 2015;107(9):djv179.
88. Muss HB, Polley MC, Berry DA, Liu H, Cirrincione CT, Theodoulou M, Mauer M, Kornblith AB, Partridge AH, Dressler LG, et al. Randomized trial of standard adjuvant chemotherapy

regimens versus capecitabine in older women with early breast cancer: 10-year update of the calgb 49,907 trial. J. Clin. Oncol. 2019;37(26):2338–48.
89. Reck M, Rodríguez-Abreu D, Robinson AG, Hui R, Csőszi T, Fülöp A, Gottfried M, Peled N, Tafreshi A, Cuffe S, O'Brien M. Pembrolizumab versus chemotherapy for pd-l1–positive non–small-cell lung cancer. N. Engl. J. Med. 2016;375(19):1823–33.
90. Brahmer JR, Rodr'ıguez-Abreu D, Robinson AG, Hui R, Csoszi T, Fulop A, Gottfried M, Peled N, Tafreshi A, Cuffe S, et al. Health-related quality-of-life results for pembrolizumab versus chemotherapy in advanced, pd-l1-positive NSCLC (keynote-024): a multicentre, international, randomised, open-label phase 3 trial. Lancet Oncol. 2017;18(12):1600–9.
91. Christensen E. Methodology of superiority vs. equivalence trials and non-inferiority trials. J. Hepatol. 2007;46(5):947–54.
92. Flight L, Julious SA. Practical guide to sample size calculations: non-inferiority and equivalence trials. Pharm. Stat. 2016;15(1):80–9.
93. Lesaffre E. Superiority, equivalence, and non-inferiority trials. Bull. NYU Hosp. Jt. Dis. 2008;66(2)
94. Vulto G. Biologicals and biosimilars in hematology: the case of rituximab. HemaSphere. 2019;3(6):e322.
95. Laster LL, Johnson MF. Non-inferiority trials: the 'at least as good as' criterion. Stat. Med. 2003;22(2):187–200.
96. START Trialists' Group, et al. The UK standardisation of breast radiotherapy (start) trial b of radiotherapy hypofractionation for treatment of early breast cancer: a randomised trial. Lancet. 2008;371(9618):1098–107.
97. J. H. Ware and E. M. Antman. Equivalence trials, 1997.
98. Montgomery AA, Peters TJ, Little P. Design, analysis and presentation of factorial randomised controlled trials. BMC Med. Res. Methodol. 2003;3(1):26.
99. Baker TB, Smith SS, Bolt DM, Loh W, Mermelstein R, Fiore MC, Piper ME, Collins LM. Implementing clinical research using factorial designs: a primer. Behav. Ther. 2017;48(4):567–80.
100. Collins LM, Dziak JJ, Kugler KC, Trail JB. Factorial experiments: efficient tools for evaluation of intervention components. Am. J. Prev. Med. 2014;47(4):498–504.
101. Cheng C. Theory of factorial design. Boca Raton: Chapman and Hall/CRC; 2016.
102. Auspurg K, Hinz T. Factorial survey experiments, vol. 175. Sage; 2014.
103. Sharifi N, Gulley JL, Dahut WL. Androgen deprivation therapy for prostate cancer. JAMA. 2005;294(2):238–44.
104. Early Breast Cancer Trialists' Collaborative Group, et al. Effects of chemotherapy and hormonal therapy for early breast cancer on recurrence and 15-year survival: an overview of the randomised trials. Lancet. 2005;365(9472):1687–717.
105. Seymour MT, Maughan TS, Ledermann JA, Topham C, James R, Gwyther SJ, Smith DB, Shepherd S, Maraveyas A, Ferry DR, et al. Different strategies of sequential and combination chemotherapy for patients with poor prognosis advanced colorectal cancer (MRC focus): a randomised controlled trial. Lancet. 2007;370(9582):143–52.
106. Mills EJ, Chan A, Wu P, Vail A, Guyatt GH, Altman DG. Design, analysis, and presentation of crossover trials. Trials. 2009;10(1):27.
107. Sibbald B, Roberts C. Understanding controlled trials crossover trials. BMJ. 1998;316(7146):1719–20.
108. Haslam A, Prasad V. When is crossover desirable in cancer drug trials and when is it problematic? Ann. Oncol. 2018;29(5):1079–81.
109. Isbary G, Staab TR, Amelung VE, Dintsios CM, Iking-Konert C, Nesurini SM, Walter M, Ruof J. Effect of crossover in oncology clinical trials on evidence levels in early benefit assessment in Germany. Value Health. 2018;21(6):698–706.
110. Ishak KJ, Proskorovsky I, Korytowsky B, Sandin R, Faivre S, Valle J. Methods for adjusting for bias due to crossover in oncology trials. PharmacoEconomics. 2014;32(6):533–46.
111. Louis TA, Philip WL, Polansky M. Crossover and self-controlled designs in clinical research. In: Pepe MS, Fleming TR, Halperin MA, editors. Medical uses of statistics. Boca Raton: CRC Press; 2019. p. 83–103. ISBN 9780367400783.
112. Morrow GR, Hickok JT, Rosenthal SN. Progress in reducing nausea and emesis: Comparisons of ondansetron (zofran), granisetron (kytril), and tropisetron (navoban). Cancer. 1995;76(3):343–57.
113. Finfer S, Cook D, Machado FR, Perner A. Clinical research: from case reports to international multicenter clinical trials. Crit. Care Med. 2021;49(11):1866–82.
114. Senn SJ, Lewis RJ. Treatment effects in multicenter randomized clinical trials. JAMA. 2019;321(12):1211–2. https://doi.org/10.1001/jama.2019.1220.
115. Tunis SR, Stryer DB, Clancy CM. Practical clinical trials: Increasing the value of clinical research for decision making in clinical and health policy. JAMA. 2003;290(12):1624–32.
116. Rothwell PM. External validity of randomised controlled trials: "to whom do the results of this trial apply?". Lancet. 2005;365(9453):82–93.
117. Fountzilas E, Tsimberidou AM. Overview of precision oncology trials: Challenges and opportunities. Expert. Rev. Clin. Pharmacol. 2018;11(8):797–804. https://doi.org/10.1080/17512433.2018.1500894.
118. Estellat C, Torgerson DJ, Ravaud P. How to perform a critical analysis of a randomised controlled trial. Best Pract. Res. Clin. Rheumatol. 2009;23(2):291–303.
119. Hortobagyi GN, Stemmer SM, Burris HA, Yap Y, Sonke GS, Paluch- Shimon S, Campone M, Petrakova K, Blackwell KL, Wunsch C, et al. Ribociclib as first-line therapy for hr-positive, advanced breast cancer. N. Engl. J. Med. 2016;375(18):1738–48.
120. Tripathy S, Im M, Colleoni F, Franke A, Bardia N, Harbeck SA, Hurvitz C, Sohn J, Lee K, et al. Ribociclib plus endocrine therapy for pre- menopausal women with hormone-receptor-positive, advanced breast cancer (monaleesa-7): a randomised phase 3 trial. N. Engl. J. Med. 2018;379(2):173–84.
121. Berry DA. Adaptive clinical trials: the promise and the caution. J. Clin. Oncol. 2011;30(25):2576–7.
122. Chow S, Chang M. Adaptive design methods in clinical trials–a review. Orphanet J. Rare Dis. 2008;3(1):11.
123. Pallmann P, Bedding AW, Choodari-Oskooei B, Dimairo M, Flight L, Hampson LV, Holmes J, Mander AP, Sydes MR, Villar SS, Wason J, Weir CJ, Wheeler GM, Yap C, Jaki T. Adaptive designs in clinical trials: why use them, and how to run and report them. BMC Med. 2018;16(1):29.
124. Calvert M, Kyte D, Mercieca-Bebber R, Slade A, Chan A, King MT. Guidelines for inclusion of patient-reported outcomes in clinical trial protocols: the spirit-pro extension. JAMA. 2018;319(5):483–94.
125. Jennison C, Turnbull BW. Group sequential methods with applications to clinical trials. Boca Raton: CRC Press; 1999.
126. Kummar S, Chen HX, Wright J, Holbeck S, Millin MD, Tomaszewski J, Zweibel J, Collins J, Doroshow JH. Utilizing targeted cancer therapeutic agents in combination: Novel approaches and urgent requirements. Nat. Rev. Drug Discov. 2010;9(11):843–56.
127. Thall PF, Wathen JK. Practical bayesian adaptive randomisation in clinical trials. Eur. J. Cancer. 2007;43(5):859–66.
128. Kim ES, Herbst RS, Wistuba II, Lee JJ, Blumenschein GR, Tsao A, Stewart DJ, Hicks ME, Erasmus J, Gupta R, et al. The battle trial: personalizing therapy for lung cancer. Cancer Discov. 2011;1(1):44–53.

129. Coates E, Biggs K, Hamasaki T, Scott JA, Ando Y, Hind D, Altman DG, ACE Consensus Group, et al. The adaptive designs consort extension (ACE) statement: a checklist with explanation and elaboration guideline for reporting randomised trials that use an adaptive design. BMJ (Clinical research ed.). 2020;369
130. Woodcock J, LaVange LM. Master protocols to study multiple therapies, multiple diseases, or both. N. Engl. J. Med. 2017;377(1):62–70.
131. Park JJH, Siden E, Zoratti MJ, Dron L, Harari O, Singer J, Thorlund K. Systematic review of basket trials, umbrella trials, and platform trials: Implications for precision oncology. BMJ. 2019;364:k563.
132. Hirsch FR, Suda K, Wiens J, Bunn PA. New and emerging targeted treatments in advanced non-small-cell lung cancer. Lancet. 2016;388(10048):1012–24.
133. Hobbs BP, Pestana RC, Zabor EC, Kaizer AM, Hong DS. Basket trials: Review of current practice and innovations for future trials. J. Clin. Oncol. 2022;40(30):3520–8.
134. Flaherty KT, Gray R, Chen A, Li S, Patton D, Hamilton SR, Williams PM, Iafrate J, Sklar J, Banks P, Gocke CD, McShane LM, Harris LN, Mitchell EP, Boyle TA, Brodie S, Costantini C, Davids M, et al. The molecular analysis for therapy choice (NCI-match) trial: lessons for genomic trial design. JNCI J. Natl. Cancer Inst. 2020;112(10):1021–9.
135. Park JJH, Harari O, Dron L, Lester RT, Thorlund K, Mills EJ. An overview of platform trials with a checklist for clinical readers. J. Clin. Epidemiol. 2020;125:1–8.
136. Barker AD, Sigman CC, Kelloff GJ, Hylton NM, Berry DA, Esserman L. I-spy 2: an adaptive breast cancer trial design in the setting of neoadjuvant chemotherapy. Clin Pharmacol Therap. 2009;86(1):97–100.
137. Delgado A, Guddati AK. Clinical endpoints in oncology—a primer. Am. J. Cancer Res. 2021;11(4):1121–31.
138. Kilickap U, Demirci N, Karadurmus M, Dogan BA, Sendur MAN. Endpoints in oncology clinical trials. J. BUON. 2018;23(7):1–6. PMID: 30722104
139. McLeod C, Norman R, Litton E, Saville BR, Webb S, Snelling TL. Choosing primary endpoints for clinical trials of health care interventions. Contemp Clin Trials Commun. 2019;16:100486. https://doi.org/10.1016/j.conctc.2019.100.486.
140. U.S. Food and Drug Administration. Clinical trial endpoints for the approval of cancer drugs and biologics. Guidance for industry. https://www.fda.gov/ media/71195/download; 2018.
141. Driscoll JJ, Rixe O. Overall survival: still the gold standard: why overall survival remains the definitive end point in cancer clinical trials. Cancer J. 2009;15(5):401–5. https://doi.org/10.1097/PPO.0b013e3181bdc2e0.
142. Royle KL, Meads D, Visser-Rogers JK, et al. How is overall survival assessed in randomised clinical trials in cancer and are subsequent treatment lines considered? A systematic review. Trials. 2023;24:708. https://doi.org/10.1186/s13063-023-07730-1.
143. Fiteni F, Westeel V, Pivot X, Borg C, Vernerey D, Bonnetain F. Endpoints in cancer clinical trials. J Visceral Surg. 2014;151(1):17–22. https://doi.org/10.1016/j.jviscsurg.2013.10.001.
144. Therasse P, Arbuck SG, Eisenhauer EA, et al. New guidelines to evaluate the response to treatment in solid tumors. J. Natl. Cancer Inst. 2000;92(3):205–16. https://doi.org/10.1093/jnci/92.3.205.
145. Dancey JE, Dodd LE, Ford R, et al. Recommendations for the assessment of progression in randomised cancer treatment trials. Eur. J. Cancer. 2009;45(2):281–9. https://doi.org/10.1016/j.ejca.2008.10.042.
146. Mauguen A, Pignon JP, Burdett S, et al. Surrogate endpoints for overall survival in chemotherapy and radiotherapy trials in operable and locally advanced lung cancer: a re-analysis of meta-analyses of individual patients' data. Lancet Oncol. 2013;14(7):619–26. https://doi.org/10.1016/S1470-2045(13)70158-X.
147. Sargent DJ, Wieand HS, Haller DG, et al. Disease-free survival versus overall survival as a primary end point for adjuvant colon cancer studies: individual patient data from 20,898 patients on 18 randomized trials. J. Clin. Oncol. 2005;23(34):8664–70. https://doi.org/10.1200/JCO.2005.01.6071.
148. Eisenhauer EA, Therasse P, Bogaerts J, et al. New response evaluation criteria in solid tumours: revised recist guideline (version 1.1). Eur. J. Cancer. 2009;45(2):228–47. https://doi.org/10.1016/j.ejca.2008.10.026.
149. Hu C, Wang M, Wu C, Zhou H, Chen C, Diede S. Comparison of duration of response vs conventional response rates and progression-free survival as efficacy end points in simulated immuno-oncology clinical trials. JAMA Network Open. 2021. ISSN 2574–3805;4(5):e218175. https://doi.org/10.1001/jamanetworkopen.2021.8175.
150. Weber H-J, Corson S, Li J, Mercier F, Roychoudhury S, Sailer MO, Sun S, Todd A, Yung G, The Industry Working Group on Estimands in Oncology. Duration of and time to response in oncology clinical trials from the perspective of the estimand framework. Pharm Statist. 2024;23(1):91–106. https://doi.org/10.1002/pst.2340. https://onlinelibrary.wiley.com/doi/abs/10.1002/pst.2340.
151. Churruca K, Pomare C, Ellis LA, Long JC, Henderson SB, Murphy LED, Leahy CJ, Braithwaite J. Patient- reported outcome measures (proms): A review of generic and condition-specific measures and a discussion of trends and issues. Health Expect. 2021;24(4):1015–24. https://doi.org/10.1111/hex.13254.
152. Weldring T, Smith SMS. Article commentary: patient-reported outcomes (pros) and patient-reported outcome measures (proms). Health Serv. Insights. 2013;6:HSI.S11093. https://doi.org/10.4137/HSI.S11093. PMID: 25114561
153. Roila F, Cortesi E. Quality of life as a primary end point in oncology. Ann. Oncol. 2001;12(Suppl 3):S3–6. https://doi.org/10.1093/annonc/12.suppl/3.s3.
154. Prentice RL. Surrogate endpoints in clinical trials: Definition and operational criteria. Stat. Med. 1989;8:431–40. https://doi.org/10.1002/sim.4780080407.
155. Prasad V, Kim C, Burotto M, Vandross A. The strength of association between surrogate end points and survival in oncology: a systematic review of trial-level meta-analyses. JAMA Intern. Med. 2015;175(8):1389–98. https://doi.org/10.1001/jamainternmed.2015.2829.
156. Walia A, Haslam A, Prasad V. FDA validation of surrogate endpoints in oncology: 2005–2022. J Cancer Pol. 2022;34:100364. https://doi.org/10.1016/j.jcpo.2022.100364. ISSN 2213–5383. https://www.sciencedirect.com/science/article/pii/S2213538322000431
157. Medina-Herrera A, Sarasquete ME, Jime'nez C, Puig N, Garc'ıa-Sanz R. Minimal residual disease in multiple myeloma: past, present, and future. Cancers (Basel). 2023;15(14):3687. https://doi.org/10.3390/cancers15143687.
158. Molero-Calafell J, Buro'n A, Castells X, Porta M. Intention to treat and per protocol analyses: differences and similarities. J Clin Epidemiol. 2024;173:111457. https://doi.org/10.1016/j.jclinepi.2024.111457. ISSN 0895–4356. https://www.sciencedirect.com/science/article/pii/S0895435624002130
159. Smith VA, Coffman CJ, Hudgens MG. Interpreting the results of intention- to-treat, per-protocol, and as-treated analyses of clinical trials. JAMA. 2021. ISSN 0098–7484;326(5):433–4. https://doi.org/10.1001/jama.2021.2825.
160. Silveira LTY, Ferreira JC, Patino CM. Mixed-effects model: a useful statistical tool for longitudinal and cluster studies. J. Bras. Pneumol. 2023;49(2):e20230137. https://doi.org/10.36416/1806-3756/e20230137.
161. Cutler SJ, Ederer F. Maximum utilization of the life table method in analyzing survival. J. Chronic Dis. 1958;8(6):699–712.

162. Kleinbaum DG, Klein M. Survival analysis: a self-learning text. 3rd ed. New York: Springer; 2012. https://doi.org/10.1007/978-1-4419-6646-9.
163. Bouliotis G, Billingham L. Crossing survival curves: alternatives to the log-rank test. Trials. 2011. ISSN 1745–6215;12(1):A137. https://doi.org/10.1186/1745-6215-12-S1-A137.
164. McDermott R. Internal and external validity. In: Druckman JN, Green DP, Kuklinski JH, Lupia A, editors. Cambridge handbook of experimental political science. Cambridge: Cambridge University Press; 2011. p. 27–40.
165. Antman K, Amato D, Wood W, Carson J, Suit H, Proppe K, Carey R, Greenberger J, Wilson R, Frei E. Selection bias in clinical trials. J. Clin. Oncol. 1985;3(8):1142–7.
166. Longford NT. Selection bias and treatment heterogeneity in clinical trials. Stat. Med. 1999;18(12):1467–74.
167. McCambridge J, Sorhaindo A, Quirk A, Nanchahal K. Patient preferences and performance bias in a weight loss trial with a usual care arm. Patient Educ. Couns. 2014;95(2):243–7.
168. Widom CS, Czaja SJ, DuMont KA. Intergenerational transmission of child abuse and neglect: Real or detection bias? Science. 2015;347(6229):1480–5.
169. Hewitt CE, Kumaravel B, Dumville JC, Torgerson DJ, Trial Attrition Study Group. Assessing the impact of attrition in randomized controlled trials. J. Clin. Epidemiol. 2010;63(11):1264–70.
170. Mant D. Can randomised trials inform clinical decisions about individual patients? Lancet. 1999;353(9154):743–6.
171. Begg CB, Carbone PP. Clinical trials and drug toxicity in the elderly: the experience of the eastern cooperative oncology group. Cancer. 1983;52(11):1986–92.
172. Fowles JB, Kind AC, Craft C, Kind EA, Mandel JL, Adlis S. Patients' interest in reading their medical record: relation with clinical and sociodemographic characteristics and patients' approach to health care. Arch. Intern. Med. 2004;164(7):793–800.
173. Pocock SJ. Clinical trials: a practical approach. Wiley; 2013.
174. Fojo T, Grady C. How much is life worth: Cetuximab, non–small cell lung cancer, and the $440 billion question. J. Natl. Cancer Inst. 2009;101(15):1044–8.
175. Korn EL, Freidlin B, Abrams JS. Overall survival as the outcome for randomized clinical trials with effective subsequent therapies. J. Clin. Oncol. 2011;29(17):2439–42.
176. Page P. Beyond statistical significance: Clinical interpretation of rehabilitation research literature. Int J Sports Phys Ther. 2014;9(5):726–36.
177. Cheng JD, Hitt J, Koczwara B, Schulman KA, Burnett CB, Gaskin DJ, Rowland JH, Meropol NJ. Impact of quality of life on patient expectations regarding phase I clinical trials. J. Clin. Oncol. 2000;18(2):421.
178. Ioannidis JPA. The proposal to lower p value thresholds to 0.005. JAMA. 2018;319(14):1429–30.
179. Glück S, Mamounas T, Klem J. Improving outcomes in early-stage breast cancer. Oncology. 2010;24(4)
180. Peng Y, Lyu P, Peng X. Improving research transparency: an interpretation of the updated consolidated standards of reporting trials 2025 guideline from the perspective of clinical trials in oncology. Cancer Pathogenesis Ther. 2025;3:E01–29.
181. Ratitch B, Bell J, Mallinckrodt C, Bartlett JW, Goel N, Molenberghs G, O'Kelly M, Singh P, Lipkovich I. Choosing estimands in clinical trials: putting the ich e9 (r1) into practice. Ther. Innov.Regul. Sci. 2020;54(2):324–41.
182. Keene ON, Lynggaard H, Englert S, Lanius V, Wright D. Why estimands are needed to define treatment effects in clinical trials. BMC Med. 2023;21(1):276.
183. Oxnard GR, Morris MJ, Hodi FS, Baker LH, Kris MG, Venook AP, Schwartz LH. When progressive disease does not mean treatment failure: reconsidering the criteria for progression. J. Natl. Cancer Inst. 2012;104(20):1534–41.
184. Ciolino JD, Kaizer AM, Bonner LB. Guidance on interim analysis methods in clinical trials. J Clin Transl Sci. 2023;7(1):e124.

Mathematical Oncology: Bridging the Gap Between Theory and Clinical Practice

12

Renee Brady-Nicholls

Introduction

Cancer is a highly complex and heterogeneous disease characterized by uncontrolled cell growth, genetic mutations, and abnormal tissue interactions. It is a multiscale process whereby genetic mutations at a subcellular level manifest themselves as functional changes at the cellular and tissue scale [1]. Tumors evolve dynamically over time, and their behavior can vary greatly across patients due to factors such as their genetic background, tumor microenvironment, response to therapy, and environmental factors. Medical oncology typically focuses on diagnosing cancer and choosing the best treatment modality among those available. This might include surgery, chemotherapy, radiation, targeted therapy, or immunotherapy and is often done using a one-size-fits-all approach among patients with the same type of cancer. Determining the most effective treatment plan for an individual patient, tailored to their specific biology, is a crucial issue that needs attention. The key lies in accurately predicting the tumor's behavior and its response to treatments over time.

The field of mathematical oncology provides valuable tools to address this critical challenge. The purpose of mathematical oncology is to use quantitative models to better understand, predict, and treat cancer [1, 2]. This is especially relevant to medical physicians and clinical oncologists as mathematical models can provide insight that complements and enhances the clinical decision-making process. This interdisciplinary field draws from mathematics, biology, and clinical practice to offer new insights into cancer biology, so much so that mathematical models have had a significant impact on cancer research in the past 20 years [3–10]. Oncologists, as well as experimentalists, are beginning to recognize the potential that mathematical models hold for delivering a more mechanistic understanding of the complex biology and how they can be integrated into clinical practice.

Grounded in biological data or observations, mathematical models can be used to represent the intricacies of cancer cell development, growth, metastasis, and therapy response across multiple scales and cancer subtypes. Modeling can be used to describe the interactions of various cell subtypes (i.e., tumor and immune cells [11]). They can also forecast how tumors grow under different conditions and how they may respond to specific treatments [12]. Researchers also use models to simulate personalized treatment plans by incorporating patient-specific data such as longitudinal tumor volumes [13], liquid biopsy data [14], or tumor spatial characteristics [15, 16], which can subsequently be used to design personalized therapies to maximize efficacy and minimize side effects. Mathematical models are used in radiation treatment planning to compute the exact radiation dosage for each tumor, reducing the risk of side effects and improving overall survival rates [17]. While models have great potential, integrating them into daily clinical practice requires educating clinicians on how to interpret and use these models effectively.

This chapter aims to introduce medical physicians and clinical oncologists to the emerging field of mathematical oncology. To demonstrate the utility of mathematical oncology in clinical practice, we will describe a general tumor growth model and demonstrate how it can be used to make response predictions. Next, we will describe the advantages and common challenges faced in the field. Finally, we will end with highlighting research that has been conducted in cancer treatment and prevention.

R. Brady-Nicholls (✉)
Integrated Mathematical Oncology Department, Moffitt Cancer Center, Tampa, FL, USA
e-mail: renee.brady@moffitt.org

J. Huang, H. S.L. Jim (eds.), *Cancer Research Guidance for Clinicians and Researchers*,
https://doi.org/10.1007/978-3-032-19175-5_12

Practical Application

Modeling Tumor Growth

With unlimited resources, cancer cells grow and proliferate uncontrollably, continuously dividing without stopping. Mathematically, we can describe this exponential growth as

$$C(t) = C_0 e^{\alpha t},$$

where $C(t)$ describes the number of cancer cells present at time t. C_0 and α represent the number of cells initially present and the growth rate, respectively. Here, $C(t)$ is the solution to the ordinary differential equation (ODE) given by

$$\frac{dC}{dt} = \alpha C. \qquad (12.1)$$

Here, $\frac{dC}{dt}$ represents the change in C over time. This change is proportional to the number of cells present, modeled as αC. The value of α determines how fast the population changes (or grows) over time (Fig. 12.1a). Mathematically, C is the variable of interest and α is the model parameter or input.

Though this may accurately describe cells growing alone in a dish under perfect conditions, we know that resources such as oxygen, nutrients, and space become limited as the tumor expands due to the complex tumor microenvironment (TME). Blood vessels supplying the tumor often become disorganized and inefficient, leading to areas of low oxygen and nutrient shortages. Other cells in the TME, such as immune cells and fibroblasts, often compete with tumor cells for these nutrients, resulting in reduced proliferation of the tumor population. Given this, we can expand Eq. 12.1 to become the logistic growth [18] equation given by

$$\frac{dC}{dt} = \alpha C\left(1 - \frac{C}{K}\right), \qquad (12.2)$$

which is modulated by the parameters α and K. Like above, α represents the population growth rate. The carrying capacity K represents the maximum number of cells that the environment can sustainably support over time, given its limited resources. In general, logistic growth has a sigmoidal, S-shaped curve where the initial growth resembles exponential growth due to the population being far from its carrying capacity. As the population grows, resources become scarcer, growth slows, and the population approaches its carrying capacity. Mathematically, as the population rises, the ratio of population to carrying capacity C/K increases, which leads to a decrease in the net growth rate. A larger growth rate α will allow the population to reach the carrying capacity sooner, while a larger K allows for a larger population in the end. Figure 12.1b shows the logistic growth dynamics and how it slows in comparison to exponential growth due to dampening from the carrying capacity.

We will illustrate how this model can be used to characterize patient-specific tumor dynamics and predict individual patient responses. It is important to note that many models can accurately describe tumor dynamics and interactions with other variables. Ordinary differential equations, like the one presented above, can capture the interactions between multiple variables over time. We have chosen to focus on the logistic growth model because of its simplicity and wide applicability. Readers interested in exploring alternative ODE models are encouraged to look into those describing tumor growth [19, 20], tumor-immune interactions [15, 21, 22], treatment-sensitive and resistant population dynamics [23], and other models mentioned throughout the chapter.

We also encourage readers to explore other model types such as partial differential equations (PDEs), which can describe the dynamics of tumor growth and evolution by considering both spatial and temporal changes [24, 25]. These models incorporate the interactions between different variables, such as cancer cell density, nutrient levels, and other factors, that evolve over time and across space. PDEs are particularly useful in modeling cancer, because they allow for the inclusion of both spatial spread (tumor invasion) and temporal progression (cell proliferation, treatment effects, etc.), providing a more comprehensive understanding of how a tumor behaves in a physical environment. Agent-based models (ABMS) can also be used to represent tumor cells and other components (e.g., immune cells, stromal cells) as individual "agents" that interact based on pre-

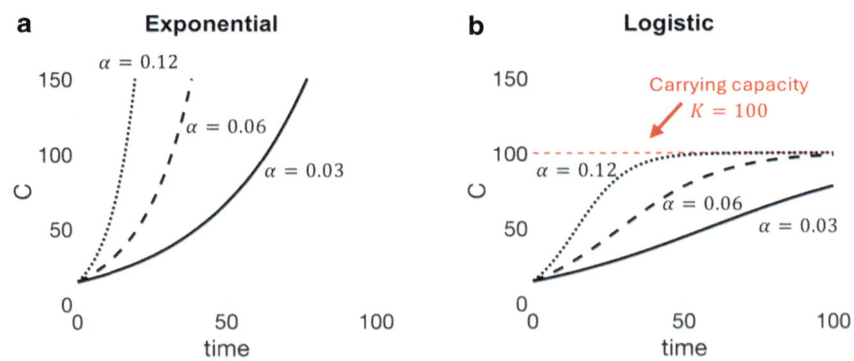

Fig. 12.1 Comparison between exponential and logistic growth dynamics. (**a**) Exponential growth with varying growth rates. (**b**) Logistic growth across varying growth rates with a carrying capacity $K = 100$. In both (**a**) and (**b**) $\alpha = 0.03$, 0.06, 0.12 for the solid, dashed, and double-dashed curves, respectively

defined rules [16]. These models simulate the behavior of each agent and its interactions with other agents, often using a discrete grid to represent the tissue.

Modeling Treatment Response

Once we have a general understanding of how the cancer population grows, we can begin to incorporate treatment and the effects it might have on individual patients. Mathematically, this can either be done explicitly, where treatment-related effects are added to the model equations, or implicitly, where treatment affects specific parameter values within the model. Here, we are going to assume that treatment affects the system implicitly by changing either the growth rate α or the carrying capacity K. To translate to data that we might observe in the clinic, we are going to consider tumor volume V as our variable of interest. Thus,

$$\frac{dV}{dt} = \alpha V\left(1 - \frac{V}{K}\right).$$

Suppose that we have tumor volumes from cancer patients undergoing treatment and we would like to use the logistic equation to analyze patient-specific dynamics to understand differences in response trends. To do this, we first need to determine parameter values for the individual patients that can be inputted into the equation above and accurately describe the dynamics seen in the data. Figure 12.2a shows the data for three representative patients. Patient 1 responds well to treatment, experiencing a consistent decrease in their tumor volume from one measurement to the next. Patient 2 does not respond well and shows an increase in tumor volume despite treatment. Patient 3 shows an overall decline in tumor volume, with a few fluctuations throughout.

We can use optimization techniques to determine appropriate values for α and K that minimize the distance between the data and the curve given by the model. It should be noted that optimization techniques are beyond the scope of this chapter. However, details on specific optimization methods can be found here [26, 27]. The model fits for Patients 1, 2, and 3 are also shown in Fig. 12.2b. While the model is able to accurately describe the dynamics for both Patients 1 and 2, it has difficulty determining parameter values for Patient 3 due to data fluctuations. By nature of its design, the logistic equation either strictly increases or decreases depending on the parameter values. It is not suited for non-monotonic dynamics and therefore cannot recapitulate unexpected increases or decreases in the data. The optimal curve for Patient 3 significantly overestimates the tumor volume at two points and underestimates at three others. Despite this, the model is still able to capture the general trend in the data. Analyzing the parameter values, we see that Patient 2 has a significantly higher growth rate and carrying capacity when compared to Patient 1 ($\alpha = 4.62E -02$, $K = 3.65$ for Patient 2 versus $\alpha = 1.34E -03$, $K = 0.1187$ for Patient 1). That is expected, given that Patient 2 is a nonresponder while Patient 1 is a responder. Patient 3 also has a low growth rate and carrying capacity ($\alpha = 1.965E -05$, $K = 0.0049$). These results demonstrate that the simple logistic model can accurately describe patient-specific dynamics.

Predicting Treatment Response

While developing models that can accurately describe trends observed in data is important, one of the most important applications in mathematical modeling is predicting how the tumor will continue to evolve over time. Brady and Enderling developed a pipeline to appropriately develop predictive models [28]. Once a model for a potential biomarker, such as tumor volume, is developed, it should be fitted to clinical data, and the results must be validated. Once these steps are completed, the model can be tested for its predictive ability. For brevity, we will skip the validation of the logistic model and instead will proceed to determine how well it can predict unseen data.

Imagine a patient has undergone three CT scans at different time points. Based on this data, the clinician wants to assess the likelihood that the patient will continue responding to treatment. A straightforward approach is to fit a model using the available data and project it forward to make a prediction. This process is shown in Fig. 12.3a for a representative patient. After fitting the model to the three available data points and projecting forward, the model predicts that the patient will continue responding until at least week 40. Now, if the patient undergoes an additional scan around week 20, showing continued response, the clinician may want to reassess whether the patient will keep responding. After fitting the model to all four data points, it predicts that progression will occur around week 35 (based on RECIST criteria, which defines progression as a 20% increase from the nadir in the sum of the longest diameters). Considering the patient's response so far and their tolerance to treatment (i.e., toxicity), the clinician can decide whether to continue or stop treatment. The model's predictions offer useful guidance in making an informed decision.

If the clinician chooses to continue treatment and the patient undergoes another scan around week 26, the model can be fitted to the five available data points, and a prediction can be made for the future. This predicts that the patient will progress around week 30. The clinician can then use this updated prediction, alongside earlier insights, to decide whether to proceed with or stop treatment. Figure 12.3b demonstrates the process for another representative patient. In this case, the model predicts that the patient will continue to respond at each prediction point.

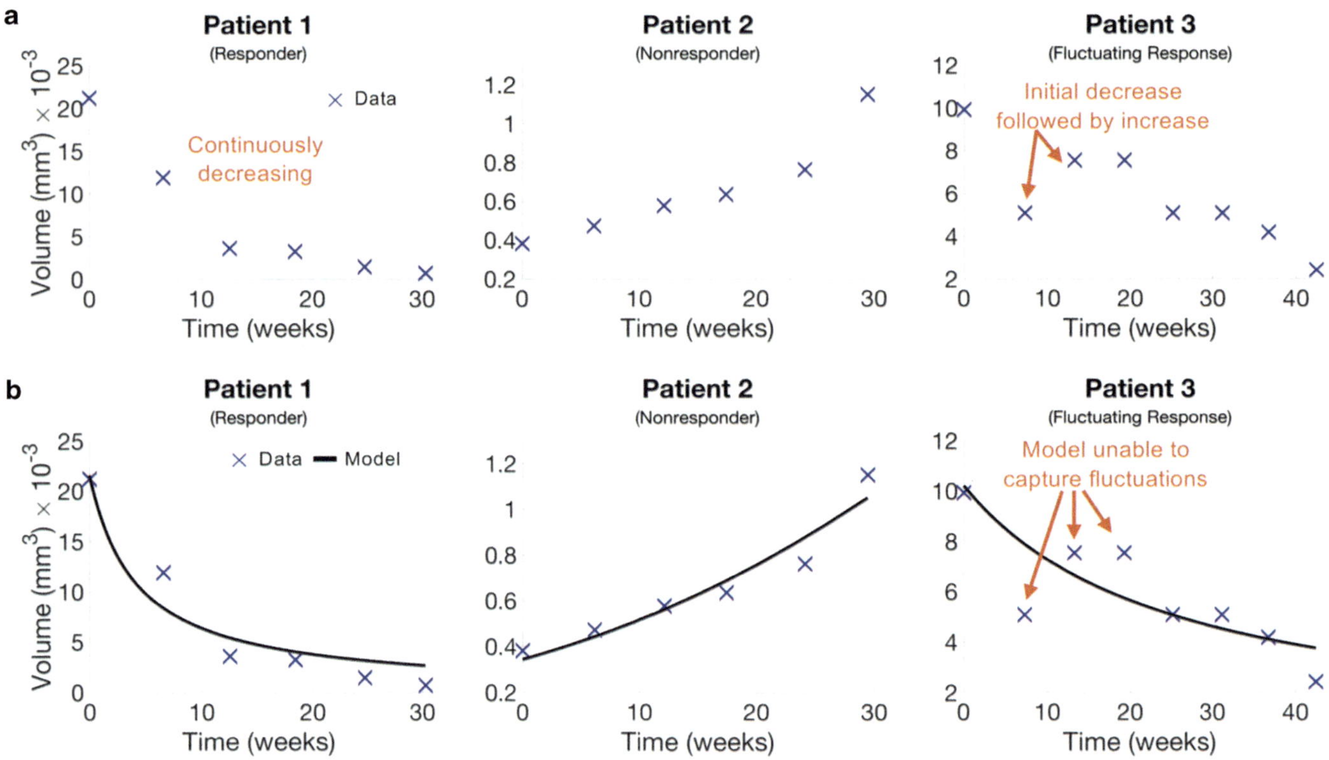

Fig. 12.2 Data and model fits for three representative patients. (**a**) Volumetric data (blue x's) for patients who (**a**) [1] respond well, (**b**) [2] do not respond, and (**c**) [3] have a fluctuating response. (**b**) Logistic equation model fits to the patient data. The model is able to describe the dynamics for the responder and nonresponder well. It is unable to capture the fluctuations in Patient 3's data due to the nature of the model

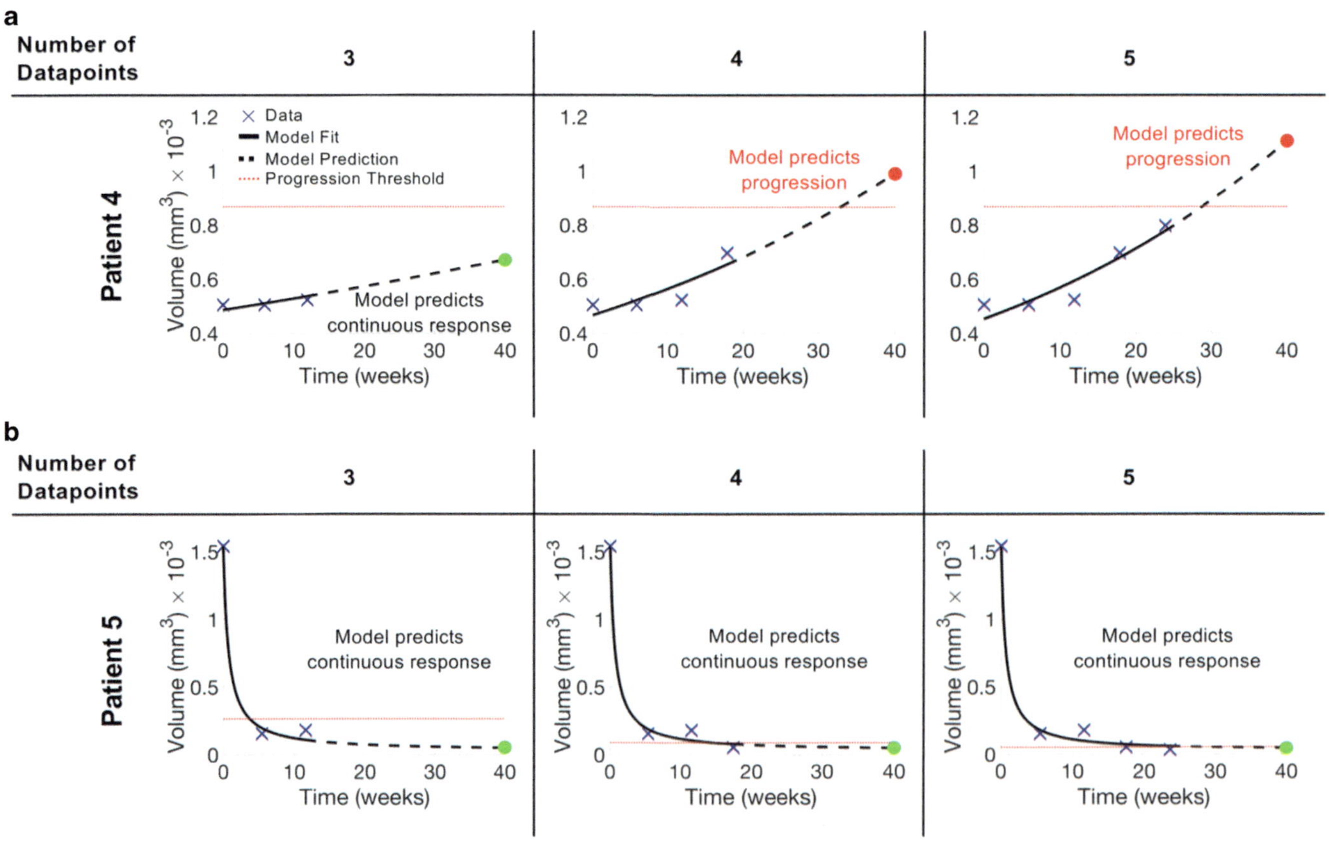

Fig. 12.3 Logistic model predictions. (**a**) Model predictions for a patient who develops progression. As more datapoints are acquired, the model is able to refine the predictions and accurately predict that the patient will develop progression. (**b**) Model predictions for a continuous responder. With just three available datapoints, the model can accurately predict that the patient will continue to respond

Benefits and Challenges of Mathematical Oncology

As we create new mathematical models to better understand and predict cancer, and as these models become more integrated into clinical practice, we begin to recognize their value and the potential impact they may have in the future. Due to the complexity and variability of cancer, it is impossible to pinpoint every pathway and cell interaction driving the disease. However, mathematical models can simulate the interactions between cancer cells, the immune system, and treatment factors, offering deeper insights into the biological processes behind cancer and the factors influencing treatment outcomes.

Moreover, mathematical models have the potential to revolutionize personalized medicine and treatment optimization. By developing models that reflect the unique dynamics of each patient, we can create treatment plans that are tailored to their specific condition and biology. These models help optimize treatment regimens by predicting the most effective dosages, combinations, or strategies to maximize the likelihood of success and minimize side effects. While clinical trials typically focus on testing a single treatment for a patient at a time, mathematical models enable the simulation of in silico trials to identify the most effective treatments or combinations on a patient-by-patient basis. These models also allow the exploration of hypothetical treatment scenarios, helping to uncover strategies that may be difficult or impractical to test directly in clinical trials, thus guiding future research and clinical studies.

It is important to recognize that the field of mathematical oncology also has its drawbacks. One issue is the reliance on simplified assumptions, which may fail to fully capture the complexity of cancer biology. Oversimplification can lead to inaccurate predictions or an incomplete understanding of disease dynamics. For instance, while the exponential and logistic models have traditionally been used to describe tumor volume dynamics, they do not account for resistance in the presence of treatment. Alternative models, such as the tumor growth inhibition model (TGI), account for resistance by allowing the effect of treatment to exponentially decay over time. This requires including an additional compartment and parameters into the model. Some models may be overly complex, making unrealistic predictions that do not align with the true biology of the disease. Another significant challenge is the limitations of available datasets. While models can be theoretically sound, they must be validated against real clinical outcomes to ensure they accurately reflect the underlying biology. This requires careful calibration and validation with clinical data. Often, the data used for model development is collected at a single time point, lacks important spatial information, is averaged across patients, or is limited to a small subset of patients, making it incomplete or noisy. In these cases, it becomes challenging to calibrate and validate models accurately, leading to uncertainties in their predictions. Striking a balance between model complexity and the quality of available data is essential.

As mathematical models become more integrated into clinical practice, it's crucial to understand that they should serve as tools to aid decision-making, not replace clinical judgment. They should never override patient preferences, overall health, or quality of life considerations. Furthermore, it's important to remain aware of the model's limitations, as it can only describe certain aspects of the complex biological processes involved. Despite these challenges, mathematical oncology remains a promising tool for enhancing cancer research and treatment.

Past and Current Contributions to Clinical Practice

Changing the Treatment Paradigm in Prostate Cancer

The evolution of resistance is a common cause of treatment failure and tumor progression across all cancer types. The conventional treatment strategy consists of continuous treatment at the maximally tolerated dose until the development of resistance. While continuous treatment can eradicate the sensitive population, it also strongly eliminates all potential competitors for the resistant population, thereby resulting in the selection for this population—a concept coined competitive release. Recognizing the flaws in such a treatment design, Zhang et al. [7] sought to change the treatment paradigm in prostate cancer. In this new design, they proposed to maintain the competition between the sensitive and resistant populations by administering treatment only until a sufficient proportion of the sensitive population were eliminated and before resistance develops, leaving enough of the sensitive population to successfully compete with the resistant population. Treatment would be withheld until the sensitive population regrew, and then treatment would begin again and continue to be cycled on and off.

Using a competition model of androgen independent, androgen dependent, and testosterone-producing phenotypes, they modeled changes in prostate-specific antigen (PSA) levels under this adaptive therapy. Model simulations demonstrated that evolutionary dynamics could be exploited to maintain the androgen dependent and testosterone-producing populations. When comparing between time to progression between adaptive and continuous therapy, they found that adaptive therapy was superior. These finding inspired a pilot trial of adaptive therapy in 17 metastatic castration-resistant prostate cancer patients. When compared to a contemporaneous cohort of 16 patients receiving continuous therapy, they found that adaptive therapy could significantly increase time to progression (33.5 months versus 14.3 months, $p < 0.001$), with less time on treatment [29].

Personalizing Radiation Therapy

In conventional clinical practice, most patients treated with radiation receive a similar dose and fractionation schedule based on the cancer type and stage, without regard for patient-specific tumor or host factors that might influence the response. While this results in favorable outcomes for some patients, others suffer from life-altering adverse events and minimal response. Given this, Prokopiou et al. aimed to determine a prognostic biomarker to personalize radiation therapy.

They started by developing a mathematical model of volumetric response to radiation therapy. The model was calibrated to longitudinal volume measurements from patients receiving radiation therapy, and the model parameters were analyzed to determine correlates with radiation response. They found that the proliferation saturation index (PSI), which is defined as the ratio of tumor volume to the host-influenced carrying capacity, was inversely correlated with treatment response. PSI is estimated from two temporally separated routine pretreatment computed tomography scans and a deterministic logistic growth tumor model. They found that larger PSI reflect a low proliferating cell fraction, and thus, treatment refractory tumors, whereas tumors with low PSI are more proliferative and radiosensitive. Model simulations demonstrated that patients with a higher PSI might benefit from hyperfractionated radiation therapy rather than conventional fractionation.

Inspired by these findings, oncologists at Moffitt Cancer Center conducted a clinical trial in 55 head and neck patients undergoing radiation therapy. Patients were stratified according to their PSI, with those with PSI greater than 0.75 receiving hyperfractionated radiation and those with PSI less than or equal to 0.75 receiving standard radiation. The primary endpoint was increasing the proportion of patients who experience a 32% or more tumor reduction by week four of treatment, which was shown to be predictive of locoregional control and disease-free survival. They reported a median 40% reduction in tumor volume by week four, with 61% of the patients achieving this [30].

Ongoing Contributions to Clinical Care

A series of clinical trials are currently underway, driven by insights from mathematical modeling. Adaptive therapy is being used to treat metastatic castration-sensitive prostate cancer [31], ovarian cancer [23], and BRAF-mutant melanoma [32]. Mathematical models describing the evolutionary dynamics of treatment [33]—whether administered individually, sequentially, or adaptively—have inspired a clinical trial for metastatic, fusion-positive rhabdomyosarcoma. In this trial, four different treatment arms are being compared, with the primary goal of improving overall survival from 6% to 35%. Trials investigating "first-strike, second-strike" sequential therapy, based on eco-evolutionary dynamics of Anthropocene extinctions [34], are being conducted in metastatic prostate cancer [35] and hormone-positive breast cancer. Additionally, an evolutionary tumor board has been developed to conduct a pilot study to develop therapeutic strategies for patients with no curative options. This interdisciplinary approach combines clinical, preclinical, and theoretical knowledge, using mathematical modeling to predict patient responses to various therapies, including novel methods grounded in eco-evolutionary principles [36].

Conclusions

From these and others, it is evident that mathematical oncology offers oncologists a powerful toolkit to better understand and treat cancer. By embracing these models, clinical oncologists can improve their ability to predict tumor behavior, personalize treatment plans, and optimize therapeutic outcomes. As the field advances, mathematical oncology will increasingly complement traditional clinical expertise, helping oncologists make more informed decisions that lead to better patient outcomes.

References

1. Anderson ARA, Maini PK. Mathematical oncology. Bull Math Biol. 2018;80(5):945–53.
2. Anderson AR, Quaranta V. Integrative mathematical oncology. Nat Rev Cancer. 2008;8(3):227–34.
3. Brady-Nicholls R, Nagy JD, Gerke TA, Zhang T, Wang AZ, Zhang J, et al. Prostate-specific antigen dynamics predict individual responses to intermittent androgen deprivation. Nat Commun. 2020;11(1):1750.
4. Poleszczuk J, Enderling H. The optimal radiation dose to induce robust systemic anti-tumor immunity. Int J Mol Sci. 2018;19(11)
5. Basanta D, Gatenby RA, Anderson AR. Exploiting evolution to treat drug resistance: combination therapy and the double bind. Mol Pharm. 2012;9(4):914–21.
6. Gatenby RA, Maini PK. Mathematical oncology: cancer summed up. Nature. 2003;421(6921):321.
7. Zhang J, Cunningham JJ, Brown JS, Gatenby RA. Integrating evolutionary dynamics into treatment of metastatic castrate-resistant prostate cancer. Nat Commun. 2017;8(1):1816.
8. Hawkins-Daarud A, Rockne R, Corwin D, Anderson AR, Kinahan P, Swanson KR. In silico analysis suggests differential response to bevacizumab and radiation combination therapy in newly diagnosed glioblastoma. J R Soc Interface. 2015;12(109):20150388.
9. Li X, Abramson RG, Arlinghaus LR, Kang H, Chakravarthy AB, Abramson VG, et al. Multiparametric magnetic resonance imaging for predicting pathological response after the first cycle of Neoadjuvant chemotherapy in breast cancer. Investig Radiol. 2015;50(4):195–204.

10. Rockne RC, Hawkins-Daarud A, Swanson KR, Sluka JP, Glazier JA, Macklin P, et al. The 2019 mathematical oncology roadmap. Phys Biol. 2019;16(4):041005.
11. Kuznetsov VA, Knott GD. Modeling tumor regrowth and immunotherapy. Math Comput Model. 2001;33(12):1275–87.
12. West J, You L, Zhang J, Gatenby RA, Brown JS, Newton PK, et al. Towards multidrug adaptive therapy. Cancer Res. 2020;80(7):1578–89.
13. Zahid MU, Mohsin N, Mohamed ASR, Caudell JJ, Harrison LB, Fuller CD, et al. Forecasting individual patient response to radiation therapy in head and neck cancer with a dynamic carrying capacity model. Int J Radiat Oncol Biol Phys. 2021;111(3):693–704.
14. Brady-Nicholls R, Zhang J, Zhang T, Wang AZ, Butler R, Gatenby RA, et al. Predicting patient-specific response to adaptive therapy in metastatic castration-resistant prostate cancer using prostate-specific antigen dynamics. Neoplasia (New York, NY). 2021;23(9):851–8.
15. Bekker RA, Kim S, Pilon-Thomas S, Enderling H. Mathematical modeling of radiotherapy and its impact on tumor interactions with the immune system. Neoplasia (New York, NY). 2022;28:100796.
16. Gallaher JA, Enriquez-Navas PM, Luddy KA, Gatenby RA, Anderson ARA. Spatial heterogeneity and evolutionary dynamics modulate time to recurrence in continuous and adaptive cancer therapies. Cancer Res. 2018;78(8):2127–39.
17. Zahid MU, Mohamed ASR, Caudell JJ, Harrison LB, Fuller CD, Moros EG, et al. Dynamics-adapted radiotherapy dose (DARD) for head and neck cancer radiotherapy dose personalization. J Pers Med. 2021;11(11)
18. Harshe I, Enderling H, Brady-Nicholls R. Predicting patient-specific tumor dynamics: how many measurements are necessary? Cancer. 2023;15(5)
19. Benzekry S, Lamont C, Beheshti A, Tracz A, Ebos JM, Hlatky L, et al. Classical mathematical models for description and prediction of experimental tumor growth. PLoS Comput Biol. 2014;10(8):e1003800.
20. Vaidya VG, Alexandro FJ Jr. Evaluation of some mathematical models for tumor growth. Int J Biomed Comput. 1982;13(1):19–36.
21. Robertson-Tessi M, El-Kareh A, Goriely A. A mathematical model of tumor-immune interactions. J Theor Biol. 2012;294:56–73.
22. Wilkie KP. A review of mathematical models of cancer-immune interactions in the context of tumor dormancy. Adv Exp Med Biol. 2013;734:201–34.
23. Strobl M, Martin AL, West J, Gallaher J, Robertson-Tessi M, Gatenby R, et al. Adaptive therapy for ovarian cancer: an integrated approach to PARP inhibitor scheduling. bioRxiv. 2023;
24. Karolak A, Markov DA, McCawley LJ, Rejniak KA. Towards personalized computational oncology: from spatial models of tumour spheroids, to organoids, to tissues. J R Soc Interface. 2018;15(138)
25. Jarrett AM, Kazerouni AS, Wu C, Virostko J, Sorace AG, DiCarlo JC, et al. Quantitative magnetic resonance imaging and tumor forecasting of breast cancer patients in the community setting. Nat Protoc. 2021;16(11):5309–38.
26. Poli R, Kennedy J, Blackwell T. Particle swarm optimization. Swarm Intelligence. 2007;1(1):33.
27. Hassan R, Cohanim B, de Weck O, Venter G. A comparison of particle swarm optimization and the genetic algorithm. In: 46th AIAA/ASME/ASCE/AHS/ASC structures, structural dynamics and materials conference. Structures, structural dynamics, and materials and co-located conferences. American Institute of Aeronautics and Astronautics; 2005.
28. Brady R, Enderling H. Mathematical models of cancer: when to predict novel therapies, and when not to. Bull Math Biol. 2019;81:3722.
29. Zhang J, Cunningham J, Brown J, Gatenby R. Evolution-based mathematical models significantly prolong response to abiraterone in metastatic castrate-resistant prostate cancer and identify strategies to further improve outcomes. elife. 2022;11:11.
30. Caudell J, Echevarria M, Yang G, Kim Y, Kirtane K, Kish J, et al. Prospective trial of personalized fractionation in low-risk HPV positive oropharyngeal cancer. ESTRO 2023 Annual Meeting [abstract]; 2023.
31. Zhang J, Gallaher J, Cunningham JJ, Choi JW, Ionescu F, Chatwal MS, et al. A phase 1b adaptive androgen deprivation therapy trial in metastatic castration sensitive prostate cancer. Cancer. 2022;14(21)
32. Kim E, Brown JS, Eroglu Z, Anderson ARA. Adaptive therapy for metastatic melanoma: predictions from patient calibrated mathematical models. Cancer. 2021;13(4)
33. Gatenby RA, Brown JS. Integrating evolutionary dynamics into cancer therapy. Nat Rev Clin Oncol. 2020;17(11):675–86.
34. Gatenby RA, Artzy-Randrup Y, Epstein T, Reed DR, Brown JS. Eradicating metastatic cancer and the eco-evolutionary dynamics of anthropocene extinctions. Cancer Res. 2020;80(3):613–23.
35. Zhang J, Gallaher J, Chatwal MS, Jain RK, Chadha J, Li R, et al. A phase IIa study of sequential ("first strike, second strike") therapies, modeled on evolutionary dynamics of anthropocene extinctions, for high-risk metastatic castration-sensitive prostate cancer. J Clin Oncol. 2024;42:TPS245.
36. Robertson-Tessi M, Brown JS, Poole MI, Johnson M, Marusyk A, Gallaher JA, et al. Feasibility of an Evolutionary Tumor Board for Generating Novel Personalized Therapeutic Strategies. medRxiv. 2023:2023.01.18.23284628.

AI and Cancer Research

13

Eungjoo Lee, Vivek Kumar Singh,
Md Mostafa Kamal Sarker, Krishna Saveri Vydyula,
and Laura J. Brattain

Introduction

Cancer remains one of the most complex and pressing global health challenges, making the search for better methods of detection, treatment, and prevention a top international priority. In recent years, artificial intelligence (AI), a powerful form of computer technology that learns from data, has emerged as a transformative tool in this effort. Far from being science fictions, AI enables computers to detect subtle patterns across vast datasets with speed and precision that surpass human capabilities. A bibliometric analysis of AI applications in cancer research from 1983 to 2022 identified 6920 relevant publications, with a surge in the last 5 years. This recent acceleration highlights the growing integration of AI into cancer research, catalyzing advances across multiple domains. Figure 13.1 illustrates the rising trend of AI-related cancer publications from 2019 to 2024, stratified by major cancer types [1]. Notably, research in breast and lung cancer has seen sharp and sustained growth, fueled by AI innovations [2–4], while colorectal cancer, brain tumors (e.g., gliomas), and liver cancer also show upward trends, though at a more moderate pace [5–7]. Figure 13.2 presents a word cloud generated from recent publications, highlighting key terms such as "machine learning," "computer vision," "convolutional neural networks," "foundation models," and "transformers," which dominate the AI cancer research landscape.

AI is now making significant contributions across the cancer care continuum, including early detection, more accurate diagnosis, treatment planning, and personalized medicine. This chapter begins by introducing the key areas where AI is driving meaningful impact in cancer care. We then provide a brief overview of core AI techniques and concepts, followed by an in-depth case study of breast cancer to demonstrate how AI is shaping real-world clinical practice. The chapter also examines the landscape of cancer-related AI datasets, again using breast cancer as a representative example. We conclude with a discussion of the major challenges facing AI in cancer research and care, followed by final reflections on the path forward.

E. Lee (✉)
Department of Electrical and Computer Engineering, University of Arizona, Tucson, AZ, USA
e-mail: eungjoolee@arizona.edu

V. K. Singh (✉) · K. S. Vydyula
Centre for Biomarkers and Biotherapeutics, Barts Cancer Institute, Queen Mary University of London, London, UK
e-mail: vivek.singh@qmul.ac.uk; k.s.vydyula@smd20.qmul.ac.uk

M. M. K. Sarker
Nuffield Department of Medicine (NDM), University of Oxford, Oxford, UK

L. J. Brattain
Department of Internal Medicine, University of Central Florida College of Medicine, Orlando, FL, USA
e-mail: laura.brattain@ucf.edu

J. Huang, H. S.L. Jim (eds.), *Cancer Research Guidance for Clinicians and Researchers*,
https://doi.org/10.1007/978-3-032-19175-5_13

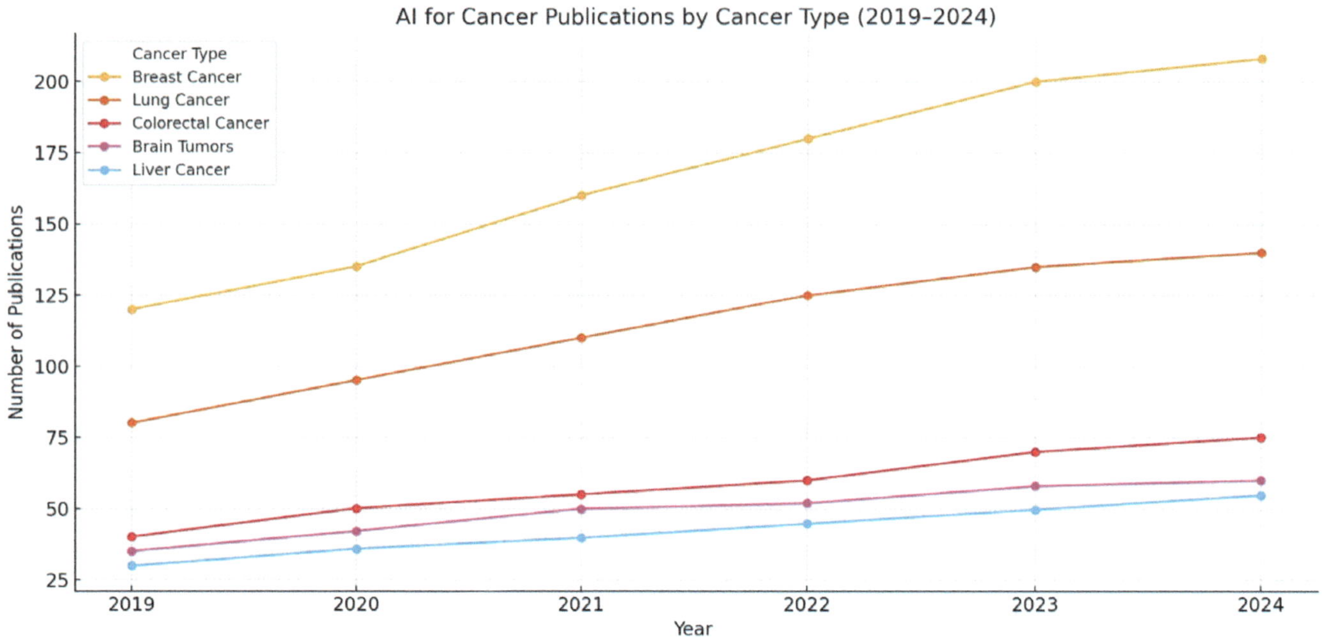

Fig. 13.1 AI cancer publications trend by type (2019–2024)

Fig. 13.2 Word cloud illustrating the prominent keywords associated with the AI in cancer research

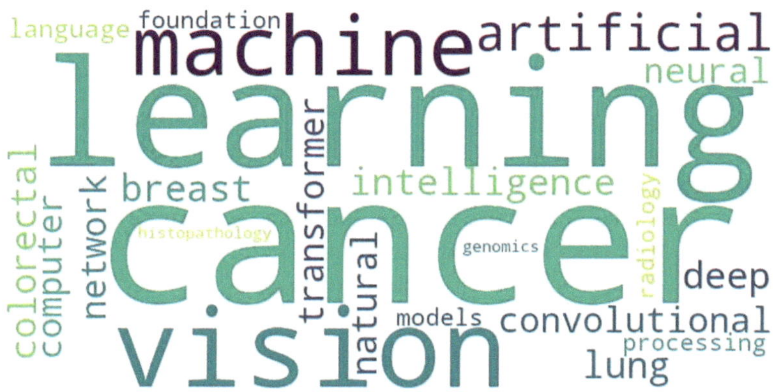

Multimodal Data in Cancer

The integration of multimodal data marks a critical advance in cancer research and clinical oncology. By synergistically combining diverse information streams, including molecular profiles (genomics, proteomics), imaging (radiology, pathology), clinical records, and lifestyle factors, this approach provides a comprehensive view of disease complexity and heterogeneity (Fig. 13.3). Such integrated analyses enhance the precision of cancer diagnosis, prognosis, and treatment prediction while also facilitating the discovery of novel biomarkers. Ultimately, multimodal data fusion is pivotal for developing highly personalized and effective therapeutic strategies, driving the paradigm shift toward precision oncology.

Medical Imaging Medical imaging serves as the primary method for the detection and diagnosis of breast cancer. Modalities such as mammography, ultrasound, magnetic resonance imaging (MRI), computed tomography (CT), and positron emission tomography (PET) provide critical information on tumor morphology, size, and functional activity. Mammography is widely used for population-based screening, especially in women over 40 years old, due to its sensitivity to detect microcalcifications and structural distortions. Ultrasound, often used as an adjunct, helps distinguish between solid and cystic lesions and is particularly valuable in women with dense breast tissue. MRI offers high-resolution soft tissue contrast and is instrumental in evaluating tumor extent, vascularity, and multifocality. PET and CT provide complementary metabolic and anatomical data, enhancing the overall understanding of disease progression. AI, particularly convolutional neural networks (CNNs), has been widely applied to imaging tasks such as the detection of lesion, tumor segmentation, and classification of benign versus malignant masses. CNNs learn hierarchical image fea-

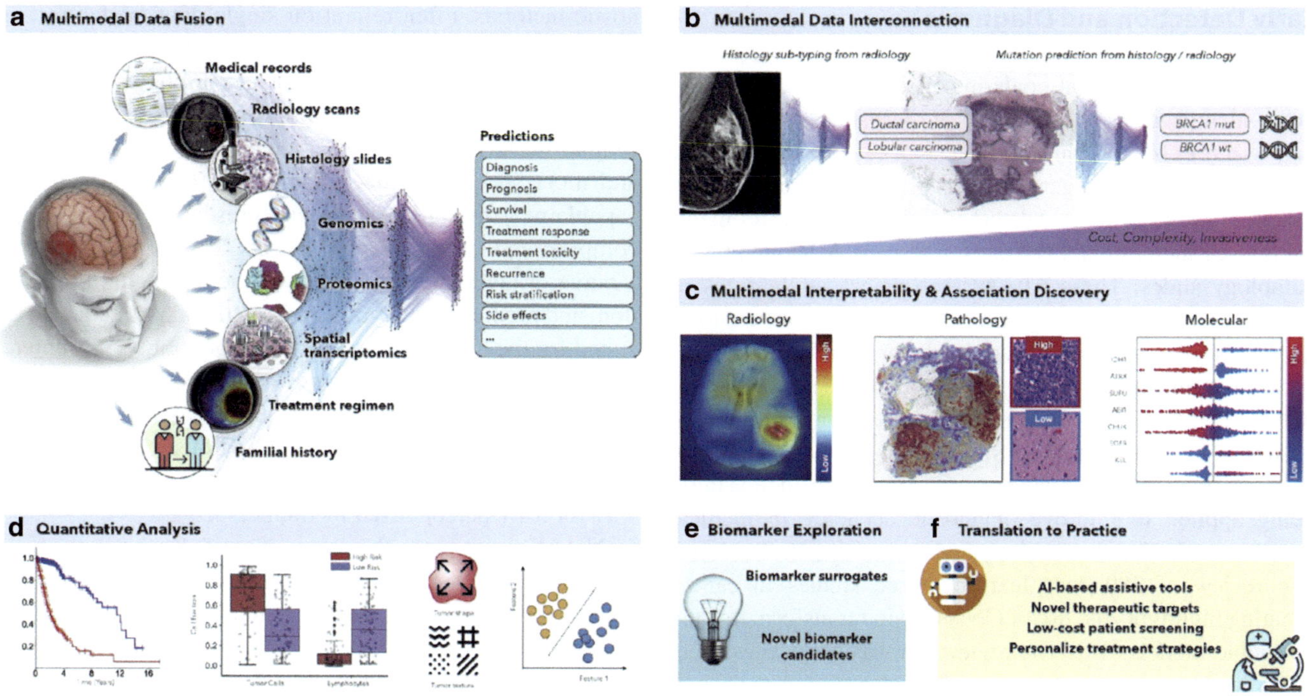

Fig. 13.3 Overview of a multimodal data fusion framework for precision medicine adapted from [8]. This shows the integration of diverse data types, their interconnectedness, analytical approaches, and potential clinical applications

tures directly from pixel data, enabling automated identification of subtle patterns that may be imperceptible to the human eye. Vision transformers (ViTs), a newer class of deep learning models, further enhance performance by capturing long-range spatial relationships within image data. These models are particularly effective in complex tasks like tumor boundary delineation and radiomic feature extraction. AI also facilitates image fusion, integrating data across imaging modalities to improve diagnostic accuracy and treatment planning.

Histopathology Histopathology remains the gold standard for the definitive diagnosis of breast cancer and the classification of molecular subtypes. The advent of whole slide imaging (WSI) has enabled the digitization of histological slides, generating high-resolution images suitable for computational analysis. Deep learning algorithms have shown remarkable success in digital pathology, performing tasks such as nuclei segmentation, mitotic count estimation, tumor classification, and histological subtype classification. CNNs and transformer-based models are employed to analyze gigapixel WSIs by breaking them into smaller patches and aggregating patch-level predictions. Self-supervised learning (SSL) techniques are gaining traction for their ability to learn robust representations from unlabeled data, addressing the scarcity of annotated pathology datasets. These models can be fine-tuned for downstream tasks such as region-of-interest (ROI) detection, stromal pattern analysis, and immune cell quantification. Digital pathology powered by AI enables objective, reproducible, and scalable histological assessments, thus reducing interobserver variability and improving diagnostic consistency.

Genomic and Transcriptomic Profiling Genomic and transcriptomic profiling provides insight into the molecular underpinnings of breast cancer, guiding the prognosis and targeting. AI models are used for a variety of tasks in this domain, including mutation detection, clustering of gene expression, pathway analysis, and prediction of the response to therapy. Deep learning architectures such as autoencoders and graph neural networks are particularly well-suited for modeling complex biological relationships within multi-omics datasets. Integrating genomics with other modalities like imaging and pathology requires sophisticated multimodal fusion techniques. Foundation models and multimodal transformers facilitate this integration by learning shared representations across different data types. AI-driven multi-omics integration enables comprehensive molecular subtyping, prediction of treatment resistance, and identification of novel biomarkers. These capabilities are critical for developing personalized therapeutic strategies and advancing the field of precision cancer.

Early Detection and Diagnosis

One of the most critical goals in cancer care is early detection—identifying the disease at its earliest stages, when treatment is more effective, and the chances of cure are significantly higher. Artificial intelligence (AI) is playing a transformative role in this area, with models being trained to interpret medical images such as mammograms, CT scans, MRI, and histopathology slides. These AI tools can detect subtle signs of cancer—sometimes even earlier than experienced radiologists or pathologists. For instance, AI can identify early-stage breast cancer, detect small lung nodules with malignant potential, and recognize atypical cell patterns in skin or colon tissues. Deep neural networks, using stages such as preprocessing, segmentation, and postprocessing, are increasingly being applied to improve diagnostic accuracy in medical imaging, including dermoscopy and radiology [9]. A systematic review of 389 deep learning-based studies in cancer imaging highlights the use of CNNs, vision transformers, and ensemble models [10]. The review emphasizes successes in classification and segmentation while also noting persistent challenges related to data quality, explainability, and model generalization. Additional surveys further describe how state-of-the-art deep learning techniques are pushing the boundaries of noninvasive cancer detection, particularly through advanced image analysis pipelines involving segmentation, feature extraction, and fusion across modalities.

In parallel, AI is also making strides in liquid biopsy analysis, a minimally invasive approach that analyzes biological fluids such as blood or urine for cancer-specific biomarkers, including circulating tumor cells (CTCs), circulating tumor DNA (ctDNA), and exosomes. This technique enables early cancer detection, monitoring of treatment response, and identification of drug targets to guide precision medicine. One notable innovation in this space is **NULISA**, a proteomic liquid biopsy platform with attomolar sensitivity. NULISA leverages DNA-barcoded antibodies and automated signal attenuation techniques to enable high-throughput, 200-plex protein quantification—dramatically enhancing the sensitivity and utility of liquid biopsies [11].

Prognosis and Risk Prediction

AI models combining imaging, genomics, and clinical data through multimodal integration can predict actionable gene mutations noninvasively, advancing precision oncology [12]. For example, breast cancer is a complex and heterogeneous disease that encompasses several molecular subtypes, including luminal A, luminal B, HER2-enriched, and triple-negative breast cancer. Each subtype differs in biological behavior, prognosis, and therapeutic response, necessitating tailored diagnostic and treatment strategies. Traditional diagnostic methods, often reliant on single data modalities, are insufficient to comprehensively characterize the multifaceted nature of the disease. This has prompted a growing interest in leveraging AI to improve diagnostic accuracy, prognostic modeling, and therapeutic decision-making. AI, and more specifically deep learning, offers powerful tools capable of learning hierarchical representations from large, complex, and heterogeneous datasets. These models excel in a range of tasks such as feature extraction, pattern recognition, and predictive analytics, making them particularly well-suited for the high-dimensional data commonly encountered in oncology. By integrating diverse data modalities including imaging, pathology, molecular profiles, and electronic health records (EHRs), AI facilitates a more holistic understanding of breast cancer biology and clinical behavior, paving the way for truly personalized medicine.

Not all cancers are the same, even if they're in the same part of the body. That's why personalized or precision medicine is so important. It means matching each person to the treatment that is most likely to work for their cancer. AI helps scientists look at a person's genes, tumor characteristics, and medical history to predict which therapies will be most effective. For example, some breast cancers respond well to hormone therapy, while others need chemotherapy. Certain lung cancers have mutations that can be targeted with special drugs. AI can quickly analyze genetic tests and match patients to clinical trials or targeted treatments, saving time and improving outcomes.

Finding a new cancer drug usually takes years and costs millions of dollars. AI can help accelerate this by predicting which molecules might fight cancer cells, identifying side effects before a drug is tested in people, and finding new uses for old drugs, such as using a medicine developed for one cancer to treat another. This means new treatments can reach patients faster, with less trial and error.

AI in Clinical Data Analysis and Decision Support EHR contain a wealth of clinical information, including demographics, comorbidities, laboratory results, treatment histories, and clinical outcomes. AI techniques, particularly natural language processing (NLP) and deep learning, are increasingly applied to structure and analyze this data for key applications such as patient stratification, risk scoring, outcome prediction, and clinical decision support. Transformer-based models like BERT and its clinical variants have proven effective in extracting relevant features from unstructured clinical text. These features can be integrated with imaging, pathology, and genomic data to create comprehensive, multimodal patient profiles. The resulting predictive models enable more personalized treatment planning, anticipate treatment toxicity, and support longitudinal monitoring. AI-driven clinical decision support tools also enhance clinician efficiency and promote evidence-based care.

AI is also helping to match patients with appropriate clinical trials, track treatment response, and anticipate disease progression. By synthesizing information from EHRs, lab results, imaging studies, and even wearable devices, AI can predict how a tumor is likely to respond, flag potential adverse effects before they become critical, and suggest timely adjustments to the care plan. Looking ahead, AI tools may also empower patients directly by helping them manage their care, ask informed questions, and stay engaged in their treatment journey.

Overview of AI Techniques

AI, Machine Learning, and Deep Learning

Recent advances in AI have led to transformative applications in cancer research and clinical care. AI is a technique that enables machines to perform tasks that typically require human intelligence, such as learning, reasoning, and problem-solving [13]. AI can simulate aspects of human thinking and behavior, such as algorithms that interpret medical images or assist in decision-making. Classic AI can include rule-based expert systems or more adaptive algorithms [14]. The key idea is that AI is an umbrella term for intelligent behavior by machines, ranging from simple automation to complex problem-solving.

Machine learning (ML) is a subset of AI focused on algorithms that learn patterns from data instead of relying on explicit programming. ML algorithms analyze large datasets to make predictions or classifications. Importantly, ML models often require human expertise to determine which data features are relevant. A traditional ML approach to predicting cancer risk might rely on handcrafted features, such as tumor size, patient age, selected by experts. ML methods include logistic regression, decision trees, random forests, and support vector machines. These algorithms can be highly effective when provided with well-chosen features and moderate-sized datasets. ML has been widely applied in cancer research for risk assessment, early diagnosis, patient prognosis estimation, and treatment selection [15].

Deep learning (DL) is a specialized subset of ML that uses artificial neural networks inspired by the human brain. These neural networks consist of many layered computations and can learn complex features from raw data in an automatic manner. Deep learning models, such as convolutional neural networks (CNNs), excel at processing unstructured data like medical images or genomic sequences. A deep neural network can process raw images or genomic data and automatically identify the important patterns without explicit human-design of features [14]. This ability to learn abstract features through multiple layers makes DL extremely powerful for tasks such as image recognition. In cancer research, Deep learning models have also been used to classify multiple cancer types from imaging and genomic data [13].

Overview of Learning Approaches

Supervised Learning AI techniques are playing an increasingly prominent role in cancer detection by enabling the analysis of complex medical data and uncovering subtle patterns indicative of disease [16]. Traditional AI systems are often built on machine learning and make future predictions by training on labeled data. This method of machine learning is known as supervised learning, where the algorithm learns to solve a task based on labeled data and helps predict outcomes for unseen data [16]. Labeled data are created by assigning labels or tags to add meaning to aspects of the data, essentially teaching the model what information is relevant to learn. However, creating labeled data by domain experts is both time-consuming and costly [17]. Since the performance of machine learning models tends to improve with more and higher-quality data, the limited availability of expert-labeled datasets remains a significant challenge in medical AI development [18]. Recent advances in access to large volumes of cancer data, including medical imaging, genomics, and clinical records, have enabled promising AI applications using supervised learning in cancer research [14].

Unsupervised Learning Unsupervised learning is a method where algorithms discover patterns or structures in data without the need for labeled examples. This approach is useful in medical imaging when annotated datasets are limited or unavailable [19]. For instance, clustering techniques can help group similar types of lesions or tissue regions, while dimensionality reduction methods can reveal hidden structures in high-dimensional patient data. This can also support anomaly detection, identifying cases that differ significantly from normal patterns, which may indicate early signs of cancer. Building upon these unsupervised approaches, the emergence of self-supervised learning (SSL) allows for large-scale models trained on vast amounts of unlabeled data, leading to increased performance while minimizing cost and time. With SSL, models learn relevant features by creating their own signals from the data without requiring human annotation [20]. SSL networks extract features by pretraining an encoder network using augmented views of unlabeled images [21]. This encoder network can then be fine-tuned using a smaller dataset for downstream tasks such as object detection or image classification, for example, by filling in missing image patches or predicting image augmentations. By mitigating the need for expert labeled data, SSL overcomes the previous challenges in developing AI models to aid medical diagnosis.

Reinforcement Learning Reinforcement learning (RL) is a technique in which a system learns by trial and error, receiving rewards or penalties for the actions it takes rather than learning directly from labeled examples [22]. An RL-based system can learn optimal strategies through experimentation and feedback [23]. In cancer detection, reinforcement learning is being explored to optimize diagnostic decision-making processes and workflows. RL has shown particular promise in dynamic treatment regimen optimization, where sequential medical decisions must be made over time. Additionally, RL can help optimize workflows, such as determining the ideal sequence of tests for high-risk patients or when to recommend additional scans. It can also adjust the AI's decision-making priorities based on clinical preferences. Ultimately, RL brings adaptive intelligence to diagnostic pathways, enabling the AI to learn how and when to act for the best clinical outcomes.

AI Architectures and Techniques in Cancer Research

In this section, we will highlight some of the leading AI architectures and techniques that have been explored for cancer research. Table 13.1 is a summary of some of the representative articles cited in this section.

Table 13.1 Examples of AI techniques applied to cancer research

AI techniques	Cancer type	Representative References
CNNs for mammogram analysis using federated learning for data privacy	Breast cancer	[43, 44]
Hybrid CNN-LSTM deep learning model for breast cancer classification	Breast cancer	[25]
A hybrid CNN-RNN approach for predicting long-term survival outcomes in lung cancer screening patients	Lung cancer	[24]
3D CNNs and transformers for CT scan segmentation, ensemble models for detection	Lung cancer	[45, 46]
Deep learning on colonoscopy images, reinforcement learning for treatment	Colorectal cancer	[47, 48]
CNN-RNN hybrids for MRI-based diagnosis, graph neural networks for grading	Brain tumors	[49, 50]
Radiomics with machine learning classifiers, GANs for synthetic data	Liver cancer	[51, 52]
Fine-tuned LLMs and transformer models for semantic patient-trial matching and eligibility criteria extraction	Any	[35–37]

CNN, RNN, and Hybrid convolutional neural networks (CNNs) are a specialized type of deep neural network, effective for image analysis. They are designed to detect visual features such as edges, textures, and shapes. In cancer detection, CNNs are widely used to interpret medical images such as mammograms, CT scans, MRIs, and digital pathology slides. For example, a CNN can identify microcalcifications in a mammogram or detect abnormal cell structures in a histology slide. CNNs support various image analysis tasks, such as tumor classification and segmentation, outlining tumor boundaries, which can serve as a reliable tool for radiologists and pathologists. Recurrent neural networks (RNNs) excel at processing sequential data and temporal dependencies. RNN-based models are particularly effective in survival analysis, where they can process irregularities in patient follow-up times and incorporate longitudinal clinical data to improve mortality prediction accuracy. Hybrid CNN-RNN approaches have demonstrated superior performance by combining CNN's imaging feature extraction capabilities with RNN's ability to investigate time series and global information [24]. These hybrid CNN-LSTM architectures enable examination of sequential characteristics in medical imaging, making them particularly advantageous for tasks requiring temporal pattern identification and video analysis [25].

Vision Transformer Vision transformers (ViTs) are a recent deep learning architecture that leverages an attention mechanism to dynamically assess the relevance of various parts of input data [26]. Vision transformers (ViTs) adapt the transformer architecture from NLP to computer vision by dividing images into patches (see example in Fig. 13.4), treating each patch as a token, and applying self-attention mechanisms [27]. The attention mechanism enables ViT to focus on multiple parts of an image and interpret information throughout the image, allowing for comprehensive spatial analysis. Unlike CNNs that use local receptive fields, ViTs can directly model relationships between distant image regions, making them effective for identifying subtle patterns that may be spatially separated [27]. This global contextual understanding is crucial for medical imaging where diagnostic features require integration of information from multiple anatomical regions. Transformers have demonstrated outstanding performance and proved to be valid alternatives to CNNs in diverse medical imaging tasks [28].

Foundation Models Foundation models (FMs) represent an area of AI trained using SSL on massive sets of data that can then be adapted to a wide range of specific tasks. The ability to process multiple modalities of data and adapt to multiple downstream tasks, such as computer vision and

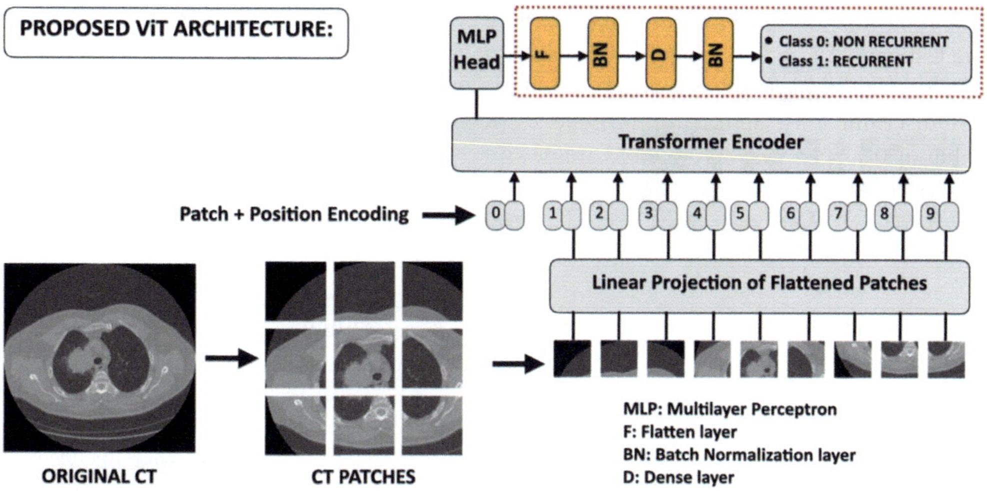

Fig. 13.4 Illustration of vision transformers (ViTs). (Adapted from [29])

natural language processing (NLP), sets foundation models apart from traditional AI methods [30]. Typically, foundation models are large-scale neural networks trained on massive datasets, employing self-supervised learning strategies to extract knowledge from multiple data modalities, mitigating the need for expert-labeled datasets (see Fig. 13.5). With billions of trainable parameters, foundation models learn rich data representations and provide a strong base for subsequent natural language processing (NLP) and computer vision applications. When used in specific downstream tasks, the pretrained model allows for greater effectiveness and accuracy, as well as adaptability. In medicine, foundation models have been used in diagnosis, reporting, and supporting medical decisions, especially in the histopathology and radiology fields [31]. Moreover, foundation models can provide a useful second opinion to professionals reviewing investigations and mitigate the need for review by multiple experts, thereby optimizing workflow and increasing the efficiency and speed of diagnosis [32].

LLM Large language models (LLMs) are trained on massive amounts of text and are capable of understanding, generating, and summarizing human language [34]. In clinical practice, LLMs can process and synthesize information from multiple clinical documents, creating comprehensive patient summaries that highlight key findings, treatment responses, and risk factors. In cancer care, LLMs are being explored for automating report generation, terminology standardization, and synthesis of complex clinical or pathology narratives. Although LLMs do not interpret images directly, they can extract critical insights from unstructured text-based data and support clinical decision-making. In this manner, LLMs enable efficient documentation of cancer research data and enhance diagnostic reasoning. LLMs are increasingly being applied to clinical trial matching through both provider-focused automated systems [35] and patient-initiated retrieval platforms [36]. Current clinical trials show promise but reveal significant implementation challenges [37]. Recent studies indicate that LLMs show promise in data analysis, patient interaction, and personalized treatment approaches in cancer care [34].

Vision-Language Models Vision-language models (VLMs) are advanced AI systems designed to jointly process images and text, enabling more natural and clinically meaningful interactions between clinicians and AI [38]. For instance, VLMs can process chest CT scans and, upon receiving a query such as "Are there any suspicious masses?," produce detailed radiology reports by automatically detecting and precisely segmenting relevant pathological findings within the scan. This bidirectional capability, understanding both visual data and natural language, makes VLMs especially valuable for streamlining workflows, improving report clarity, and enhancing explainability. The interactive nature of VLMs allows for clarification and elaboration, enabling clinicians to investigate further into specific findings or request additional analysis of particular image regions. By acting as AI interpreters that translate visual data into clinical language, these models align with how practitioners communicate and make decisions [39].

Transfer Learning Transfer learning is a technique where a pretrained AI model, originally trained on a large, general dataset, is adapted to a new, more specific task with much less data. This is especially useful in oncology, where acquiring large, labeled datasets for rare cancers is often impractical. For example, a model trained on thousands of general pathology images can be fine-tuned to detect a rare tumor type using only a few hundred images. Since the model already understands basic visual patterns such as tissue structure and tumor appearance, it can quickly adapt, saving time and improving performance. This approach is widely used in cancer research for tasks such as tumor classification, segmentation, and prediction of treatment outcomes. It

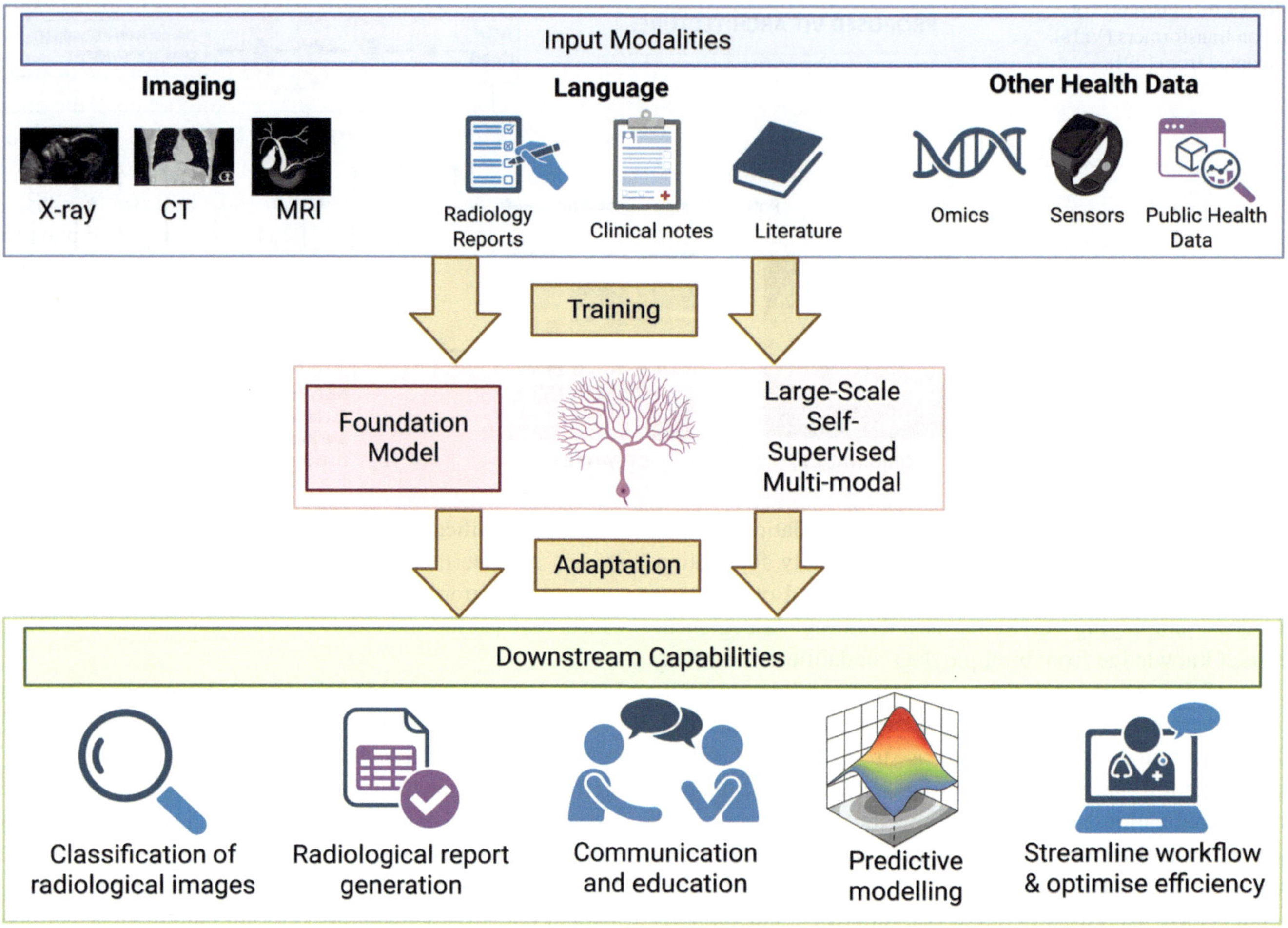

Fig. 13.5 Diverse capabilities of foundation models (FMs) in radiology and health care. FMs can train on multiple input modalities including imaging (X-ray mammography, ultrasound, and MRI scans), language sources, and other health data. FMs are large-scale, self-supervised models that can be used in a variety of downstream tasks including image classification, report generation, predictive modeling, and communication and education. FMs have the potential to streamline workflow and revolutionize medical diagnostics. Illustration motivated from [33]

enables researchers to develop accurate models even when data is limited, which is especially important for rare cancers or underrepresented populations [40].

Federated Learning Federated learning allows multiple hospitals to train a shared AI model without exchanging patient data. Each institution keeps its data locally and trains the model on-site. Only model updates, not raw data, are shared and aggregated to create a stronger global model [41]. This method is ideal for cancer research, where privacy concerns limit data sharing. Federated learning leverages distributed computation to ensure that individual data contributions remain confidential. Model updates are typically sent in encrypted form to a central server, where they are combined using algorithms that prevent the reconstruction of any individual participant's data. This process not only protects sensitive health information but also addresses the regulatory and ethical concerns associated with data sharing. This approach has proven successful in international collaborations for brain tumor segmentation, demonstrating its practical value in clinical research [42].

AI Development Pipeline

The development of AI systems for cancer care follows a multistage pipeline, beginning with rigorous data preparation. High-quality, diverse, and well-annotated datasets are the foundation of any successful AI model. This stage often involves aggregating multimodal data—such as imaging (e.g., mammograms, CT, MRI), pathology slides, genomics, and electronic health records (EHRs)—followed by cleaning, normalization, de-identification, and harmonization across sources.

For imaging data, preprocessing may include segmentation, resolution standardization, and contrast enhancement, while text data often requires natural language processing (NLP) techniques to extract structured features from unstructured clinical notes. Properly splitting datasets into training, validation, and testing cohorts, along with careful management of class imbalance and batch effects, is critical to avoid bias and overfitting.

Once data preparation is complete, the focus shifts to model development and validation. This phase includes selecting appropriate AI architectures (e.g., convolutional neural networks for image tasks, transformers for text), tuning hyperparameters, and iterating through training cycles. Techniques such as cross validation, data augmentation, and ensemble modeling are commonly employed to enhance robustness. Model interpretability, fairness, and generalizability must be addressed throughout the process, especially when targeting high-stakes clinical decisions. The final stage—clinical translation—involves external validation on independent datasets, prospective trials, regulatory approval, and integration into clinical workflows. Key considerations here include interoperability with existing health IT systems, user interface design for clinician adoption, and ongoing performance monitoring in real-world settings. Effective clinical translation ensures that AI not only demonstrates technical accuracy but also delivers measurable improvements in patient outcomes, safety, and equity. Figure 13.6 illustrates the three major steps described above.

AI for Cancer Care Use Case

AI is transforming cancer care by enabling more accurate, efficient, and personalized approaches across the clinical continuum, from screening and diagnosis to prognosis and treatment planning. Breast cancer, one of the most prevalent and well-studied cancers worldwide, serves as an ideal use case to illustrate the roles of AI, its clinical impact and challenges of integration. With large, annotated imaging datasets (e.g., mammography, ultrasound, MRI), rich genomic profiles, and well-defined care pathways, breast cancer has become a focal point for developing and validating AI models. These tools have demonstrated promising results in enhancing radiologist performance, stratifying risk, identifying subtypes, and predicting treatment response, highlighting the potential of AI to augment clinical decision-making and improve patient outcomes in real-world oncology settings. In this section, we will use breast cancer care as a use case to illustrate the key roles of AI in the continuum of cancer care (see example Fig. 13.7).

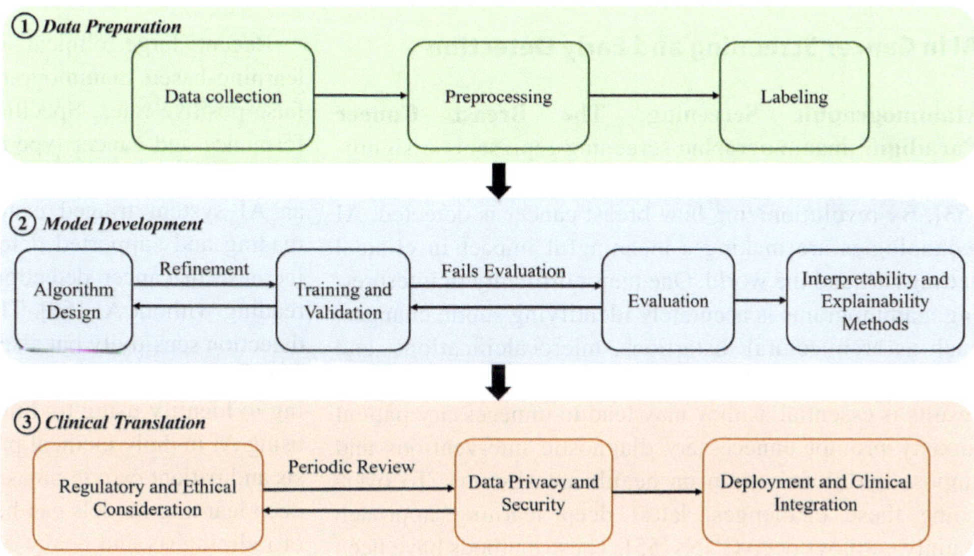

Fig. 13.6 AI development pipeline showing the three key steps starting from data preparation to model development and clinical translation

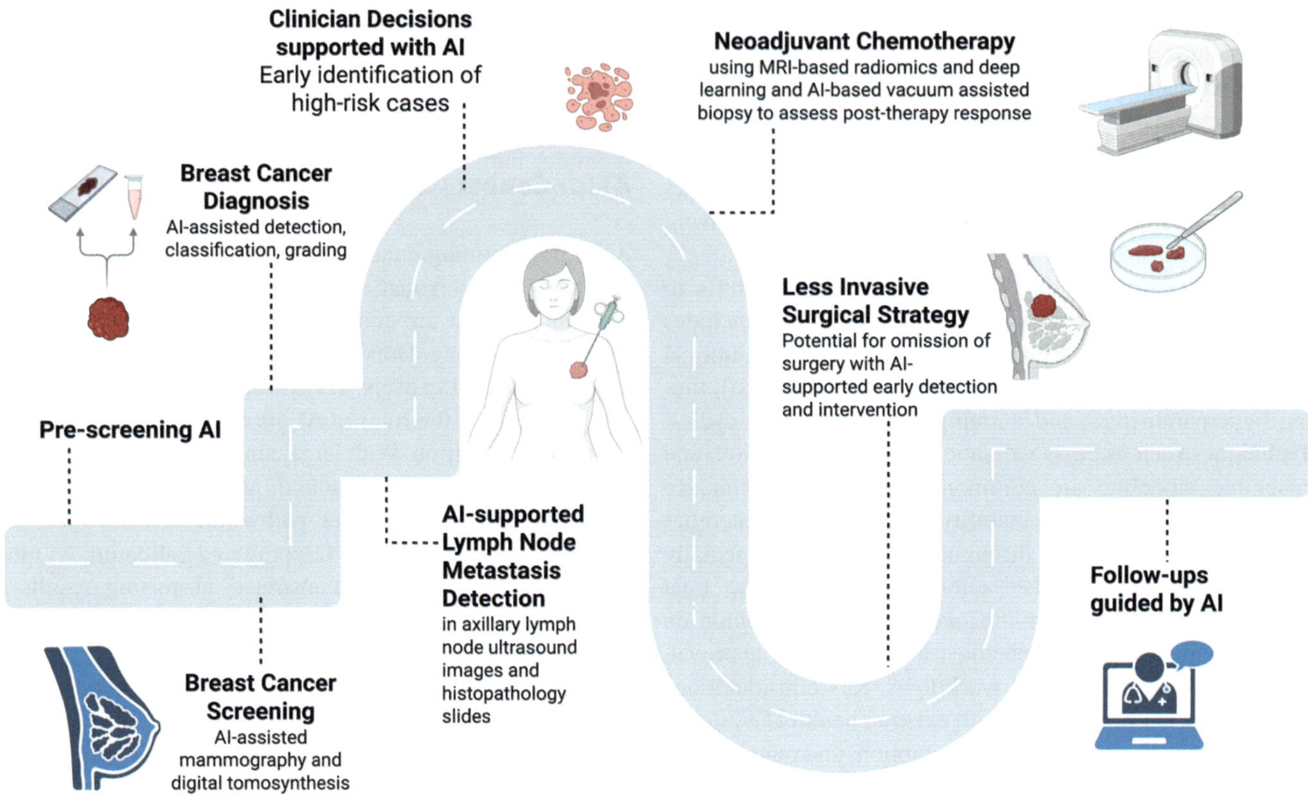

Fig. 13.7 A detailed overview of AI applications that shows complete breast cancer patient pathway, encompassing screening, diagnosis, neoadjuvant chemotherapy, and surgical de-escalation

AI in Cancer Screening and Early Detection

Mammographic Screening: The Breast Cancer Paradigm mammographic screening represents a significant advancement in the use of AI within breast cancer care [53]. By revolutionizing how breast cancer is detected, AI technologies are making a meaningful impact in clinical settings around the world. One major difficulty in interpreting mammograms is accurately identifying subtle changes, such as architectural distortions, microcalcifications, and mass lesions [54]. Moreover, minimizing false positive results is essential as they may lead to unnecessary patient anxiety prompt unnecessary diagnostic interventions and impose additional strain on healthcare systems. To overcome these challenges, latest deep learning approach mainly employs deep CNNs [55]. These methods have been trained on large-scale datasets that included hundreds of thousands of mammographic images enriched with clinical outcomes and expert annotations. As a result, they demonstrate high accuracy in identifying suspicious lesions with sensitivity and specificity levels that often overcome those of experienced radiologists. This performance is particularly notable in challenging cases such as those involving dense breast tissue or subtle abnormalities, and it highlights the potential of these methods to enhance the early detection of breast cancer.

Recent large clinical studies demonstrate that deep learning-based mammogram screening effectively reduces false-positive rates. Specifically, analysis of screening performance and cancer type and stage in the Mammography Screening with Artificial Intelligence (MASAI) trial, where an AI system triaged examinations for single or double reading and supported detection, shows a significant 29% increase in cancer detection compared to standard double reading without AI [56]. These methods not only maintain detection sensitivity but also frequently improve it and prove especially effective for early-stage cancers that are challenging to identify using traditional techniques. This shows that using AI in daily medical practice can help improve diagnosis and patient care in breast cancer and means AI especially deep learning models can help with problems like shortages of radiologists and heavy workloads in health care. Among these models, CNNs stand out as some of the most effective algorithms for analyzing mammograms, because they autonomously identify complex patterns related to breast cancer. Noteworthy architectures such as Inception and ResNet further enhance diagnostic accuracy by capturing features at multiple resolutions and enabling the training of deeper networks without loss of effectiveness [57]. Advancements in deep learning have significantly enhanced mammographic screening by employing transfer learning to tailor pretrained models to specific mammography datasets, thereby improving accuracy even when labeled data are scarce [58]. Furthermore, hybrid techniques that integrate deep leaning approaches with traditional radiology workflows have increased efficiency by utilizing generative adversarial networks to generate synthetic images that enrich training datasets and strengthen model performance [59]. Collectively, these methods contribute to more accurate and efficient breast cancer detection while enabling radiologists to dedicate their expertise to complex cases.

Risk Stratification and Personalized Screening There is increasing recognition of the potential that machine learning techniques offer in advancing breast cancer risk prediction [60]. Models such as CNNs and recurrent neural networks (RNNs) have demonstrated strong capabilities in analyzing complex datasets that include demographic variables, family history, genetic markers, and breast density measurements [61]. These systems support the development of individualized risk profiles by accounting for both biological predispositions and environmental influences. When imaging data processed by CNNs is combined with genomic and clinical data analyzed through RNNs or ensemble methods like random forests, the result is a powerful and holistic approach to risk stratification that overcome the accuracy of traditional models. The clinical integration of AI-derived risk assessments has enabled more personalized and effective breast cancer screening strategies [62]. Deep learning frameworks support data-driven decisions regarding screening intervals and imaging modalities, thereby facilitating individualized recommendations that optimize diagnostic sensitivity while minimizing unnecessary radiation exposure and resource consumption [63]. For individuals identified as high risk, more intensive surveillance involving advanced imaging techniques such as digital breast tomosynthesis (DBT) or automated breast ultrasound may be appropriate, whereas those at lower risk can be screened less frequently without compromising safety [64]. These advancements allow for better stratification of patients by risk, improving cancer detection rates and supporting more equitable and cost-effective prevention programs. Importantly, such models not only enhance clinical outcomes but also contribute to resource optimization in overstretched healthcare systems.

Multimodal Data Integration Deep learning has become an essential tool in the development of advanced methods for cancer diagnostics, particularly in the analysis of medical imaging. These methods enable the integration of information from multiple imaging modalities, including mammography, ultrasonography, MRI, and CT, thereby supporting a more comprehensive evaluation of disease [65, 66]. Neural network architectures such as CNNs with attention mechanisms and transformer-based models are widely used to process and interpret complex, multimodal imaging and genomic data [67]. These models significantly improve the early detection and diagnosis of cancer. By leveraging multimodal imaging and genomic data, these models significantly enhance diagnostic accuracy, precision, and reliability. The complementary nature of the integrated modalities enables more accurate discrimination between benign and malignant lesions, reduces diagnostic errors, and supports informed clinical decision-making. This improved diagnostic performance facilitates earlier intervention and contributes to better long-term patient outcomes.

AI in Cancer Diagnosis and Staging

Pathological Diagnosis Enhancement Digital pathology involves utilizing whole-slide imaging (WSI) to digitize and analyze tissue samples using a computer that combined with AI has transformed cancer diagnosis by enabling more accurate and efficient analysis [68, 69]. Deep learning models, including CNNs and vision transformers as well as the use of foundation models, can process high-resolution WSIs to identify complex morphological patterns in cancer tissues [70–72]. In recent years, advances in AI have led to the emergence of foundation models as transformative tools in digital pathology. These models leverage large-scale pretraining and self-supervised learning to overcome long-standing challenges in histopathological image analysis. Some prominent foundation models and platforms in this domain include COBRA, Phikon-v2, TissueConcepts, HIBOU, Virchow2, OmniScreen, Prov-GigaPathV, Kaiko-ai, UNI, Virchow, BROW, and Phikon [73]. By training on diverse and extensive histopathological datasets, these models exhibit remarkable performance across diagnostic and prognostic tasks [74], effectively generalizing across different tissue types, staining protocols, and institutional variations. Foundation models employ advanced self-supervised learning techniques, such as contrastive learning and masked image modeling, which allow them to extract meaningful features from vast amounts of unlabeled histopathological images [73]. This training strategy mitigates the limitations imposed by scarce annotated data, enabling the models to develop a robust understanding of tissue architecture. Consequently, they are highly adaptable to a wide spectrum of diagnostic applications across various cancer types and clinical contexts [75]. Importantly, beyond facilitating early diagnosis, foundation models demonstrate significant potential in the precise staging of cancer. By integrating comprehensive histopathological information, these models can accurately assess tumor characteristics including size, invasiveness, and lymph node involvement. Such detailed staging is critical for optimizing treatment strategies and improving prognostic assessments, thereby contributing to enhanced patient management and outcomes.

AI in Treatment Planning and Precision Medicine

Genomic Analysis and Molecular Profiling The exponential expansion of high-throughput genomic sequencing technologies in oncological practice has generated unprecedented volumes of molecular data, necessitating advanced deep learning architectures for clinical interpretation and actionable insight extraction [76]. Deep neural networks demonstrate good capacity for processing high-dimensional genomic datasets through multilayer perceptron architectures, CNNs, and transformer models that employ hierarchical feature learning to identify clinically actionable mutations and predict therapeutic response patterns [77, 78]. In breast cancer molecular profiling, deep learning frameworks utilize autoencoders for dimensionality reduction of genomic data, followed by deep feedforward networks and RNNs that analyze comprehensive tumor genomic landscapes to predict chemotherapeutic efficacy through learned representations. These deep learning approaches employ attention mechanisms and residual connections to decode intricate genomic signatures, while graph neural networks model gene interaction networks and pathway relationships that correlate with clinical outcomes [79, 80]. Advanced deep learning architectures integrate variational autoencoders with generative adversarial networks to augment limited genomic datasets, enabling robust training of deep models for evidence-based treatment selection and therapeutic decision-making optimization. This deep learning-driven computational paradigm represents a fundamental advancement in precision oncology, implementing end-to-end learning pipelines that automatically extract hierarchical features from raw genomic data and optimize therapeutic matching through deep neural network-based decision support systems, ultimately advancing the clinical translation of deep learning-guided cancer care.

Treatment Response Prediction Predicting treatment responses in breast cancer has improved significantly, thanks to advanced models that combine data from imaging, genetics, and clinical information. These AI-based systems can accurately predict how patients will respond to neoadjuvant chemotherapy, identify those likely to achieve a complete pathological response, and help doctors adjust treatments early for better outcomes [81]. Radiomics plays a crucial role in this process by extracting quantitative features from medical images using AI algorithms, providing valuable predictive biomarkers for treatment response. By analyzing pretreatment mammographic, ultrasound, or MRI features, these models can predict chemotherapy responses with accuracy comparable to traditional invasive molecular testing [82, 83]. This noninvasive strategy enhances personalized treatment approaches while reducing the burden on patients. Moreover, integrating longitudinal imaging data through AI analysis allows for a dynamic evaluation of treatment responses. These systems can detect subtle changes in tumor characteristics throughout the course of treatment, enabling the early identification of nonresponders and supporting timely modifications to the treatment plan.

Radiation Therapy Planning and Optimization Recent advancements in radiation therapy planning have brought about significant transformations, particularly through the integration of AI. These innovations include the automation of contouring procedures, optimization of dose distributions, and prediction of treatment-related toxicity [84]. In breast cancer radiation therapy, for instance, AI systems can automatically delineate target volumes and identify organs at risk, which streamlines the planning process while enhancing both consistency and accuracy [85]. Furthermore, deep learning algorithms trained on expert contoured cases can generate high-quality treatment plans that meet or exceed the standards of manual planning methods. These AI-optimized treatment plans achieve superior dose distributions while reducing radiation exposure to critical structures, such as the heart and lungs. In addition, predictive models for radiation toxicity are developed through the AI analysis of dosimetric parameters and patient characteristics, enabling a more personalized approach to treatment. These models facilitate a balance between effective tumor control and the risk of toxicity, helping clinicians make informed decisions regarding fractionation schedules, dose prescriptions, and the use of advanced techniques such as proton therapy.

Treatment Monitoring and Assessment To improve treatment monitoring, AI plays a crucial role in facilitating the continuous assessment of patient responses. By analyzing serial imaging studies, laboratory results, and patient reported outcomes, AI provides valuable information on the efficacy of treatment [86]. Specifically, in breast cancer management, AI systems are utilized to evaluate tumor responses during neoadjuvant therapy, delivering quantitative assessments that guide treatment decisions. In addition, digital biomarkers obtained from wearable devices and mobile health applications offer expanded monitoring capabilities. Generally, AI algorithms analyze activity patterns, activity patterns, sleep quality, and various physiological tolerances to treatment. Consequently, the integration of various monitoring modalities through AI analysis leads to the development of comprehensive treatment dashboards that improve clinical decision-making. These sophisticated systems provide early warning of potential treatment failures, the onset of toxicity, or disease progression, enabling timely interventions designed to optimize patient outcomes.

AI in Survivorship and Long-Term Care

Surveillance and Recurrence Detection Long-term surveillance of cancer survivors presents unique challenges in terms of resource utilization and cost-effectiveness. AI systems support efficient surveillance strategies by stratifying patients' risks, optimizing imaging schedules, and detecting early signs of recurrence. In breast cancer survivors, AI algorithms analyze surveillance imaging to detect local recurrence, contralateral breast cancer, and distant metastases. These systems can identify subtle changes that may indicate recurrence before they become clinically apparent, potentially improving treatment outcomes through early intervention. Predictive models for recurrence risk, developed using artificial intelligence analysis of treatment response data, pathological characteristics, and genomic profiles, guide the intensity and duration of surveillance. These models support personalized surveillance strategies that balance the benefits of early detection with the costs and potential harms of intensive monitoring.

Toxicity Management and Quality of Life AI systems support long-term toxicity management by analyzing patient-reported results, clinical evaluations, and physiological data to identify survivors at risk of late effects. In breast cancer survivors, AI algorithms can predict risk for cardiac toxicity, secondary malignancies, and psychosocial complications. Natural language processing of clinical notes and patient communications enables automated detection of symptom clusters and quality of life issues. These systems can trigger appropriate interventions, referrals, or support services to address survivor needs proactively. The integration of wearable device data provides continuous monitoring of survivor health status. AI analysis of activity patterns, heart rate variability, and sleep quality can detect early signs of fatigue, depression, or physical decline, enabling timely interventions to maintain quality of life.

Challenges for AI in Breast Cancer Care

Despite significant progress, several challenges hinder the widespread adoption of AI in breast cancer care. Data quality and diversity remain major concerns, as many models are trained on datasets that lack demographic and clinical heterogeneity, resulting in biased and non-generalizable predictions. Limited availability of annotated data, particularly in genomics and digital pathology, restricts the development of high-performing models. Standardization of data acquisition, labeling, and preprocessing across institutions is essential to improve reproducibility and facilitate external validation. Interpretability remains a critical issue, as many deep learning models function as black boxes, providing predictions without clear explanations. This lack of transparency can undermine clinician trust and pose ethical and legal risks. Furthermore, integrating AI systems into clinical workflows requires robust infrastructure, interoperability with existing health IT systems, and training for healthcare professionals. The deployment of AI in clinical settings raises several ethical and legal concerns. Issues related to patient privacy, data ownership, informed consent, and algorithmic accountability must be carefully addressed. Regulatory bodies are increasingly developing frameworks to ensure the safe and effective use of AI in health care, emphasizing transparency, explainability, and fairness. The use of sensitive patient data necessitates robust data protection measures and compliance with legal standards such as HIPAA and GDPR. Efforts should also be made to develop interpretable AI models and establish audit trails for decision-making processes. The integration of AI into clinical practice offers substantial potential for advancing healthcare delivery. Nonetheless, it demands thorough consideration of clinicians' roles in the development and validation of AI models.

Cancer Datasets for AI

Datasets are the backbone of AI cancer research, providing the raw material from which models learn to detect patterns, make predictions, and support clinical decision-making. These datasets, ranging from medical images and pathology slides to genomic sequences and electronic health records, enable the development of algorithms that can replicate or augment expert-level performance across various tasks, such as tumor classification, risk stratification, and treatment response prediction. The quality, diversity, and scale of these datasets directly impact the accuracy, generalizability, and fairness of AI models. For example, training a model on a narrow or biased dataset may lead to poor performance in real-world, heterogeneous patient populations, potentially exacerbating disparities in care.

Moreover, well-curated cancer datasets facilitate benchmarking, reproducibility, and transparency in AI research. The National Cancer Institute (NCI), part of the NIH, maintains several comprehensive data repositories that are essential for advancing cancer research. One of the most prominent is the Cancer Research Data Commons (CRDC), which offers access to a range of high-quality, harmonized datasets across genomics, proteomics, imaging, clinical, and epidemiological domains. Notable resources include The Cancer Genome Atlas (TCGA) for genomic and clinical data and The Cancer Imaging Archive (TCIA) for radiological images linked to clinical and molecular annotations. These repositories promote open science by enabling researchers worldwide to develop, benchmark, and validate AI models on standardized datasets, accelerating innovation and reproducibility in cancer research. Other publicly available datasets such as BRATS (Brain Tumor Segmentation Challenge), and CBIS-DDSM (for breast mammography), have become foundational resources that enable the broader research community to compare methods and validate findings. These datasets also drive innovation by fostering data challenges and collaborations across institutions.

In the use case of AI for breast cancer, high-quality, diverse, and large number of images are required to build a robust AI model capable of detecting cancers at the clinical level. Breast cancer occurs most frequently in the breast milk glands, known as lobules, and the tubes that carry milk to the nipple, known as ducts. Clinically, breast structures can be visualized using multiple imaging modalities, all of which are used in the detection, classification, and staging of breast lesions. Most breast tumors are detected on mammographic images through screening programs, which aim to detect and treat breast cancer early through regular imaging of the breasts. Mammography is an imaging technique that sends low-dose X-ray waves through breast tissue to produce a digital image of the structures within, including the density of tissue, areas of asymmetry, and any masses or calcifications. While mammograms are often the first port of call for breast lesion detection, ultrasound scans are also used as an adjunct, particularly in those who cannot be exposed to X-rays. This handheld technique uses sound waves and has the advantage of being able to be performed at the bedside, with both the clinician and the patient able to see structures within the breast tissue in real time. US is more sensitive to fluid than mammography and is often used to differentiate between benign, fluid-filled cysts and solid masses. Similarly, MRI uses magnetic fields to produce very high-quality images of soft tissue structures, especially the lobules and ducts where cancer is not only the most common but also the most aggressive. Due to its high cost and lack of availability, MRI is often reserved for high-risk or complex cases. Images from these investigations are often stored in the standardized international medical image format, DICOM. Finally, cancer is confirmed and graded through biopsy, which uses a needle to collect cell samples from the breast lesion. The cell samples are stained and looked under a microscope to confirm the presence of cancerous cells. Biopsy samples are scanned and stored digitally as WSI, and breast imaging results are classified and communicated about using the international Breast Imaging Reporting and Data System (BI-RADS).

The detection, grading, and staging of breast cancer require multiple components and multiple clinicians working together. The images produced because of these investigations require careful labeling by experts and ethical approval to be shared as public datasets. Here, we collate a total of 17 multimodal breast cancer datasets, including 7 mammography datasets, 4 ultrasound datasets, 3 WSI datasets, and 3 MRI datasets. These datasets include images from patients taken in different views and contain multiple types of breast lesions including benign and malignant tumors, calcifications, and other masses. Images are further classed based on radiologists' assessments, BI-RADS data, and molecular subtype. Additionally, most of the datasets also include image masks, which is useful in isolating relevant parts of the image for AI model deployment.

Data diversity is essential for ensuring the generalizability and fairness of AI models in cancer care. When selecting datasets for model development, careful attention must be paid to patient demographics and population characteristics.

For instance, while the datasets listed in the accompanying table are sourced from various countries, the largest among them—CSAW-CC, which includes over 1 million images derived from cancer screening programs in Sweden. As a result, the data may reflect region-specific clinical practices and population traits, which could limit the model's applicability to more diverse or global populations (Table 13.2).

Table 13.2 Major public breast cancer datasets by imaging modality

Dataset	Modality	Sample size	Data type	Labels	Key features/source
CBIS-DDSM [87]	Mammography	3102 cases, 10,239 images	2D images, ROI masks	Benign/malignan pathology, ROI contours	Curated DDSM sub-Set, TCIA
INbreast [88]	Mammography	115 cases, 410 images	2D images, contours	BI-RADS, density, lesion contours	High-quality, full-field digital, Portugal
KAU-BCMD [89]	Mammography	1416 cases, 2206 images	2D images, metadata	Density, BI-RADS, pathology	Saudi Arabia, diverse population
CMMD [90]	Mammography	1775 patients, 5202 images	2D images, Clinical	Molecular subtype, pathology	Chinese cohort, subtype info
RSNA screening Mammography [91]	Mammography	20,000 patients, 54,705 images	DICOM images	BI-RADS, density, case difficulty	Large-scale, annotated, RSNA
VinDr-Mammo [92]	Mammography	5000 exams, 20,000 images	2D images, lesion-level annotation	Mass, calcification, BI-RADS	Vietnamese population, open access
CSAW-CC [93]	Mammography	1,000,000+ images	2D images, metadata	Cancer outcome, radiologist assessment	Swedish screening, longitudinal

(continued)

Table 13.2 (continued)

Dataset	Modality	Sample size	Data type	Labels	Key features/source
BUSI [94]	Ultrasound	780 images, 600+ lesions	Images (PNG), masks	Benign, malignant, normal, Segmentation masks	Public, Egypt, Kaggle/ ScienceDirect
BrEaST [95]	Ultrasound	1048 images, 625 lesions	Images, annotation	Benign, malignant, normal,BI-RADS	Curated, nature scientific data
BUS-UCLM [96]	Ultrasound	683 images, 38 patients	Images (PNG), masks	Benign, malignant, normal, segmentation masks	Spain, Mendeley Data
BUS (AAPM/Wiley, 2023) [97]	Ultrasound	1600 images, 625 patients	Images, masks	Tumor segmentation, benign/malignant	Multi-institutional, AAPM/Wiley
BreastDCEDL [98]	MRI	2070 patients	3D MRI (NIfTI), clinical metadata	Tumor annotation, pCR, HR, HER2 status	Pretreatment DCE-MRI, arXiv
TCGA-BRCA [99]	MRI, WSI, genomics	~1100 patients	MRI, WSI, multi-omics, clinical	Genomics, histopathology, outcomes	TCGA/nature, multi-modal
RV-Cherry-Picker [100]	MRI	2035 subjects	DICOM MRI, clinical	Harmonized, searchable, FAIR	TCIA/PMC11001841
BCSS [101]	WSI (histopathology)	151 images, 20,000+ annotations	WSI, segmentation masks	Tissue region segmentation	TCGA, papers with Code
BreakHis [102]	WSI (histopathology)	7909 images	Images, 4 magnifications	Benign, malignant, 8 classes	Brazil, Kaggle

Challenges in AI for Cancer Research

AI has shown great promise in cancer research and care, but several key challenges remain that limit its widespread clinical adoption and impact. Table 13.3 summarizes the above challenges and suggests potential AI solutions to mitigate the issues.

The first challenge is data quality and availability. Cancer data often are heterogeneous and fragmented, because they usually come from multiple sources (e.g., pathology, imaging, genomics, EHR), stored in inconsistent formats across institutions. High-quality labeled data (e.g., tumor segmentations, mutation annotations) require expert input, which is time-consuming and costly. Patient data privacy regulations, e.g., HIPAA (Health Insurance Portability and Accountability Act) and GDPR (General Data Protection Regulation), restrict data sharing, hindering large-scale model training. Combining data from genomics, imaging, pathology, and clinical notes requires advanced architectures and harmonized preprocessing pipelines. In real-world settings, patients often lack one or more data types, which complicates model training and deployment. Emerging techniques like federated learning and synthetic data generation offer promising solutions to these barriers, enabling collaborative model training without compromising patient privacy.

Another critical issue is the lack of fairness and generalizability in many AI models. Training datasets often overrepresent certain demographics or single cancer types, leading to models that underperform on underrepresented populations. Furthermore, models trained on data from a single institution frequently fail to generalize to others due to variations in clinical protocols, imaging equipment, and population characteristics. Addressing these limitations requires the development of more inclusive datasets, as well as the adoption of fairness-aware algorithms and domain adaptation techniques. Additionally, many clinicians remain skeptical of AI

Table 13.3 AI for cancer: challenges, descriptions, and potential solutions

Challenge	Description	Potential solutions
Data quality and availability	Incomplete, noisy, or siloed data; expensive annotation; privacy concerns	Federated learning, synthetic data, data harmonization, annotation tools
Bias and generalizability	Models overfit to specific populations or institutions	Diverse datasets, fairness aware learning, domain Adaptation
Interpretability & Trust	Clinicians distrust "Blackbox" models	Explainable AI (XAI), attention maps, uncertainty quantification
Clinical integration	Poor fit with existing workflows; limited usability	Human-centered design Clinician-in-the-loop systems
Reproducibility & Validation	Few studies validate models across sites or in real-world conditions	External validation cohorts, open benchmarks, reproducible pipelines
Multimodal integration	Complex data fusion; missing modalities in real-world data	Robust multimodal architectures, Imputation methods, cross-modal training
Ethical and legal	Accountability, transparency, and regulatory compliance issues	Model documentation (e.g., datasheets), regulatory frameworks, open-source ethics audits

tools due to the "black-box" nature of deep learning models. In high-stakes environments like oncology, trust hinges on interpretability. Thus, explainable AI (XAI) methods, such as attention maps, uncertainty quantification, and model reasoning interfaces, are essential to foster clinical trust and accountability.

Integration into clinical workflows also poses practical challenges. Many AI tools are not designed with end users in mind, making them difficult to adopt in fast-paced clinical environments. Regulatory pathways, such as FDA approval, require rigorous validation and documentation, often slowing down deployment. Human-centered design, with clinicians involved throughout development, is key to creating usable, trustworthy systems. Finally, legal and ethical questions remain unresolved, such as who bears responsibility if an AI system makes a harmful recommendation: the developer, the institution, or the clinician? Proprietary models that lack transparency further complicate oversight and accountability. Moreover, many AI studies rely solely on internal test sets and do not validate performance on external or real-world datasets. The lack of standardized benchmarks also hampers meaningful comparison between models. To advance clinical translation, the field must prioritize open, diverse benchmarking datasets, robust validation protocols, and engagement with evolving regulatory frameworks.

Conclusion

AI is rapidly reshaping the landscape of cancer research, diagnosis, and treatment. From early detection to personalized treatment optimization and multiomics integration, AI-driven methods are enabling more precise, timely, and scalable approaches to cancer care. AI models have demonstrated remarkable accuracy in pathology, radiology, and genomics, often matching or exceeding expert level performance. Furthermore, their ability to integrate complex datasets from diverse sources is laying the foundation for a new era of precision cancer care.

Despite these advances, significant challenges remain. AI models sometimes are trained on limited datasets, compromising their generalizability across populations and institutions. The black-box nature of many deep learning models continues to raise concerns about interpretability, safety, and clinician trust. Regulatory hurdles, data privacy restrictions, and inconsistent validation further hinder the transition from research prototypes to real-world clinical tools. In addition, the fusion of multimodal data from radiological images and histopathology to genomic and clinical records remains a technical and operational hurdle, especially in resource-limited settings.

Looking ahead, the future of AI in cancer care will depend on three key pillars: collaboration, transparency, and clinical integration. Multi-institutional efforts to share and harmonize high-quality, diverse datasets will be essential to building robust and fair models. Advances in explainable AI and uncertainty quantification will help bridge the gap between algorithmic insight and clinical reasoning. Equally important, AI tools must be designed with direct input from patients, oncologists, and care teams to ensure they are practical, interpretable, and ethically sound.

Ultimately, AI is not a replacement for human expertise but a powerful tool to augment decision-making, reduce disparities, and accelerate innovation in cancer research. With continued interdisciplinary effort, regulatory clarity, and ethical foresight, AI has the potential to transform cancer care from reactive and generalized to proactive, personalized, and equitable.

References

1. Lin L, Liang L, Wang M, Huang R, Gong M, Song G, Hao T. A bibliometric analysis of worldwide cancer research using machine learning methods. Cancer Innov. 2023;2(3):219–32.
2. Sun W, Tseng T-LB, Qian W, Zhang J. Ai applications in breast cancer: a bibliometric analysis (2000–2023). Cancer. 2023;15(17):4455.
3. Davor Topalovic and et al. Artificial intelligence in lung cancer screening: a systematic review. Eur Respir Rev, 31(165):220075, 2022.
4. Ardila D, et al. End-to-end lung cancer screening with three dimensional deep learning on low-dose chest computed tomography. Nat Med. 2019;25(6):954–61.
5. Yuan Q, et al. Ai applications in colorectal cancer diagnosis and detection: a review. Front Oncol. 2023;13:1187137.
6. Ali HM, et al. Bibliometric analysis of artificial intelligence applications in glioblastoma research. Front Oncol. 2023;13:1189924.
7. Li Y, et al. A bibliometric analysis of artificial intelligence applications in liver cancer research from 2013 to 2023. Front Oncol. 2023;13:1223490.
8. Lipkova J, Chen RJ, Chen B, Lu MY, Barbieri M, Shao D, Vaidya AJ, Chen C, Zhuang L, Williamson DFK, et al. Artificial intelligence for multimodal data integration in oncology. Cancer Cell. 2022;40(10):1095–110.
9. Munir K, Siddiqui MS, Dengel A, Ahmed S, et al. Cancer diagnosis using deep learning: a bibliographic review. Comput Biol Med. 2019;104:103–15. Publisher: Elsevier
10. Wu C, Lin W, Zhang X, Zhang Y, Xie W, Wang Y. PMC-LLaMA: toward building open-source language models for medicine. J Am Med Inform Assoc. 2024:ocae045.
11. W. Feng, X. Li, H. Wang, and others. NULISA: a proteomic liquid biopsy platform with Attomolar sensitivity. Nat Commun, 14(1):2450, 2023.
12. Shao J, Wang Y, Qian Z. Predicting gene mutation status via AI based on multimodal integration. NPJ Precision Oncol. 2023;7:34.
13. Bhinder B, Gilvary C, Madhukar NS, Elemento O. Artificial intelligence in cancer research and precision medicine. Cancer Discov. 2021;11(4):900–15.
14. Koh D-M, Papanikolaou N, Bick U, Illing R, Kahn CE Jr, Kalpathi-Cramer J, Matos C, Mart'ıBonmat'ı L, Miles A, Mun

SK, et al. Artificial intelligence and machine learning in cancer imaging. Commun Med. 2022;2(1):133.
15. Kourou K, Exarchos KP, Papaloukas C, Sakaloglou P, Exarchos T, Dimitrios IF. Applied machine learning in cancer research: a systematic review for patient diagnosis, classification and prognosis. Comput Struct Biotechnol J. 2021;19:5546–55.
16. Gayathri B, Vidyasagar KE, Mudigonda M, Saikia MJ. Cancer detection using artificial intelligence: a paradigm in early diagnosis. Arch Comput. Methods Eng. 2025:1–39.
17. Iqbal MJ, Javed Z, Sadia H, Qureshi IA, Irshad A, Ahmed R, Malik K, Raza S, Abbas A, Pezzani R, et al. Clinical applications of artificial intelligence and machine learning in cancer diagnosis: looking into the future. Cancer Cell Int. 2021;21(1):270.
18. Zhang B, Shi H, Wang H. Machine learning and AI in cancer prognosis, prediction, and treatment selection: a critical approach. J Multidiscip Healthc. 2023;16:1779–91.
19. Shih-Cheng Huang, Anuj Pareek, Malte Jensen, Matthew P Lungren, Serena Yeung, Akshay S Chaudhari. Self-supervised learning for medical image classification: a systematic review and implementation guidelines. NPJ Digit Med. 2023;6(1):74.
20. Carl N, Schramm F, Haggenmuller S, Kather JN, Hetz MJ, Wies C, Michel MS, Wessels F, Brinker TJ. Large language model use in clinical oncology. NPJ Precis Oncol. 2024;8(1):240.
21. Singh P, Chukkapalli R, Chaudhari S, Chen L, Chen M, Pan J, Smuda C, Cirrone J. Shifting to machine supervision: annotation-efficient semi and self-supervised learning for automatic medical image segmentation and classification. Sci Rep. 2024;14(1):10820.
22. Eckardt J-N, Wendt K, Bornhaeuser M, Middeke JM. Reinforcement learning for precision oncology. Cancer. 2021;13(18):4624.
23. Khajuria R, Sarwar A. Review of reinforcement learning applications in segmentation, chemotherapy, and radiotherapy of cancer. Micron. 2024;178:103583.
24. Lu Y, Aslani S, Zhao A, Shahin A, Barber D, Emberton M, Alexander DC, Jacob J. A hybrid CNN-RNN approach for survival analysis in a lung cancer screening study. Heliyon. 2023;9(8)
25. Kaddes M, Ayid YM, Elshewey AM, Fouad Y. Breast cancer classification based on hybrid CNN with LSTM model. Sci Rep. 2025;15(1):4409.
26. Boehm KM, Khosravi P, Vanguri R, Gao J, Shah SP. Harnessing multimodal data integration to advance precision oncology. Nat Rev Cancer. 2022;22(2):114–26.
27. Shamshad F, Khan S, Zamir SW, Khan MH, Hayat M, Khan FS, Fu H. Transformers in medical imaging: a survey. Med Image Anal. 2023;88:102802.
28. Parvaiz A, Khalid MA, Zafar R, Ameer H, Ali M, Fraz MM. Vision transformers in medical computer vision—a contemplative retrospection. Eng Appl Artif Intell. 2023;122:106126.
29. Fanizzi A, Fadda F, Comes MC, Bove S, Catino A, Di Benedetto E, Milella A, Montrone M, Nardone A, Soranno C, et al. Comparison between vision transformers and convolutional neural networks to predict non-small lung cancer recurrence. Sci Rep. 2023;13(1):20605.
30. Bommasani R, Hudson DA, Adeli E, Altman R, Arora S, von Arx S, Bernstein MS, Bohg J, Bosselut A, Brunskill E, et al. On the opportunities and risks of foundation models. arXiv preprint arXiv:2108.07258; 2021.
31. Azad B, Azad R, Eskandari S, Bozorgpour A, Kazerouni A, Rekik I, Merhof D. Foundational models in medical imaging: A comprehensive survey and future vision. arXiv preprint arXiv:2310.18689; 2023.
32. Zhang S, Metaxas D. On the challenges and perspectives of foundation models for medical image analysis. Med Image Anal. 2024;91:102996.
33. Paschali M, Chen Z, Blankemeier L, Varma M, Youssef A, Bluethgen C, Langlotz C, Gatidis S, Chaudhari A. Foundation models in radiology: what, how, when, why and why not. Publisher: arXiv Version Number: 2; 2024.
34. Thirunavukarasu AJ, Ting DSJ, Elangovan K, Gutierrez L, Tan TF, Ting DSW. Large language models in medicine. Nat Med. 2023;29(8):1930–40.
35. Gupta S, Basu A, Nievas M, Thomas J, Wolfrath N, Ramamurthi A, Taylor B, Kothari AN, Schwind R, Miller TM, et al. Prism: patient records interpretation for semantic clinical trial matching system using large language models. Npj Digit Med. 2024;7(1):305.
36. Datta S, Lee K, Huang L-C, Paek H, Gildersleeve R, Gold J, Pillai D, Wang J, Higashi MK, Shi L, et al. Patient2trial: From patient to participant in clinical trials using large language models. Inform Med Unlocked. 2025:101615.
37. Omar M, Nadkarni GN, Klang E, Glicksberg BS. Large language models in medicine: a review of current clinical trials across healthcare applications. PLoS Digit Health. 2024;3(11):e0000662.
38. Hartsock I, Rasool G. Vision-language models for medical report generation and visual question answering: a review. Front Artif Intell. 2024;7:1430984.
39. Tanno R, Barrett DGT, Sellergren A, Ghaisas S, Dathathri S, See A, Welbl J, Lau C, Tu T, Azizi S, et al. Collaboration between clinicians and vision– language models in radiology report generation. Nat Med. 2025;31(2):599–608.
40. Bi WL, Hosny A, Schabath MB, Giger ML, Birkbak NJ, Mehrtash A, Allison T, Arnaout O, Abbosh C, Dunn IF, et al. Artificial intelligence in cancer imaging: clinical challenges and applications. CA Cancer J Clin. 2019;69(2):127–57.
41. Luchini C, Pea A, Scarpa A. Artificial intelligence in oncology: current applications and future perspectives. Br J Cancer. 2022;126(1):4–9.
42. Nguyen DC, Pham Q-V, Pathirana PN, Ding M, Seneviratne A, Lin Z, Dobre O, Hwang W-J. Federated learning for smart healthcare: a survey. ACM Comput Surveys (Csur). 2022;55(3):1–37.
43. Rodrigues MA, et al. Federated learning for breast cancer diagnosis via mammograms in a multi-institutional setting. Artif Intell Med. 2021;112:102003.
44. Gao Y, et al. Privacy-preserving federated learning for mammography image classification. Nat Commun. 2022;13:1234.
45. Xiaoming Zhou, Yusheng Wang. Artificial intelligence in medical imaging of the lungs. Front Med. 2020;7:204. Publisher: Frontiers
46. Lin J, et al. Transformer-based models for lung cancer detection in CT scans. IEEE Trans Med Imaging. 2023;42(4):998–1010.
47. Kather JN, et al. Deep learning can predict microsatellite instability directly from histology in gastrointestinal cancer. Nat Med. 2019;25:1054–6.
48. Bilal M, et al. Development and validation of deep learning algorithms for detecting colorectal polyps. Lancet Digit Health. 2021;3(12):e715–23.
49. Nie D, et al. Automatic brain tumor segmentation using cascaded CNN and RNN. Med Image Anal. 2021;67:101842.
50. Senders JT, et al. Graph neural networks for brain tumor grading with multi-parametric MRI. Neuro-oncol. 2022;24(3):482–93.
51. Chen Y, et al. Radiomics-based machine learning for liver cancer diagnosis and prognosis. Hepatology. 2020;71:1116–28.
52. Hu Z, Ma L, Ding Y, Zhao X, Shi X, Lu H, Liu K. Enhancing the accuracy of lymph-node-metastasis prediction in gynecologic malignancies using multimodal federated learning: integrating CT, MRI, and PET/CT. Cancer. 2023;15(21):5281.
53. Frazer HML, Pen˜a-Solorzano CA, Kwok CF, Elliott MS, Chen Y, Wang C, BRAIx Team Al-Qershi Osamah, Fox Samantha K, Brendan H, Ravishankar K, Katrina K, Shuai L, Enes M, Nguyen Tuong L, Basnayake RP, Daniel S, Weideman Prue C, Lippey JF, Hopper JL, Brotchie P, et al. Comparison of AI-integrated pathways with human-ai interaction in population mammographic screening for breast cancer. Nat Commun. 2024;15(1):7525.

54. Azam S, Eriksson M, Sjolander A, Gabrielson M, Hellgren R, Czene K, Hall P. Mammographic microcalcifications and risk of breast cancer. Br J Cancer. 2021;125(5):759–65.
55. Wu N, Huang Z, Shen Y, Park J, Phang J, Makino T, Kim SG, Cho K, Heacock L, Moy L, et al. Reducing false-positive biopsies using deep neural networks that utilize both local and global image context of screening mammograms. J Digit Imaging. 2021;34:1414–23.
56. Hernstr¨om V, Josefsson V, Sartor H, Schmidt D, Larsson A-M, Hofvind S, Andersson I, Rosso A, Hagberg O, Lang K. Screening performance and characteristics of breast cancer detected in the mammography screening with artificial intelligence trial (masai): a randomised, controlled, parallel-group, non-inferiority, single-blinded, screening accuracy study. Lancet Digit Health. 2025;
57. Aly GH, Marey MAE-R, Amin SES. Mammograms with ResNet and inception. In: Advanced machine learning technologies and applications: proceedings of AMLTA 2021, vol. 1339; 2021. p. 145.
58. Garrucho L, Kushibar K, Jouide S, Diaz O, Igual L, Lekadir K. Domain generalization in deep learning based mass detection in mammography: a large-scale multi-center study. Artif Intell Med. 2022;132:102386.
59. Shen T, Hao K, Gou C, Wang F-Y. Mass image synthesis in mammogram with contextual information based on gans. Comput Methods Prog Biomed. 2021;202:106019.
60. Hussain S, Ali M, Naseem U, Nezhadmoghadam F, Jatoi MA, Gulliver TA, TamezPen˜a JG. Breast cancer risk prediction using machine learning: a systematic review. Front Oncol. 2024;14:1343627.
61. Maurizio C'e, Elena C, Maria E P, Mariachiara B, Adriana S, Deborah F, Giancarlo O, Michaela C. Artificial intelligence in breast cancer imaging: risk stratification, lesion detection and classification, treatment planning and prognosis—a narrative review. Exploration of targeted anti-tumor therapy. 2022;3(6):795.
62. Yala A, Mikhael PG, Lehman C, Lin G, Strand F, Wan Y-L, Hughes K, Satuluru S, Kim T, Banerjee I, et al. Optimizing risk-based breast cancer screening policies with reinforcement learning. Nat Med. 2022;28(1):136–43.
63. Yala A, Schuster T, Miles R, Barzilay R, Lehman C. A deep learning model to triage screening mammograms: a simulation study. Radiology. 2019;293(1):38–46.
64. McKinney SM, Sieniek M, Godbole V, Godwin J, Antropova N, Ashrafian H, Back T, Chesus M, Corrado GS, Darzi A, et al. International evaluation of an AI system for breast cancer screening. Nature. 2020;577(7788):89–94.
65. Sushanki S, Bhandari AK, Singh AK. A review on computational methods for breast cancer detection in ultrasound images using multi-image modalities. Arch Comput Methods Eng. 2024;31(3):1277–96.
66. Xu Z, Wang Y, Chen M, Zhang Q. Multi-region radiomics for artificially intelligent diagnosis of breast cancer using multimodal ultrasound. Comput Biol Med. 2022;149:105920.
67. Sangeetha SKB, Mathivanan SK, Muthukumaran V, Cho J, Easwaramoorthy SV. An empirical analysis of transformer-based and convolutional neural network approaches for early detection and diagnosis of cancer using multimodal imaging and genomic data. IEEE Access. 2024;
68. Zhang DY, Venkat A, Khasawneh H, Sali R, Zhang V, Pei Z. Implementation of digital pathology and artificial intelligence in routine pathology practice. Lab Invest. 2024:102111.
69. McGenity C, Clarke EL, Jennings C, Matthews G, Cartlidge C, Freduah-Agyemang H, Stocken DD, Treanor D. Artificial intelligence in digital pathology: a systematic review and meta-analysis of diagnostic test accuracy. NPJ Digit Med. 2024;7(1):114.
70. Hu W, Li X, Li C, Li R, Jiang T, Sun H, Huang X, Grzegorzek M, Li X. A state-of-the-art survey of artificial neural networks for whole-slide image analysis: from popular convolutional neural networks to potential visual transformers. Comput Biol Med. 2023;161:107034.
71. Katayama A, Aoki Y, Watanabe Y, Horiguchi J, Rakha EA, Oyama T. Current status and prospects of artificial intelligence in breast cancer pathology: convolutional neural networks to prospective vision transformers. Int J Clin Oncol. 2024;29(11):1648–68.
72. Waqas A, Bui MM, Glassy EF, El Naqa I, Borkowski P, Borkowski AA, Rasool G. Revolutionizing digital pathology with the power of generative artificial intelligence and foundation models. Lab Investig. 2023;103(11):100255.
73. Bilal M, Raza M, Altherwy Y, Alsuhaibani A, Abduljabbar A, Almarshad F, Golding P, Rajpoot N, et al. Foundation models in computational pathology: a review of challenges, opportunities, and impact. arXiv preprint arXiv:2502.08333. 2025;
74. Li D, Wan G, Wu X, Wu X, Nirmal AJ, Lian CG, Sorger PK, Semenov YR, Zhao C. A survey on computational pathology foundation models: Datasets, adaptation strategies, and evaluation tasks. arXiv preprint arXiv:2501.15724. 2025;
75. Xu H, Usuyama N, Bagga J, Zhang S, Rao R, Naumann T, Wong C, Gero Z, Gonz'alez J, Gu Y, et al. A whole-slide foundation model for digital pathology from real-world data. Nature. 2024;630(8015):181–8.
76. Khalsan M, Machado LR, Al-Shamery ES, Ajit S, Anthony K, Mu M, Agyeman MO. A survey of machine learning approaches applied to gene expression analysis for cancer prediction. IEEE Access. 2022;10:27522–27,534.
77. Umakanthan S. Role of molecular-genetic profiling and artificial intelligence in breast cancer diagnosis and insight into targeted pharmacotherapeutics. London J. Med. Health Res. 2024;24(10):1–25.
78. Yang Z, Guo C, Li J, Li Y, Zhong L, Pu P, Shang T, Cong L, Zhou Y, Qiao G, et al. An explainable multimodal artificial intelligence model integrating histopathological microenvironment and EHR phenotypes for germline genetic testing in breast cancer. Adv Sci. 2025:e02833.
79. Guo H, Lv X, Li Y, Li M. Attention-based GCN integrates multi-omics data for breast cancer subtype classification and patient-specific gene marker identification. Brief Funct Genomics. 2023;22(5):463–74.
80. Choi SR, Lee M. Transformer architecture and attention mechanisms in genome data analysis: a comprehensive review. Biology. 2023;12(7):1033.
81. Amkrane Y, El Adoui M, Benjelloun M. Towards breast cancer response prediction using artificial intelligence and radiomics. In: 2020 5th International Conference on Cloud Computing and Artificial Intelligence: Technologies and Applications (CloudTech). IEEE; 2020. p. 1–5.
82. Skarping I, Larsson M, D F¨ornvik. Analysis of mammograms using artificial intelligence to predict response to neoadjuvant chemotherapy in breast cancer patients: proof of concept. Eur Radiol. 2022:1–11.
83. Romeo V, Accardo G, Perillo T, Basso L, Garbino N, Nicolai E, Maurea S, Salvatore M. Assessment and prediction of response to neoadjuvant chemotherapy in breast cancer: a comparison of imaging modalities and future perspectives. Cancer. 2021;13(14):3521.
84. Dodington DW, Andrew L, Sami T, Majid M, Ali S-N, Tran WT, Fang-I L. Analysis of tumor nuclear features using artificial intelligence to predict response to neoadjuvant chemotherapy in high-risk breast cancer patients. Breast Cancer Res Treat. 2021;186:379–89.

85. Poortmans PMP, Takanen S, Marta GN, Meattini I, Kaidar-Person O. Winter is over: the use of artificial intelligence to individualise radiation therapy for breast cancer. Breast. 2020;49:194–200.
86. Moser EC, Narayan G. Improving breast cancer care coordination and symptom management by using AI driven predictive toolkits. Breast. 2020;50:25–9.
87. Lee RS, Gimenez F, Hoogi A, Miyake KK, Gorovoy M, Rubin DL. A curated mammography data set for use in computer-aided detection and diagnosis research. Sci Data. 2017;4(1):1–9.
88. Moreira IC, Amaral I, Domingues I, Cardoso A'o, Cardoso MJ, Cardoso JS. Inbreast: toward a full-field digital mammographic database. Acad Radiol. 2012;19(2):236–48.
89. Alsolami AS, Shalash W, Alsaggaf W, Ashoor S, Refaat H, Elmogy M. King abdulaziz university breast cancer mammogram dataset (kau-BCMD). Data. 2021;6(11):111.
90. Cui C, Li L, Cai H, Fan Z, Zhang L, Dan T, Li J, Wang J. The Chinese mammography database (CMMD): an online mammography database with biopsy confirmed types for machine diagnosis of breast. Cancer Imaging Arch. 2021;1
91. Carr C, Kitamura F, Kalpathy-Cramer J, Mongan J, Andriole K, Vazirabad M, Riopel M, Ball R, Dane S. RSNA screening mammography breast cancer detection. Kaggle; 2022.
92. Nguyen HT, Nguyen HQ, Pham HH, Lam K, Le LT, Dao M, Vu V. Vindr-mammo: a large-scale benchmark dataset for computer-aided diagnosis in full-field digital mammography. Sci Data. 2023;10(1):277.
93. Strand F. Csaw-cc (mammography)—a dataset for AI research to improve screening, diagnostics and prognostics of breast cancer, version 1. Karolinska Institutet; 2022.
94. Al-Dhabyani W, Gomaa M, Khaled H, Fahmy A. Dataset of breast ultrasound images. Data Brief. 2020;28:104863.
95. Pawlowska A, Cwierz-Pien'kowska A, Domalik A, Jagu's D, Kasprzak P, Matkowski R, Fura L, Nowicki A, Zolek N. Curated benchmark dataset for ultrasound based breast lesion analysis. Sci Data. 2024;11(1):148.
96. Vallez N, Bueno G, Deniz O, Rienda MA, Pastor C. Bus-UCLM: breast ultrasound lesion segmentation dataset. Sci Data. 2025;12(1):242.
97. Thomas C, Byra M, Marti R, Yap MH, Zwiggelaar R. Bus-set: a benchmark for quantitative evaluation of breast ultrasound segmentation networks with public datasets. Med Phys. 2023;50(5):3223–43.
98. Fridman N, Solway B, Fridman T, Barnea I, Goldshtein A. Breastdcedl: Curating a comprehensive DCE-MRI dataset and developing a transformer implementation for breast cancer treatment response prediction. arXiv preprint arXiv:2506.12190. 2025;
99. Thennavan A, Beca F, Xia Y, Garcia-Recio S, Allison K, Collins LC, Tse GM, Chen Y-Y, Schnitt SJ, Hoadley KA, et al. Molecular analysis of TCGA breast cancer histologic types. Cell Geno. 2021;1(3):100067.
100. Kilintzis V, Kalokyri V, Kondylakis H, Joshi S, Nikiforaki K, D'ıaz O, Lekadir K, Tsiknakis M, Marias K. Public data homogenization for AI model development in breast cancer. Eur Radiol Exp. 2024;8(1):42.
101. Amgad M, Elfandy H, Hussein H, Atteya LA, Elsebaie MAT, Abo Elnasr LS, Sakr RA, Salem HSE, Ismail AF, Saad AM, et al. Structured crowdsourcing enables convolutional segmentation of histology images. Bioinformatics. 2019;35(18):3461–7.
102. Spanhol FA, Oliveira LS, Petitjean C, Heutte L. A dataset for breast cancer histopathological image classification. IEEE Trans Biomed Eng. 2015;63(7):1455–62.

Part III

Special Topics

14 Research on Neurological Cancer

Emily M. Pearson, Kevin L. Pham, and James K. C. Liu

Abbreviations

5-ALA	5-aminolevulinic acid
ACTH	Adrenocorticotropic hormone
ALK	Anaplastic lymphoma kinase
BBB	Blood-brain barrier
BM	Brain metastases
BRAF	B-Raf proto-oncogene
CAFÉ	Cancer Patient Fracture Evaluation
CEBRT	Conventional external-beam radiation therapy
CNS	Central nervous system
CTLA-4	Cytotoxic T-lymphocyte antigen 4
DCVax-L	Dendritic cell vaccine
EGFR	Epidermal growth factor receptor
FSRT	Fractionated stereotactic radiotherapy
GBM	Glioblastoma
GH	Growth hormone
GTR	Gross total resection
HER2	Human epidermal growth factor receptor 2
ICI	Immune checkpoint inhibitors
IDH	Isocitrate dehydrogenase
NCCN	National Comprehensive Cancer Network
NF2	Neurofibromin 2
NSCLC	Non-small cell lung cancer
OS	Overall survival
PCV	Procarbazine, lomustine, vincristine
PD-1	Programmed cell death protein 1
PFS	Progression-free survival
PitNETs	Pituitary neuroendocrine tumors
RT	Radiation therapy
SBRT	Stereotactic body radiation therapy
SINS	Spine Instability Neoplastic Score
SM	Spinal metastases
SRS	Stereotactic radiosurgery
SSTR2A	Somatostatin receptor 2A
STR	Subtotal tumor resection
TKI	Tyrosine kinase inhibitor
TMZ	Temozolomide
TSH	Thyroid-stimulating hormone
TTF	Tumor-treating fields
VEGF	Vascular endothelial growth factor
VEGFα	Vascular endothelial growth factor α
WBRT	Whole-brain radiation therapy
WHO	World Health Organization

Introduction

Neoplasms in the central nervous system (CNS) can be best categorized based on primary versus metastatic malignancies. Metastatic tumors of the brain and spine are much more commonly encountered due to the variety of malignancies that have a propensity for metastasizing to the brain. The treatment for metastatic disease typically involves a multidisciplinary approach, consisting of a combination of surgical, radiation, and medical therapies. Although surgery and radiation have been the predominant therapies used for the treatment of brain and spinal metastases, emerging systemic therapies have demonstrated effectiveness in the treatment of malignancies targeting specific mutations and receptors and have enhanced the options for treatment. Primary tumors within the brain can be categorized as benign or malignant. Among the two most common benign primary malignancies are meningiomas and pituitary neuroendocrine tumors, formerly pituitary adenomas. The most common malignant primary tumor is adult diffuse-type gliomas, which include low-grade and high-grade astrocytomas, oligodendrogliomas, and glioblastomas (GBM). These tumors can be challenging to treat and require a multidisciplinary approach.

E. M. Pearson
Morsani School of Medicine, University of South Florida, Tampa, FL, USA

K. L. Pham · J. K. C. Liu (✉)
Neurosurgical Oncology, Department of Neuro-Oncology, Moffitt Cancer Center, Tampa, FL, USA
e-mail: James.liu@moffitt.org

J. Huang, H. S.L. Jim (eds.), *Cancer Research Guidance for Clinicians and Researchers*,
https://doi.org/10.1007/978-3-032-19175-5_14

Here we will review common primary brain tumors followed by malignant and metastatic tumors of the brain and spine.

Meningiomas

Meningiomas are the most common form of primary intracranial tumors in adults, making up nearly 40.8% of all primary brain tumors and 56.2% of nonmalignant tumors [1]. These tumors arise from the meningeal layers of the brain and spinal cord originating from arachnoid cap cells [2]. Meningiomas can occur in a variety of anatomical locations, from the cortical surface to the base of the skull. Meningiomas occur in 9.73 per 100,000 individuals. They are more common in adults in comparison to children (ages 0–19), with a mean age of 66 years old. Females are more frequently affected than males with a ratio of 2.3:1. Among all other spinal cord tumors, these neoplasms account for the largest proportion of brain tumors contributing to 39.9% for patients ages 20 years and older [1].

These tumors are generally sporadic in nature and may consist of one or more focal chromosomal deletions. Among them is the functional loss of neurofibromin 2 (*NF2*) which is found in nearly 40–60% of those with meningiomas. A known risk factor associated with the development of meningiomas is a history of ionizing radiation [3]. The 2021 World Health Organization (WHO) classification of CNS tumors defines 15 distinct subtypes of meningiomas based on histopathological features [4]. These subtypes are graded from 1 to 3 based on prognosis and molecular biomarkers. Grade 1 meningiomas are the most prevalent and encompass roughly 80% of all meningiomas, whereas grades 2 and 3 make up approximately 15–20% and 1–3% of such tumors, respectively [5].

Depending on the location of the meningioma, symptoms can range from headaches to focal neurological deficits such as decreased strength, loss of coordination, and difficulty with speech. Meningiomas located at the base of the skull may result in symptoms affecting cranial nerves, including visual changes and facial motor or sensory asymmetry.

Treatment for meningiomas depends on the size, growth rate, and presence of neurological symptoms. Since most meningiomas are grade 1 and considered benign, incidentally found lesions that are asymptomatic are managed conservatively with serial imaging. Tumors that demonstrate marked growth and are causing significant mass effect or neurological symptoms can be treated. The mainstay treatment for meningioma is surgery. The extent of surgical resection of meningiomas is categorized using the Simpson grading scale. Simpson grades 1–3 are gross total resections (GTR) of the tumor with varying amounts of dura and bone resection, grade 4 is a subtotal tumor resection (STR), and grade 5 is a biopsy [6]. Even with GTR, recurrence rates can be up to 23% for grade 1, 55% for grade 2, and 78% for grade 3 tumors [7]. Intraoperative technologies have been employed to improve tumor visualization for high-grade meningiomas that may demonstrate infiltration into the adjacent brain parenchyma. 5-aminolevulinic acid (5-ALA; Gleolan, NX Development Corps, Lexington, USA) is an indirect fluorophore that allows for the visualization of tumor cells under fluorescent light and has been approved for use in malignant gliomas [8]. Building on the knowledge that meningiomas are also known to fluoresce, the NXDC-MEN-301 study was a multicenter trial that examined the utility of 5-ALA-induced tumor fluorescence during meningioma resection. This phase 3, single-arm study enrolled 88 patients across 15 sites as of May 2022 [9]. The LUMINA phase I/II trial recruited 25 patients to explore the possibility of highlighting meningiomas using bevacizumab, an antibody against vascular endothelial growth factor α (VEGFα), with a fluorescent label. Because VEGFα is highly expressed in the tumor but not in the dura mater, bevacizumab-IRDye800CW allowed visualization of the tumor margins as well as meningioma infiltration into adjacent dural matter and bone [10].

Radiation therapy (RT) is often used for residual tumors, surgically inaccessible tumors, or as an adjunct for grade 2 or 3 meningiomas. Adjuvant radiotherapy has been shown to increase progression-free survival (PFS) and overall survival (OS), decrease recurrence, and improve local control [11, 12]. The RTOG 0539 trial broadly sought to evaluate PFS among patients with meningiomas of all WHO grades. Among the low-risk cohort, 60 patients with grade 1 meningiomas were observed following GTR or STR without adjuvant therapies. PFS was higher for the GTR group (94.3% at 3 years, 87.6% at 10 years) than the STR group (83.1% at 3 years, 72.7% at 10 years), suggesting that optimization of adjuvant therapies is necessary to improve outcomes among low-risk patients who undergo STR [13]. The intermediate-risk cohort included 48 patients with either recurrent grade 1 meningioma after resection or a new grade 2 meningioma who underwent GTR. Each patient received an RT dosage of 54 Gy in 30 fractions. The cohort showed a PFS of 93.8% over 3 years, supporting the role of adjuvant RT in the management of intermediate-risk meningiomas [14]. The high-risk cohort included 51 evaluable patients with either recurrent grade 2 meningiomas, new grade 2 meningiomas after STR, or any grade 3 meningioma. All patients in this cohort received an RT dosage of 60 Gy in 30 fractions. This cohort showed a PFS of only 58.8% over 3 years, emphasizing the need for more effective treatment of high-grade meningiomas [15]. Current National Comprehensive Cancer Network (NCCN) guidelines for CNS tumors recommend RT for grade 2 meningioma undergoing STR or any grade 3 meningiomas regardless of the extent of resection [16].

Numerous types of systemic therapies have been applied to meningiomas, but none have demonstrated significant effectiveness. Chemotherapeutic agents that are recommended for use for meningiomas by the NCCN guideline include vascular endothelial growth factor (VEGF) inhibitors and somatostatin receptor agonists. A phase II trial of sunitinib, a VEGF inhibitor, for grade 2/3 recurrent meningiomas demonstrated a 6-month progression-free survival (PFS-6) of 42% among the 36 patients [17]. In another phase II trial with 50 patients, bevacizumab, also a VEGF inhibitor, demonstrated PFS-6 of 87%, 77%, and 46% for grade 1, 2, and 3 meningiomas, respectively, and has demonstrated evidence of tumor regression [18].

Currently, ongoing research for meningioma consists of attempts to establish chemotherapeutic options, especially for high-grade tumors. The CEVOREM trial was a phase II trial evaluating the coadministration of octreotide, a somatostatin receptor 2A (SSTR2A) agonist, and everolimus, an mTOR inhibitor, that demonstrated promising antitumor results. In this trial, 20 patients underwent administration of these agents which resulted in more than a 50% growth decrease in 78% of tumors [19]. Other chemotherapeutic options have demonstrated less efficacy in exploratory testing. Trabectedin, a chemotherapeutic alkylating agent, was evaluated in 90 patients with recurrent grade 2 or 3 meningiomas in a phase II clinical trial. Patients were randomly assigned to trabectedin treatment or the local standard of care. Trabectedin failed to significantly improve the primary endpoint of PFS and was associated with an increased rate of adverse events [20].

Trials assessing the utility of additional systemic therapies are ongoing. A phase II randomized-controlled study initiated in 2023 is evaluating the utility of abemaciclib, a cyclin-dependent kinase 4/6 inhibitor. An estimated 72 patients with newly diagnosed grade 3 meningiomas will be randomly assigned to treatment with abemaciclib or placebo after receiving standard RT, with the PFS measured over 2 years as the primary outcome [21]. The MIRAGE trial (NCT06275919) was initiated in 2024 to test the efficacy of regorafenib, a multi-kinase inhibitor currently approved for the treatment of cancers including hepatocellular carcinoma and colorectal cancer. This randomized-controlled phase II trial in Italy will recruit an estimated 104 patients with recurrent grade 2 and 3 meningiomas and randomly assign them to regorafenib or local standard-of-care treatment. The primary outcome will be PFS measured over a period of 36 months [22].

Pituitary Neuroendocrine Tumors

Previously referred to as pituitary adenomas, these tumors are now classified as pituitary neuroendocrine tumors (PitNETs) in the 2022 5th edition of the WHO Classification of Endocrine and Neuroendocrine Tumors [23]. This nomenclature change took place to provide a more accurate representation of these types of tumors which are not all benign, as would be implied by the term "adenoma." PitNETs are among the most prevalent types of primary brain tumors, making up roughly 17.2% of all primary brain tumors [1]. Incidence rates of PitNETs are 4.54 per 100,000 population. The median age of diagnosis is 51 years old. These tumors are more commonly found in females with a male-to-female incidence rate ratio of 0.77 and are more prevalent in African American individuals when compared to Caucasians [1]. The pathogenesis of these tumors remains unknown, and they arise sporadically. Genetic mutations are rare; however, mutations in multiple endocrine neoplasia types 1 and 4 have the potential to form tumors in the pituitary glands [24].

PitNETs are defined as a clonal neoplastic proliferation of hormone-producing cells from the anterior pituitary gland. They are generally considered benign and slow-growing, with rare aggressive and malignant cases. Classification is based on the size, cell of origin, and whether they are functioning or nonfunctioning. Functional tumors are characterized by the increased secretion of one or more hormones, most commonly prolactin, followed by growth hormone (GH), adrenocorticotropic hormone (ACTH), and thyroid-stimulating hormone (TSH). Nonfunctional tumors do not secrete hormones but have the potential to cause neurological deficits due to their size and compression of the adjacent neural structures. They can also cause hormone deficiencies due to compression of the anterior pituitary gland [25].

Small nonfunctional PitNETs are generally asymptomatic. Larger tumors that extend into the suprasellar space or cavernous sinus can cause mass effect on the adjacent cranial nerves resulting in visual field defects (bitemporal hemianopsia) or pupil/extraocular muscle disorders. Functional tumors result in endocrinologic abnormalities depending on the type of hormone being oversecreted. Prolactin-secreting tumors result in amenorrhea-galactorrhea in women and impotence in men. GH secretion results in acromegaly, ACTH-secreting tumors result in Cushing's disease, and TSH results in symptoms consistent with hyperthyroidism.

Treatment for PitNETs depends on the size and functional status of the tumor. Small nonfunctional tumors that are asymptomatic and do not cause mass effect on adjacent neural structures can be observed with serial imaging. For tumors that cause mass effect on the adjacent neural structures, surgical resection is the optimal treatment and is often performed through an endoscopic transnasal transsphenoidal approach [26]. A transcranial approach is an alternative for larger tumors or tumors that extend above the sella.

For all functional PitNETs except prolactin-secreting tumors, surgical resection is the first-line treatment. Prolactin-secreting tumors can be treated with dopamine agonists such as cabergoline or bromocriptine [27]. For prolactinomas that are refractory to medical therapy or in patients who are unable to tolerate systemic therapy, surgical resection is an effective option and achieves remission in up to 72% of patients [28]. GH-secreting tumors that persist despite surgical resection can be treated with somatostatin receptor ligands such as octreotide or lanreotide [29]. Pegvisomant, a GH receptor antagonist, has also been demonstrated to be effective for the treatment of acromegaly. The ACROSTUDY included 2221 patients treated with pegvisomant followed for a median of 7.4 years. Over 60% of the participants achieved insulin-like growth factor-1 normalization by the conclusion of the study [30]. ACTH-secreting tumors refractory to surgical treatment can be treated with pasireotide, a multi-receptor somatostatin analog that inhibits ACTH secretion. A phase III clinical trial included 162 patients with ACTH-secreting tumors randomly assigned to treatment with different dosages of pasireotide. The results demonstrated a measurable decrease in pituitary tumor size among 75% of patients in the higher-dose group as well as 44% of patients in the lower-dose group [31].

Systemic options are limited for nonfunctioning tumors. There has been some evidence of the effective use of chemotherapies for PitNETs, most notably temozolomide (TMZ) [32]. In a study of 100 patients, TMZ therapy showed a 55% response rate for aggressive PitNETs [33]. Furthermore, the use of cabergoline in the management of nonfunctioning pituitary adenomas has been controversial. A 2022 meta-analysis including 5 relevant studies encompassing 187 patients with nonfunctioning PitNETs demonstrated modest efficacy of cabergoline. Pooled proportions of tumor shrinkage and prevention of tumor progression were 19% and 50%, respectively [34].

Novel medical approaches are undergoing evaluation, mostly in small-scale trials. Lapatinib, a tyrosine kinase inhibitor (TKI) targeting the epidermal growth factor receptor and receptor tyrosine-protein kinase, demonstrated potential as a treatment for prolactinomas. A small phase IIa trial applied lapatinib treatment to four patients with aggressive prolactinomas resistant to dopamine agonist therapy. Three patients showed stable disease after 6 months of treatment, though no patients reached the primary endpoint of a 40% reduction in tumor burden [35]. A phase III trial in Japan focused on the treatment of TSH-secreting tumors with lanreotide. Among the 13 patients with TSH-secreting tumors, tumor size decreased by an average of 23.82% [36].

Adult-Type Diffuse Gliomas

Each year, over 86,000 individuals are diagnosed with a primary brain tumor. Roughly 28% of these tumors are considered malignant, and 26.3% are considered gliomas [1]. Gliomas are neuroepithelial tumors originating from glial cells found within the CNS. They are among the most prevalent forms of primary brain tumors affecting the CNS, affecting 6 per 100,000 individuals annually in the United States. Though no definite underlying causes for gliomas have been identified, one established risk factor for these tumors includes exposure to ionizing radiation, especially for the treatment of other cancers such as leukemia [37].

The 2021 5th edition of the WHO Classification of Tumors of the Central Nervous System introduced significant changes to glioma classification by incorporating molecular profiling. Previous classifications focused heavily on histological analysis to determine grading or degree of malignancy [38]. The updated version considers molecular classification to more accurately classify CNS neoplasms to allow grouping for similar behavior and outcomes. The most common type of glioma tumors is adult-type diffuse gliomas, which consist of three main types of tumors: astrocytoma, oligodendroglioma, and glioblastoma (Fig. 14.1) [4]. Astrocytomas are classified based on the presence of isocitrate dehydrogenase (IDH) gene mutations and are graded from 2 to 3. Oligodendrogliomas, classified as WHO grade 2 or 3, are defined by the presence of an IDH mutation and 1p/19q codeletion. GBM are IDH-wild-type tumors and are grade 4. Grade 2 tumors are considered low-grade tumors, whereas grades 3 and 4 are high grade.

Primary diffuse gliomas most commonly present with headaches secondary to increased intracranial pressure. Depending on the location of the tumor, symptoms can also include focal neurological deficits such as motor and sensory symptoms, as well as speech aphasias. Tumors may also present with focal or generalized seizures, a common initial presenting symptom in low-grade gliomas [39].

Treatment for diffuse gliomas typically involves a combination of surgery, radiation, and chemotherapy, depending on the type and grade of the tumor. Maximal safe surgical resection is recommended for both low-grade and high-grade adult diffuse-type gliomas. Surgery allows for the establishment of a pathologic diagnosis, alleviation of symptoms from mass effect and cerebral edema, and tumor cytoreduction to enhance the effectiveness of adjuvant radiation therapy. GTR is ideal as the extent of resection, including the residual tumor volume, has been demonstrated to correlate with overall survival [40–42]. Therefore, whenever possible, maximal safe resection is favored as first-line treatment over biopsy alone.

Treatment of low-grade tumors consists of surgical resection followed by observation or adjuvant therapy, depending on the amount of residual tumor or the presence of risk factors for recurrence. For grade 2 oligodendrogliomas (IDH-mut, 1p/19q co-deleted), treatment consists of surgical resection followed by observation if a complete resection was performed. In the presence of residual tumor, adjuvant therapy with radiation followed by procarbazine, lomustine,

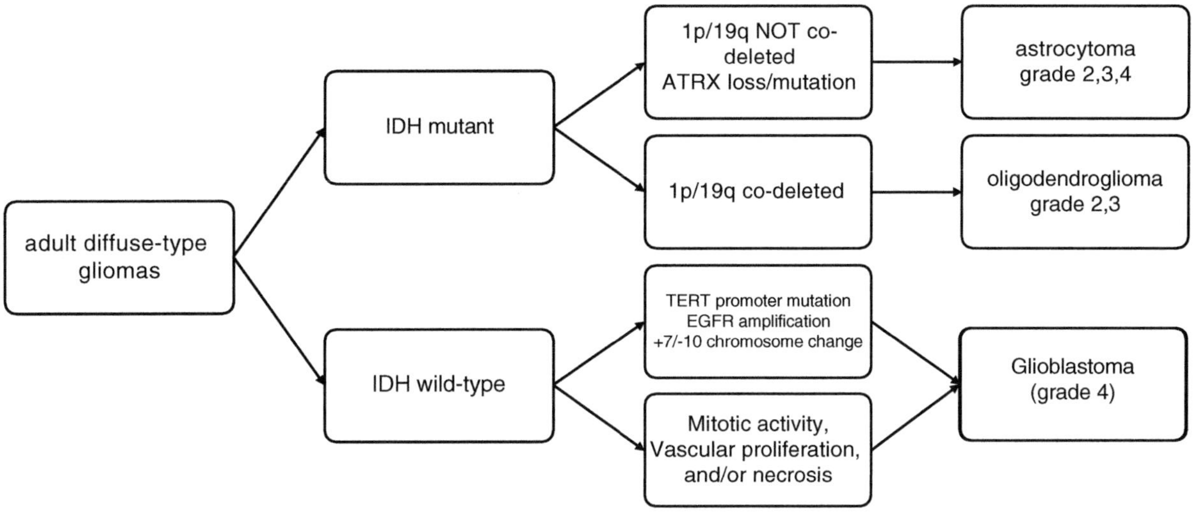

Fig. 14.1 Summary of 2021 WHO CNS Tumor Classification of adult diffuse-type gliomas. The 2021 WHO CNS Tumor classification identifies astrocytoma, oligodendrogliomas, and glioblastoma based on molecular profiling

and vincristine (PCV) is recommended. RTOG 9802, a phase III randomized trial with 251 patients, demonstrated that adjuvant PCV following radiation therapy can improve OS and PFS in IDH-mutant tumors [43].

For grade 3 oligodendrogliomas, several studies have demonstrated that the addition of adjuvant PCV following RT resulted in a significant increase in overall survival [44]. The CODEL trial evaluated radiation alone, TMZ alone, or a combination in the treatment of newly diagnosed grade 3 oligodendroglioma. The combination of RT with TMZ resulted in improved PFS and OS [45]. A follow-up to this study evaluated RT with PCV versus TMZ in grade 3 oligodendroglioma [46]. In this study of 305 newly diagnosed grade 3 oligodendroglioma patients, it was found that there was improved OS with PCV and RT compared to TMZ and RT.

Treatment for high-grade (3 and 4) astrocytoma (IDH-mutant) is similar to GBM, consisting of maximal safe surgical resection followed by concurrent chemoradiation therapy and adjuvant systemic therapy. The CATNON trial, a phase III randomized trial with 751 patients, demonstrated that the addition of adjuvant TMZ, but not concurrent TMZ with radiation, significantly improved OS and PFS [47].

For GBM, first-line treatment includes adjuvant therapy with 6 weeks of concurrent TMZ and radiation therapy followed by maintenance TMZ therapy [48]. Studies have demonstrated that shorter courses of radiation administered over 3 weeks, or even 1 week, can be an effective alternative for older patients who may not tolerate a 6-week course [49, 50]. Since this protocol for the treatment of GBM was introduced in 2005, there has been little progress except for the addition of tumor-treating fields (TTF) as part of the standard of care maintenance therapy following concurrent chemoradiation therapy [51]. TTF creates an alternating electrical field in the intracranial space that disrupts cell division. In a phase III randomized trial of 695 patients with newly diagnosed GBM, the group that received TTF therapy as part of their maintenance TMZ therapy demonstrated a statistically significant PFS advantage of 6.7 months compared to 4.0 months for the group that received TMZ alone [52].

One recent study that has led to a significant advance in the treatment of adult-type diffuse gliomas is the INDIGO trial. This was a phase III randomized clinical trial consisting of 331 patients with grade 2 astrocytomas, IDH-mutant, that were treated with vorasidenib, an IDH inhibitor, versus placebo. PFS was significantly higher in the vorasidenib group compared to the placebo group (27.7 vs. 11.1 months) [53].

Additional studies have focused on the utilization of the immune system to treat GBMs. A phase III trial evaluated the use of a dendritic cell vaccine (DCVax-L) versus the standard of care for newly diagnosed and recurrent GBM [54]. Although the study demonstrated improvement in OS in newly diagnosed and recurrent GBM, changing the primary endpoint from PFS to OS and the use of an external control arm questioned the validity of the study [55]. Follow-up studies are in progress to further validate the effectiveness of the vaccine.

Metastatic Brain Tumors

Metastatic brain tumors are the most common type of brain tumor [56]. An estimated range of 70,000–400,000 new cases of brain metastases (BM) are identified yearly in the United States [57]. BMs are rare in children, and risk is highest among adults in the fifth and sixth decades of life [58]. Lung cancer is the most common primary malignancy to metastasize to the brain followed by breast, melanoma, and renal cell carcinomas with some variation by patient race

[57, 59] (Fig. 14.2). The most common locations for BMs are the frontal lobes and cerebellum [60] (Fig. 14.3).

The treatment approach for metastatic brain tumors encompasses a multidisciplinary approach which can include surgical resection, radiation, and medical therapies. The decision toward which modality is best for the patient depends on several factors, including the number, size, and location of lesions, associated neurological symptoms, primary malignancy, and overall oncologic status.

Surgical resection allows for immediate removal of the tumor and reduction in peritumoral edema. Surgery is indicated for solitary lesions which may improve overall survival. Surgery may also be indicated where there is significant mass effect from the tumor resulting in neurological deficits and increased intracranial pressure requiring immediate decompression. Surgical resection of brain metastases is typically followed by adjuvant radiation to the cavity to decrease the chance of local recurrence.

Metastatic lesions that do not require surgical resection can be treated with RT consisting of either whole brain radiation therapy (WBRT) or stereotactic radiosurgery (SRS). WBRT allows for radiation of multiple sites of metastases but has been associated with memory loss [61]. Hippocampal-sparing techniques along with the administration of memantine have demonstrated protective effects [62]. SRS or fractionated stereotactic radiotherapy (FSRT) consists of conformal high-dose radiation targeted at specific lesions in one to five fractions [63]. SRS and FSRT regimens have been preferred in patients with low numbers of BMs because of the more favorable side effect profile due to the conformal nature of the radiation minimizing radiation to unaffected brain regions [64]. A randomized phase III clinical trial compared long-term outcomes between adjuvant SRS and WBRT treatments for 54 patients who had one to four BMs and had undergone resection. At 12 months, 81.5% of WBRT patients achieved intracranial control compared to only 40.7% of SRS patients. However, WBRT was associated with lower measures of cognitive function and quality of life compared to SRS [65]. Regarding patients with greater metastatic burden, a prospective nonrandomized controlled single-arm trial used propensity score matching to compare 40 SRS patients to 70 WBRT patients, all of whom had 4 to 10 BMs. Though OS was greater for SRS patients compared to WBRT patients at 10.4 months versus 6.5 months, respectively, this difference was not found to be significant [66].

Systemic treatments were thought to be of minimal use in CNS malignancy due to the relative impermeability of the blood-brain barrier (BBB). Targeted therapies in several different cancers have demonstrated success in controlling brain metastases. Epidermal growth factor receptor (EGFR) inhibitors have shown efficacy against *EGFR*-mutated non-small cell lung cancer (NSCLC) patients. The FLAURA trial

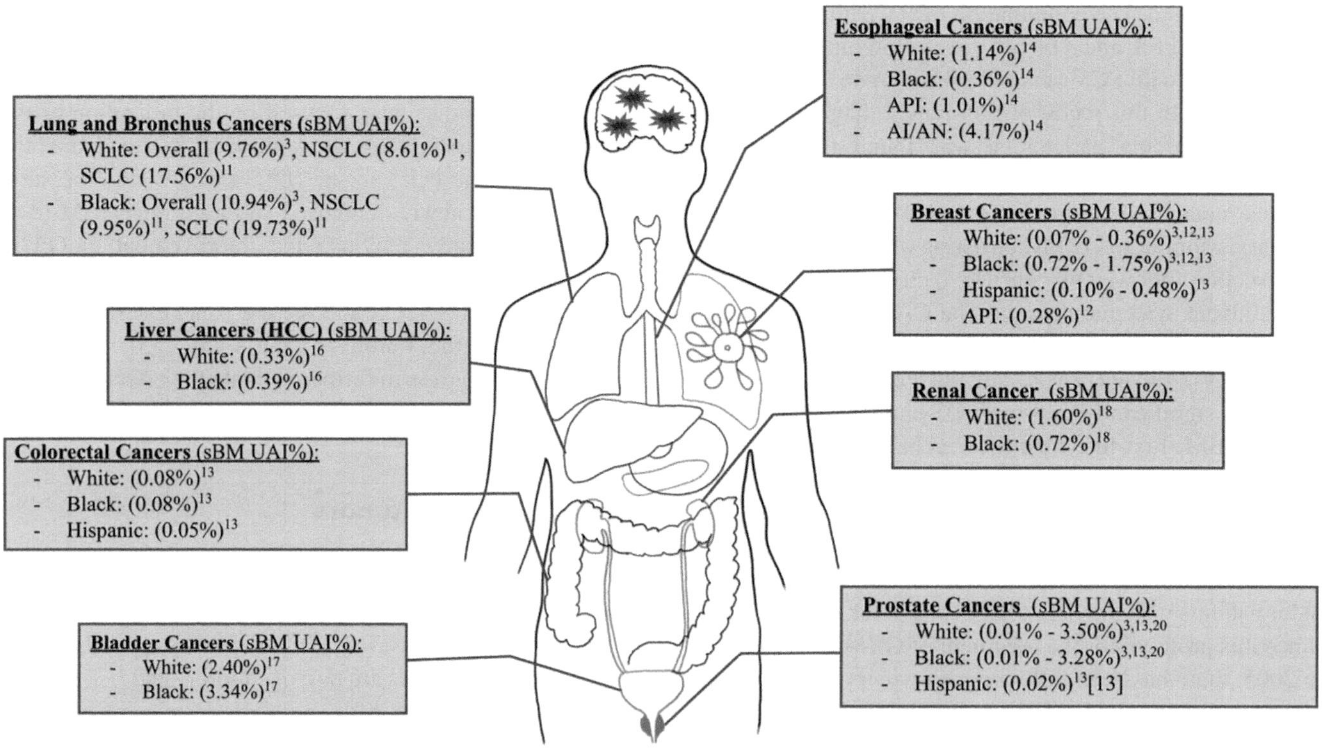

Fig. 14.2 Epidemiology of origins of brain metastases. Unadjusted incidence percentage (UAI%) of brain metastases, separated by patient race and type of primary cancer (Source: Gomez et al. [59])

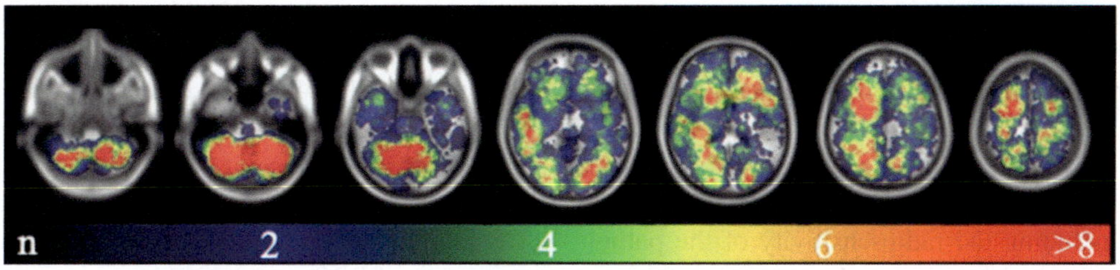

Fig. 14.3 Distribution of brain metastases. Probability map showing the distribution of brain metastases based on MRI data from 369 patients. Blue represents areas where only one metastasis was detected, while green, yellow, and red represent areas with progressively higher numbers. Brain slices are ordered from caudal (left) to cranial (right) (Source: Schroeder et al. [60])

was a phase III randomized control trial in which 556 patients with untreated *EGFR*-mutant NSCLC were randomized to osimertinib, a third-generation EGFR inhibitor, or first-generation EGFR inhibitors such as gefitinib and erlotinib [67]. PFS was significantly increased among patients in the osimertinib group. This survival benefit was shared by the subset of patients with known CNS metastases at the onset of the study, which comprised 21% of the patient sample. In the FLAURA2 trial, 557 *EGFR*-positive NSCLC patients, with 41% of patients having known CNS metastases, were treated with osimertinib with or without chemotherapy [68]. At 2.5 years of follow-up, the combination of osimertinib with chemotherapy demonstrated a PFS benefit for the subset of patients with CNS metastases. In NSCLC patients with anaplastic lymphoma kinase (ALK) rearrangements, alectinib, an ALK inhibitor, has become first-line therapy. In the J-ALEX trial, a randomized phase III clinical trial comparing alectinib to crizotinib, alectinib was found to demonstrate significant improvement in PFS [69].

Specific targeted therapies have also demonstrated effectiveness in other malignancies. Trastuzumab is a commonly used agent in cases of human epidermal growth factor receptor 2 (HER2) positive breast cancer and continues to play a role in the management of BMs, often in combination with other systemic agents [70]. The HER2CLIMB trial enrolled 613 patients with HER2-positive breast cancer refractory to previous therapy, including 291 patients with BMs [71]. Among the BM subgroup, the addition of tucatinib to trastuzumab and capecitabine significantly improved overall and progression-free survival compared to the placebo group. In melanoma patients, vemurafenib and dabrafenib, inhibitors of B-Raf proto-oncogene (BRAF), have demonstrated effectiveness against *BRAF*-mutant melanoma brain metastases [72, 73].

Immune checkpoint inhibitors (ICIs) have also been shown to be effective against BMs. Among the note notable trials is the CheckMate 204 trial in which a combination of ipilimumab, an anti-cytotoxic T lymphocyte antigen 4 (CTLA-4) antibody, and nivolumab, anti-programmed cell death protein 1 (PD-1) antibody, was tested in a multicenter phase II study for metastatic melanoma patients with at least one BM. In 94 patients with a mean follow-up of 14.0 months, the study demonstrated a clinical benefit of 57% and a complete response rate of 26% [74]. Utilizing the abscopal effect in which local radiation treatment results in enhanced antitumor response systemically, ICIs have been combined with SRS to demonstrate treatment benefits. Current studies are underway to evaluate combination ICI and SRS therapy in a variety of malignancies [75, 76].

Metastatic Spine Tumors

The most common type of spinal column tumor is metastatic [77]. Autopsy studies suggest that over 30% of deceased cancer patients develop spinal metastases (SM) over the course of their disease [78]. Lung, breast, kidney, and prostate cancers are among the most frequent primary malignancies that disseminate to the spine [79]. As systemic therapies improve, resulting in longer life spans for cancer patients, the prevalence of SMs has also increased [79].

Metastatic spread to the spine is hematogenous and occurs most frequently in the thoracic spine, followed by the lumbar and cervical. The most common manifestation of SMs is axial back pain which can occur in different forms. Oncologic back pain is a result of inflammatory markers released from cancer cells within the bone. This type of pain is worse at night due to the body's natural decrease in cortisol levels in the evening. Mechanical back pain is pain that is exacerbated with movement and relieved with rest. Mechanical back pain results from the destruction of the bony spine causing spinal instability. SMs can also cause radicular pain, which is pain in the distribution of a specific dermatome. Radicular pain is often secondary to nerve root compression which indicates epidural extension of the tumor.

Spinal instability can increase movement-related pain, cause physical deformity, or contribute to neural deficits, ultimately decreasing quality of life among SM patients. The Spine Instability Neoplastic Score (SINS) was designed by the Spine Oncology Study Group in 2010 as a means of defining the degree of instability secondary to SMs [80]. SINS evaluates spinal stability based on the location of the lesion, presence of back pain, lytic or blastic bony lesion, radiographic spinal alignment, percentage of vertebral body collapse, and involvement of the posterior spinal elements (Fig. 14.4).

Treatment of SMs is performed with a combination of surgical and/or radiation strategies and is also dependent on several factors including the radiosensitivity of the pathology, the degree of spinal instability, the presence of neurological compression or symptoms, and the overall oncologic status of the patient. Multiple algorithms have been devised to consider these factors to suggest the most optimal treatment [81, 82].

Radiation therapy plays a significant role in the treatment of SMs. Currently the most effective means of achieving local tumor control, radiation therapy represents a mainstay in SM treatment either in the form of conventional external-beam radiation therapy (cEBRT), which delivers low doses of radiation over 10–20 fractions over a large field, or conformal radiation therapy in the form of stereotactic body radiation (SBRT) or SRS [81, 82]. For radiosensitive tumors such as hematological malignancies, breast, and prostate cancer, cEBRT is effective in providing durable local control [83]. For radioresistant tumors, SBRT or SRS is required to provide effective local control [81, 84].

Several studies have compared the efficacy of cEBRT to SRS. The NRG/RTOG 0631 compared SRS to cEBRT for

SINS Element	Score
Location	
Junctional (C1-2, C7-T2, T11-L1, L5-S1)	3
Mobile (C3-6, L2-4)	2
Semi-rigid (T3-10)	1
Rigid (S2-S5)	0
Pain	
Mechanical	3
Occasional, not mechanical	1
None	0
Bone lesion type	
Lytic	2
Mixed	1
Blastic	0
Spinal alignment	
Subluxation	4
Deformity (kyphosis/scoliosis)	2
Normal	0
Vertebral body collapse	
>50%	3
<50%	2
No collapse, >50% body involved	1
None	0
Posterolateral involvement	
Bilateral	3
Unilateral	1
None	0
0-6: stable; 7-12: indeterminate; 13-18: unstable	

Fig. 14.4 Spinal Instability Neoplastic Score summary. Overview of all SINS elements with corresponding score values and total score designations (Adapted from Fisher [80])

pain control and spinal cord complications. 339 patients with 1 to 3 SMs were assigned to treatment groups with either SRS or cEBRT. While no difference was found between groups in terms of adverse effects, cEBRT was superior in terms of pain response at 3 months post-intervention, with 60.5% of patients reporting pain relief compared to 41.3% of SRS patients [85]. Similar studies have demonstrated the superiority of SRS over cEBRT for pain control at 3 months [86, 87]. Multiple clinical trials are underway to fine-tune the use of SRS and SBRT in terms of dosage and timing with surgery. The ALLSTAR trial will assess the importance of SRS fractionation on long-term tumor control and safety by randomly assigning patients with one to three SMs to treatment groups receiving either a single dose or two doses of SRS [88].

Surgical treatment of SM is reserved for the presence of significant spinal cord compression and/or neurological deficits in radioresistant tumors. Patchell et al. demonstrated the advantage of circumferential surgical decompression of SMs resulting in improved ambulatory status over radiation alone [89]. Surgical strategies have evolved to allow for spinal stabilization and adequate epidural tumor resection that enables safe administration of SBRT or SRS without having to perform extensive spinal reconstruction, termed "separation surgery" [90]. For certain SMs which do not require open surgical decompression for tumor resection, minimally invasive strategies such as percutaneous pedicle screw fixation allow for spinal stabilization through smaller incisions with adjuvant radiation providing local tumor control [91]. A retrospective study of open and percutaneous pedicle screw fixation for the treatment of SMs in 273 patients demonstrated a trend toward decreased postoperative hospital stay and higher performance status at 1 year for patients undergoing percutaneous versus open fixation [92]. The use of minimally invasive strategies provides the opportunity for lower complication rates, shorter hospital length of stay, and decreased blood loss which allows for the quicker recovery and continuation of systemic therapy [93].

Cement augmentation, or kyphoplasty, is an alternative minimally invasive strategy that can provide pain relief for pathologic compression fractures. The Cancer Patient Fracture Evaluation (CAFÉ) trial randomized 134 patients to either kyphoplasty or nonsurgical management for pathologic compression fractures and demonstrated decreased pain and improved functionality with cement augmentation [94].

Although systemic therapies are not utilized directly for treating SMs, the presence of favorable or actionable mutations or markers within the primary cancer for which targeted therapies are available may allow for the potential of favorable prognosis and influence surgical or radiation treatment decision-making for SMs. Patients with SMs and the presence of mutations such as EGFR and EML4-ALK in lung cancer and HER2-positive status in breast cancer in which targeted therapies are available have demonstrated improved survival [95].

Conclusion

Treatment for CNS malignancies often involves a multidisciplinary approach that combines surgical, radiation, and systemic treatments. While benign tumors such as meningiomas and pituitary adenomas are often manageable through surgical resection and monitoring, malignant gliomas and metastatic brain and spine tumors pose greater treatment challenges. Emerging molecular-targeted therapies and advanced radiological techniques are transforming the management of these conditions, offering additional options for treatment.

References

1. Ostrom QT, Price M, Neff C, Cioffi G, Waite KA, Kruchko C, et al. CBTRUS statistical report: primary brain and other central nervous system tumors diagnosed in the United States in 2016–2020. Neuro-Oncol. 2023;25(12 Suppl 2):iv1–iv99.
2. Maggio I, Franceschi E, Tosoni A, Nunno VD, Gatto L, Lodi R, et al. Meningioma: not always a benign tumor. A review of advances in the treatment of meningiomas. CNS Oncol. 2021;10(2):CNS72.
3. Szulzewsky F, Thirimanne HN, Holland EC. Meningioma: current updates on genetics, classification, and mouse modeling. Ups J Med Sci. 2024;129:e10579.
4. Louis DN, Perry A, Wesseling P, Brat DJ, Cree IA, Figarella-Branger D, et al. The 2021 WHO classification of tumors of the central nervous system: a summary. Neuro-Oncology. 2021;23(8):1231–51.
5. Azab MA, Cole K, Earl E, Cutler C, Mendez J, Karsy M. Medical management of meningiomas. Neurosurg Clin. 2023;34(3):319–33.
6. Simpson D. The recurrence of intracranial meningiomas after surgical treatment. J Neurol Neurosurg Psychiatry. 1957;20(1):22.
7. Buerki RA, Horbinski CM, Kruser T, Horowitz PM, James CD, Lukas RV. An overview of meningiomas. Future Oncol. 2018;14(21):2161–77.
8. Lakomkin N, Hadjipanayis CG. Fluorescence-guided surgery for high-grade gliomas. J Surg Oncol. 2018;118(2):356–61.
9. Stummer W, Holling M, Bendok BR, Vogelbaum MA, Cox A, Renfrow SL, et al. The NXDC-MEN-301 study on 5-ALA for meningiomas surgery: an innovative study design for the assessing the benefit of intra-operative fluorescence imaging. Brain Sci. 2022;12(8):1044.
10. Dijkstra B, Cordia QC, Nonnekens J, Meersma GJ, Donthu VS, Wagemakers M, et al. Fluorescence guided surgery for the detection of meningioma using bevacizumab-IRDye800CW (LUMINA trial)-a single center phase I/II study. Brain Spine. 2023;3:102138.
11. Kaur G, Sayegh ET, Larson A, Bloch O, Madden M, Sun MZ, et al. Adjuvant radiotherapy for atypical and malignant meningiomas: a systematic review. Neuro-Oncology. 2014;16(5):628–36.
12. Aizer AA, Arvold ND, Catalano P, Claus EB, Golby AJ, Johnson MD, et al. Adjuvant radiation therapy, local recurrence, and the need for salvage therapy in atypical meningioma. Neuro-Oncology. 2014;16(11):1547–53.
13. Rogers CL, Pugh SL, Vogelbaum MA, Perry A, Ashby LS, Modi JM, et al. Low-risk meningioma: initial outcomes from NRG oncology/RTOG 0539. Neuro Oncol. 2023;25(1):137–45.
14. Rogers L, Zhang P, Vogelbaum MA, Perry A, Ashby LS, Modi JM, et al. Intermediate-risk meningioma: initial outcomes from NRG oncology RTOG 0539. J Neurosurg. 2018;129(1):35–47.
15. Rogers CL, Won M, Vogelbaum MA, Perry A, Ashby LS, Modi JM, et al. High-risk meningioma: initial outcomes from NRG oncology/RTOG 0539. Int J Radiat Oncol Biol Phys. 2020;106(4):790–9.
16. Central Nervous System Cancers. National Comprehensive Cancer Network; 2025 March 18.
17. Kaley TJ, Wen P, Schiff D, Ligon K, Haidar S, Karimi S, et al. Phase II trial of sunitinib for recurrent and progressive atypical and anaplastic meningioma. Neuro Oncol. 2015;17(1):116–21.
18. Kumthekar P, Grimm SA, Aleman RT, Chamberlain MC, Schiff D, Wen PY, et al. A multi-institutional phase II trial of bevacizumab for recurrent and refractory meningioma. Neuro-oncol Adv. 2022;4(1):vdac123.
19. Graillon T, Sanson M, Campello C, Idbaih A, Peyre M, Peyrière H, et al. Everolimus and octreotide for patients with recurrent meningioma: results from the phase II CEVOREM trial. Clin Cancer Res. 2020;26(3):552–7.
20. Preusser M, Silvani A, Le Rhun E, Soffietti R, Lombardi G, Sepulveda JM, et al. Trabectedin for recurrent WHO grade 2 or 3 meningioma: a randomized phase II study of the EORTC Brain Tumor Group (EORTC-1320-BTG). Neuro Oncol. 2022;24(5):755–67.
21. Abemaciclib in Newly Diagnosed Meningioma Patients [Internet]. 2023. Available from: https://clinicaltrials.gov/study/NCT05940493
22. Regorafenib for Recurrent Grade 2 and 3 Meningioma (MIRAGE Trial) (MIRAGE) [Internet]. 2024. Available from: https://clinicaltrials.gov/study/NCT06275919
23. Asa SL, Mete O, Perry A, Osamura RY. Overview of the 2022 WHO classification of pituitary tumors. Endocr Pathol. 2022;33(1):6–26.
24. Ferrante E, Ferraroni M, Castrignano T, Menicatti L, Anagni M, Reimondo G, et al. Non-functioning pituitary adenoma database: a useful resource to improve the clinical management of pituitary tumors. Eur J Endocrinol. 2006;155(6):823–9.
25. Tsukamoto T, Miki Y. Imaging of pituitary tumors: an update with the 5th WHO classifications—part 1. Pituitary neuroendocrine tumor (PitNET)/pituitary adenoma. Jpn J Radiol. 2023;41(8):789–806.
26. Varlamov EV, McCartney S, Fleseriu M. Functioning pituitary adenomas–current treatment options and emerging medical therapies. Eur Endocrinol. 2019;15(1):30.
27. Auriemma RS, Pirchio R, Pivonello C, Garifalos F, Colao A, Pivonello R. Approach to the patient with prolactinoma. J Clin Endocrinol Metab. 2023;108(9):2400–23.
28. Mehta GU, Lonser RR. Management of hormone secreting pituitary adenomas. Neuro Oncol. 2017;19(6):762–73.
29. Fleseriu M, Langlois F, Lim DST, Varlamov EV, Melmed S. Acromegaly: pathogenesis, diagnosis, and management. Lancet Diabetes Endocrinol. 2022;10(11):804–26.
30. Fleseriu M, Führer-Sakel D, van der Lely AJ, De Marinis L, Brue T, van der Lans-Bussemaker J, et al. More than a decade of real-world experience of pegvisomant for acromegaly: ACROSTUDY. Eur J Endocrinol. 2021;185(4):525–38.
31. Lacroix A, Gu F, Schopohl J, Kandra A, Pedroncelli AM, Jin L, et al. Pasireotide treatment significantly reduces tumor volume in patients with Cushing's disease: results from a Phase 3 study. Pituitary. 2020;23(3):203–11.
32. Lin AL, Sum MW, DeAngelis LM. Is there a role for early chemotherapy in the management of pituitary adenomas? Neuro-Oncology. 2016;18(10):1350–6.
33. Bruno OD, Juárez-Allen L, Christiansen SB, Manavela M, Danilowicz K, Vigovich C, et al. Temozolomide therapy for aggres-

sive pituitary tumors: results in a small series of patients from Argentina. Int J Endocrinol. 2015;2015:587893.
34. Botelho MS, Franzini ÍA, Nunes-Nogueira VS, Boguszewski CL. Treatment of non-functioning pituitary adenoma with cabergoline: a systematic review and meta-analysis. Pituitary. 2022;25(6):810–8.
35. Cooper O, Bonert VS, Rudnick J, Pressman BD, Lo J, Salvatori R, et al. EGFR/ErbB2-targeting lapatinib therapy for aggressive prolactinomas. J Clin Endocrinol Metab. 2021;106(2):e917–25.
36. Shimatsu A, Nakamura A, Takahashi Y, Fujio S, Satoh F, Tahara S, et al. Preoperative and long-term efficacy and safety of lanreotide autogel in patients with thyrotropin-secreting pituitary adenoma: a multicenter, single-arm, phase 3 study in Japan. Endocr J. 2021;68(7):791–805.
37. Yoshikawa MH, Rabelo NN, Telles JPM, Figueiredo EG. Modifiable risk factors for glioblastoma: a systematic review and meta-analysis. Neurosurg Rev. 2023;46(1):143.
38. Louis DN, Perry A, Reifenberger G, von Deimling A, Figarella-Branger D, Cavenee WK, et al. The 2016 World Health Organization classification of tumors of the central nervous system: a summary. Acta Neuropathol. 2016;131(6):803–20.
39. Lapointe S, Perry A, Butowski NA. Primary brain tumours in adults. Lancet. 2018;392(10145):432–46.
40. Grabowski MM, Recinos PF, Nowacki AS, Schroeder JL, Angelov L, Barnett GH, et al. Residual tumor volume versus extent of resection: predictors of survival after surgery for glioblastoma. J Neurosurg. 2014;121(5):1115–23.
41. Chaichana KL, Jusue-Torres I, Navarro-Ramirez R, Raza SM, Pascual-Gallego M, Ibrahim A, et al. Establishing percent resection and residual volume thresholds affecting survival and recurrence for patients with newly diagnosed intracranial glioblastoma. Neuro Oncol. 2014;16(1):113–22.
42. McGirt MJ, Chaichana KL, Attenello FJ, Weingart JD, Than K, Burger PC, et al. Extent of surgical resection is independently associated with survival in patients with hemispheric infiltrating low-grade gliomas. Neurosurgery. 2008;63(4):700–7; author reply 7–8.
43. Buckner JC, Shaw EG, Pugh SL, Chakravarti A, Gilbert MR, Barger GR, et al. Radiation plus procarbazine, CCNU, and vincristine in low-grade glioma. N Engl J Med. 2016;374(14):1344–55.
44. van den Bent MJ, Brandes AA, Taphoorn MJ, Kros JM, Kouwenhoven MC, Delattre JY, et al. Adjuvant procarbazine, lomustine, and vincristine chemotherapy in newly diagnosed anaplastic oligodendroglioma: long-term follow-up of EORTC brain tumor group study 26951. J Clin Oncol. 2013;31(3):344–50.
45. Jaeckle KA, Ballman KV, van den Bent M, Giannini C, Galanis E, Brown PD, et al. CODEL: phase III study of RT, RT+ TMZ, or TMZ for newly diagnosed 1p/19q codeleted oligodendroglioma. Analysis from the initial study design. Neuro-Oncology. 2021;23(3):457–67.
46. Kacimi SEO, Dehais C, Feuvret L, Chinot O, Carpentier C, Bronnimann C, et al. Survival outcomes associated with first-line procarbazine, CCNU, and vincristine or temozolomide in combination with radiotherapy in IDH-mutant 1p/19q-codeleted grade 3 oligodendroglioma. J Clin Oncol. 2025;43(3):329–38.
47. van den Bent MJ, Tesileanu CMS, Wick W, Sanson M, Brandes AA, Clement PM, et al. Adjuvant and concurrent temozolomide for 1p/19q non-co-deleted anaplastic glioma (CATNON; EORTC study 26053-22054): second interim analysis of a randomised, open-label, phase 3 study. Lancet Oncol. 2021;22(6):813–23.
48. Stupp R, Mason WP, van den Bent MJ, Weller M, Fisher B, Taphoorn MJ, et al. Radiotherapy plus concomitant and adjuvant temozolomide for glioblastoma. N Engl J Med. 2005;352(10):987–96.
49. Roa W, Brasher PM, Bauman G, Anthes M, Bruera E, Chan A, et al. Abbreviated course of radiation therapy in older patients with glioblastoma multiforme: a prospective randomized clinical trial. J Clin Oncol. 2004;22(9):1583–8.
50. Roa W, Kepka L, Kumar N, Sinaika V, Matiello J, Lomidze D, et al. International Atomic Energy Agency randomized phase III study of radiation therapy in elderly and/or frail patients with newly diagnosed glioblastoma multiforme. J Clin Oncol. 2015;33(35):4145–50.
51. Stupp R, Taillibert S, Kanner A, Read W, Steinberg D, Lhermitte B, et al. Effect of tumor-treating fields plus maintenance temozolomide vs maintenance temozolomide alone on survival in patients with glioblastoma: a randomized clinical trial. JAMA. 2017;318(23):2306–16.
52. Stupp R, Hegi ME, Idbaih A, Steinberg DM, Lhermitte B, Read W, et al. Abstract CT007: tumor treating fields added to standard chemotherapy in newly diagnosed glioblastoma (GBM): final results of a randomized, multi-center, phase III trial. Cancer Res. 2017;77(13_Supplement):CT007.
53. Mellinghoff IK, van den Bent MJ, Blumenthal DT, Touat M, Peters KB, Clarke J, et al. Vorasidenib in IDH1- or IDH2-mutant low-grade glioma. N Engl J Med. 2023;389(7):589–601.
54. Liau LM, Ashkan K, Brem S, Campian JL, Trusheim JE, Iwamoto FM, et al. Association of autologous tumor lysate-loaded dendritic cell vaccination with extension of survival among patients with newly diagnosed and recurrent glioblastoma: a phase 3 prospective externally controlled cohort trial. JAMA Oncol. 2023;9(1):112–21.
55. Preusser M, van den Bent MJ. Autologous tumor lysate-loaded dendritic cell vaccination (DCVax-L) in glioblastoma: breakthrough or fata morgana? Neuro Oncol. 2023;25(4):631–4.
56. Ostrom QT, Wright CH, Barnholtz-Sloan JS. Brain metastases: epidemiology. Handb Clin Neurol. 2018;149:27–42.
57. Lamba N, Wen PY, Aizer AA. Epidemiology of brain metastases and leptomeningeal disease. Neuro Oncol. 2021;23(9):1447–56.
58. Cagney DN, Martin AM, Catalano PJ, Redig AJ, Lin NU, Lee EQ, et al. Incidence and prognosis of patients with brain metastases at diagnosis of systemic malignancy: a population-based study. Neuro Oncol. 2017;19(11):1511–21.
59. Gomez D, Feng JJ, Cheok S, Shah I, Dicharry H, Cote DJ, et al. Incidence of brain metastasis according to patient race and primary cancer origin: a systematic review. J Neuro Oncol. 2024;169(3):457–67.
60. Schroeder T, Bittrich P, Kuhne J, Noebel C, Leischner H, Fiehler J, et al. Mapping distribution of brain metastases: does the primary tumor matter? J Neuro Oncol. 2020;147:229–35.
61. Chang EL, Wefel JS, Hess KR, Allen PK, Lang FF, Kornguth DG, et al. Neurocognition in patients with brain metastases treated with radiosurgery or radiosurgery plus whole-brain irradiation: a randomised controlled trial. Lancet Oncol. 2009;10(11):1037–44.
62. Westover KD, Mendel JT, Dan T, Kumar K, Gao A, Pulipparacharuv S, et al. Phase II trial of hippocampal-sparing whole brain irradiation with simultaneous integrated boost for metastatic cancer. Neuro Oncol. 2020;22(12):1831–9.
63. Minniti G, D'Angelillo RM, Scaringi C, Trodella LE, Clarke E, Matteucci P, et al. Fractionated stereotactic radiosurgery for patients with brain metastases. J Neuro Oncol. 2014;117:295–301.
64. Aizer AA, Lamba N, Ahluwalia MS, Aldape K, Boire A, Brastianos PK, et al. Brain metastases: a Society for Neuro-Oncology (SNO) consensus review on current management and future directions. Neuro Oncol. 2022;24(10):1613–46.
65. Palmer JD, Klamer BG, Ballman KV, Brown PD, Cerhan JH, Anderson SK, et al. Association of long-term outcomes with stereotactic radiosurgery vs whole-brain radiotherapy for resected brain metastasis: a secondary analysis of the N107C/CEC. 3 (Alliance for Clinical Trials in Oncology/Canadian Cancer Trials Group) randomized clinical trial. JAMA Oncol. 2022;8(12):1809–15.
66. Bodensohn R, Kaempfel AL, Boulesteix AL, Orzelek AM, Corradini S, Fleischmann DF, et al. Stereotactic radiosurgery versus whole-brain radiotherapy in patients with 4-10 brain metastases: a nonrandomized controlled trial. Radiother Oncol. 2023;186:109744.

67. Soria J-C, Ohe Y, Vansteenkiste J, Reungwetwattana T, Chewaskulyong B, Lee KH, et al. Osimertinib in untreated EGFR-mutated advanced non–small-cell lung cancer. N Engl J Med. 2018;378(2):113–25.
68. Planchard D, Jänne PA, Cheng Y, Yang JC-H, Yanagitani N, Kim S-W, et al. Osimertinib with or without chemotherapy in EGFR-mutated advanced NSCLC. N Engl J Med. 2023;389(21):1935–48.
69. Hida T, Nokihara H, Kondo M, Kim YH, Azuma K, Seto T, et al. Alectinib versus crizotinib in patients with ALK-positive non-small-cell lung cancer (J-ALEX): an open-label, randomised phase 3 trial. Lancet. 2017;390(10089):29–39.
70. Rostami R, Mittal S, Rostami P, Tavassoli F, Jabbari B. Brain metastasis in breast cancer: a comprehensive literature review. J Neuro-Oncol. 2016;127:407–14.
71. Murthy RK, Loi S, Okines A, Paplomata E, Hamilton E, Hurvitz SA, et al. Tucatinib, trastuzumab, and capecitabine for HER2-positive metastatic breast cancer. N Engl J Med. 2020;382(7):597–609.
72. McArthur GA, Maio M, Arance A, Nathan P, Blank C, Avril MF, et al. Vemurafenib in metastatic melanoma patients with brain metastases: an open-label, single-arm, phase 2, multicentre study. Ann Oncol. 2017;28(3):634–41.
73. Long GV, Stroyakovskiy D, Gogas H, Levchenko E, de Braud F, Larkin J, et al. Dabrafenib and trametinib versus dabrafenib and placebo for Val600 BRAF-mutant melanoma: a multicentre, double-blind, phase 3 randomised controlled trial. Lancet. 2015;386(9992):444–51.
74. Tawbi HA, Forsyth PA, Algazi A, Hamid O, Hodi FS, Moschos SJ, et al. Combined nivolumab and Ipilimumab in melanoma metastatic to the brain. N Engl J Med. 2018;379(8):722–30.
75. Ahmed KA, Kim Y, Arrington JA, Kim S, DeJesus M, Soyano AE, et al. Nivolumab and stereotactic radiosurgery for patients with breast cancer brain metastases: a nonrandomized, open-label phase 1b study. Adv Radiat Oncol. 2021;6(6):100798.
76. Altan M, Wang Y, Song J, Welsh J, Tang C, Guha-Thakurta N, et al. Nivolumab and ipilimumab with concurrent stereotactic radiosurgery for intracranial metastases from non-small cell lung cancer: analysis of the safety cohort for non-randomized, open-label, phase I/II trial. J Immunother Cancer. 2023;11(7):e006871.
77. Kumar N, Tan WLB, Wei W, Vellayappan BA. An overview of the tumors affecting the spine—inside to out. Neuro Oncol Pract. 2020;7(Supplement 1):i10–i7.
78. Costa F, Restelli F, Innocenti N, Zileli M, Vaishya S, Zygourakis C, et al. Incidence, epidemiology, radiology, and classification of metastatic spine tumors: WFNS Spine Committee recommendations. Neurosurg Rev. 2024;47(1):1–12.
79. Van den Brande R, Cornips EM, Peeters M, Ost P, Billiet C, Van de Kelft E. Epidemiology of spinal metastases, metastatic epidural spinal cord compression and pathologic vertebral compression fractures in patients with solid tumors: a systematic review. J Bone Oncol. 2022;35:100446.
80. Fisher CG, DiPaola CP, Ryken TC, Bilsky MH, Shaffrey CI, Berven SH, et al. A novel classification system for spinal instability in neoplastic disease: an evidence-based approach and expert consensus from the Spine Oncology Study Group. Spine (Phila Pa 1976). 2010;35(22):E1221–9.
81. Laufer I, Rubin DG, Lis E, Cox BW, Stubblefield MD, Yamada Y, et al. The NOMS framework: approach to the treatment of spinal metastatic tumors. Oncologist. 2013;18(6):744–51.
82. Spratt DE, Beeler WH, de Moraes FY, Rhines LD, Gemmete JJ, Chaudhary N, et al. An integrated multidisciplinary algorithm for the management of spinal metastases: an International Spine Oncology Consortium report. Lancet Oncol. 2017;18(12):e720–30.
83. Gerszten PC, Mendel E, Yamada Y. Radiotherapy and radiosurgery for metastatic spine disease: what are the options, indications, and outcomes? Spine (Phila Pa 1976). 2009;34(22 Suppl):S78–92.
84. Guo L, Xu Q, Ke L, Wu Z, Zeng Z, Chen L, et al. The impact of radiosensitivity on clinical outcomes of spinal metastases treated with stereotactic body radiotherapy. Cancer Med. 2023;12(12):13279–89.
85. Ryu S, Deshmukh S, Timmerman RD, Movsas B, Gerszten P, Yin F-F, et al. Stereotactic radiosurgery vs conventional radiotherapy for localized vertebral metastases of the spine: phase 3 results of NRG oncology/RTOG 0631 randomized clinical trial. JAMA Oncol. 2023;9(6):800–7.
86. Sprave T, Verma V, Förster R, Schlampp I, Bruckner T, Bostel T, et al. Randomized phase II trial evaluating pain response in patients with spinal metastases following stereotactic body radiotherapy versus three-dimensional conformal radiotherapy. Radiother Oncol. 2018;128(2):274–82.
87. Sahgal A, Myrehaug SD, Siva S, Masucci GL, Maralani PJ, Brundage M, et al. Stereotactic body radiotherapy versus conventional external beam radiotherapy in patients with painful spinal metastases: an open-label, multicentre, randomised, controlled, phase 2/3 trial. Lancet Oncol. 2021;22(7):1023–33.
88. Pratapneni A, Klebaner D, Soltys SG, Rahimy E, Gibbs IC, Chang SD, et al. Single-versus multi-fraction spine stereotactic radiosurgery (ALL-STAR) for patients with spinal metastases: a randomized phase III trial protocol. BMC Cancer. 2025;25(1):323.
89. Patchell RA, Tibbs PA, Regine WF, Payne R, Saris S, Kryscio RJ, et al. Direct decompressive surgical resection in the treatment of spinal cord compression caused by metastatic cancer: a randomised trial. Lancet. 2005;366(9486):643–8.
90. Laufer I, Iorgulescu JB, Chapman T, Lis E, Shi W, Zhang Z, et al. Local disease control for spinal metastases following "separation surgery" and adjuvant hypofractionated or high-dose single-fraction stereotactic radiosurgery: outcome analysis in 186 patients. J Neurosurg Spine. 2013;18(3):207–14.
91. Barzilai O, Fisher CG, Bilsky MH. State of the art treatment of spinal metastatic disease. Neurosurgery. 2018;82(6):757–69.
92. Bilenkin A, Barnes A, Brisco A, Whiting J, Tran ND, Beer-Furlan A, et al. Comparison of open and percutaneous instrumented fixation for the treatment of spinal metastases. Neurosurg Focus. 2025;58(5):E12.
93. Pranata R, Lim MA, Vania R, Bagus Mahadewa TG. Minimal invasive surgery instrumented fusion versus conventional open surgical instrumented fusion for the treatment of spinal metastases: a systematic review and meta-analysis. World Neurosurg. 2021;148:e264–74.
94. Berenson J, Pflugmacher R, Jarzem P, Zonder J, Schechtman K, Tillman JB, et al. Balloon kyphoplasty versus non-surgical fracture management for treatment of painful vertebral body compression fractures in patients with cancer: a multicentre, randomised controlled trial. Lancet Oncol. 2011;12(3):225–35.
95. Goodwin CR, De la Garza Ramos R, Bettegowda C, Barzilai O, Shreyaskumar P, Fehlings MG, et al. Overview of molecular prognostication for common solid tumor histologies – what the surgeon should know. Glob Spine J. 2025;15(1_suppl):6s–15s.

Research on Head Neck Cancer I: Oral and Oropharyngeal Cancer—Part I

15

John Mills and Deepa Danan

Background

In 2024, nearly 60,000 new cases of cancer of the oral cavity and oropharynx are expected to be diagnosed in the United States, with over 12,000 anticipated deaths [1]. Squamous cell carcinoma (SCC) comprises the vast majority of these cases [2]. Globally, the incidence of oral cavity SCC has been decreasing, likely due to a reduction in tobacco use. However, oropharyngeal SCC cases are on the rise, largely driven by human papillomavirus (HPV) infections [3–6]. The total incidence rate for these cancers is 12.1 per 100,000 people, with the rate for men double that for women [1]. The median age for diagnosis is 64 for men and 66 for women [7].

The National Comprehensive Cancer Network (NCCN) Guidelines recommend a multidisciplinary approach to managing these cancers, with treatment options that may include surgery, radiotherapy (RT), chemotherapy, immunotherapy, or a combination of these modalities. For primary oral cavity cancers, surgical excision is often the preferred treatment, while oropharyngeal tumors may initially be treated with surgery or radiotherapy, depending on the expertise of the treatment team [8]. Multiple techniques are available for tumor removal, including a direct transoral approach, neck or facial incisions, and minimally invasive transoral robotic surgery (TORS) [2, 9]. For locally or regionally advanced tumors, multimodality therapy is often employed.

The 5-year relative survival rate for oral cavity and oropharyngeal cancers, including all stages of disease at time of diagnosis, is 69.0% [1, 7]. For localized disease, the 5-year relative survival rate is more favorable at 87%, dropping to 69% for regional diseas and 39% for distant metastasis [1, 7]. Ongoing research has steadily improved survival rates over time.

J. Mills · D. Danan (✉)
Moffitt Cancer Center, Tampa, FL, USA
e-mail: deepa.danan@moffitt.org

Prevention

Risk Factors

Tobacco and alcohol are major risk factors for the development of head and neck cancers. Both have been independently shown to increase this risk, with smoking demonstrating a clear dose-response relationship with duration [10–12]. Importantly, a synergistic effect has been observed with the combined use of alcohol and tobacco, particularly for oral cavity and oropharyngeal cancers. For example, a case control study that analyzed tobacco and alcohol use in 1114 individuals and 1268 controls demonstrated those who smoked 2 or more packs per day and consumed more than 4 drinks daily had a 35-fold increased risk [13].

Specifically, for oropharyngeal cancer, HPV status plays a critical role in pathogenesis, staging, treatment, and survival. HPV-positive and HPV-negative oropharyngeal cancers are considered distinct entities. Among the hundreds of identified HPV subtypes, types 16 and 18 are the most oncogenic, with type 16 implicated in up to 80% of oropharyngeal SCC, according to a systematic review that included 5046 cancer specimens from 60 studies [14]. Pathogenesis involves the development of E6 and E7 proteins that disrupt cell cycle regulation.

Screening

Currently, no screening tests exist for head and neck cancers of the oral cavity or oropharynx. These cancers are often incidental findings, such as an oral cavity mass or ulceration, during routine physical or dental examinations. Patients may also present with symptoms such as dysphagia, odynophagia, otalgia, dysphonia, or lateral neck lymphadenopathy. Such findings warrant a referral to an otolaryngologist for a thorough head and neck examination, typically involving

J. Huang, H. S.L. Jim (eds.), *Cancer Research Guidance for Clinicians and Researchers*,
https://doi.org/10.1007/978-3-032-19175-5_15

flexible laryngoscopy (a "scope" exam). Further evaluation includes imaging, such as contrast-enhanced computed tomography (CT) of the head, neck, and chest, and PET imaging for regional or distant metastasis.

A definitive diagnosis requires a pathological specimen, which can be obtained through various methods, including direct laryngoscopy biopsy under general anesthesia. Alternatively, less invasive same-day procedures, such as in-office biopsies, fine-needle aspiration, and ultrasound-guided core needle biopsy, may reduce the time to diagnosis [15]. Prompt diagnosis is critical, as delays in treatment initiation may increase the risk of local recurrence, as demonstrated in a meta-analysis of 20 studies (relative risk: 1.15; 95% CI: 1.02–1.29 per month of increased wait time for definitive RT) [16].

All pathology samples should be reviewed by a pathologist for histologic features and HPV testing for oropharyngeal cancers, either through direct DNA or RNA detection using PCR or surrogate testing with P16 immunohistochemical staining [17]. Testing for circulating cell-free tumor DNA as a liquid biomarker has shown a high sensitivity (95.7%) and specificity (97.8%) for oropharyngeal SCC, based on a prospective diagnostic test study including 138 patients who initially presented with a lateral neck mass [18]. This is particularly useful for cases presenting as isolated lateral neck masses without an obvious primary tumor site. These nodes are often cystic in nature compared to other head and neck cancers, complicating tissue sampling for definitive diagnosis.

Once diagnosis is confirmed, staging is established during a multidisciplinary tumor board discussion using the AJCC TNM staging system [19]. Data has shown improved outcomes for patients treated at high-volume surgical centers offering multidisciplinary care. In a randomized trial including 471 subjects, patients treated at institutions with less experience had worse overall survival compared to those treated at high-volume centers (5-year survival: 51.0% vs. 69.1%; $P = 0.002$) [20]. HPV status is essential for oropharyngeal cancers, as a separate staging system exists for these cases due to alternative treatment protocols and generally better outcomes. Treatment decisions are made based on staging and tumor board recommendations.

Vaccination

HPV vaccination is the only existing primary prevention for certain head and neck cancers. Vaccination has been shown to reduce the risk of other HPV-related diseases, such cervical carcinoma. In an observational prospective cohort study comparing 849 vaccinated women with 849 controls, only 1 vaccinated individual required treatment for abnormal cervical pathology, compared to 8.4% in the unvaccinated group [21]. CDC guidelines recommend vaccination at ages 11 or 12 with a 2- or 3-dose series. Older individual (ages 27–45) may also be eligible based on clinical decision-making, but benefits may be reduced due to prior HPV exposure [22]. Vaccination rates remain low; one cross-sectional retrospective study reported only 33.6% of females and 24.5% of males completed the HPV vaccine series, far short of Health People 2030 goal of 80% [23]. Given the increasing incidence of HPV-positive oropharyngeal SCC and new research implicating HPV in a small percentage of oral cavity (3.9% of 12,612 total cases) and laryngeal cancers (2.8% of 11,170 total cases) based on a retrospective study using 2016–2020 US Cancer Statistics data, vaccination will become even more important [24].

Treatment

Surgical

Proper surgical planning using radiographic imaging prior to resection is critical. Depending on the size and depth of the tumor, en bloc resection of the primary tumor with clear pathological margins is preferred [25]. This of course is balanced with preserving reasonable cosmetic and functional outcomes. The compact and complex anatomical reality of the head and neck region makes this balancing act especially challenging.

Cancers that have spread locally through lymph nodes typically require removal through a neck dissection. The extent of surgical resection is determined based on evidence of local metastasis to neck nodes, usually occurring on the ipsilateral side of the primary tumor [25]. This procedure has evolved to be more selective in tissue removal to reduce morbidity over time. It is also used as a preemptive measure in early-stage, clinically node-negative oral cancers, targeting lymph nodes that appear free of cancer. Known as elective neck dissection, this procedure is performed during the initial tumor removal. Evidence from a randomized control trial compared 245 patients who received elective surgery with 255 patients who underwent observation followed by therapeutic surgery. The elective group had improved 3-year overall survival (80.0%; 95% CI: 74.1–85.8) compared with the therapeutic dissection group (67.5%, 95% CI: 61.0–73.9) [26]. These findings were further substantiated with a Cochrane review, which suggested that elective neck dissection can improve overall survival compared to observation and delayed neck dissection performed for nodal recurrence (HR 0.64; 95% CI: 0.50–0.83; 4 trials, 883 participants) [27].

Robotic-assisted surgery has emerged as a leading surgical technique for HPV-positive oropharyngeal cancers.

Initially adapted for transoral use in the 2000s, TORS had become a mainstay of therapy for oropharyngeal SCC due to its favorable approach without making incisions in the face or neck [28]. The use of TORS for resection of oropharyngeal tumors has been shown to be an effective treatment in clinical trials comparing postoperative patients who receive standard adjuvant chemotherapy with those receiving de-intensified or reduced dosage adjuvant chemoradiation [9]. The ECOG 3311 phase 2 multicenter study included 443 patients undergoing TORS who were stratified based on risk assessment for different levels of postoperative radiotherapy. The intermediate-risk group with de-intensified radiotherapy was found to have similar 2-year progression-free survival to the standard-of-care treatment group (94.9% versus 96.0%) but significantly lower toxicity (14% vs. 24%) [29].

Consensus for the use of sentinel lymph node biopsy (SLNB) in head and neck cancer remains unclear [30]. Currently, the NRG-HN006 trial is a prospective randomized control trial, with an estimated 618 patients enrolled, comparing SLNB versus elective neck dissections in patients with early-stage oral cavity cancer (T1-T2, N0, or clinically node negative necks). Outcomes of this trial might offer clarity to the utility of this procedure.

Most head and neck cancer patients require complex reconstruction. Free flap reconstruction using skin, fasciocutaneous, myocutaneous, or osseomyocutaneous donor sites is preferred over local or rotational flaps. These reconstructions, while complex, are essential for both functional and aesthetic outcomes.

Radiotherapy

RT can be used alone or with chemotherapy. While surgery is the preferred treatment for oral cavity cancers, national guidelines suggest that surgery alone or RT alone can be used for stage I or II oropharyngeal cancers [8]. Historically, oropharyngeal cancers were treated with chemoradiation, but its associated morbidity has led to investigations into minimally invasive alternatives, such as previously discussed TORS or de-escalation chemoradiation. The choice in treatment often depends on institutional preferences and anatomical considerations, with multimodality approaches frequently employed.

Following surgical resection, restaging is performed using AJCC pathological guidelines, considering features like number and laterality of malignant cervical nodes, node size, and the presence of extranodal extension [19]. High-risk features may necessitate adjuvant radiation or chemoradiation to address the risk of micrometastasis not cleared during surgical resection.

Chemotherapy

Systemic therapy for head and neck cancer are typically cisplatin-based regimens. Chemotherapy alone is usually reserved for palliative treatment in advanced, unresectable cases. Most chemotherapy regimens are used in addition to radiotherapy for definitive management.

Neoadjuvant chemotherapy does not appear to benefit surgical candidates with oral cavity disease. A systematic review of 2 randomized control trials including 451 patients with T1-T4, N1-N2 oral cavity disease found no survival benefit from neoadjuvant chemotherapy prior to surgery (n = 226) versus upfront surgery alone (n = 225) [31]. However, a recent multicenter retrospective cohort study of 342 patients with stage III and IV HPV-positive oropharyngeal cancers found that neoadjuvant cisplatin therapy followed by TORS with neck dissection reduced distant metastasis compared to traditional radiotherapy with concurrent chemotherapy (1% vs. 14.3%) [32]. These results warrant further investigation through randomized controlled trials.

Immunotherapy

The use of PD-1/PD-L1 immunotherapy in cancer treatment has been a major breakthrough in recent years and represents the leading future direction in cancer therapy. Several clinical trials have evaluated immunotherapy for head and neck cancer with varying success. The KEYNOTE-412 randomized clinical trial evaluated pembrolizumab, a PD-1 monoclonal antibody, combined with chemoradiation (n = 402) versus chemoradiation alone (n = 402) for the treatment of locally advanced head and neck SCC. However, no significant benefit in event-free survival was demonstrated [33]. Pembrolizumab proved more effective in treating recurrent or metastatic head and neck cancer during the KEYNOTE-048 trial. Results indicated that pembrolizumab, both as monotherapy and in combination with additional chemotherapy, improved overall survival for recurrent or metastatic head and neck SCC when compared to cetuximab with chemotherapy (HR 0.61; 95% CI: 0.45–0.83 and HR 0.77; 95% CI: 0.63–0.93, respectively) [34]. Additionally, the CheckMate 141 trial showed promising results for nivolumab, a PD-1 receptor antibody, which demonstrated improved survival among patients with platinum-refractory recurrent cancer compared to standard therapy. In this open-label phase 3 trial, 240 patients with recurrent SCC were given nivolumab and compared to 161 patients given standard single-agent chemotherapy, with the former group showing improved overall survival (7.5 months vs. 5.1 months) [35].

Survival

Overall survival rates for patients with oral cavity and oropharyngeal head and neck cancer have been improving over time with advances in treatment regimens. The 5-year relative survival rate, including all stages of disease at time of diagnosis, is 69.0% and has been steadily increasing over the last few decades [1, 7]. Current clinical trials are not only focusing on improving overall survival but also on reducing adverse effects caused by treatment. This includes efforts to de-escalate chemoradiation, develop immunotherapy with reduced adverse effect profiles, and perform reconstruction to address functional and aesthetic defects caused by surgical resection. For patients with metastatic or recurrent disease, promising immunotherapy options are available to prolong survival in cases of aggressive disease. The future of treatment for oral cavity and oropharyngeal cancer remains robust.

Summary

Head and neck cancer of the oral cavity and oropharynx are common and typically are first discovered by primary care providers or dental practitioners. Prompt referral to an otolaryngologist is essential to ensure timely diagnosis, staging, and treatment. Tobacco and alcohol cessation, along with HPV vaccination, are effective preventative measures for patients in your community. Initial treatment involves surgery, chemotherapy, radiation, or a combination of these modalities, as determined by a multidisciplinary tumor board. Future research is focused on understanding DNA changes in tumor cells and refining treatment modalities. Recent studies show promise in reducing morbidity without impacting survival through de-intensified radiotherapy after robotic resection of oral cavity tumors. Future studies on SLNB may further reduce morbidity compared to a neck dissection, while systemic immunotherapy as adjuvant therapy may expand treatment options.

References

1. American Cancer Society. 2024. https://cancerstatisticscenter.cancer.org/?_gl=1*18px229*_ga*NjY2MDIyNzU2LjE2OTg3ODAwNTg.*_ga_12CJLLFFQT*MTcxMjU4MjgxMS4yLjEuMTcxMjU4Mjg4OC40Ni4wLjA.&_ga=2.46094244.1830919746.1712582797-666022756.1698780058
2. Mody MD, Rocco JW, Yom SS, Haddad RI, Saba NF. Head and neck cancer. Lancet. 2021;398(10318):2289–99. https://doi.org/10.1016/s0140-6736(21)01550-6.
3. Chaturvedi AK, Anderson WF, Lortet-Tieulent J, et al. Worldwide trends in incidence rates for oral cavity and oropharyngeal cancers. J Clin Oncol. 2013;31(36):4550–9. https://doi.org/10.1200/jco.2013.50.3870.
4. Chaturvedi AK, Engels EA, Anderson WF, Gillison ML. Incidence trends for human papillomavirus-related and -unrelated oral squamous cell carcinomas in the United States. J Clin Oncol. 2008;26(4):612–9. https://doi.org/10.1200/jco.2007.14.1713.
5. Gillison ML, Broutian T, Pickard RK, et al. Prevalence of oral HPV infection in the United States, 2009–2010. JAMA. 2012;307(7):693–703. https://doi.org/10.1001/jama.2012.101.
6. Mehanna H, Beech T, Nicholson T, et al. Prevalence of human papillomavirus in oropharyngeal and nonoropharyngeal head and neck cancer—systematic review and meta-analysis of trends by time and region. Head Neck. 2013;35(5):747–55. https://doi.org/10.1002/hed.22015.
7. SEER Database. 2024. https://seer.cancer.gov/statistics-network/explorer/application.html?site=3&data_type=4&graph_type=2&compareBy=sex&chk_sex_3=3&chk_sex_2=2&relative_survival_interval=5&race=1&age_range=1&stage=101&advopt_precision=1&advopt_show_ci=on&hdn_view=0&advopt_show_apc=on&advopt_display=1
8. Pfister DG, Spencer S, Adelstein D, et al. Head and neck cancers, Version 2.2020, NCCN clinical practice guidelines in oncology. J Natl Compr Cancer Netw. 2020;18(7):873–98. https://doi.org/10.6004/jnccn.2020.0031.
9. Howard J, Dwivedi RC, Masterson L, Kothari P, Quon H, Holsinger FC. De-intensified adjuvant (chemo)radiotherapy versus standard adjuvant chemoradiotherapy post transoral minimally invasive surgery for resectable HPV-positive oropharyngeal carcinoma. Cochrane Database Syst Rev. 2018;12(12):Cd012939. https://doi.org/10.1002/14651858.CD012939.pub2.
10. Wyss A, Hashibe M, Chuang SC, et al. Cigarette, cigar, and pipe smoking and the risk of head and neck cancers: pooled analysis in the International Head and Neck Cancer Epidemiology Consortium. Am J Epidemiol. 2013;178(5):679–90. https://doi.org/10.1093/aje/kwt029.
11. Hammond EC, Horn D. Smoking and death rates: report on forty-four months of follow-up of 187,783 men. 2. Death rates by cause. J Am Med Assoc. 1958;166(11):1294–308. https://doi.org/10.1001/jama.1958.02990110030007.
12. Hashibe M, Brennan P, Benhamou S, et al. Alcohol drinking in never users of tobacco, cigarette smoking in never drinkers, and the risk of head and neck cancer: pooled analysis in the International Head and Neck Cancer Epidemiology Consortium. J Natl Cancer Inst. 2007;99(10):777–89. https://doi.org/10.1093/jnci/djk179.
13. Blot WJ, McLaughlin JK, Winn DM, et al. Smoking and drinking in relation to oral and pharyngeal cancer. Cancer Res. 1988;48(11):3282–7.
14. Kreimer AR, Clifford GM, Boyle P, Franceschi S. Human papillomavirus types in head and neck squamous cell carcinomas worldwide: a systematic review. Cancer Epidemiol Biomarkers Prev. 2005;14(2):467–75. https://doi.org/10.1158/1055-9965.Epi-04-0551.
15. Ahn D, Lee GJ, Sohn JH. Time and cost of ultrasound-guided fine-needle aspiration biopsy/Core-needle biopsy for primary laryngohypopharyngeal squamous cell carcinoma. Otolaryngol Head Neck Surg. 2021;164(3):602–7. https://doi.org/10.1177/0194599820945953.
16. Chen Z, King W, Pearcey R, Kerba M, Mackillop WJ. The relationship between waiting time for radiotherapy and clinical outcomes: a systematic review of the literature. Radiother Oncol. 2008;87(1):3–16. https://doi.org/10.1016/j.radonc.2007.11.016.
17. Lewis JS Jr, Beadle B, Bishop JA, et al. Human papillomavirus testing in head and neck carcinomas: guideline from the College of American Pathologists. Arch Pathol Lab Med. 2018;142(5):559–97. https://doi.org/10.5858/arpa.2017-0286-CP.
18. Ferrandino RM, Barlow J, Gold B, et al. Diagnostic accuracy of circulating tumor HPV DNA testing in patients with a lateral neck

mass. JAMA Otolaryngol Head Neck Surg. 2024;150(12):1089–96. https://doi.org/10.1001/jamaoto.2024.2702.
19. Zanoni DK, Patel SG, Shah JP. Changes in the 8th edition of the American Joint Committee on Cancer (AJCC) staging of head and neck cancer: rationale and implications. Curr Oncol Rep. 2019;21(6):52. https://doi.org/10.1007/s11912-019-0799-x.
20. Wuthrick EJ, Zhang Q, Machtay M, et al. Institutional clinical trial accrual volume and survival of patients with head and neck cancer. J Clin Oncol. 2015;33(2):156–64. https://doi.org/10.1200/jco.2014.56.5218.
21. Paraskevaidis E, Athanasiou A, Paraskevaidi M, et al. Cervical pathology following HPV vaccination in Greece: a 10-year HeCPA observational cohort study. In Vivo. 2020;34(3):1445–9. https://doi.org/10.21873/invivo.11927.
22. CDC Vaccines & Immunizations. 2024. https://www.cdc.gov/vaccines/vpd/hpv/hcp/recommendations.html
23. Khalil L, Russo E, Venkatakrishnan K, Mazul AL, Zevallos JP. Barriers to human papillomavirus vaccination initiation and completion among adults aged 18–26 years in a large healthcare system. Cancers (Basel). 2023;15(17) https://doi.org/10.3390/cancers15174243.
24. Kava CM, Chaturvedi AK, Senkomago V, et al. The role of HPV16 in oral cavity and laryngeal cancers in the United States. J Natl Cancer Inst. 2024. https://doi.org/10.1093/jnci/djae320.
25. Simon C, Nicolai P, Paderno A, Dietz A. Best practice in surgical treatment of malignant head and neck tumors. Front Oncol. 2020;10:140. https://doi.org/10.3389/fonc.2020.00140.
26. D'Cruz AK, Vaish R, Kapre N, et al. Elective versus therapeutic neck dissection in node-negative oral cancer. N Engl J Med. 2015;373(6):521–9. https://doi.org/10.1056/NEJMoa1506007.
27. Worthington HV, Bulsara VM, Glenny AM, Clarkson JE, Conway DI, Macluskey M. Interventions for the treatment of oral cavity and oropharyngeal cancers: surgical treatment. Cochrane Database Syst Rev. 2023;8(8):Cd006205. https://doi.org/10.1002/14651858.CD006205.pub5.
28. Rinaldi V, Pagani D, Torretta S, Pignataro L. Transoral robotic surgery in the management of head and neck tumours. Ecancermedicalscience. 2013;7:359. https://doi.org/10.3332/ecancer.2013.359.
29. Ferris RL, Flamand Y, Weinstein GS, et al. Phase II randomized trial of transoral surgery and low-dose intensity modulated radiation therapy in resectable p16+ locally advanced oropharynx cancer: an ECOG-ACRIN cancer research group trial (E3311). J Clin Oncol. 2022;40(2):138–49. https://doi.org/10.1200/jco.21.01752.
30. Schilling C, Stoeckli SJ, Vigili MG, et al. Surgical consensus guidelines on sentinel node biopsy (SNB) in patients with oral cancer. Head Neck. 2019;41(8):2655–64. https://doi.org/10.1002/hed.25739.
31. Marta GN, Riera R, Bossi P, et al. Induction chemotherapy prior to surgery with or without postoperative radiotherapy for oral cavity cancer patients: systematic review and meta-analysis. Eur J Cancer. 2015;51(17):2596–603. https://doi.org/10.1016/j.ejca.2015.08.007.
32. Sadeghi N, Subramaniam T, Richardson K, Mascarella M, Zeitouni A, Shenouda G, Sultanem K, Mlynarek A, Caglar D, Esfahani K, Joshi A, Siegel R, Goodman J, Thakkar P, Lee E, Golabi N, Ramanakumar AV, Hier M, Bouganim N. Neoadjuvant Chemotherapy and Transoral Robotic Surgery for Human Papillomavirus-Related Oropharyngeal Cancer. JAMA Otolaryngol Head Neck Surg. 2025 Feb 1;151(2):128-134. https://doi.org/10.1001/jamaoto.2024.3303. PMID: 39636629; PMCID: PMC11622064.
33. Machiels JP, Tao Y, Licitra L, et al. Pembrolizumab plus concurrent chemoradiotherapy versus placebo plus concurrent chemoradiotherapy in patients with locally advanced squamous cell carcinoma of the head and neck (KEYNOTE-412): a randomised, double-blind, phase 3 trial. Lancet Oncol. 2024;25(5):572–87. https://doi.org/10.1016/s1470-2045(24)00100-1.
34. Burtness B, Harrington KJ, Greil R, et al. Pembrolizumab alone or with chemotherapy versus cetuximab with chemotherapy for recurrent or metastatic squamous cell carcinoma of the head and neck (KEYNOTE-048): a randomised, open-label, phase 3 study. Lancet. 2019;394(10212):1915–28. https://doi.org/10.1016/s0140-6736(19)32591-7.
35. Ferris RL, Blumenschein G Jr, Fayette J, et al. Nivolumab for recurrent squamous-cell carcinoma of the head and neck. N Engl J Med. 2016;375(19):1856–67. https://doi.org/10.1056/NEJMoa1602252.

16 Research on Head and Neck Cancer II: Laryngeal Cancer—Part II

Mahnoor Khan and Deepa Danan

Introduction

Laryngeal cancer makes up about a third of head and neck cancers [1]. The rate of new cases of laryngeal cancer is 2.6 per 100,000 men and women per year [2]. The larynx has multiple subsites which may be involved including the supraglottis, glottis, and subglottis, each influencing the disease's presentation, spread patterns, and treatment options. Squamous cell carcinoma (SCCa), in particular, accounts for 85–95% of laryngeal cancers [1]. Other laryngeal malignancies include spindle cell carcinoma and chondrosarcoma, although rare, only comprising 2–5% of laryngeal tumors [3]. There is a preponderance of laryngeal cancer in men, with a male to female ratio of 3.8:1. This is likely related to increased exposure to the known risk factors of significant tobacco and alcohol use, which may have a synergistic relationship in the development of laryngeal cancer [1, 4]. Laryngopharyngeal reflux also moderately increases risk of pathology in the larynx.

Glottic SCCa is slightly more common than supraglottic SCCa in the USA, comprising 70% of laryngeal cancers [5]. Subglottic SCCa is very rare and is only seen in 1% of laryngeal cancers, although it indicates a poor prognosis [6].

Presentation of laryngeal cancer may be dependent on the site involved:

- Supraglottic SCCa:
  - Structures: epiglottis, aryepiglottic folds, arytenoids, false vocal cords.
  - SCCa commonly presents in advanced stage with neck disease due to bilateral lymphatic drainage.
  - Symptoms: dysphonia, dysphagia, odynophagia, otalgia, dyspnea, and stridor.
- Glottic SCCa:
  - Structures: true vocal cords, including the anterior and posterior commissures.
  - SCCa more commonly presents at early stage due to decreased lymphatic drainage.
  - Symptoms: dysphonia, dyspnea, stridor.
- Subglottic SCCa:
  - Structure/location: lower border of glottis to inferior border of cricoid cartilage.
  - SCCa presents at a later stage with distant metastases, commonly, the paratracheal nodes.

Depending on the pathology, site, and stage, patient may be offered surgical intervention including organ preservation approaches including endoscopic CO_2 laser surgery, partial laryngectomies, or total laryngectomy. Medical management may involve radiation therapy (RT), concurrent chemoradiotherapy (CRT), and, in some cases, immunotherapy. The choice of therapy depends not only on clinical features of the cancer but also on the patient in terms of age, comorbidities, preference, and socio-family background.

Prevention

Risk Factors

The development of laryngeal SCCa is multistep process. Carcinogenesis initially starts from an epithelial precursor lesion which is a result of architectural and cytologic alterations, including dysplasia and intraepithelial lesions [3]. There are several factors which are associated with the development of cancer. As previously mentioned, smoking tobacco is the most significant risk factor for laryngeal SCCa. About 95% of laryngeal cancer patients in the USA are smokers [7]. In an 8-year long frequency matched case-controlled study with 527 patients, the odds ratio (OR) for laryngeal cancer in comparison to never smokers was found to be 19.8 for current smokers, 7.0 for ex-smokers, and 1.2

M. Khan · D. Danan (✉)
Moffitt Cancer Center, Tampa, FL, USA
e-mail: deepa.danan@moffitt.org

J. Huang, H. S.L. Jim (eds.), *Cancer Research Guidance for Clinicians and Researchers*,
https://doi.org/10.1007/978-3-032-19175-5_16

for people exposed to second hand smoke [4, 8]. Drinking poses as a significant risk factor for laryngeal SCCa, as well. More recent publications posit that alcohol has a dose-dependent effect. The same frequency match case-controlled study noted heavy consumption (>56 drinks per week) resulted in 5.9-fold increase in risk [4]. Alternatively, Bagnardi et al. noted in their meta-analysis of 486,538 cancer cases, a significant increase in risk only in moderate and heavy drinkers (⩽50 g but >12 g per day as moderate and >50 g per day of alcohol as heavy), with RRs of 1.44 (95% CI 1.25–1.66) and 2.65 (95% CI 2.19–3.19), respectively [9]. Combined alcohol and tobacco consumption showed a 177-fold increase in risk, thus suggesting a multiplicative effect on the risk for laryngeal cancer [4].

HPV and its role in oropharyngeal cancer and genital dysplasia/cancer has been well established; however, its role in laryngeal cancer is still being explored [10]. A meta-analysis looking at 55 studies found that the overall HPV prevalence in tissue with laryngeal cancer was 28%, of those, subtype HPV-16 was most frequently observed with prevalence of 19.8% [11]. However, other case series noted significantly less (<10%) HPV DNA in laryngeal SCCa [10]. Serologic testing of E6/E7 antibodies revealed odds ratios between two and five suggesting a small contribution of high-risk HPV infection in the development of laryngeal cancer [10]. The relationship between HPV infection and the risk of laryngeal cancer does not appear to be influenced by factors that contribute to prevalence of HPV. Further research is needed to show a clear association of HPV infection and laryngeal cancer risk. EBV has also been suggested to play a possible role as a cofactor in the development and progression of laryngeal cancer [12]. Unfortunately, there is not yet strong data to definitively establish a link.

Certain environmental pollutants such as Agent Orange, a herbicide commonly used during the Vietnam war in the 1960s, has been an area of developing research in the veteran population. The chemic contains 2,3,7,8-tetra-chlorodibenzo-p-dioxin (TCDD) which is a well-documented carcinogen [6]. In 2020, a retrospective cohort analysis out of the Veterans Affairs Corporate Data Warehouse (VA CDW) showed that among the 22% of veterans who self-reported exposure during the Vietnam Ware, the relative risk of developing laryngeal cancer was 1.1 [6]. Of note, Agent Orange exposure was associated with improved 10-year overall survival in upper aerodigestive tract cancer patients [6].

Screening

Because of the relatively low incidence, regular screening is not standard of care per American Head and Neck Society/American Academy of Otolaryngology Head and Neck Surgery and the American Cancer Society. Currently, there are not any screening tests for laryngeal cancer.

Symptoms including dysphonia, persistent hoarseness, otalgia, persistent cough, hemoptysis, odynophagia, dysphagia, shortness of breath, stridor, and unexplained weight loss are often the first signs of laryngeal cancer.

Nasopharyngolaryngoscopy is often performed by an otolaryngologist in the clinic to view your laryngeal structures and assess for possible supra glottic, glottis, and subglottis lesions which may be contributing to the previously mentioned symptoms.

Depending on clinic resources and patient factors, a channel scope biopsy may be performed if patient is amenable. This entails the use of a small biopsy forceps which is fed into the nasopharyngolaryngoscope and aimed at the lesion in question [13]. If an obvious node is palpable, a fine-needle aspiration may also be completed in the clinic setting. Often time, otolaryngologists will take biopsies under general anesthesia by performing a direct laryngoscopy for an adequate biopsy of the tissue and full examination of the surrounding areas including the hypopharynx.

Radiological imaging is an important part of the evaluation for a possible laryngeal malignancy. If possible, CT neck with contrast, CT chest with contrast, and fluorodeoxyglucose positron emission tomography/CT are completed before biopsy to obtain images before possible edema and distortion from the surgery. Imaging is ordered to assess the extent of the disease, presence of lymphadenopathy, and possible secondary primary tumors. The CT chest and PET/CT are ordered to assess for pulmonary lesions, as the lungs are the most likely area for metastasis for laryngeal squamous cell cancer and may change patient management.

Biomarkers

Current research efforts on the topic are centered on finding biomarkers to allow earlier diagnosis. Based on the recently identified mutations in laryngeal squamous cell cancer, the major pathologic pathways implicated in its tumorigenesis include the dysregulation of some key processes, such as cellular survival and proliferation (Tp53 and EGFR), cell-cycle control, and cellular differentiation (NOTCH1) pathways [1, 3].

Tp53: p53 plays a crucial role as a tumor suppressor protein, thus regulating cell division. It plays a part in oncogenesis in different tumors; however, in head and neck, the *TP53* mutation was noted with an incidence ranging from 50% to 80% [14]. In a prospective multi-institute study involving 560 head and neck squamous cell carcinoma patients who were treated surgically with curative intent, *TP53* mutations were noted in 53.3% of patients. The study also showed decreased overall survival (OS) compared with the wild-type ones [14]. Another study analyzed the genetic changes associated with the transformation-progression of 94 tissue samples by multiple ligation-dependent probe amplification

(MLPA)—it showed a copy number variation for 37 genes, the most common being *TP53* [15].

Bcl 2: The Bcl 2 members regulate apoptotic cell death. It has been proven that p53/Bcl-2 co-expression was significantly associated with poor differentiation, tumor extension, LNM, and advanced clinical stage of laryngeal squamous cell carcinoma [3]. In a study published in 2019, tissue samples of patients with primary laryngeal squamous cell cancer were collected over the span of 7 years which were immunohistochemically evaluated for the protein expression of BCL2; the Kaplan–Meier survival curves of the 78 patients with advanced laryngeal squamous cell cancer who had BCL2L12-positive tumors were shown to have significantly longer OS time and a lower risk of death, suggesting that BCL2L12 protein expression could be used as a favorable prognostic tissue biomarker in patients with advanced cancer [16].

EGFR: EGFR pathway induces cell transformation and EGFR overexpression by gene amplification can alter the transcriptional mechanism of survival. EGFR overexpression is frequently observed in LSCC combined with low ALK levels, thus suggesting possible targeted therapeutic strategies for patients with a high EGFR/ALK ratio [17].

NOTCH1: NOTCH signaling contributes to cell growth and survival. Sun et al. performed DNA copy number, methylation, expression, and mutation analysis among head and neck cancer SCCa patients compared to those with normal mucosa. The ligand receptor copy number was noted to be increased in HNSCC subsets when compared to the control [18]. Regarding the biomarker properties of this gene, a retrospective study showed that NOTCH1 expression in the LSCC tissues of 106 patients was significantly associated with clinical stage, supporting the role of NOTCH1 in the malignant progression of laryngeal cancer [19].

Table 16.1 Glottic cancer treatment by stage per NCCN guidelines

Clinical stage of **glottic** cancer	Recommendation treatment of primary and neck
Carcinoma in situ	Endoscopic resection (preferred) or RT
Amenable to larynx-preserving (conservation) surgery (T1–T2,N0 or select T3,N0)	RT or partial laryngectomy/endoscopic or open resection as indicated and neck dissection as indicated
T3 requiring (amenable to) total laryngectomy (N0–1)	Concurrent systemic therapy/RT or RT if patient not candidate for systemic therapy/RT or Surgery (laryngectomy) N0: Ipsilateral thyroidectomy (as indicated), pretracheal and ipsilateral paratracheal lymph node dissection N1: Also ipsilateral or bilateral neck dissection or induction chemotherapy
T3 requiring (amenable to) total laryngectomy (N2–3)	Concurrent systemic therapy/RT or Surgery (laryngectomy, thyroidectomy, ipsilateral or bilateral neck dissection, pretracheal and ipsilateral paratracheal lymph node dissection) or Induction chemotherapy
T4a,N0–3	Surgery ➔ Total laryngectomy N0: thyroidectomy ± unilateral or bilateral neck dissection, pretracheal and ipsilateral paratracheal lymph node dissection N1: thyroidectomy, ipsilateral or bilateral neck dissection, pretracheal and ipsilateral paratracheal lymph node dissection N2–3: total laryngectomy with thyroidectomy, ipsilateral or bilateral neck dissection, pretracheal and ipsilateral paratracheal lymph node dissection
T4b	Clinical trial preferred Standard therapy PS 0–1: concurrent ST/RT or induction ST + RT or ST/RT PS 2: RT or concurrent ST/RT PS 3: palliative RT, single-agent ST, or best supportive care

Treatment

There are different surgical and nonsurgical strategies to manage laryngeal cancer. The goals in treatment of laryngeal cancer include curing the patient, preserving the larynx (or maintaining a functional larynx), and minimizing morbidity (see Tables 16.1 and 16.2).

The histologic diagnosis, site of origin, and the stage of disease dictate the therapeutic decision-making.

Surgery and Radiation

In those with early-stage cancers, like T1-2N0/CIS glottic cancer, management with a single modality therapy is preferred. Surgery can be offered, especially to patients with a functional larynx and those whose cancer can be adequately approached/resected via endoscopic techniques (transoral laser microsurgery or transoral robotic surgery) (see Table 16.1). Early-stage cancer like T1-2N0 may also be treated with primary radiation. In a randomized trial looking at 56 patients with early-stage laryngeal squamous cell cancer, the overall survival and disease-specific survival between surgical management vs. radiation therapy (RT) management were shown to be superior with surgery [20, 21].

Advanced cancers, including T3-4N1-3 disease, require multimodal therapy which entails surgery followed by radiation therapy or a combination of chemotherapy and radiation therapy. If surgically resectable, these patients will generally require a total laryngectomy. Definitive radiation concurrent with cisplatin chemotherapy remains an option for laryngeal preservation in patients who would like to defer surgery or

Table 16.2 Supraglottic cancer treatment by stage per NCCN guidelines

Clinical stage of **supraglottic** cancer	Recommendation treatment of primary and neck
T1–2,N0; selected T3 patients	Endoscopic resection + neck dissection or Open partial supraglottic laryngectomy + neck dissection or definitive RT
T3,N0	Concurrent systemic therapy/RT or RT if patient not candidate for systemic therapy/RT or surgery (laryngectomy + neck dissection) or induction chemotherapy
Amenable to larynx-preserving (conservation) surgery(T1–2,N+ and selected T3, N1)	Concurrent systemic therapy/RT or definitive RT for low-volume disease (T1–2,N1) or partial supraglottic laryngectomy and neck dissection or induction chemotherapy
Requiring (amenable to) total laryngectomy (most T3,N1–N3)	Concurrent systemic therapy/RT or laryngectomy, ipsilateral thyroidectomy with neck dissection or Induction chemotherapy
T4a,N0–3	Laryngectomy, thyroidectomy as indicated with ipsilateral or bilateral neck dissection

who are unsuitable candidates for operative intervention [22]. Combined chemotherapy and radiation have demonstrated improved locoregional control and larynx preservation in patients with a functional larynx and without cartilage erosion. A chart review of 221 patients with T4 disease demonstrated similar locoregional control rates but improved overall survival in those who underwent laryngectomy and adjuvant radiation therapy when compared to chemoradiation and salvage surgery [23].

Like early-stage glottic cancers, early supraglottic cancers can be managed with either larynx-sparing surgery or RT. In patients who cannot be successfully oncologically resected endoscopically, primary radiation therapy is the preferred option due to the morbidity of operative interventions. Surgical approaches include endoscopic resection and open partial laryngectomy for T1-2 and low-volume T3 disease, with neck dissections often indicated in T2 or T3 lesions (see Table 16.2). Unlike the glottis, however, there is more lymphatic drainage of the supraglottis and increased risk of nodal metastasis; thus, the management of the cervical lymph nodes is managed differently [24]. Adjuvant radiation therapy is given to many patients, with common indications including positive nodal disease, extracapsular extension, and positive surgical margins [24].

Chemotherapy and Immunotherapy

Chemotherapy and immunotherapy play a large role in advanced stage cancer, although neither alone is administered with curative intent as they are generally for palliative treatment. Platinum-based chemotherapeutic agents like cisplatin and carboplatin are the first-line choice in combination with 5-fluorouracil, paclitaxel, docetaxel, or methotrexate [25]. Immunotherapy agents such as cetuximab, pembrolizumab, and nivolumab are offered when patients are not ideal candidates for chemotherapy [25].

Induction chemotherapy before surgery and/or radiation aims to shrink the tumor to a size which may allow resection to be possible in a previously unresectable cancer. Gao et al. performed a meta-analysis of randomized controlled trials (1985–2017) investigating the effect of induction chemotherapy on survival, disease control, larynx-preserving surgery, and disease-free survival; the study found an overall survival benefit in using induction chemotherapy for patients with resectable laryngeal cancer [26]. Chemotherapy is currently more often used in the adjuvant setting with radiation after surgical resection of the tumor with poor prognostic factors including histology, positive surgical margins, perineural invasion, lymphovascular invasion, and extracapsular spread or matted nodal disease.

The tables below show the updated NCCN guidelines for laryngeal cancer based on subsite.

Survival

The prognosis of laryngeal cancer is linked to the stage of disease at the time of treatment and the subsite involved; however, the overall 5-year survival rate for laryngeal cancer in the USA is 61% [27].

The overall 5-year survival rate for glottic SCCa is 77%. If confined to the larynx (stage I and II), the 5-year survival rate is 84% [28]. This drops to 52% if lymph node metastases are present and further to 45% in the setting of distant metastases [28].

The overall 5-year survival rate for supraglottic squamous cell carcinoma is 45%. If the disease is confined to the larynx (stages I and II), the 5-year survival rate is 61% [29]. With nodal metastasis, it drops to 46% and further decreases to 30% in the setting of distant metastases [28].

The overall 5-year survival rate for subglottic squamous cell carcinoma is 49%. If the disease is confined to the larynx (stages I and II), the 5-year survival rate is 59%. With nodal metastasis, it drops to 38% and further decreases to 44% in the setting of distant metastases [30].

Summary

Laryngeal cancer makes up about a third of head and neck cancers. Due to the vague and sometimes nonspecific symptoms, laryngeal cancer is often found in a later phase, resulting in delayed treatment and poor prognosis. Depending on the subsite affected, stage, and patient factors, management can vary including surgical and nonsurgical therapies. Major pathologic pathways implicated in the tumorigenesis of laryngeal squamous cell cancer including cellular survival and proliferation, cell-cycle control, and cellular differentiation may play a key in allowing early diagnosis and allow for organ preservation.

References

1. Falco M, Tammaro C, Takeuchi T, Cossu AM, Scafuro G, Zappavigna S, Itro A, Addeo R, Scrima M, Lombardi A, Ricciardiello F, Irace C, Caraglia M, Misso G. Overview on molecular biomarkers for laryngeal cancer: looking for new answers to an old problem. Cancers (Basel). 2022;14(7):1716.
2. SEER cancer stat facts: laryngeal cancer. National Cancer Institute, Bethesda. https://seer.cancer.gov/statfacts/html/laryn.html
3. Liberale C, Soloperto D, Marchioni A, Monzani D, Sacchetto L. Updates on larynx cancer: risk factors and oncogenesis. Int J Mol Sci. 2023;24(16):12913.
4. Talamini R, Bosetti C, La Vecchia C, Dal Maso L, Levi F, Bidoli E, Negri E, Pasche C, Vaccarella S, Barzan L, Franceschi S. Combined effect of tobacco and alcohol on laryngeal cancer risk: a case-control study. Cancer Causes Control. 2002;13(10):957–64.
5. Arboleda LPA, Neves AB, Kohler HF, Vartanian JG, Candelária LM, Borges MF, Fernandes GA, de Carvalho GB, Kowalski LP, Brennan P, Santos-Silva AR, Curado MP. Overview of glottic laryngeal cancer treatment recommendation changes in the NCCN guidelines from 2011 to 2022. Cancer Rep (Hoboken). 2023;6(8):e1837.
6. Mowery A, Conlin M, Clayburgh D. Increased risk of head and neck cancer in Agent Orange exposed Vietnam era veterans. Oral Oncol. 2020;100:104483.
7. Ramsey T, Guo E, Svider PF, Lin H, Syeda S, Raza SN, Fribley AM. Laryngeal cancer: global socioeconomic trends in disease burden and smoking habits. Laryngoscope. 2018;128:2039–53.
8. Ramroth H, Dietz A, Becher H. Environmental tobacco smoke and laryngeal cancer: results from a population-based case-control study. Eur Arch Otorrinolaringol. 2008;265(11):1367–71.
9. Bagnardi V, Rota M, Botteri E, Tramacere I, Islami F, Fedirko V, Scotti L, Jenab M, Turati F, Pasquali E, Pelucchi C, Galeone C, Bellocco R, Negri E, Corrao G, Boffetta P, La Vecchia C. Alcohol consumption and site-specific cancer risk: a comprehensive dose-response meta-analysis. Br J Cancer. 2015;112(3):580–93.
10. Wittekindt C, Wuerdemann N, Gattenlöhner S, Brobeil A, Wierzbicka M, Wagner S, Klußmann JP. The role of high-risk human papillomavirus infections in laryngeal squamous cell carcinoma. Eur Arch Otorrinolaringol. 2017;274(11):3837–42.
11. Li X, Gao L, Li H, Gao J, Yang Y, Zhou F, Gao C, Li M, Jin Q. Human papillomavirus infection and laryngeal cancer risk: a systematic review and meta-analysis. J Infect Dis. 2013;207:479–88.
12. De Lima MAP, Silva ÁDL, do Nascimento Filho ACS, Cordeiro TL, Bezerra JPdS, Rocha MAB, Pinheiro SdFL, Pinheiro Junior RFF, Gadelha MdSV, da Silva CGL. Epstein-Barr virus-associated carcinoma of the larynx: a systematic review with meta-analysis. Pathogens. 2021;10:1429.
13. Shah MD, Johns MM 3rd. Office-based laryngeal procedures. Otolaryngol Clin N Am. 2013;46(1):75–84. https://doi.org/10.1016/j.otc.2012.08.019.
14. Poeta ML, Manola J, Goldwasser MA, Forastiere A, Benoit N, Califano JA, Ridge JA, Goodwin J, Kenady D, Saunders J, et al. TP53 mutations and survival in squamous-cell carcinoma of the head and neck. N Engl J Med. 2007;357:2552–61.
15. Marcos CÁ, Alonso-Guervós M, Prado NR, Gimeno TS, Iglesias FD, Hermsen M, Llorente JL. Genetic model of transformation and neoplastic progression in laryngeal epithelium. Head Neck. 2011;33:216–24.
16. Giotakis AI, Lazaris AC, Kataki A, Kontos CK, Giotakis EI. Positive BCL2L12 expression predicts favorable prognosis in patients with laryngeal squamous cell carcinoma. Cancer Biomark. 2019;25:141–9.
17. Politi A, Tsiambas E, Mastronikolis NS, Peschos D, Asproudis I, Kyrodimos E, Armata IE, Chrysovergis A, Asimakopoulos A, Papanikolaou VS, et al. Combined EGFR/ALK expression analysis in laryngeal squamous cell carcinoma. In Vivo. 2019;33:815–9.
18. Sun W, Gaykalova DA, Ochs MF, Mambo E, Arnaoutakis D, Liu Y, Loyo M, Agrawal N, Howard J, Li R, et al. Activation of the NOTCH pathway in head and neck cancer. Cancer Res. 2014;74:1091–104.
19. Li D, Dong P, Wu C, Cao P, Zhou L. Notch1 overexpression associates with poor prognosis in human laryngeal squamous cell carcinoma. Ann Otol Rhinol Laryngol. 2014;123:705–10.
20. Pakkanen P, Irjala H, Ilmarinen T, Halme E, Lindholm P, Mäkitie A, Wigren T, Aaltonen LM. Survival and larynx preservation in early glottic cancer: a randomized trial comparing laser surgery and radiation therapy. Int J Radiat Oncol Biol Phys. 2022;113(1):96–100.
21. Sungur AC, Bayır Ö, Toptaş G, Aksoy Ş, Karahan S, Yücel V, Tatar EÇ, Saylam G, Korkmaz MH. Retrospective analysis of laryngeal cancer patients in a tertiary referral center. Turk Arch Otorhinolaryngol. 2024;62(1):21–9.
22. Forastiere AA, Ismaila N, Lewin JS, Nathan CA, Adelstein DJ, Eisbruch A, Fass G, Fisher SG, Laurie SA, Le QT, O'Malley B, Mendenhall WM, Patel S, Pfister DG, Provenzano AF, Weber R, Weinstein GS, Wolf GT. Use of larynx-preservation strategies in the treatment of laryngeal cancer: American Society of Clinical Oncology clinical practice guideline update. J Clin Oncol. 2018;36(11):1143–69.
23. Rosenthal DI, Mohamed AS, Weber RS, Garden AS, Sevak PR, Kies MS, Morrison WH, Lewin JS, El-Naggar AK, Ginsberg LE, Kocak-Uzel E, Ang KK, Fuller CD. Long-term outcomes after surgical or nonsurgical initial therapy for patients with T4 squamous cell carcinoma of the larynx: A 3-decade survey. Cancer. 2015;121(10):1608–19.
24. Prasad A, Carey RM, Panara K, Rajasekaran K, Cannady SB, Newman JG, Brant JA, Brody RM. Nodal metastasis in surgically treated laryngeal squamous cell carcinoma. Head Neck. 2023;45(9):2303–12.
25. Campbell G, Glazer TA, Kimple RJ, Bruce JY. Advances in organ preservation for laryngeal cancer. Curr Treat Options in Oncol. 2022;23(4):594–608.
26. Gao P, Gong L, Wang X. Induction chemotherapy in patients with resectable laryngeal cancer: a meta-analysis. Mol Clin Oncol. 2018;9(2):155–62.
27. Steuer CE, El-Deiry M, Parks JR, Higgins KA, Saba NF. An update on larynx cancer. CA Cancer J Clin. 2017;67(1):31–50.
28. Li MM, Zhao S, Eskander A, Rygalski C, Brock G, Parikh AS, Haring CT, Swendseid B, Zhan KY, Bradford CR, Teknos TN, Carrau RL, VanKoevering KK, Seim NB, Old MO, Rocco JW, Puram SV, Kang SY. Stage migration and survival trends in laryngeal cancer. Ann Surg Oncol. 2021;28(12):7300–9.
29. Nahavandipour A, Jakobsen KK, Grønhøj C, Hebbelstrup Jensen D, Kim Schmidt Karnov K, Klitmøller Agander T, Specht L, von Buchwald C. Incidence and survival of laryngeal cancer in Denmark: a nation-wide study from 1980 to 2014. Acta Oncol. 2019;58(7):977–82.
30. Yang F, He L, Rao Y, Feng Y, Wang J. Survival analysis of patients with subglottic squamous cell carcinoma based on the SEER database. Braz J Otorhinolaryngol. 2022;88 Suppl 4(Suppl 4):S70–80.

Research on Thoracic Cancer: Lung Cancer

17

Kerry Calkins, Tianyu Jiang, and Jeffrey Huang

Introduction

Lung cancer continues to represent a major health burden, accounting for approximately 12% of all cancer diagnoses globally and 19% of cancer deaths worldwide [1]. In 2025, in the United States alone, an estimated 226,650 new cases and 124,730 deaths are projected, with age-adjusted incidence rates of 47.8 per 100,000 population [2]. The disease demonstrates significant geographic variation, with the highest age-standardized rates observed in Eastern Asia, Eastern Europe, and Northern America [1].

Histologic Subtypes

The histologic landscape of lung cancer has evolved over recent decades. Adenocarcinoma now represents the predominant subtype globally, comprising 45% of cases overall and showing enrichment in never-smokers and Asian populations [3, 4]. Lung cancer in never-smokers, representing 10–25% of cases, demonstrates distinct molecular characteristics [4–6]. Lung cancer in never-smokers disproportionately affects women and younger patients, underscoring the need for comprehensive molecular profiling regardless of smoking history [7]. Prevalence of lung cancer is organized by histological subtype in Table 17.1. Non-small cell lung cancers (NSCLC) constitute most cases, including adenocarcinoma, squamous cell carcinoma, and large cell carcinoma [8, 9]. Histologic subtype carries profound implications for treatment, as adenocarcinomas harbor higher frequencies of targetable driver mutations; molecular heterogeneity within histologic subtypes has led to a shift from histology-based to biomarker-driven treatment selection [10]. Notably, small cell lung cancer (SCLC) has declined from 17% to 13% of cases over time [2, 5].

K. Calkins
The Ohio State University College of Medicine,
Columbus, OH, USA

T. Jiang
Department of Anesthesiology and Perioperative Medicine,
University of Rochester School of Medicine, Rochester, NY, USA

J. Huang (✉)
Anesthesiology and Critical Care, Moffitt Cancer Center,
Tampa, FL, USA
e-mail: jeffrey.huang@moffitt.org

J. Huang, H. S.L. Jim (eds.), *Cancer Research Guidance for Clinicians and Researchers*,
https://doi.org/10.1007/978-3-032-19175-5_17

Table 17.1 Major lung cancer subtypes and their clinical associations [2, 5]

Histologic subtype	Overall prevalence [5]	Male prevalence[a] [5]	Female prevalence[a] [5]	Key associations [2]
Adenocarcinoma	~45–50%	~39%	~55–60%	Never-smokers, Asian populations
Squamous cell	~20–21%	~25%	~10–12%	Smokers, central location
Small cell	~13–15%	~11%	~9%	Heavy smokers, rapid progression
Large cell	~6-8%	~8%	~6%	Poor differentiation

[a]Percentages reflect within-sex distribution and vary by country and region. These categories are not exhaustive.

Risk Factors

Tobacco smoking is the leading cause of lung cancer, accounting for 80–90% of cases; smokers have a 15- to 30-fold higher risk of dying from lung cancer compared with never-smokers [11]. The risk of lung cancer increases with the duration of tobacco exposure. Importantly, smoking cessation provides lasting health benefits, although the risk remains elevated for 15 years or more after quitting [4, 12]. In addition to tobacco, environmental exposures contribute substantially to lung cancer burden; radon, asbestos, arsenic, chromium, and diesel exhaust are all established carcinogens that raise risk [11, 13]. Recently, air pollution has been linked specifically to adenocarcinoma, acting through pathways independent of direct mutagenesis [4, 5, 14].

Prognosis and Survival Trends

Overall 5-year relative survival for lung cancer has improved from about 12% in 1975 to 28% in 2022, largely due to earlier detection, advances in molecular profiling, and new therapeutic strategies [15]. Survival outcomes vary greatly by stage at diagnosis: Between 2015 and 2021, the National Cancer Institute (NCI) reported 5-year survival rates of 64.7% for localized disease, 37.1% for regional disease, and 9.7% for distant disease [15]. Beyond staging, molecular markers have become increasingly important prognostic indicators; for example, patients with resected, early-stage EGFR-mutated NSCLC achieve 5-year survival in the range of two-thirds to three quarters [16, 17].

Prevention Strategies

Primary prevention through smoking cessation remains the most impactful strategy for reducing lung cancer burden [11]. Comprehensive tobacco control policies including taxation, smoke-free legislation, and cessation support services have contributed to declining smoking rates and subsequent reductions in lung cancer incidence [11]. Population-level interventions addressing environmental exposures, particularly radon mitigation and air quality improvements, represent additional prevention opportunities [11].

Screening Guidelines

The 2021 United States Preventive Services Task Force (USPSTF) guidelines expanded lung cancer screening by expanding eligibility criteria to adults aged 50–80 years with a 20 pack-year smoking history who currently smoke or quit within the past 15 years [18]. This represented an expansion from previous criteria, which recommended screening for persons aged 55–80, with 30 pack-year smoking history; it nearly doubles the eligible population and is projected to save 30,000–60,000 additional lives annually [18, 19]. The National Comprehensive Cancer Network (NCCN) further expanded recommendations by eliminating the 15-year quit limit, recognizing that lung cancer risk persists beyond this arbitrary cutoff [20]. This change increases eligibility for those aged 50–80 who ever smoked [20]. Medicare coverage slightly narrows the age range to 50–77 years while maintaining other USPSTF criteria (Table 17.2) [21]. Implementation challenges persist, with approximately 1 out of every 5 eligible individuals currently screened [18, 22]. There are several explanations for implementation challenges, which include but are not limited to geographic disparities, provider training, distrust in healthcare systems, and policy landscape factors [23].

Table 17.2 Comparison of USPSTF 2021 vs. NCCN 2025 lung cancer screening guidelines

Feature	USPSTF 2021 [18]	NCCN 2025 [20]
Age range	50–80 years	≥50 years (no upper age limit)
Pack-year history	≥20 pack-years	≥20 pack-years
Smoking cessation window	Quit within past 15 years	No time limit since quitting
Additional risk factors	Not included	Optional inclusion of other risk factors
Screening modality	Annual low-dose CT	Annual low-dose CT
Medicare coverage	Official USPSTF: age 50–80; in practice, Medicare coverage stops at 77	NCCN criteria are broader but Medicare coverage follows USPSTF

Artificial Intelligence (AI) in Lung Cancer Screening

In parallel, AI offers tools to overcome some of these barriers from screening to treatment selection. The Sybil model predicts lung cancer risk 1–6 years from a single low-dose CT (LDCT) scan with remarkable accuracy [24]. Critically, this deep learning model requires only LDCT images without clinical data or radiologist annotations, enabling real-time risk stratification in diverse populations including never-smokers [24]. Beyond screening tools like Sybil, AI-based models used in digital pathology now achieve >90% accuracy in histologic classification and biomarker quantification [25]. In addition, clinical decision support systems integrate molecular profiles with clinical data to generate treatment recommendations and match patients to clinical trials [26, 27]. Several commercial AI solutions have achieved FDA approval and clinical implementation. One example is the Optellum Virtual Nodule Clinic, which is an AI model that analyzes CT scans to provide a malignancy risk score for each nodule and has been implemented in the National Health Service (NHS), Wake Forest Baptist Health, and Vanderbilt Lung Institute [28]. In a 2025 Precision Oncology review, authors map where AI is already helping across the lung cancer pathway and why clinical translation still lags: data sharing, bias/fairness, interpretability, and reproducibility [29]. The next leap in advancements will come from generalist, multimodal AI that fuses radiology, pathology, genomics, and longitudinal biosignals, paired with stricter standards and prospective, multisite validation [29].

Application of LDCT, PET-CT, and Liquid Biopsy

While maintaining diagnostic quality, modern LDCT protocols have transformed lung cancer screening by reducing radiation exposure to approximately 2 mSv, which is less than a third of standard chest CT's 7 mSv dose [30, 31]. The shift from diameter-based to volume-based nodule assessment, validated through the NELSON trial, has revolutionized screening accuracy [32, 33]. In a 2020 publication in the New England Journal of Medicine, Koning et al. further solidified this finding after analyzing over 22,600 CT scans and finding that volume-based approaches achieved a significant reduction in lung cancer mortality with a remarkably low false-positive rate of 1.2% [34]. Volume doubling time (VDT) calculations now provide superior prognostic value, while semiautomated volumetric analysis has reduced inter-reader variability of small lung nodules [35].

While FDG-PET assesses general metabolic activity, novel tracers are expanding diagnostic and surveillance capabilities. ^{89}Zr-labeled atezolizumab (anti-PD-L1) imaging of tracer uptake demonstrated a strong predictor of response to the treatment [36]. For immunotherapy response assessment, modified criteria such as iRECIST or iPERCIST account for unique patterns including pseudoprogression and mixed responses [37, 38]. Quantitative PET metrics have advanced beyond maximum standardized uptake value (SUVmax) to include measures such as metabolic tumor volume (MTV) and total lesion glycolysis (TLG), which offer more comprehensive and informative assessments [39].

Next-generation liquid biopsy approaches analyze not only circulating tumor DNA (ctDNA) but also additional biomarkers such as exosomes and proteins [40, 41]. Enhanced sensitivity through deeper sequencing and analytical methods such as fragmentomics enable earlier cancer detection [42]. Population-level screening trials including the ongoing SUMMIT study are validating multi-cancer early detection strategies in high-risk populations [43]. The FDA has approved several liquid biopsies such as FoundationOne Liquid CDx which covers 300+ genes and demonstrates comparable sensitivity to tissue-based testing for actionable mutations [44]. Beyond mutation detection, ctDNA can identify minimal residual disease (MRD), and assays can detect mutant molecules [41, 45]. Postsurgical MRD detection identifies 94% of patients with recurrence, with ctDNA positivity preceding radiographic progression by a median of 5.2 months [41, 46]. It is clear that liquid biopsy technologies can enable risk-stratified surveillance and help guide adjuvant therapy decisions.

Treatment

Surgery

In early-stage lung cancer, surgical resection remains the treatment of choice. The extent of surgery is determined by tumor size, location, and the patient's preoperative pulmonary function.

Displayed in Table 17.3, the American College of Chest Physicians recently published their new guidelines of management of early-stage non-small cell lung cancer [47].

Targeted Therapies and Immunotherapy

An improved understanding of the lung microbiome's influence on treatment response opens new therapeutic avenues through microbiome modulation [48]. In advanced NSCLC, targeted therapies and immunotherapies have significantly improved clinical outcomes for a substantial subset of patients.

Table 17.3 American College of Chest Physicians 2025 guidelines

NSCLC stage	Surgery methods
Clinical stage I and II	Minimally invasive approaches (video-assisted thoracic surgery [VATS]/robotic-assisted thoracic surgery) over thoracotomy
Peripherally located, or <2 cm, stage I	Lobectomy, segmentectomy, or sublobar nonanatomic (wedge) resection
Centrally located or >2 cm, stage I	Lobectomy
Stage II	Lobectomy
Stage I and II	Systematic lymph node sampling or dissection
NSCLC adjuvant therapy recommendations	
Stage I, completely resected	Do not recommend routine adjuvant chemotherapy or immunotherapy
Stage II, completely resected	Recommend adjuvant chemotherapy
Stage II, resected, with EGFR or ALK alterations	Recommend adjuvant targeted therapy following chemotherapy
Stage II, resected, without EGFR or ALK alterations	Suggest adjuvant immunotherapy following chemotherapy

Molecular Pathogenesis and Biomarkers of Lung Cancer

The molecular landscape of lung cancer has diverged into distinct therapeutic paradigms for NSCLC and SCLC. While NSCLC has evolved into a precision oncology success story with multiple targetable oncogenic drivers, SCLC remains largely defined by transcriptional subtypes and immunotherapeutic approaches. This dichotomy reflects fundamental differences in genomic architecture: NSCLC frequently harbors mutually exclusive oncogenic drivers amenable to targeted therapy, whereas SCLC is characterized by RB1/TP53 inactivation and high tumor mutational burden [49, 50].

NSCLC: Targetable Driver Mutations

In NSCLC, oncogenic driver mutations are typically mutually exclusive, enabling prediction of targeted therapy response and facilitating treatment selection for each patient's specific mutation. Table 17.4 displays that fusion oncogenes (ALK, ROS1, RET), and EGFR mutations are more common in never-smokers, while KRAS mutations predominate in smokers [4, 7, 52].

NSCLC: Immunotherapy Biomarkers

Programmed death-ligand 1 (PD-L1) is a cell-surface protein that, when bound to its receptor PD-1, suppresses T-cell activity and allows PD-L1 expressing cells to evade immune surveillance. Tumors with higher PD-L1 expression are more likely to benefit from immune checkpoint inhibitors. The PD-L1 tumor proportion score (TPS), assessed with the 22C3 pharmDx assay, stratifies NSCLC patients into high (≥50%, ~30%), positive (1–49%, ~40%), and negative (<1%, ~30%) expression groups. Corresponding 5-year overall survival rates with pembrolizumab monotherapy, a monoclonal antibody that targets PD-1, are 31.9%, 19.4%, and 16.6%, respectively [59]. Another emerging biomarker is tumor mutational burden (TMB), which reflects the total number of mutations within a tumor genome. High TMB has been linked to improved responses to immunotherapy and improved survival, although its routine clinical use remains limited by cost, variability among assays, and lack of standardization.

NSCLC: Negative Predictive Biomarkers

Loss of STK11 is associated with "cold" tumor biology characterized by poor response to immune checkpoint inhibitors, with median progression-free survival of 1.8 versus 4.8 months [59]. Similarly, KEAP1 mutations, present in approximately 15–20% of NSCLC, are linked to adverse outcomes across treatment modalities [59].

SCLC: Molecular Landscape

SCLC is characterized by near-universal inactivation of TP53 (>90%) and RB1 (>70%), along with a relatively high tumor mutational burden (median 8–10 mutations/Mb) [50]. Molecular profiling further delineates four major transcriptional subtypes: ASCL1 (~70%), NEUROD1 (~11%), POU2F3 (~7%), and YAP1 (~2%), in addition to an inflamed subtype present in approximately 10% of cases [50].

SCLC Immunotherapy

First-line atezolizumab or durvalumab plus platinum-etoposide improves median overall survival from 10.3 to 12.3–13.0 months [62]. Neither PD-L1 nor TMB predict benefit in SCLC; this is because high mutational burden paradoxically fails to enhance immunotherapy efficacy due to low MHC-I expression [63, 64]. Tarlatamab, a DLL3-CD3 bispecific, achieved 40% ORR and 9.7-month median duration of response in pretreated patients [60]. Additional DLL3-directed therapies and subtype-specific approaches are under investigation (Table 17.5).

Table 17.4 Targetable driver mutations in NSCLC

Driver mutation	Overall frequency	Never-smoker enrichment	ORR (1L)	Median PFS (months)	FDA approval year
EGFR (Ex19del/L858R) [51]	~10–15% (US) ~30–50% (Asia)	~40–60%	~80–85%	18.9	2018 (osimertinib)
ALK rearrangement [52]	~3–5%	~20–34%	~82%	NR (60% at 5 year)	2024 (lorlatinib)
ROS1 rearrangement [53]	~1–2%	~39–77%	~72–77%	15.7–19.2	2019 (entrectinib)
RET rearrangement [54]	~1–2%	~60–75%	~85%	22.0	2020 (selpercatinib)
BRAF V600E [54]	~1–2%	~50–60%	~64%	10.9	2017 (dabrafenib/trametinib)
MET exon 14 skipping [55]	~2–4%	~30–40%	~68%	12.4	2020 (capmatinib)
HER2 mutations [56]	~2–3%	~57–83%	~55%	8.2	2022 (T-DXd)
KRAS G12C [53, 57]	~10–13%	~2–5%	~37–43%	6.5–6.8	2021 (sotorasib)
NTRK fusions [54, 58]	~0.1–0.2%	~Equal	~75–80%	28–35	2018 (larotrectinib)

NR not reached, *ORR* objective response rate, *1L* first-line, *T-DXd* trastuzumab deruxtecan, *PFS* progression-free survival

Table 17.5 Molecular targets and biomarkers in SCLC

Target/biomarker	Frequency	Clinical application	Therapeutic agent	Efficacy	FDA status
DLL3 [60]	75–94%	Surface antigen	Tarlatamab (BiTE)	ORR 40%, mPFS 4.9 mon	2024 approved (2L)
MYC amplification [50]	20–30%	Prognostic	None approved	Poor prognosis	Research only
PD-L1* [61]	18%	Not used	Atezolizumab/durvalumab	See below	Not required
TMB-high (≥10 mut/Mb) [61]	40–50%	Not predictive	Checkpoint inhibitors	Not predictive	Not used
Transcriptional subtypes [50]	100%**	Research	Subtype-specific trials	Variable	Investigational

BiTE bispecific T-cell engager, *CPS* combined positive score, *2L* second line, *ORR* overall response rate, *mPFS* median progression-free survival, *PD-L1 expression is generally low on tumor cells; assay-dependent, **All tumors classifiable; proportions vary by cohort, Note: Frequency column is approximate.

Emerging Therapies and Clinical Implementation Challenges

Antibodies and Vaccines

Antibody-drug conjugates (ADCs) are emerging as a promising therapeutic class. Trastuzumab deruxtecan achieved a 55% response rate in HER2-mutant NSCLC with a median overall survival of 17.8 months [56]. Datopotamab deruxtecan, the first TROP2-targeted ADC in lung cancer, showed a 45% response rate in EGFR-mutated disease progressing on prior therapy [65]. Bispecific antibodies such as amivantamab (EGFR/MET) act through multiple mechanisms, including ligand blocking, receptor degradation, and antibody-dependent cytotoxicity. When combined with chemotherapy, amivantamab has demonstrated efficacy in EGFR exon 20 insertion-mutant tumors and in post-osimertinib progression [66]. In immunotherapy, mRNA cancer vaccines represent a new frontier. Moderna's mRNA-4157/V940, which encodes up to 34 patient-specific neoantigens, has shown encouraging activity in combination with pembrolizumab [67].

Challenges and Future Directions

The rapid expansion of precision medicine and immunotherapy underscores a widening gap between innovation and real-world implementation. While clinical trials increasingly demonstrate remarkable survival gains, translation into routine practice is constrained by variability in access to genomic profiling, liquid biopsy adoption, and standardized biomarker testing [10, 20, 42]. Turnaround times, cost, and uneven availability across health systems continue to delay the initiation of targeted therapies and limit the reach of advances to underserved populations [23, 27].

Another major challenge is ensuring equitable access to screening and early detection. Despite expanded eligibility criteria, uptake of LDCT remains strikingly low, with fewer than one in five eligible individuals screened in the United States [18, 22]. This shortfall disproportionately affects rural populations and racial minorities, reinforcing long-standing survival disparities. Addressing provider training, health system infrastructure, and patient trust will be as important as expanding guidelines.

Looking forward, next-generation technologies hold the promise of reshaping lung cancer management. Liquid biopsy enables earlier detection of minimal residual disease and recurrence, often preceding radiographic progression by months [41, 46]. Artificial intelligence has shown the capacity to integrate imaging, pathology, and molecular data to support individualized decision-making, yet issues of bias, reproducibility, and regulatory oversight slow adoption [24, 29]. Previously mentioned emerging modalities such as ADCs, bispecific antibodies, and mRNA vaccines add to the therapeutic arsenal, but their cost and complexity may exacerbate inequities without deliberate policy and infrastructure solutions [56, 68–70]. Ultimately, the future of lung cancer care will depend not only on continued innovation but also on narrowing implementation gaps. Efforts to expand equitable access to screening, accelerate biomarker-driven therapy, and standardize integration of novel technologies will determine whether recent scientific breakthroughs translate into population-level survival gains.

Summary

Lung cancer research and treatment have undergone a remarkable transformation through the integration of precision medicine, immunotherapy advances, and innovative technologies. However, realizing the full potential of these advances requires addressing persistent disparities in access and standardization of screening, biomarker testing, and novel therapies. As we move toward increasingly personalized treatment approaches, the integration of artificial intelligence, liquid biopsy technologies, and innovative trial designs will further accelerate progress against this devastating disease. Sustained progress will depend on bridging innovation with equity, ensuring that every patient, regardless of background or setting, can benefit from the transformative advances in lung cancer care.

References

1. Bray F, et al. Global cancer statistics 2022: GLOBOCAN estimates of incidence and mortality worldwide for 36 cancers in 185 countries. CA Cancer J Clin. 2024;74(3):229–63.
2. Siegel LR, et al. Cancer statistics, 2025. CA Cancer J Clin. 2025;75(1):10–45.
3. Lopiccolo J, et al. Lung cancer in patients who have never smoked—an emerging disease. Nat Rev Clin Oncol. 2024;21(2):121–46.
4. Landi TM, et al. Tracing lung cancer risk factors through mutational signatures in never-smokers. Am J Epidemiol. 2021;190(6):962–76.
5. Zhang Y, et al. Global variations in lung cancer incidence by histological subtype in 2020: a population-based study. Lancet Oncol. 2023;24(11):1206–18.
6. Zhang T, et al. Genomic and evolutionary classification of lung cancer in never smokers. Nature Genetics. 2021;53:1348–59.
7. Cho J, et al. Proportion and clinical features of never-smokers with non-small cell lung cancer. Chin J Cancer. 2017;36(1):20.
8. National Cancer Institute. Cancer stat facts: lung and bronchus cancer. National Cancer Institute: Surveillance, Epidemiology, and End Results Program. 2023. Available from: https://seer.cancer.gov/statfacts/html/lungb.html
9. National Cancer Institute. Non-small cell lung cancer treatment. 2025. Available from: https://www.cancer.gov/types/lung/hp/non-small-cell-lung-treatment-pdq
10. Owen HD, et al. Therapy for stage IV non–small cell lung cancer with driver alterations: ASCO living guideline, Version 2024.1. J Clin Oncol. 2024;42(20):e44–59.
11. National Cancer Institute. Lung cancer prevention (PDQ) health professional version lung cancer prevention (PDQ) health professional version. 2025. Available from: https://www.cancer.gov/types/lung/hp/lung-prevention-pdq?utm_source
12. Tindle AH, et al. Lifetime smoking history and risk of lung cancer: results from the Framingham heart study. J Natl Cancer Inst. 2018;110(11):1201–7.
13. CDC. Lung cancer risk factors. Atlanta: CDC; 2025.
14. Díaz-Gay M, et al. The mutagenic forces shaping the genomes of lung cancer in never smokers. Nature. 2025;644:133–44.
15. NCI SEER. Lung and bronchus recent trends in SEER age-adjusted incidence rates, 2000–2022. 2022. Available from: https://seer.cancer.gov/statistics
16. Wu Y-L, et al. Osimertinib in resected EGFR-mutated non–small-cell lung cancer. N Engl J Med. 2020;383(18):1711–23.
17. Tsuboi M, et al. Overall survival with osimertinib in resected EGFR-mutated NSCLC. N Engl J Med. 2023;389(2):137–47.
18. US Preventive Services Task Force, et al. Screening for lung cancer: US Preventive Services Task Force recommendation statement. JAMA. 2021;325(10):962–70.
19. Meza R, et al. USPSTF modeling study: benefits and harms of lung cancer screening with LDCT. JAMA. 2021;325(10):991–993
20. NCCN. NCCN clinical practical guidelines in oncology (NCCN guidelines): lung cancer screening. 2025. Available from: https://www.nccn.org
21. CMMS. Screening for lung cancer with low dose computed tomography (LDCT). Centers for Medicare & Medicaid Services; 2022. Available from: https://www.cms.gov/medicare
22. Poghosyan H, et al. A brief report of lung cancer screening utilization before, during, and in the later stages of the COVID-19 pandemic in the United States. JTO Clin Res Rep. 2024;5(9):100705.
23. Bandi P, et al. Lung cancer screening in the US, 2022. JAMA Intern Med. 2024;184(8):882.
24. Mikhael GP, et al. Sybil: a validated deep learning model to predict future lung cancer risk from a single low-dose chest computed tomography. J Clin Oncol. 2023;41(12):2191–200.
25. Mcgenity C, et al. Artificial intelligence in digital pathology: a systematic review and meta-analysis of diagnostic test accuracy. NPJ Digit Med. 2024;7(1):114.
26. Tamborero D, et al. The molecular tumor board portal supports clinical decisions and automated reporting for precision oncology. Nat Cancer. 2022;3(2):251–61.
27. Farhangfar JC, et al. Impact of a clinical genomics program on trial accrual for targeted treatments: practical approach overcoming bar-

riers to accrual for underserved patients. JCO Clin Cancer Informat. 2022;6:e2200011.
28. O'Dowd E, et al. Determining the impact of an artificial intelligence tool on the management of pulmonary nodules detected incidentally on CT (DOLCE) study protocol: a prospective, non-interventional multicentre UK study. BMJ Open. 2024;14(1):e077747.
29. Zhu E, et al. Progress and challenges of artificial intelligence in lung cancer clinical translation. NPJ Precision Oncology. 2025;9(1):210.
30. Larke JF, et al. Estimated radiation dose associated with low-dose chest CT of average-size participants in the National Lung Screening Trial. Am J Roentgenol. 2011;197(5):1165–9.
31. Iball RG, et al. An evaluation of CT radiation doses within the Yorkshire Lung Screening Trial. Br J Radiol. 2024;97(1154):469–76.
32. Xu MD, et al. Nodule management protocol of the NELSON randomised lung cancer screening trial. Lung Cancer. 2006;54(2):177–84.
33. van Klaveren RJ, et al. Management of lung nodules detected by volume CT scanning. N Engl J Med. 2009;361(23):2221–9.
34. Koning DJH, et al. Reduced lung-cancer mortality with volume CT screening in a randomized trial. N Engl J Med. 2020;382(6):503–13.
35. Zacharias F, Svahn MT. Interobserver variability in manual versus semi-automatic CT assessments of small lung nodule diameter and volume. Tomography. 2024;10(12):2087–99.
36. Bensch F, et al. 89Zr-atezolizumab imaging as a non-invasive approach to assess clinical response to PD-L1 blockade in cancer. Nat Med. 2018;24(12):1852–8.
37. Seymour L, et al. iRECIST: guidelines for response criteria for use in trials testing immunotherapeutics. Lancet Oncol. 2017;18(3):e143–52.
38. Ito K, et al. 18F-FDG PET/CT for monitoring of Ipilimumab therapy in patients with metastatic melanoma. J Nucl Med. 2019;60(3):335–41.
39. Chen WHH, et al. Prognostic value of whole-body total lesion glycolysis at pretreatment FDG PET/CT in non-small cell lung cancer. Radiology. 2012;264(2):559–66.
40. Abbosh C, et al. Phylogenetic ctDNA analysis depicts early-stage lung cancer evolution. Nature. 2017;545(7655):446–51.
41. Wu M, et al. Research progress on postoperative minimal/molecular residual disease detection in lung cancer. Chronic Dis Transl Med. 2022;8(2):83–90.
42. Rolfo C, et al. Liquid biopsy for advanced NSCLC: a consensus statement from the International Association for the Study of Lung Cancer. J Thorac Oncol. 2021;16(10):1647–62.
43. University College, London. The SUMMIT study: a cancer screening study (SUMMIT). 2024. Clinicaltrials.gov
44. Woodhouse R, et al. Clinical and analytical validation of FoundationOne Liquid CDx, a novel 324-gene blood-based comprehensive genomic profiling assay. J Clin Oncol. 2020;38(15_suppl):e13685.
45. Wang Y, et al. Clinical application of minimal residual disease detection by ctDNA testing in non-small cell lung cancer: a narrative review. Transl Lung Cancer Res. 2025;14(3):1007–20.
46. Chaudhuri AA, et al. Early detection of molecular residual disease in localized lung cancer by circulating tumor DNA profiling. Cancer Discov. 2017;7(12):1394–403.
47. Howington J, et al. Management of patients with early-stage non-small cell lung cancer: an American College of Chest Physicians clinical practice guideline. Chest. 2025;168:810–27.
48. Li R, Li J, Zhou X. Lung microbiome: new insights into the pathogenesis of respiratory diseases. Signal Transduct Targeted Ther. 2024;9(1):19.
49. George J, et al. Comprehensive genomic profiles of small cell lung cancer. Nature. 2015;524(7563):47–53.
50. Rudin MC, et al. Molecular subtypes of small cell lung cancer: a synthesis of human and mouse model data. Nat Rev Cancer. 2019;19(5):289–97.
51. Ramalingam SS, et al. Overall survival with osimertinib in untreated, EGFR – mutated advanced NSCLC. N Engl J Med. 2020;382(1):41–50.
52. Solomon JB, et al. Lorlatinib versus crizotinib in patients with advanced ALK-positive non-small cell lung cancer: 5-year outcomes from the Phase III CROWN Study. J Clin Oncol. 2024;42(29):3400–9.
53. Dziadziuszko R, et al. Updated integrated analysis of the efficacy and safety of entrectinib in locally advanced or metastaticROS1fusion–positive non-small-cell lung cancer. J Clin Oncol. 2021;39(11):1253–63.
54. Planchard D, et al. Phase 2 study of dabrafenib plus trametinib in patients with BRAF V600E-mutant metastatic NSCLC: updated 5-year survival rates and genomic analysis. J Thorac Oncol. 2022;17(1):103–15.
55. Wolf J, et al. Capmatinib in MET exon 14-mutated or MET-amplified non-small-cell lung cancer. N Engl J Med. 2020;383(10):944–57.
56. Li TB, et al. Trastuzumab deruxtecan in HER2 – mutant non-small-cell lung cancer. N Engl J Med. 2022;386(3):241–51.
57. Jänne AP, et al. Adagrasib in non-small-cell lung cancer harboring a KRAS G12C mutation. N Engl J Med. 2022;387(2):120–31.
58. Drilon A, et al. Efficacy of larotrectinib in TRK fusion-positive cancers in adults and children. N Engl J Med. 2018;378(8):731–9.
59. Skoulidis F, et al. STK11/LKB1 mutations and PD-1 inhibitor resistance in KRAS-mutant lung adenocarcinoma. Cancer Discov. 2018;8(7):822–35.
60. Ahn M-J, et al. Tarlatamab for patients with previously treated small-cell lung cancer. N Engl J Med. 2023;389(22):2063–75.
61. Hellmann DM, et al. Tumor mutational burden and efficacy of nivolumab monotherapy and in combination with ipilimumab in small-cell lung cancer. Cancer Cell. 2018;33(5):853–61.e4.
62. Liu VS, et al. Updated overall survival and PD-L1 subgroup analysis of patients with extensive-stage small-cell lung cancer treated with atezolizumab, carboplatin, and etoposide (IMpower133). J Clin Oncol. 2021;39(6):619–30.
63. Dolkar T, et al. New developments in immunotherapy for SCLC. J Immunother Cancer. 2025;13(1):e009667.
64. Mahadevan RN, et al. Intrinsic immunogenicity of small cell lung carcinoma revealed by its cellular plasticity. Cancer Discov. 2021;11(8):1952–69.
65. Smit FE, et al. Trastuzumab deruxtecan in patients with metastatic non-small-cell lung cancer (DESTINY-Lung01): primary results of the HER2-overexpressing cohorts from a single-arm, phase 2 trial. Lancet Oncol. 2024;25(4):439–54.
66. Zhou C, et al. Amivantamab plus chemotherapy in NSCLC with EGFR exon 20 insertions. N Engl J Med. 2023;389(22):2039–51.
67. Weber SJ, et al. Individualised neoantigen therapy mRNA-4157 (V940) plus pembrolizumab versus pembrolizumab monotherapy in resected melanoma (KEYNOTE-942): a randomised, phase 2b study. Lancet. 2024;403(10427):632–44.
68. Lindeman IN, et al. Updated molecular testing guideline for the selection of lung cancer patients for treatment with targeted tyrosine kinase inhibitors: guideline from the College of American Pathologists, the International Association for the Study of Lung Cancer, and the Association for Molecular Pathology. Arch Pathol Lab Med. 2018;142(3):321–46.
69. Ganti PKA, et al. Small cell lung cancer, Version 2.2022, NCCN clinical practice guidelines in oncology. J Natl Compr Cancer Netw. 2021;19(12):1441–64.
70. Gu Y, Benavente AC. Landscape and treatment options of shape-shifting small cell lung cancer. J Clin Med. 2024;13(11):3120.

Research on Gastrointestinal Cancer I (Esophagus, Stomach, Small Intestine, Colon)

18

Pratik Patel and Shaffer Mok

Abbreviations

AI	Artificial intelligence
BE	Barrett's esophagus
CADe	Computer-aided detection
CAR	Chimeric antigen receptor
CEA	Carcinoembryonic antigen
cfDNA	Cell-free DNA
CI	Confidence interval
CNN	Convolutional neuronal networks
CRC	Colorectal cancer
CTC	Circulating tumor cell
ctDNA	Circulating tumor DNA
DLBCL	Diffuse large B-cell lymphoma
DM	Diabetes mellitus
EAC	Esophageal adenocarcinoma
EC	Esophageal cancer
EFTR	Endoscopic full-thickness resection
EGFR	Epidermal growth factor receptor
EMR	Endoscopic mucosal resection
ESD	Endoscopic submucosal dissection
EUS	Endoscopic ultrasound
FAP	Familial adenomatous polyposis
FDA	Food and Drug Administration
FGFR	Fibroblast growth factor receptor
FIT	Fecal immunochemical test
FOBT	Fecal occult blood test
GAC	Gastric adenocarcinoma
GERD	Gastroesophageal reflux disease
GIST	Gastrointestinal stromal tumor
GLP1	Glucagon-like peptide 1
HDGC	Hereditary diffuse gastric cancer
HGD	High-grade dysplasia
HPV	Human papillomavirus
HR2A	Histamine-2-receptor antagonists
IBD	Inflammatory bowel disease
IHC	Immunohistochemistry
ISH	In situ hybridization
LGD	Low-grade dysplasia
MALT	Mucosa-associated lymphoid tissue
MMR	Mismatch repair
MSA	Magnetic sphincter augmentation
MSI	Microsatellite instability
NBI	Narrow-band imaging
NET	Neuroendocrine tumor
OR	Odds ratio
PCAB	Potassium-competitive acid blocker
PCR	Polymerase chain reaction
PDL1	Programmed cell death ligand 1
PJS	Peutz-Jeghers syndrome
PPI	Proton pump inhibitor
PRRT	Peptide receptor radionucleotide therapy
RFA	Radiofrequency ablation
RNYGB	Roux-en-Y gastric bypass
SCE	Squamous cell carcinoma of the esophagus
SEL	Subepithelial lesion
TEP	Tumor-educated platelets
TIF	Transoral incisionless fundoplication
TKI	Tyrosine kinase inhibitor
TNT	Total neoadjuvant therapy
TXI	Texture and color enhancement imaging
USPSTF	United States Preventative Services Task Force

P. Patel · S. Mok (✉)
Department of Gastroenterology, Moffitt Cancer Center, Tampa, FL, USA
e-mail: Shaffer.mok@moffitt.org

J. Huang, H. S.L. Jim (eds.), *Cancer Research Guidance for Clinicians and Researchers*,
https://doi.org/10.1007/978-3-032-19175-5_18

Esophagus

Introduction

Esophageal cancer (EC) ranks as the 7th most common cancer and the 6th highest cause of cancer death worldwide [1] and the 14th most common cancer and the 11th leading cause of cancer death in the United States [2, 3]. EC can be further classified into esophageal adenocarcinoma (EAC) and squamous cell carcinoma of the esophagus (SCE), the two most common histologic subtypes. EAC and SCE have distinct risk factors, clinical presentation, and treatment. Risk factors for EAC include gastroesophageal reflux disease (GERD), Barrett's esophagus (BE), tobacco use, obesity, male sex, diet, and genetic factors [4].

The strongest risk factor for SCE is tobacco use, while diet and consumption of alcohol and hot beverages as well as human papillomavirus (HPV) infection also play a role in the development of SCE [5]. SCE is more commonly diagnosed in Eastern countries such as China, where up to 90% of cases of EC are SCE [6]. On the other hand, EAC is more often diagnosed in Western countries, such as the United States [7]. Geographic differences such as these have resulted in screening programs for EAC in the United States and for SCE in China over the past few decades. Despite improvements in screening, surgical and endoscopic resection methods, and the advent of newer chemo and immunotherapeutic agents, the overall 5-year survival of EC remains low [8]. Thus, continued efforts through research and innovation are required to improve overall outcomes of EC.

Prevention and Screening

Prevention for EC depends on the histologic subtype of the cancer. For EAC, the primary goal involves both the management of GERD and the early diagnosis of BE with long-term endoscopic surveillance programs. The treatment of GERD is multifactorial and involves initial lifestyle modifications such as weight loss, tobacco, and alcohol cessation, avoiding spicy and acetic foods, and elevation of the head after meals among others [9]. When lifestyle modifications fail to work, medications aimed at lowering esophageal acid exposure such as histamine-2-receptor antagonists (H2RAs) and proton pump inhibitors (PPIs) have shown benefit. Endoscopic and surgical options for severe cases include fundoplication, magnetic sphincter augmentation (MSA), Roux-en-Y gastric bypass (RNYGB), and transoral incisionless fundoplication (TIF) [9]. Obesity plays a major role in the development of GERD symptoms and progression to BE and EAC. While the recent advent of glucagon-like peptide 1 (GLP1) receptor agonists may help with obesity, they have been noted to increase GERD given delayed gastric emptying [10]. Similarly, sleeve gastrectomy increases esophageal acid exposure; therefore, RNYGB may be the preferred weight loss surgery for patients with severe GERD, esophagitis, or Barrett's esophagus [11].

While many interventions exist for the prevention of EAC, the same is not true for SCE. The primary aim for prevention of SCE involves the cessation of tobacco and alcohol use as the risk of developing SCE increases up to sevenfold in tobacco users and up to fivefold in alcohol drinkers [12, 13]. Other modifiable risk factors include the consumption of hot liquids and diet. Studies have shown that a diet rich in fruits and vegetables may also decrease the risk of development of SCE [14]. While no studies exist to date, the HPV vaccine may provide some benefit in reducing the risk of development of SCE.

In the United States, robust endoscopic screening and surveillance programs currently exist for BE as highlighted by guidelines from major societies such as the American College of Gastroenterology (ACG) and American Society for Gastrointestinal Endoscopy (ASGE) [15, 16]. These guidelines help to stratify which patients are at high risk for BE and would qualify for endoscopic screening programs. Surveillance intervals for BE depend on the length of BE, presence of low-grade dysplasia (LGD), high-grade dysplasia (HGD), or EAC. Recent advances in endoscopic therapies including radiofrequency ablation (RFA), cryoablation, endoscopic mucosal resection (EMR), and endoscopic submucosal dissection (ESD) have played a significant role in the prevention of progression of BE into EAC [17–19]. While BE represents the precursor lesion for EAC, esophageal squamous dysplasia is the precursor lesion for SCE. Unlike with EAC, screening programs for SCE are scarce. Some studies have shown that screening for SCE in high-risk populations may be cost-effective [20]; however, robust screening programs do not currently exist in the United States.

Diagnosis

The diagnosis of esophageal cancer is typically made through biopsies taken on upper endoscopic examination either performed for screening purposes or for diagnostic purposes given underlying symptoms. Unfortunately, symptoms are typically not seen in EC until the later stages of the disease. As a result, nearly 50% of patients diagnosed with EC in North America have cancer that extends beyond the locoregional confines of the tumor at the time of diagnosis [2]. Once the diagnosis is made, it is imperative to obtain accurate staging of the cancer which will assist with guiding treatment plans. Staging of both EAC and SCE involves initial upper endoscopy with biopsy, PET-CT scan, and in some cases endoscopic ultrasound (EUS). Accuracy is especially critical in early stages as some of these lesions may be endoscopically resectable, preventing the patient from a surgical procedure that carries a high morbidity [21]. Once the diagnosis is made, further testing of the tissue sample through immunohistochemistry (IHC), in situ hybridization (ISH), and polymerase chain reaction (PCR) can be performed. These additional tests can evaluate for biomarkers and genetic alterations such as HER2, microsatellite instability (MSI), mismatch repair (MMR), programmed cell death ligand 1 (PDL1), and TP53 mutations, among others. This information can help identify the most appropriate chemo/immunotherapeutic regimen for the patient [2]. Another diagnostic tool that has gained steam over the past few years is circulating tumor DNA (ctDNA). Assays that can detect ctDNA are now commonly used in practice; however, its utility in the diagnosis of EC remains to be seen. Recent studies show the value of ctDNA for diagnosis only in late stages of the disease. Nonetheless, it is being used effectively in a variety of malignancies, including EC, to monitor response to treatment [22]. One study involving 42 patients with SCE showed a significantly better overall survival for patients with lower ctDNA post initial cycle of chemotherapy [23].

Treatment

The treatment of EC depends on multiple factors including histologic subtype, stage of the disease, molecular profile of the tumor, as well as underlying patient comorbidities. For early-stage EAC and SCE, the most important distinction is the depth of invasion of the tumor. A T1a tumor indicates invasion into the mucosa, lamina propria, or muscularis mucosa, while T1b indicates invasion into the submucosa of the esophagus. Per the National Comprehensive Cancer Network (NCCN) Guidelines from 2024, for EAC, both T1a and T1b lesions strategies for esophageal cancer can be resected endoscopically. However, for SCE, endoscopic resection is only recommended for T1a lesions, given high risk of lymph node metastasis. The latest ASGE guidelines for ESD of the upper gastrointestinal tract, released in 2024, indicate curative resection for EAC if submucosal invasion does not exceed 500 μm (SM1). Whereas for SCE, invasion into the submucosa carries a high risk of lymph node metastasis, and endoscopic resection should only be considered in patients with less than 200 μm of submucosal invasion [24].

For EAC staged T1b to T2N0 and considered a low-risk lesion (<3 cm and well differentiated), the recommendation is for esophagectomy in surgically fit patients. Treatment strategies for EAC staged higher than T2N0 (low-risk) include pre- or perioperative chemotherapy +/− radiation followed by esophagectomy or neoadjuvant or perioperative immune checkpoint inhibitor if the tumor is MSI-high or MMR deficient. Stage T4b indicates invasion into adjacent structures such as aorta, airway, or vertebral body, and these tumors are only candidates for definitive chemotherapy +/− radiation.

For SCE staged T1bN0 to T2N0 and considered a low-risk lesion (<3 cm and well differentiated), the recommendation is for esophagectomy in surgically fit patients. Treatment for SCE staged higher than T2N0 (low risk) includes preoperative chemoradiation or definitive chemoradiation. Definitive chemoradiation or chemotherapy alone remains the mainstay of treatment for T4b disease (invasion into adjacent structures such as aorta, airway, or vertebral body).

Finally, a few treatment options are available for palliation in patients with advanced disease. These include esophageal stenting, placement of gastrostomy or jejunostomy tube for nutrition, external beam radiation therapy, and brachytherapy [25].

Future Research

The aim of future research in EC targets prevention and early diagnosis through effective screening programs as well as improvements in molecular profiling of the tumor and resection. For EAC, prevention is targeted at reduction of esophageal acid exposure and avoidance of risk factors such as tobacco. While H2RAs and PPIs have remained the mainstay of therapy for GERD for many years, the recent introduction of potassium competitive acid blockers (PCABs) as an effective medication for GERD and erosive esophagitis may play a role in the prevention of BE and thus progression into EAC. One prospective RCT in 2023 involving 1024 patients comparing vonoprazan, a PCAB, to lansoprazole, a proton pump inhibitor (PPI) showed that vonoprazan was noninferior to PPI in healing and superior to PPI in maintenance of healing of erosive esophagitis [26]. The increasing use of ctDNA can potentially provide insights into the molecular profile of a tumor, allowing for the use of more targeted systemic therapies and clinical prognostication [22]. One cohort study involving 1630 patients showed that postoperative ctDNA was significantly associated with inferior disease-free survival [27].

Nimotuzumab is a monoclonal antibody that targets the epidermal growth factor receptor (EGFR) pathway. One RCT (107 patients) in treatment naïve patients with unresectable EC compared chemoradiation alone to chemoradiation plus Nimotuzumab. Median survival for the Nimotuzumab arm was 15.9 months compared to 11.5 for the control [28]. Anti-PD1 antibodies such as pembrolizumab and camrelizumab have also shown some promise in the treatment of EC. The KEYNOTE-590, a randomized, placebo-controlled, double-blind study involving 749 patients with advanced EC and Siewert 1 gastroesophageal junction cancer compared pembrolizumab plus chemotherapy to chemotherapy alone in treatment naïve patients. On 5-year follow-up, the median overall survival was 12.3 months for pembrolizumab plus chemotherapy and 9.8 months for control (HR 0.72 [95% CI 0.62–0.84]) with 5-year overall survival rates of 10.6% and 3.0%, respectively [29]. The ESCORT-1st study, a multicenter, randomized, double-blind, placebo-controlled trial (596 patients) compared camrelizumab plus chemotherapy vs. placebo plus chemotherapy as a first-line treatment in advanced or metastatic esophageal squamous cell carcinoma. Overall survival for the camrelizumab group was 15.3 months (95% CI, 12.8–17.3; 135 deaths) vs. 12.0 months (95% CI, 11.0–13.3; 174 deaths) for the control (hazard ratio [HR] for death, 0.70 [95% CI, 0.56–0.88]) [30].

In addition to pharmacotherapy, minimally invasive procedures for the treatment of early stage EAC and SCE such as EMR and ESD are becoming more widely accepted and performed. These procedures have the potential to provide patients with an organ sparing, curative resection. Advances in endoscopic therapy along with the implementation of artificial intelligence (AI) in endoscopy and surgery may also help assist in both the prevention and management of EC.

Stomach

Introduction

The most common gastric tumors include adenocarcinoma, subepithelial lesions (SELs), neuroendocrine tumors (NETs), and lymphoma. Gastric adenocarcinoma (GAC) accounts for approximately 95% of gastric malignancies. GAC is the fifth most common cancer worldwide and the third leading cause of cancer mortality worldwide [31]. GAC is further classified depending on location (proximal or distal) as well as histologic subtype (diffuse or intestinal). The 5-year survival rate for GAC remains low in the United States despite a decline in the intestinal subtype of GAC over the past few decades; this may partly be due to the increasing incidence of the diffuse subtype in addition to most cases being diagnosed in later stages [32]. GAC presents such a significant challenge to the healthcare system in Eastern countries such as Japan, South Korea, and China that these countries have developed a robust population wide screening program [32]. Major risk factors contributing to the epidemiology of GAC include diet, tobacco use, and *H. pylori* infection. Gastric lymphoma, SELs, and NETs are much less commonly seen and oftentimes are diagnosed incidentally at the time of upper endoscopy performed for another indication. Most of these tumors are slow to progress and typically carry a much better prognosis than GAC.

Prevention/Screening

Helicobacter pylori was designated a class I carcinogen by the World Health Organization (WHO) International Agency for Research on Cancer (IARC) in 1994. The decision was made in part due to epidemiologic data from Japan given high rates of GAC [33]. It is now known that infection with *H. pylori* can carry a two- to sixfold risk of developing GAC and an approximately twofold risk of developing gastric mucosa-associated lymphoid tissue (MALT) lymphoma [34, 35]. Prevention of GAC and MALT lymphoma through *H. pylori* eradication is well studied and highly effective, particularly in high-risk countries such as Japan [36]. Dietary modification such as increased fruit/vegetable intake and decreased salt intake along with tobacco and alcohol cessation also has been shown to reduce the risk of gastric cancer [37]. Finally, for patients with pathogenic CDH1 mutation, which is associated with hereditary diffuse gastric cancer (HDGC), prophylactic gastrectomy can prevent the development of GAC.

Screening for GAC in the absence of a pathogenic mutation is currently not recommended in the United States. Routine screening for gastric NETs, SELs, and lymphoma is also not recommended. However, in countries with high incidence of GAC such as Japan, screening programs have been present for over a decade [38]. Screening programs for *H. pylori* infection have also existed for over a decade in Japan [39].

Diagnosis

The diagnosis of gastric malignancies is dependent on the type of lesion. GAC, Gastric NETs, and lymphoma can typically be diagnosed via upper endoscopy with biopsies. For gastric NETs, serum chromogranin A and fasting gastrin levels can help aid with diagnosis. Elevated fasting serum gastrin levels are seen in Type I and II gastric NETs. Type III gastric NET typically has normal fasting gastrin levels. Type I gastric NET has an association with atrophic gastritis, and Type II gastric NET has an association with Zollinger-Ellison syndrome. Chromogranin A is typically elevated in all three types of gastric NETs [40]. The diagnosis of gastric SELs can typically be obtained via EUS-guided fine needle aspiration or biopsy. Immunohistochemistry can help differentiate the different types of SELs. For instance, gastrointestinal stromal tumors (GISTs) stain positive for CD117 and DOG1, whereas Leiomyomas stain positive for desmin and smooth muscle actin [41]. Once a diagnosis is made, EUS, PET-CT, and, in certain indications, laparoscopy can be performed for staging purposes.

Treatment

Treatment for gastric malignancy depends on the histologic subtype, staging, and patient comorbidities. The treatment of GAC can range from endoscopic resection to palliative chemoradiation. Techniques for endoscopic resection include EMR, ESD, and endoscopic full-thickness resection (EFTR). Lesions staged T1b and lower may be amenable to endoscopic resection if the tumor involves less than 500 μm of the submucosa [24]. The treatment for tumors staged higher than T1b ranges from surgical resection to preoperative chemoradiation or immunotherapy to chemoradiation if not fit for surgery. Systemic therapy or chemoradiation may be used in the case of metastatic disease. For GISTs, surgical/endoscopic resection is recommended if any of the following are present: symptomatic, size >2 cm, presence of high-risk features (irregular borders, cystic features, echogenic foci, ulceration, heterogenous appearance and tumor progression) [42, 43]. Tyrosine kinase inhibitors are used for unresectable or metastatic GISTs [44]. Management of gastric NETs is dependent on tumor grade and stage, ranging from endoscopic resection to systemic therapies, including somatostatin analogs, everolimus, and peptide receptor radionucleotide therapy (PRRT). Approximately 80% of cases of MALT lymphoma achieve remission with successful eradication of *H. pylori* [45]. In refractory cases, radiation therapy or rituximab can be used [46, 47].

Future Research

The focus of future research in the field of gastric malignancies relies on improving techniques for diagnosis and identifying targets for directed therapies. As with other malignancies, the utility of ctDNA is being investigated in gastric cancer. Additionally, targets for therapy thorough molecular genetics, such as PD-1, HER2, MSI, fibroblast growth factor receptor (FGFR), and chimeric antigen receptor (CAR)-T cells, are currently being investigated [48].

The standard of care for gastric adenocarcinoma has shifted to a standard of perioperative chemotherapy. A landmark RCT study (716 patients) compared perioperative FLOT (fluorouracil, leucovorin, oxaliplatin, and docetaxel) to the standard ECF/ECX regimen (epirubicin, cisplatin, and fluorouracil/capecitabine) for gastric cancer patients with cT2 or higher and nodal positive disease. Overall survival was increased in the FLOT group compared with the ECF/ECX group (hazard ratio [HR] 0.77; 95% CI; [0.63–0.94]). Median survival was 50 months vs. 35 months [49]. Another recent open label, RCT involving 187 patients comparing trastuzumab deruxtecan (anti-HER2 antibody) to physician's choice for HER2+ gastric adenocarcinoma, showed significantly improved median OS with trastuzumab deruxtecan (12.5 months vs. 8.4 months; HR: 0.59, 95% CI: 0.39–0.88) [50]. A multicenter, double-blind, placebo-controlled, randomized trial involving 2409 patients comparing pembrolizumab (anti-PD-1) plus chemotherapy to placebo plus chemotherapy showed longer overall survival in pembrolizumab group (12.9 months [95% CI 11.9–14.0] vs. 11.5 months [10.6–12.1]) [51].

AI will be key in improving outcomes for gastric cancer and may soon be utilized in endoscopy, pathology, and radiology to augment diagnostic accuracy [52]. One study comparing a deep learning approach using convolutional neuronal networks (CNNs) to endoscopists at diagnostic accuracy of atrophic gastritis (a gastric premalignant condition) revealed a 93% diagnostic accuracy of the deep learning approach, which was significantly higher than the accuracy of the endoscopists [53]. In endoscopy, technology to improve visualization through texture and color enhancement imaging (TXI), narrow-band imaging (NBI), and near focus/zoom magnification may also help improve diagnostic accuracy of gastric lesions. One trial involving 6 endoscopists comparing TXI to standard white light for 52 known gastric cancer lesions revealed significantly improved visibility scale for TXI mode compared to standard white light [54]. Finally, more widespread use of minimally invasive methods such as ESD can provide a curative resection through an organ-sparing technique for early-stage lesions [24].

Small Intestine

Introduction

The small intestine malignancy is quite rare, only accounting for approximately 3% of primary gastrointestinal tract malignancies [55]. The four common subtypes of small intestinal malignancies include adenocarcinoma, NET, lymphoma, and sarcoma. Diagnosis of small intestinal malignancy remains difficult as most cases do not present with symptoms until later stages. Given this, the 5-year survival rate of small intestinal malignancy remains low. Additionally, the incidence of small intestinal malignancies appears to be on the rise [56]. Of the four most common small intestinal malignancies, adenocarcinoma carries the worst prognosis. Risk factors for the development of small intestinal malignancies include tobacco and alcohol consumption, obesity, diabetes mellitus (DM), and red meat intake. Crohn's disease, celiac disease, and some hereditary cancer syndromes also increase the risk for small intestinal malignancy [56]. Improving outcomes in small intestinal malignancies remains difficult due to the rarity of the disease.

Prevention/Screening

Prevention of small intestinal malignancies remains a challenge; however, some strategies do currently exist. Modifiable risk factors such as tobacco and alcohol consumption and dietary modification can be effective in preventing many types of malignancies including in the small intestine. Reduction of small intestinal inflammation in conditions such as Crohn's disease and celiac disease can also decrease the development of small intestinal malignancy. Many therapeutic options are now available for Crohn's disease, and research is ongoing for medications to treat celiac disease [57, 58]. For now, avoidance of gluten remains the mainstay of treatment and is highly effective in most patients with celiac disease.

Due to the low incidence of small intestinal malignancies, screening is currently not recommended for the general population. Screening programs for the development of small intestinal adenocarcinoma do exist for patients with certain hereditary cancer syndromes such as Lynch syndrome, familial adenomatous polyposis (FAP) syndrome, and Peutz-Jeghers syndrome (PJS). Screening methods may include endoscopy, capsule endoscopy, and/or small intestinal imaging such as CT or MR enterography [59, 60]. Currently, there are no screening recommendations for small intestinal NETs, lymphomas, or sarcomas.

Diagnosis

Diagnosis of small intestinal malignancies generally involves endoscopic evaluation with targeted biopsies and histopathologic examination. Small intestinal lesions that involve areas distal to the duodenum may require deep enteroscopy techniques (single or double balloon). In some cases, due to difficulty in accessing the lesion via endoscopy, surgical or interventional radiology techniques may be required for sampling tissue. Once tissue is obtained, the molecular and genetic profile of the tumor can be assessed to help target treatment options. PET-CT scan is commonly used for staging purposes after initial diagnosis. For NETs, 68Ga-DOTATATE PET/CT scan has recently become the primary imaging modality for diagnosis and staging due to superior sensitivity and specificity compared to 111In-octreotide scintigraphy (Octreoscan) [61].

Treatment

For small intestinal adenocarcinoma, the treatment depends on the location of the tumor, ampullary involvement, staging, and patient comorbidities. Management after staging either involves observation or chemotherapy. If the lesion is unresectable or metastatic, immunotherapy can be considered if MSI high or MMR deficient. For ampullary adenocarcinoma, the treatment for localized disease is pancreaticoduodenectomy and for advanced stages either systemic chemotherapy, chemoradiation, or palliative radiation therapy [62, 63].

For NETs, treatment depends on the stage of disease. Localized disease is typically managed with surgical resection. Somatostatin analogues are the mainstay of treatment for metastatic NETs. Advanced and unresectable disease may also be treated with PRRT. PRRT involves combining a radionucleotide with a somatostatin analogue to allow for targeted treatment at the site of tumor [64]. Other options for advanced stage NETs may include everolimus and sunitinib [65].

Multiple subtypes of lymphoma can present in the small intestine and treatment varies depending on the histology. The most common histology of small intestinal lymphoma is diffuse large B-cell lymphoma (DLBCL) and MALT lymphoma. Management of small intestinal MALT lymphoma, similar to gastric MALT lymphoma, centers around the treatment and eradication of *H. pylori* infection. Refractory cases can be treated with chemotherapy and radiation. The mainstay of treatment for DLBCL is R-CHOP (rituximab, cyclophosphamide, doxorubicin, vincristine, and prednisone) [66].

The treatment of small intestinal sarcomas primarily involves surgical resection of the lesion. In advanced cases, treatment typically involves a tyrosine-kinase inhibitor (TKI) such as imatinib or sunitinib. While TKIs have shown benefit in GISTs, the same is not true with leiomyosarcomas, where surgical resection is the primary treatment [42, 67].

Future Research

Future direction in the diagnosis and management of small intestinal malignancies is focused on improvements in diagnostic imaging modalities and outcomes through targeted therapies. Diagnosis of small bowel tumors, particularly subepithelial lesions remains challenging. Recent advances in AI may potentially improve diagnostic accuracy of capsule endoscopy thorough the use of a CNN [68]. One study trained a CNN model using 158,235 images of the small bowel on capsule endoscopy. After training, the CNN algorithm was at least 99.8% sensitive at detecting abnormal capsule endoscopy findings on a series of 113,426,569 images compared to approximately 75% sensitivity for gastroenterologists [69]. As described previously, advances in imaging, specifically the 68Ga-DOTATATE PET/CT scan, have been a game changer in the diagnosis and staging of NETs [61]. Another recent study noted positive results with the use of AI and deep learning for the diagnosis of small intestinal carcinoid tumors using CT scans. The deep learning method achieved an area under the curve of 0.86, sensitivity of 78% and specificity of 82% using a series of 33 patients with surgically proven small bowel carcinoid tumors [70].

Small intestinal adenocarcinoma is a rare malignancy; thus, clinical trials for management are limited. Nonetheless, molecular profiling for mutations in ERBB2, BRCA1/2, and C-KIT may help target specific chemotherapeutic regimens. Tumors that have high MSI and tumor mutational burden may also be good candidates for immunotherapy [71]. The Zebra trial, a multicenter RCT (40 patients) evaluated the response of pembrolizumab for patients with previously treated small intestinal adenocarcinoma. The results showed that the median OS was higher (28.5 months) in patients with MSI-H status compared to patients with MSS/MSI-l status (17.5 months) [72]. For small intestinal DLBCL, new therapies are being studied including CAR-T therapy, immunotherapy, and polatuzumab vedotin [66, 73].

Colon

Introduction

Colorectal cancer (CRC) is the third most common cancer among both men and women and ranks second in overall mortality among all cancers. Given increasing usage of screening modalities over the past few decades, the incidence of CRC in adults >55 years of age has steadily declined. However, mortality from CRC in adults <55 years of age has increased by approximately 1% per year [74]. In light of these findings, the American Cancer Society (ACS) decreased the age to initiate CRC screening in average risk individuals to 45 in 2018. The United States Preventative Services Task Force (USPSTF) followed suit in 2021.

Risk factors for the development of CRC include tobacco and alcohol use, consumption of red meat/processed foods, obesity and physical inactivity, diabetes mellitus, personal history of inflammatory bowel disease (IBD), family history of CRC, and certain genetic mutations [75, 76]. Five-year survival for CRC ranges from approximately 90% for localized disease to as low as 12% for distant disease [77]. Significant strides in CRC screening and treatment have been made over the past few decades. Further research hopes to aim at the continued improvement in prevention, diagnosis, and survival of CRC.

Prevention/Screening

The most important strategy for the prevention of colorectal cancer involves the reduction of modifiable risk factors including tobacco/alcohol use, diet, obesity, and sedentary lifestyle. A recent systematic review and meta-analysis of 188 studies found a relative risk of CRC of 1.14 (95% CI 1.10–1.18) for current smokers and also showed that quitting smoking reduced the risk of CRC [78]. Another recent cohort study found that alcohol consumption increased the risk of CRC with an odds ratio (OR) of 1.79 (95% CI: 1.23–2.61) [79]. Obesity plays a major role in many different cancers, including CRC. One study from the using Mendelian randomization of a CRC consortium found that obesity was associated with an increased risk of CRC in men OR 1.23 (95% CI: 1.08–1.38) and a higher waist to hip ratio was associated with CRC in women OR 1.25 (95% CI: 1.08–1.43). Physical activity has also been shown to significantly reduce the risk of CRC [80]. Aspirin use has also been shown to have a chemoprotective effect with regard to the development of CRC [81, 82].

Screening for CRC has become an incredibly important component of routine health maintenance for patients in the United States. Screening began as a stool test over 60 years ago, but the major change in the landscape of CRC screening came in the late 1990s and early 2000s. The passing of the Balanced Budget Act in 1997 allowed for Medicare coverage for colonoscopy as a screening modality in 2001 [83]. Current approved tests for CRC screening include fecal occult blood testing (FOBT), fecal immunochemical testing (FIT), stool and blood DNA tests, sigmoidoscopy, colonoscopy, and CT colonography. Guidelines now recommend initiation of screening at the age of 45 for all average risk individuals with earlier screening for higher-risk individuals [84]. In 2024, the Food and Drug Administration (FDA) approved a blood test that measures cell-free DNA (cfDNA) for the screening of CRC in average-risk individuals. The approval was largely due to a prospective, observational, multicenter study involving more than 10,000 individuals that showed an 83% sensitivity of cfDNA for the detection of colorectal cancer and 90% specificity for advanced neoplasia [85].

Diagnosis

The diagnosis of CRC predominantly relies on colonoscopy with biopsies and histopathologic analysis. Once the diagnosis is made, staging can be obtained through CT, MRI, EUS, and PET scans. MRI and EUS are more commonly used for the staging of rectal cancer. Carcinoembryonic antigen (CEA) is a serum blood test that is commonly used in CRC, although elevation alone is not enough for a diagnosis of CRC. CEA is often used to assess treatment response [86]. Once the diagnosis of CRC is confirmed, molecular testing for markers such as BRAF, KRAS, NRAS, as well as assessing for TMB, MSI, and MMR status can provide a roadmap for which therapeutic decisions [87, 88]. Circulating tumor DNA (ctDNA) is also helpful in assessing treatment response and can provide additional information for early-stage CRC with regard to the initiation of adjuvant chemotherapy [89].

Treatment

The treatment algorithm of CRC is quite complex and depends on the location (rectal vs. colon), type of lesion, staging, molecular profile of the tumor, as well as patient comorbidities. A malignant polyp is defined as a polyp that contains cancer that invades into the submucosa (pT1). Favorable histology for resected malignant polyp includes grade 1 or 2 histology, no lymphovascular invasion, negative resection margin >1 mm, and low tumor budding. For pedunculated polyps in the rectum that contain invasive cancer with favorable histology, pT1 lesions that are completely resected with negative margins can be observed.

Sessile lesions in the rectum staged pT1 with favorable histology may also be observed or can proceed with transanal excision or transabdominal resection after EUS or MRI. For T1 rectal cancer without metastasis, the current recommendation is either ESD or transanal local excision depending on local expertise. T2 lesions of the rectum should undergo transabdominal resection and, if confirmed pT2N0M0, can be observed. Upstaging on pathologic examination would require adjuvant chemotherapy +/− radiation. Rectal tumors that are MMR deficient or MSI high are candidates for immunotherapy [90].

For colon cancer (proximal to the rectum), management can range from observation (if R0 resection) to surgical resection +/− chemo or immunotherapy for advanced stages. Therapeutic options differ based on MMR and MSI status along with molecular profile and mutation status. Immunotherapy may be used in select cases with MMR-deficient and MSI high tumors as well as tumors with POLE/POLD1 mutations. Alleviation of obstructing lesions can be pursued through palliative stenting or ostomy creation [90].

Future Research

Research in colon cancer likely exceeds that of all other cancers of the gastrointestinal tract due to the tremendous impact the disease presents to public health. Research is aimed at improving screening and diagnostic methods to improve patient compliance, novel tumor molecular markers that can help individualize therapy, and the development of new drugs.

As previously mentioned, the FDA approved a "liquid biopsy" blood test that detects cfDNA for the screening of CRC in 2024. This was based on a large cohort study involving 10,258 patients who were average risk for colon cancer. The cfDNA test has a 83% sensitivity for colon cancer and 90% specificity for advanced neoplasia [85]. Research into blood tests for circulating tumor cells (CTCs), ctDNA, and tumor-educated platelets (TEPs) for CRC screening and diagnosis is currently being conducted and may begin to become more widely accepted [85]. One prospective RCT (455 patients) involving the use of ctDNA to guide adjuvant chemotherapy for stage II CRC showed decreased utilization of chemotherapy with ctDNA guidance with no significant difference of 2-year recurrence-free survival [89].

Molecular biomarkers play a large role in the selection of chemo/immunotherapy. Medications such as cetuximab and panitumumab are examples of the expanding role of personalized medicine through identifiable genetic mutations [91, 92]. Greater understanding of CRC tumor biology and genetics will further expand the armamentarium for the management of CRC. For rectal cancer, a recent paradigm shift toward total neoadjuvant therapy (TNT) for locally advanced mid/low rectal cancers has shown promise, particularly for organ preservation. The landmark PRODIGE-23 study, a multicenter, randomized open-label, phase III trial (461 patients) compared neoadjuvant chemotherapy vs. standard-of-care group for patients with T3-T4, nonmetastatic rectal cancer. At long-term follow-up of 82.2 months, the 7-year disease-free survival rates were 67.6% (95% CI, 61–74) in the neoadjuvant chemotherapy group and 62.5% (56–69) in the standard-of-care group [93, 94].

Computer-aided detection (CADe) devices are now on the market to assist with polyp detection during colonoscopy. One meta-analysis of 7 studies and over 5000 colonoscopies showed that CADe-assisted colonoscopies demonstrated an 80% increase in adenomas detected per patient as compared to conventional colonoscopy [95]. Improvement in CADe devices and AI in the coming years may help decrease rates of missed polyps and post colonoscopy colon cancer. A variety of image enhancement technologies are now also available in the latest versions of most commercially available endoscopes/colonoscopes. The most used include TXI, NBI, and near focus. This technology helps endoscopists more closely examine lesions to assess for covert signs of malignancy and deep submucosal invasion, assisting with stratification of resection strategies for polyps [96]. The future of polyp detection and classification will likely also involve deep learning through convolutional neural networks [97–99].

References

1. Kamangar F, Nasrollahzadeh D, Safiri S, Sepanlou S, Fitzmaurice C, et al. The global, regional, and national burden of oesophageal cancer and its attributable risk factors in 195 countries and territories, 1990–2017: a systematic analysis for the Global Burden of Disease Study 2017. Lancet Gastroenterol Hepatol. 2020;5(6):582–97. https://doi.org/10.1016/S2468-1253(20)30007-8.

2. Ajani JA, D'Amico TA, Bentrem DJ, Cooke D, Corvera C, et al. Esophageal and esophagogastric junction cancers, Version 2.2023, NCCN clinical practice guidelines in oncology. J Natl Compr Cancer Netw. 2023;21(4):393–422.
3. Morgan E, Soerjomataram I, Rumgay H, Coleman HG, Thrift AP, et al. The global landscape of esophageal squamous cell carcinoma and esophageal adenocarcinoma incidence and mortality in 2020 and projections to 2040: new estimates from GLOBOCAN 2020. Gastroenterology. 2022;163(3):649–58.e2.
4. Huang FL, Yu SJ. Esophageal cancer: risk factors, genetic association, and treatment. Asian J Surg. 2018;41(3):210–5. https://doi.org/10.1016/j.asjsur.2016.10.005.
5. Tarazi M, Chidambaram S, Markar SR. Risk factors of esophageal squamous cell carcinoma beyond alcohol and smoking. Cancers (Basel). 2021;13(5):1009.
6. Liu CQ, Ma YL, Qin Q, Wang PH, Luo Y, Xu PF, Cui Y. Epidemiology of esophageal cancer in 2020 and projections to 2030 and 2040. Thorac Cancer. 2023;14(1):3–11.
7. Caspa Gokulan R, Garcia-Buitrago MT, Zaika AI. From genetics to signaling pathways: molecular pathogenesis of esophageal adenocarcinoma. Biochim Biophys Acta Rev Cancer. 2019;1872(1):37–48.
8. An L, Zheng R, Zeng H, Zhang S, Chen R, Wang S, Sun K, Li L, Wei W, He J. The survival of esophageal cancer by subtype in China with comparison to the United States. Int J Cancer. 2023;152(2):151–61.
9. Katz PO, Dunbar KB, Schnoll-Sussman FH, Greer KB, Yadlapati R, Spechler SJ. ACG clinical guideline for the diagnosis and management of gastroesophageal reflux disease. Am J Gastroenterol. 2022;117(1):27–56.
10. Liu BD, Udemba SC, Liang K, Tarabichi Y, Hill H, Fass R, Song G. Shorter-acting glucagon-like peptide-1 receptor agonists are associated with increased development of gastro-oesophageal reflux disease and its complications in patients with type 2 diabetes mellitus: a population-level retrospective matched cohort study. Gut. 2024;73(2):246–54.
11. DuPree CE, Blair K, Steele SR, Martin MJ. Laparoscopic sleeve gastrectomy in patients with preexisting gastroesophageal reflux disease: a national analysis. JAMA Surg. 2014;149(4):328–34.
12. Yang CS, Chen X, Tu S. Etiology and prevention of esophageal cancer. Gastrointest Tumors. 2016;3(1):3–16.
13. Freedman ND, Abnet CC, Leitzmann MF, Mouw T, Subar AF, Hollenbeck AR, Schatzkin A. A prospective study of tobacco, alcohol, and the risk of esophageal and gastric cancer subtypes. Am J Epidemiol. 2007;165(12):1424–33.
14. Castro C, Peleteiro B, Lunet N. Modifiable factors and esophageal cancer: a systematic review of published meta-analyses. J Gastroenterol. 2018;53(1):37–51.
15. Qumseya B, Sultan S, Bain P, Jamil L, Jacobson B, Anandasabapathy S, et al. ASGE guideline on screening and surveillance of Barrett's esophagus. Gastrointest Endosc. 2019;90(3):335–59.e2.
16. Shaheen NJ, Falk GW, Iyer PG, Souza RF, Yadlapati RH, Sauer BG, Wani S. Diagnosis and management of Barrett's esophagus: an updated ACG guideline. Am J Gastroenterol. 2022;117(4):559–87.
17. Schembre DB, Huang JL, Lin OS, Cantone N, Low DE. Treatment of Barrett's esophagus with early neoplasia: a comparison of endoscopic therapy and esophagectomy. Gastrointest Endosc. 2008;67(4):595–601.
18. Zehetner J, DeMeester SR, Hagen JA, Ayazi S, Augustin F, Lipham JC, DeMeester TR. Endoscopic resection and ablation versus esophagectomy for high-grade dysplasia and intramucosal adenocarcinoma. J Thorac Cardiovasc Surg. 2011;141(1):39–47.
19. Rubenstein JH, Sawas T, Wani S, Eluri S, Singh S, Chandar AK, et al. AGA clinical practice guideline on endoscopic eradication therapy of Barrett's esophagus and related neoplasia. Gastroenterology. 2024;166(6):1020–55.
20. Yang J, Wei WQ, Niu J, Liu ZC, Yang CX, Qiao YL. Cost-benefit analysis of esophageal cancer endoscopic screening in high-risk areas of China. World J Gastroenterol. 2012;18(20):2493–501.
21. Low DE, Kuppusamy MK, Alderson D, Cecconello I, Chang AC, Darling G, et al. Benchmarking complications associated with esophagectomy. Ann Surg. 2019;269(2):291–8.
22. Min J, Zhou H, Jiang S, Yu H. A review of circulating tumor DNA in the diagnosis and monitoring of esophageal cancer. Med Sci Monit. 2022;28:e934106.
23. Fujisawa R, Iwaya T, Endo F, Idogawa M, Sasaki N, Hiraki H, et al. Early dynamics of circulating tumor DNA predict chemotherapy responses for patients with esophageal cancer. Carcinogenesis. 2021;42(10):1239–49.
24. Al-Haddad MA, Elhanafi SE, Forbes N, Thosani NC, Draganov PV, Othman MO, et al. American Society for Gastrointestinal Endoscopy guideline on endoscopic submucosal dissection for the management of early esophageal and gastric cancers: methodology and review of evidence. Gastrointest Endosc. 2023;98(3):285–305.e38.
25. National Comprehensive Cancer Network. Esophageal and esophagogastric junction cancers. Version 3.2025. https://www.nccn.org/professionals/physician_gls/pdf/esophageal.pdf. Accessed 10 Mar 2025.
26. Laine L, DeVault K, Katz P, Mitev S, Lowe J, Hunt B, Spechler S. Vonoprazan versus lansoprazole for healing and maintenance of healing of erosive esophagitis: a randomized trial. Gastroenterology. 2023;164(1):61–71.
27. Maron SB, Chase LM, Lomnicki S, Kochanny S, Moore KL, Joshi SS, et al. Circulating tumor DNA sequencing analysis of gastroesophageal adenocarcinoma. Clin Cancer Res. 2019;25(23):7098–112.
28. de Castro Junior G, Segalla JG, de Azevedo SJ, Andrade CJ, Grabarz D, de Araújo Lima França B, Del Giglio A, et al. A randomised phase II study of chemoradiotherapy with or without nimotuzumab in locally advanced oesophageal cancer: NICE trial. Eur J Cancer. 2018;88:21–30.
29. Shah MA, Sun JM, Shen L, Kato K. First-line pembrolizumab (pembro) plus chemotherapy (chemo) for advanced esophageal cancer: 5-year outcomes from the phase 3 KEYNOTE-590 study. J Clin Oncol. 2024;42:250.
30. Luo H, Lu J, Bai Y, Mao T, Wang J, Fan Q, Zhang Y, Zhao K, et al. Effect of camrelizumab vs placebo added to chemotherapy on survival and progression-free survival in patients with advanced or metastatic esophageal squamous cell carcinoma: the ESCORT-1st randomized clinical trial. JAMA. 2021;326(10):916–25.
31. Ajani JA, D'Amico TA, Bentrem DJ, Chao J, Cooke D, Corvera C, Das P, et al. Gastric cancer, Version 2.2022, NCCN clinical practice guidelines in oncology. J Natl Compr Cancer Netw. 2022;20(2):167–92.
32. Sitarz R, Skierucha M, Mielko J, Offerhaus GJA, Maciejewski R, Polkowski WP. Gastric cancer: epidemiology, prevention, classification, and treatment. Cancer Manag Res. 2018;10:239–48.
33. Asaka M, Kudo M, Kato M, Sugiyama T, Takeda H. Review article: long-term helicobacter pylori infection—from gastritis to gastric cancer. Aliment Pharmacol Ther. 1998;12(Suppl 1):9–15.
34. Ishikura N, Usui Y, Ito H, Kasugai Y, Oze I, Kato S, Yatabe Y, Nakamura S, Matsuo K. Helicobacter pylori (HP) infection alone, but not HP-induced atrophic gastritis, increases the risk of gastric lymphoma: a case-control study in Japan. Ann Hematol. 2019;98(8):1981–7.
35. Crowe SE. Helicobacter pylori infection. N Engl J Med. 2019;380(12):1158–65.
36. Kowada A, Asaka M. Economic and health impacts of introducing helicobacter pylori eradication strategy into national gastric cancer policy in Japan: a cost-effectiveness analysis. Helicobacter. 2021;26(5):e12837.

37. Norwood DA, Montalvan-Sanchez E, Dominguez RL, Morgan DR. Gastric cancer: emerging trends in prevention, diagnosis, and treatment. Gastroenterol Clin N Am. 2022;51(3):501–18.
38. Mabe K, Inoue K, Kamada T, Kato K, Kato M, Haruma K. Endoscopic screening for gastric cancer in Japan: current status and future perspectives. Dig Endosc. 2022;34(3):412–9.
39. Asaka M, Kato M, Sakamoto N. Roadmap to eliminate gastric cancer with helicobacter pylori eradication and consecutive surveillance in Japan. J Gastroenterol. 2014;49(1):1–8.
40. Vinik AI, Woltering EA, Warner RR, Caplin M, O'Dorisio TM, Wiseman GA, Coppola D, Go VL, North American Neuroendocrine Tumor Society (NANETS). NANETS consensus guidelines for the diagnosis of neuroendocrine tumor. Pancreas. 2010;39(6):713–34.
41. Faulx AL, Kothari S, Acosta RD, Agrawal D, Bruining DH, Chandrasekhara V, et al. The role of endoscopy in subepithelial lesions of the GI tract. Gastrointest Endosc. 2017;85(6):1117–32.
42. Jacobson BC, Bhatt A, Greer KB, Lee LS, Park WG, Sauer BG, Shami VM. ACG clinical guideline: diagnosis and management of gastrointestinal subepithelial lesions. Am J Gastroenterol. 2023;118(1):46–58.
43. Sharzehi K, Sethi A, Savides T. AGA clinical practice update on management of subepithelial lesions encountered during routine endoscopy: expert review. Clin Gastroenterol Hepatol. 2022;20(11):2435–43.e4.
44. von Mehren M, Kane JM, Riedel RF, Sicklick JK, Pollack SM, Agulnik M, Bui MM, et al. NCCN Guidelines® insights: gastrointestinal stromal tumors, Version 2.2022. J Natl Compr Canc Netw. 2022;20(11):1204–14.
45. Evans JA, Chandrasekhara V, Chathadi KV, Decker GA, Early DS, Fisher DA, Foley K, et al. The role of endoscopy in the management of premalignant and malignant conditions of the stomach. Gastrointest Endosc. 2015;82(1):1–8.
46. Matysiak-Budnik T, Priadko K, Bossard C, Chapelle N, Ruskoné-Fourmestraux A. Clinical management of patients with gastric MALT lymphoma: a gastroenterologist's point of view. Cancers (Basel). 2023;15(15):3811.
47. Kiesewetter B, Ferreri AJ, Raderer M. Chemoimmunotherapy for mucosa-associated lymphoid tissue-type lymphoma: a review of the literature. Oncologist. 2015;20(8):915–25.
48. Ratti M, Orlandi E, Toscani I, Vecchia S, Anselmi E, Hahne JC, Ghidini M, Citterio C. Emerging therapeutic targets and future directions in advanced gastric cancer: a comprehensive review. Cancers (Basel). 2024;16(15):2692.
49. Al-Batran SE, Homann N, Pauligk C, Goetze TO, Meiler J, Kasper S, Kopp HG, et al. Perioperative chemotherapy with fluorouracil plus leucovorin, oxaliplatin, and docetaxel versus fluorouracil or capecitabine plus cisplatin and epirubicin for locally advanced, resectable gastric or gastro-oesophageal junction adenocarcinoma (FLOT4): a randomised, phase 2/3 trial. Lancet. 2019;393(10184):1948–57.
50. Shitara K, Bang YJ, Iwasa S, Sugimoto N, Ryu MH, Sakai D, Chung HC, et al. Trastuzumab deruxtecan in previously treated HER2-positive gastric cancer. N Engl J Med. 2020;382(25):2419–30.
51. Rha SY, Oh DY, Yañez P, Bai Y, Ryu MH, Lee J, Rivera F, Alves GV, et al. Pembrolizumab plus chemotherapy versus placebo plus chemotherapy for HER2-negative advanced gastric cancer (KEYNOTE-859): a multicentre, randomised, double-blind, phase 3 trial. Lancet Oncol. 2023;24(11):1181–95.
52. Niu PH, Zhao LL, Wu HL, Zhao DB, Chen YT. Artificial intelligence in gastric cancer: application and future perspectives. World J Gastroenterol. 2020;26(36):5408–19.
53. Guimarães P, Keller A, Fehlmann T, Lammert F, Casper M. Deep-learning based detection of gastric precancerous conditions. Gut. 2020;69(1):4–6.
54. Futakuchi T, Dobashi A, Horiuchi H, Furuhashi H, Matsui H, Hara Y, et al. Texture and color enhancement imaging improves the visibility of gastric neoplasms: clinical trial with image catalogue assessment using conventional and newly developed endoscopes. BMC Gastroenterol. 2023;23(1):389.
55. Siegel RL, Miller KD, Jemal A. Cancer statistics, 2020. CA Cancer J Clin. 2020;70(1):7–30.
56. Huang J, Chan SC, Fung YC, Mak FY, Lok V, Zhang L, et al. Incidence, risk factors, and temporal trends of small intestinal cancer: a global analysis of cancer registries. Gastroenterology. 2023;165(3):600–12.
57. Cockburn E, Kamal S, Chan A, Rao V, Liu T, Huang JY, Segal JP. Crohn's disease: an update. Clin Med (Lond). 2023;23(6):549–57.
58. Ghazanfar H, Javed N, Lee S, Shaban M, Cordero D, Acherjee T, et al. Novel therapies for celiac disease: a clinical review article. Cureus. 2023;15(5):e39004.
59. Giardiello FM, Allen JI, Axilbund JE, Boland CR, Burke CA, Burt RW, Church JM, et al. Guidelines on genetic evaluation and management of lynch syndrome: a consensus statement by the US Multi-Society Task Force on colorectal cancer. Gastroenterology. 2014;147(2):502–26.
60. Syngal S, Brand RE, Church JM, Giardiello FM, Hampel HL, Burt RW, American College of Gastroenterology. ACG clinical guideline: genetic testing and management of hereditary gastrointestinal cancer syndromes. Am J Gastroenterol. 2015;110(2):223–62.
61. Deppen SA, Liu E, Blume JD, Clanton J, Shi C, Jones-Jackson LB, Lakhani V, et al. Safety and efficacy of 68Ga-DOTATATE PET/CT for diagnosis, staging, and treatment management of neuroendocrine tumors. J Nucl Med. 2016;57(5):708–14.
62. National Comprehensive Cancer Network. Small bowel adenocarcinoma (Version 3.2025). https://www.nccn.org/professionals/physician_gls/pdf/small_bowel.pdf. Accessed 10 Mar 2025.
63. National Comprehensive Cancer Network. Ampullary adenocarcinoma (Version 2.2025). https://www.nccn.org/professionals/physician_gls/pdf/ampullary.pdf. Accessed 10 Mar 2025.
64. Merola E, Grana CM. Peptide receptor radionuclide therapy (PRRT): innovations and improvements. Cancers (Basel). 2023;15(11):2975.
65. Daskalakis K, Tsoli M, Angelousi A, Kassi E, Alexandraki KI, Kolomodi D, Kaltsas G, Koumarianou A. Anti-tumour activity of everolimus and sunitinib in neuroendocrine neoplasms. Endocr Connect. 2019;8(6):641–53.
66. Sehn LH, Salles G. Diffuse large B-cell lymphoma. N Engl J Med. 2021;384(9):842–58.
67. Shenoy S. Small bowel sarcoma: tumor biology and advances in therapeutics. Surg Oncol. 2015;24(3):136–44.
68. Kim SH, Lim YJ. Artificial intelligence in capsule endoscopy: a practical guide to its past and future challenges. Diagnostics (Basel). 2021;11(9):1722.
69. Ding Z, Shi H, Zhang H, Meng L, Fan M, Han C, Zhang K, Ming F, Xie X, Liu H, Liu J, Lin R, Hou X. Gastroenterologist-level identification of small-bowel diseases and normal variants by capsule endoscopy using a deep-learning model. Gastroenterology. 2019;157(4):1044–54.e5.
70. Shin SY, Shen TC, Wank SA, Summers RM. Fully-automated detection of small bowel carcinoid tumors in CT scans using deep learning. Med Phys. 2023;50(12):7865–78.
71. Schrock AB, Devoe CE, McWilliams R, Sun J, Aparicio T, Stephens PJ, Ross JS, Wilson R, Miller VA, Ali SM, Overman MJ. Genomic profiling of small-bowel adenocarcinoma. JAMA Oncol. 2017;3(11):1546–53.
72. Pedersen KS, Foster NR, Overman MJ, Boland PM, Kim SS, Arrambide KA, Jaszewski BL, Bekaii-Saab T, Graham RP, Welch J, Wilson RH, McWilliams RR. ZEBRA: a multicenter phase II study of pembrolizumab in patients with advanced small-bowel adenocarcinoma. Clin Cancer Res. 2021;27(13):3641–8.

73. Tilly H, Morschhauser F, Sehn LH, Friedberg JW, Trněný M, Sharman JP, Herbaux C, et al. Polatuzumab vedotin in previously untreated diffuse large B-cell lymphoma. N Engl J Med. 2022;386(4):351–63.
74. Siegel RL, Wagle NS, Cercek A, Smith RA, Jemal A. Colorectal cancer statistics, 2023. CA Cancer J Clin. 2023;73(3):233–54.
75. Lewandowska A, Rudzki G, Lewandowski T, Stryjkowska-Góra A, Rudzki S. Risk factors for the diagnosis of colorectal cancer. Cancer Control. 2022;29:10732748211056692.
76. Islami F, Goding Sauer A, Miller KD, Siegel RL, Fedewa SA, Jacobs EJ, McCullough ML, et al. Proportion and number of cancer cases and deaths attributable to potentially modifiable risk factors in the United States. CA Cancer J Clin. 2018;68(1):31–54.
77. Rawla P, Sunkara T, Barsouk A. Epidemiology of colorectal cancer: incidence, mortality, survival, and risk factors. Prz Gastroenterol. 2019;14(2):89–103.
78. Botteri E, Borroni E, Sloan EK, Bagnardi V, Bosetti C, Peveri G, Santucci C, Specchia C, van den Brandt P, Gallus S, Lugo A. Smoking and colorectal cancer risk, overall and by molecular subtypes: a meta-analysis. Am J Gastroenterol. 2020;115(12):1940–9.
79. Zhou X, Wang L, Xiao J, Sun J, Yu L, Zhang H, Meng X, et al. Alcohol consumption, DNA methylation and colorectal cancer risk: results from pooled cohort studies and Mendelian randomization analysis. Int J Cancer. 2022;151(1):83–94.
80. Roshandel G, Ghasemi-Kebria F, Malekzadeh R. Colorectal cancer: epidemiology, risk factors, and prevention. Cancers (Basel). 2024;16(8):1530.
81. Garcia-Albeniz X, Chan AT. Aspirin for the prevention of colorectal cancer. Best Pract Res Clin Gastroenterol. 2011;25(4–5):461–72.
82. Guo CG, Ma W, Drew DA, Cao Y, Nguyen LH, Joshi AD, Ng K, Ogino S, et al. Aspirin use and risk of colorectal cancer among older adults. JAMA Oncol. 2021;7(3):428–35.
83. Montminy EM, Karlitz JJ, Landreneau SW. Progress of colorectal cancer screening in United States: past achievements and future challenges. Prev Med. 2019;120:78–84.
84. Shaukat A, Kahi CJ, Burke CA, Rabeneck L, Sauer BG, Rex DK. ACG clinical guidelines: colorectal cancer screening 2021. Am J Gastroenterol. 2021;116(3):458–79.
85. Chung DC, Gray DM 2nd, Singh H, Issaka RB, Raymond VM, Eagle C, Hu S, Chudova DI, Talasaz A, Greenson JK, Sinicrope FA, Gupta S, Grady WM. A cell-free DNA blood-based test for colorectal cancer screening. N Engl J Med. 2024;390(11):973–83.
86. Duffy MJ. Carcinoembryonic antigen as a marker for colorectal cancer: is it clinically useful? Clin Chem. 2001;47(4):624–30.
87. Sepulveda AR, Hamilton SR, Allegra CJ, Grody W, Cushman-Vokoun AM, et al. Molecular biomarkers for the evaluation of colorectal cancer: guideline from the American Society for Clinical Pathology, College of American Pathologists, Association for Molecular Pathology, and American Society of Clinical Oncology. J Mol Diagn. 2017;19(2):187–225.
88. Bosch LJ, Carvalho B, Fijneman RJ, Jimenez CR, Pinedo HM, van Engeland M, Meijer GA. Molecular tests for colorectal cancer screening. Clin Colorectal Cancer. 2011;10(1):8–23.
89. Tie J, Cohen JD, Lahouel K, Lo SN, Wang Y, Kosmider S, Wong R, Shapiro J, Lee M, Harris S, Khattak A, Burge M, Harris M, Lynam J, Nott L, Day F, et al. Circulating tumor DNA analysis guiding adjuvant therapy in stage II colon cancer. N Engl J Med. 2022;386(24):2261–72.
90. Benson AB, Venook AP, Al-Hawary MM, Azad N, Chen YJ, Ciombor KK, et al. Rectal cancer, Version 2.2022, NCCN clinical practice guidelines in oncology. J Natl Compr Cancer Netw. 2022;20(10):1139–67.
91. Saoudi González N, Ros J, Baraibar I, Salvà F, Rodríguez-Castells M, Alcaraz A, García A, Tabernero J, Élez E. Cetuximab as a key partner in personalized targeted therapy for metastatic colorectal cancer. Cancers (Basel). 2024;16(2):412.
92. Kasi PM, Afable MG, Herting C, Lukanowski M, Jin Z. Anti-EGFR antibodies in the management of advanced colorectal cancer. Oncologist. 2023;28(12):1034–48.
93. Conroy T, Bosset JF, Etienne PL, Rio E, François É, Mesgouez-Nebout N, et al. Neoadjuvant chemotherapy with FOLFIRINOX and preoperative chemoradiotherapy for patients with locally advanced rectal cancer (UNICANCER-PRODIGE 23): a multicentre, randomised, open-label, phase 3 trial. Lancet Oncol. 2021;22(5):702–15.
94. Conroy T, Castan F, Etienne PL, Rio E, Mesgouez-Nebout N, Evesque L, et al. Total neoadjuvant therapy with mFOLFIRINOX versus preoperative chemoradiotherapy in patients with locally advanced rectal cancer: long-term results of the UNICANCER-PRODIGE 23 trial. Ann Oncol. 2024;35(10):873–81.
95. Sivananthan A, Nazarian S, Ayaru L, Patel K, Ashrafian H, Darzi A, Patel N. Does computer-aided diagnostic endoscopy improve the detection of commonly missed polyps? A meta-analysis. Clin Endosc. 2022;55(3):355–64.
96. Nagai M, Suzuki S, Minato Y, Ishibashi F, Mochida K, Ohata K, Morishita T. Detecting colorectal lesions with image-enhanced endoscopy: an updated review from clinical trials. Clin Endosc. 2023;56(5):553–62.
97. Zachariah R, Samarasena J, Luba D, Duh E, Dao T, Requa J, Ninh A, Karnes W. Prediction of polyp pathology using convolutional neural networks achieves "resect and discard" thresholds. Am J Gastroenterol. 2020;115(1):138–44.
98. Tanwar S, Vijayalakshmi S, Sabharwal M, Kaur M, AlZubi AA, Lee HN. Detection and classification of colorectal polyp using deep learning. Biomed Res Int. 2022;2022:2805607.
99. Ozawa T, Ishihara S, Fujishiro M, Kumagai Y, Shichijo S, Tada T. Automated endoscopic detection and classification of colorectal polyps using convolutional neural networks. Ther Adv Gastroenterol. 2020;13:1756284820910659.

Research on GI Cancer (Hepato-Pancreato-Biliary (HPB) Cancers)

19

Shane Zhang, Arnav Chavda, and Ji Fan

Introduction

Liver cancer is the sixth most common cancer in the world and the third most common cause of cancer death [1]. HCC is the most common form of liver cancer and also the most lethal liver tumor with only 18% 5-year survival rate [2]. By 2025, over 1 million individuals are estimated to be affected by liver cancer annually [3]. Although there is a decline in viral causes of HCC, other causes such as NASH are now one of the fastest-growing etiologies of developing HCC [4]. Regardless of the etiology, progression to cirrhosis is the strongest risk factor for developing HCC, and over 90% of HCC cases occur in the setting of chronic liver disease [3].

Pancreatic ductal adenocarcinoma (PDAC) has become the third most common cancer death in the USA [34]. PDAC is also an extremely deadly cancer with 5-year survival rates at only approximately 12% [34]. More concerningly, PDAC is projected to overtake colorectal cancer before 2040, moving only behind lung cancer as a leading cause of cancer-related mortality [34].

Similar to HCC and PDAC, cholangiocarcinoma is also an extremely deadly cancer as it is typically diagnosed at a late stage. Cholangiocarcinoma (CCA) is a rare cancer with an incidence of 1.26 per 100,000 people, and these patients typically die within 3–4 months if untreated [44].

This chapter aims to focus on diagnosing and advancements in treatment therapy for HPB, PDAC, and cholangiocarcinoma. Data on emerging technologies and treatments will also be discussed.

Prevention and Advancements in Imaging Tools to Diagnose HPB Malignancies

Hepatocellular Carcinoma Imaging

90% of HCC cases arise from liver cirrhosis, and those at high risk of developing HCC defined as greater than 1.5% per year could benefit from screening studies [1]. The most cost-effective method of screening is abdominal ultrasound, and other benefits of utilizing ultrasound include its wide availability and its well-tolerated [1]. Drawbacks of utilizing ultrasound include performing poorly in the early detection of HCC lesions, uneven quality, and interobserver variability [1]. CT and MRI can, however, be used to overcome the limitations of ultrasound in diagnosing HCC, and both have a higher sensitivity and specificity [1]. MRI has a sensitivity and specificity over 90% for HCC lesions greater than 2 cm in diameter [1]. Even though MRI has an excellent diagnostic capability, it isn't a first-line screening modality as there is restricted availability and isn't cost-effective, thus relegating MRI as a second-line HCC screening tool [1]. Another second-line imaging modality is using multiphase CT [1]. Even though its diagnostic accuracy is lower than that of extracellular contrast-enhanced MRI, it remains a viable alternative for HCC diagnosis because of its lower cost, faster imaging times, and lower technical complexity [1].

The original version of the chapter has been revised. A correction to this chapter can be found at https://doi.org/10.1007/978-3-032-19175-5_35

S. Zhang
University of South Florida, Morsani College of Medicine, Tampa, FL, USA

A. Chavda
University of South Florida, Tampa, FL, USA

J. Fan (✉)
University of South Florida, Morsani College of Medicine, Tampa, FL, USA

Moffitt Cancer Center, Tampa, FL, USA
e-mail: Ji.Fan@moffitt.org

J. Huang, H. S.L. Jim (eds.), *Cancer Research Guidance for Clinicians and Researchers*,
https://doi.org/10.1007/978-3-032-19175-5_19

Hepatocellular Carcinoma Biomarkers

Alpha-fetoprotein (AFP) is commonly used as a biomarker for the detection of HCC. Elevated AFP can be detected in 60–80% of HCCs when using 20 ng/mL plasma concentration as a pathological threshold for diagnosis [1, 2]. AFP measurements are conducted in conjunction with ultrasound imaging, and the two tests completed together have a higher sensitivity rate than only conducting ultrasound for any-stage HCC [1, 3]. It's important to note that AFP measurements aren't recommended as a solitary screening test for HCC due to limitations including a relatively inadequate sensitivity and specificity for surveillance, low positive predictive value, and inadequate diagnostic accuracy for early-stage HCC [1]. Another biomarker AFP-L3 has shown to have higher specificity for HCC than AFP and to have a superior diagnostic efficacy when combined with AFP measurements [1, 4]. In addition, AFP-L3 levels to be predictive of early HCC even in the absence of elevated AFP [1, 5]. AFP-L3 is currently approved by the Food and Drug Administration FDA for the assessment of liver cancer risk as a part of the GALAD score [1].

Pancreatic Ductal Adenocarcinoma Ultrasound

Multidetector-row contrast-enhanced CT of the abdominal cavity is recommended to diagnose patients with PDAC [6]. Multidetector-row CT has high sensitivity; however, the sensitivity decreases for lesions smaller than 1.5 cm [6]. The CT is also crucial in evaluation of the disease stage and prediction of tumor unresectability. This examination allows one to accurately determine the size of the tumor, its localization, infiltration of large vessels, involvement of lymph nodes, and presence of distant metastases [6, 7].

Endoscopic ultrasound (EUS) is one of the most accurate methods for the detection of pancreatic focal lesions [6, 8]. EUS is more sensitive than CT diagnosing PDAC, particularly for small lesions of diameter smaller than 2 cm. Endoscopic ultrasound is indicated in tumor staging, particularly in patients with an unclear result of a CT examination [6].

Pancreatic Ductal Adenocarcinoma Biomarker

CA19-9 antigen is a recognized PDAC marker and is the most common marker applied in PDAC diagnostics [6]. CA19-9 antigen does not appear to be useful in early diagnostics or PDAC screening as the antigen is typically not elevated in the early stages of PDAC [6]. However, it could be useful as a prognostic and predictive PDAC marker [6]. An increased serum level of CA19-9 serum indicates advanced malignancy, and its increased preoperative level is associated with worse postoperative prognosis [6]. The marker may be useful in the evaluation of treatment efficacy because a postoperative CA19-9 decrease and normalization after implementation of adjuvant therapy are associated with better prognosis [6, 9]. In addition, a postoperative level of CA19-9 < 90 U/ml was associated with a better response to gemcitabine adjuvant chemotherapy and higher median survival [6]. Lastly, according to ESMO guidelines, in patients with a high preoperative CA19-9 level, after the operation, this marker should be monitored every 3 months for 2 years, along with an abdominal CT scan every 6 months [6].

Cholangiocarcinoma Imaging

Computed tomography is considered the standard imaging modality for the characterization and staging of CCA [10]. Ancillary findings such as delayed enhancement, capsular retraction, vascular invasion, or satellite nodules are highly suggestive of iCCA [10]. In lesions smaller than 1 cm or in the presence of cirrhosis or atypical features, the characterization is challenging [10, 11].

Magnetic resonance imaging has a similar accuracy to CT for diagnosis and staging of CCA with the advantage of the use of hepato-specific contrast media, dedicated sequences to obtain MRI cholangiopancreatography (MRCP), and diffusion-weighted imaging (DWI) helpful for the differentiation between HCC and iCCA [10]. In addition, MRI is as accurate as CT to estimate resectability of pCCA (sensitivity 94%), since it can evaluate portal vein (sensitivity 79%) and bile ducts (accuracy 71%) involvement [10].

Advancements in Perioperative Therapy of HPB Cancers

Adjuvant Therapy for Clear Cell Hepatocellular Carcinoma

Patients who are eligible for surgical resection to treat HCC still have 50–70% of recurrence in 5 years [12, 13]. Previously, two phase 3 trials, STORM and PATRON, were conducted as adjuvant therapy post-resection or ablation [14]. The STORM trial randomly assigned 556 patients in sorafenib group and 558 patients in placebo group. Sorafenib group received the addition of 400 mg sorafenib twice daily as adjuvant HCC therapy. STORM trial found no difference in median recurrence-free survival between sorafenib and placebo [14, 15]. The PATRON trial randomized (1:1) a total of 520 HCC patients and compared the efficacy of muparfostat to placebo following surgical resection of HCC. Similarly, the PATRON trial found no significant difference in efficacy of disease-free survival [14, 16]. Currently, there are no adjuvant treatments that have been established for patients who are at high risk of HCC recurrence [14]. Recently, however, several phase 3 clinical trials are ongoing investigating immunotherapy as adjuvant therapy post curative intent resection or ablation, including IMbrave050, ESMERALD-2, CHECKMATE-9DX, and KEYNOTE 937 which show promise as adjuvant therapy [12, 14]. The IMbrave050 phase 3 trial enrolled 668 patients and investigated the efficacy of atezolizumab (anti-PDL1) plus bevacizumab versus active surveillance as adjuvant therapy in patients who are at high risk of HCC recurrence [14]. Treatment was 1200 mg intravenous atezolizumab plus intravenous bevacizumab 15 mg/kg every 3 weeks for up to 12 months or 17 cycles, whichever occurred first [14]. The primary endpoint was recurrence-free survival (RFS), and it was significantly improved in atezolizumab and bevacizumab treatment group compared to surveillance only [14]. The IMbrave050 trial is the first trial to show the benefit of HCC adjuvant therapy, and other trials investigating other immune checkpoint inhibitors are still ongoing [14]. These positive results have led to the development of atezolizumab and bevacizumab combination as the standard of care for adjuvant therapy in HCC [17].

Microvascular invasion (MVI) occurs in about 30–50% of HCC patients [17]. MVI is also a significant risk factor for early recurrence of HCC after surgical resection [17]. Because of this, there is interest in using adjuvant therapy in the MVI population to prevent HCC recurrence. A phase 3 multicenter trial involving 315 patients was conducted to investigate the safety and efficacy of postoperative adjuvant hepatic arterial infusion chemotherapy (HAIC) with FOLFOX (leucovorin, 5-FU, oxaliplatin) in HCC patients [17]. The research group found that postoperative adjuvant HAIC with FOLFOX significantly improved the DFS benefits with acceptable toxicities in HCC patients with MVI [17]. These results show that HAIC FOLFOX could eventually become the standard of care adjuvant therapy for HCC patients with MVI.

Adjuvant Therapy for Pancreatic Ductal Adenocarcinoma (PDAC)

Approximately 20% of patients diagnosed with PDAC have surgically resectable disease; unfortunately, most of those patients will develop recurrent disease [18]. In patients with metastatic cancer, FOLFIRINOX (fluorouracil, leucovorin, irinotecan, and oxaliplatin) leads to longer overall survival than gemcitabine therapy [19]. Investigators wanted to investigate if FOLFIRINOX would be efficacious as adjuvant PDAC therapy post-resection. A phase 3 multicenter randomized open-label trial was conducted with 493 patients who had resected PDAC that utilized FOLFIRINOX as adjuvant therapy compared to gemcitabine, and the primary endpoint was disease-free survival (DFS) [19]. DFS was significantly improved in FOLFIRINOX group compared to gemcitabine monotherapy [19]. DFS rates at 1 year, 2 years, and 3 years were 69.0%, 47%, and 39.7% in FOLFIRINOX group compared to 53.7%, 30.7%, and 21.4% in the gemcitabine group [19]. In addition, the median overall survival (54.4 months) and median metastasis-free survival (30.4 months) were significantly improved in FOLFIRIOX group than in the gemcitabine treatment group [19]. The positive results from this study have now made FOLFIRINOX first-line adjuvant therapy as the standard of care for PDAC [18].

Adjuvant Therapy for Cholangiocarcinoma

Similar to HCC and PDAC, recurrence of cholangiocarcinoma is common after surgical resection [20]. Adjuvant therapy can help reduce recurrence, and the current standard of care adjuvant therapy is capecitabine postsurgical resection as recommended by ASCO practice guidelines [20]. BILCAP was a multicentered phase 3 randomized controlled trial that included 447 patients and compared the efficacy of capecitabine adjuvant therapy to observation in cholangiocarcinoma [20, 21]. The primary endpoint of the study was overall survival which was 51.1 months in capecitabine group compared to 36.4 months was not statistically significant [21]. However, the sensitivity analyses of this population, the per-protocol overall survival, and recurrence-free survival analyses showed benefit, and the overall survival effect size of 14.7 months is clinically meaningful [21].

Novel Treatments in Treating Advanced HPB Cancers

TKI and Advanced Hepatocellular Carcinoma

One of the biggest breakthroughs in treating advanced HCC was the development of sorafenib, a tyrosine kinase inhibitor, which blocks VEGF and PDGF. Sorafenib was approved as a first-line therapy for HCC in 2007 following the phase 3 randomized controlled SHARP trial, which randomly assigned 602 patients with advanced HCC and demonstrated the superiority of sorafenib to placebo (overall survival, 10.7 months versus 7.9 months) [22, 23]. Subsequent retrospective studies further showed the benefits of sorafenib in treating advanced HCC. Patidar et al. evaluated retrospectively the clinical data of 78 patients with Barcelona Clinic Liver Cancer (BCLC) stage C HCC who received either TACE-sorafenib (TS) combination therapy or TACE monotherapy and found significantly higher OS with the TACE-sorafenib (10.1 months) compared to transarterial chemoembolization (TACE) alone (7.8 months) [24, 25]. Mulyadi et al. conducted a systematic review which compiled four retrospective studies and compared the Overall

Survival (OS) of 401 patients with TACE-Sorafenib to TACE-alone [24]. The systematic review showed that sorafenib and TACE combination therapy not only improved overall survival but also improved disease control rate (DCR), the time to progression (TTP), and progression-free survival (PFS) [24]. This systemic review demonstrates that combination TACE and sorafenib is superior to TACE monotherapy in overall survival, time to progression, disease control rate, and progression-free survival without significantly increasing significant adverse events in BCLC-C HCC patients.

For over 10 years, sorafenib was the standard of care for advanced HCC until lenvatinib became approved. Lenvatinib was approved in 2018 as first-line therapy for advanced HCC after the REFLECT trial. The REFLECT trial was a global open-label randomized phase III study that included 954 patients and demonstrated the non-inferiority of lenvatinib compared to sorafenib [24, 26]. The primary endpoint was overall survival, measured from the date of randomization until the date of death from any cause [26]. Median survival time for lenvatinib of 13·6 months was non-inferior to sorafenib 12.3 months [26]. The safety and tolerability profiles of lenvatinib were consistent with those previously observed, which include hypertension, diarrhea, and decreased appetite [26]. The REFLECT trial found lenvatinib to be non-inferior to sorafenib; however, recent systematic reviews have found lenvatinib monotherapy to be superior to sorafenib in treating unresectable HCC. Wang et al. conducted a systematic review on 24 studies comparing lenvatinib with sorafenib and found that lenvatinib provided better tumor responses and survival benefits and similar incidence of adverse events. 23 studies included were retrospective studies which include important data from a real-world setting and 1 phase 3 randomized clinical trial [27]. Pooled median OS was 11.36 months, and pooled median PFS was 6.68 months for lenvatinib patients [27]. 11 studies compared OS of lenvatinib to sorafenib [28]. The pooled hazard ratio (HR) of those studies was 0.85 where lenvatinib mediated significantly better overall survival than sorafenib [27]. PFS was also significantly improved in lenvatinib treatment group from a meta-analysis of eight studies where the pooled HR was 0.72 [27]. Objective response rate (ORR) was investigated in ten studies and similarly showed lenvatinib with a significantly higher overall response rate than sorafenib where the pooled analysis showed an odds ratio (OR) of 4.25 [27]. Another group, Hu et al. conducted a similar systematic review investigating lenvatinib as monotherapy compared to sorafenib in hepatocellular cancer. Their systematic review incorporated nine studies, eight of which were nonrandomized studies and one randomized controlled trial, which looked at OS, PFS, ORR, and DCR [28]. Similar to Wang's systematic review, OS was increased in lenvatinib treatment group compared to sorafenib where the HR was 0.87, PFS was increased with lenvatinib therapy based on pooled results of eight studies HR 0.67 [28]. ORR was reported in eight studies; the meta-analysis indicated that lenvatinib provided significantly higher ORR than sorafenib OR: 7.50 [28]. Lastly, lenvatinib was associated with a significantly higher DCR than sorafenib OR: 7.50 [28]. Both Hu and Wang's systematic review give us good data on the effectiveness and safety of lenvatinib and sorafenib in a real-world setting which builds upon the REFLECT trial. The data from the two systematic reviews point toward the superiority of lenvatinib over sorafenib, where patients can benefit from increased OS, PFS, ORR, and DCR. The results of these studies show that there is potential for lenvatinib to be preferred over sorafenib to treat unresectable HCC in the future.

The benefit of lenvatinib can also be seen in its combination with TACE to treat advanced HCC. Liu et al. conducted a systematic review and examined 6 studies which included 1 randomized controlled trial and 5 cohort studies that encompassed 598 patients which compared lenvatinib and TACE combination to sorafenib and TACE combination therapy [29]. The lenvatinib and TACE combination demonstrated a superior efficacy compared to sorafenib and TACE treatment group [8]. In the lenvatinib and TACE group, ORR, OS, PFS, TTP, and DCR were all improved compared to sorafenib and TACE [29]. Here Liu's systematic review again shows the benefits of incorporating lenvatinib into treating advanced HCC over sorafenib when combined with TACE.

TKI and Immunotherapy for Treating HCC

Immunotherapy has become a cornerstone in treating many solid tumors, and it has been utilized to treat HCC as well. The IMbrave150 was an open-label phase 3 trial included 336 patients, which investigated the efficacy of atezolizumab (anti PD-L1) combined with bevacizumab compared to sorafenib monotherapy in treating unresectable HCC [30]. The coprimary end points were OS and PFS [30]. Both OS and PFS were significantly improved in the atezolizumab and bevacizumab treatment group compared to sorafenib [30]. OS at 12 months was 67.2% (with atezolizumab plus bevacizumab and 54.6% with sorafenib [30]. Median progression-free survival was 6.8 months with atezolizumab plus bevacizumab and 4.3 months with sorafenib [30].

Apatinib/rivoceranib is a TKI currently approved for treating advanced HCC in China, and in 2024, the FDA accepted a new drug application for rivoceranib in combination with camrelizumab (anti-PD-1) to treat unresectable or metastatic hepatocellular carcinoma in 2024 [31]. CARES-310 is a randomized, open-label, international phase 3 trial which included 543 patients and compared the combination therapy of camrelizumab-rivoceranib to sorafenib monotherapy to treat unresectable or metastatic HCC. The primary endpoint of PFS was significantly improved in camrelizumab-rivoceranib group [32]. PFS in camrelizumab-rivoceranib was 5.6 months compared to 3.7 months in sorafenib treatment [32]. In addition, overall survival was also significantly improved with camrelizumab-rivoceranib treatment at 22.1 months compared to 15.2 months [32]. Camrelizumab plus rivoceranib showed a statistically significant and clinically meaningful benefit in PFS and OS compared with sorafenib for patients with unresectable hepatocellular carcinoma and could be a new and effective first-line treatment option.

As previously discussed, lenvatinib monotherapy, when in combination with TACE, shows significantly improved outcomes in treating HCC. Recently, investigators have conducted cohort studies that examined the combination of lenvatinib with different immunotherapies to treat HCC. Zhang et al. conducted a systematic review which included six cohort studies that evaluated the benefits of lenvatinib in combination with various PD-1/PD-L1 inhibitors which included camrelizumab, nivolumab (anti-PD-1), toripalimab (anti-PD-1), sintilimab (anti-PD-1), tislelizumab (anti-PD-1), and pembrolizumab (anti-PD-1) [33]. This study found the ORR, DCR, partial response of combined lenvatinib, and PD-1/PD-L1 inhibitor therapy were significantly higher than those of lenvatinib monotherapy [33]. Subgroup DCR analysis showed that combination therapy using lenvatinib and nivolumab was significantly higher than that of lenvatinib monotherapy (OR, 2.20) [33]. Pooled results also showed that combination of lenvatinib plus immunotherapy was safe, and there weren't significant difference in the incidence rate of hand-foot skin reaction, hypertension, decreased platelet count, and diarrhea. This systematic review demonstrated the improved outcomes for HCC patients when lenvatinib was combined with immunotherapy. These recent trials clearly demonstrate that immunotherapy will have an important role to play in treating advanced HCC.

Metastatic PDAC and Chemotherapy

The current standard of care chemotherapy for PDAC is either FOLFIRINOX, which is a combination of 5-fluorouracil (5-FU), leucovorin, irinotecan, and oxaliplatin, or a combination of gemcitabine and nab-paclitaxel (GEM-NABP) [34, 35]. Patients may progress on either FOLFIRINOX or GEM-NABP as first-line therapy and can be switched to the chemotherapy that they weren't on as second-line therapy; i.e., patient started on FOLFIRINOX and experienced disease progression, or intolerable side effects can be switched to GEM-NABP or vice versa [34]. In addition to FOLFIRINOX and GEM-NABP, a third alternative systemic chemotherapy regimen has recently arisen as first-line therapy for PDAC. NAPOLI 3 is a phase 3 randomized controlled trial that enrolled 770 patients and aimed to compare the efficacy and safety of NALIRIFOX versus nab-paclitaxel and gemcitabine as first-line therapy for metastatic pancreatic ductal adenocarcinoma [36]. NALIRIFOX is a chemotherapy regimen which includes liposomal irinotecan, oxaliplatin, leucovorin, and fluorouracil [36]. The primary endpoint was OS in the intention-to-treat population and was evaluated when at least 543 events were observed across the two treatment groups [36]. Median OS was significantly improved at 11.1 months with NALIRIFOX versus 9.2 months with nab-paclitaxel-gemcitabine [36]. In addition to the NAPOLI 3 trials, NALIRIFOX was further investigated, and a systematic review conducted by Nichetti et al. conducted a systematic review comparing NALIRIFOX, FOLFIRINOX, and GEM-NABP [37]. A total of 7 trials with data on 2581 patients were analyzed, including 383 patients treated with NALIRIFOX, 433 patients treated with FOLFIRINOX, and 1756 patients treated with GEM-NABP [16]. Median PFS was 7.4 months for NALIRIFOX, 5.7 months for GEM-NABP, and 7.3 months for FOLFIRINOX [37]. The GEM-NABP group had worse PFS (HR 1.45), while no statistically significant difference was observed for the FOLFIRINOX group (HR 1.21) [37]. NALIRIFOX also had an excellent hematologic safety profile compared to the other regimens. NALIRIFOX had significantly lower incidence of thrombocytopenia compared with both other regimens (1.6% vs. 11.8% with FOLFIRINOX and 10.8% with GEM-NABP) and of anemia and neutropenia compared with GEM-NABP [37]. The reduced incidence of thrombocytopenia and anemia is important as they could be a significant side effect which ultimately limits the use of FOLFIRINOX and GEM-NABP in PDAC patients. Nichetti's meta-analysis showed NALIRIFOX improved efficacy in PFS and a favorable toxicity profile compared to GEM-NABP which further supports its use as first-line therapy in treating advanced PDAC.

PDAC and KRAS Inhibitor

In addition to systemic chemotherapy, recent clinical trials are investigating KRAS inhibition as a potential treatment for PDAC as it's mutated in 90% of PDAC patients [38]. Recently, two novel KRAS G12C inhibitors, sotorasib and adagrasib, were approved for NSCLC. Sotorasib was subsequently investigated in a phase 1/2 trial (CodeBreak 100) to assess the safety and efficacy of sotorasib treatment in 38 patients with KRAS p.G12C-mutated pancreatic cancer who had received at least one previous systemic therapy [38, 39]. The primary endpoint for phase 2 was a centrally confirmed objective response (defined as a complete or partial response) [39]. The results from that study were positive as partial response was seen in 21% of the patients, with an 84% DCR [38, 39]. The median PFS and overall survival were 4.0 and 6.9 months, respectively [38, 39]. KRYSTAL 1, a phase 1/2 trial, included 21 metastatic PDAC patients and investigated the efficacy of adagrasib at treating it [38, 40]. Similar to sotorasib, PDAC patients also benefited from adagrasib. A partial response was seen in 33% of patients with a 81% DCR, and the median progression-free survival and overall survival were 5.4 and 8.0 months, respectively [38, 40]. Unfortunately, KRAS G12C mutations only account for 1% of KRAS mutations in PDAC; therefore, adagrasib and sotorasib could only benefit that small select group of PDAC patients [38]. The majority of KRAS mutations in PDAC are G12D which accounts for 39–41% of patients [38]. Following the success of adagrasib, Mirati therapeutics, the developer of adagrasib, is currently developing a KRAS G12D inhibitor (MRTX1133) to treat PDAC, and it is currently undergoing phase 1/2 trial [39]. Hopefully Mirati's new KRAS G12D medication can follow the success of its predecessor and become standard of care in treating PDAC.

Metastatic PDAC and PARP Inhibitor

PARP inhibitors are a type of targeted therapy that interferes with cancer cells' abilities to repair their own DNA. PARP inhibitors were previously approved for breast and ovarian cancer, but after the phase 3 POLO study, olaparib, a PARP inhibitor, was approved for maintenance treatment of adult patients with BRCA-mutated metastatic pancreatic adenocarcinoma in 2019. The POLO study included 154 PDAC patients, and its primary endpoint was PFS. The patients who received olaparib as active maintenance therapy experienced a significantly longer median PFS compared to placebo (7.4 months vs. 3.8 months; HR 0.54) while preserving quality of life [41–43]. Other PARP inhibitors besides olaparib are currently under investigation to treating PDAC. Rucaparib recently showed promise in a phase 2 trial which treated patients with somatic or germline variants in BRCA or PALB2, advanced pancreatic cancer [42, 43]. The study found the median PFS was 13.1 months, with a 6-month PFS of 59.5% and a 12-month PFS of 54.8% [43]. The median OS was 23.5 months, with eight patients alive more than 2 years after enrollment [43].

Cholangiocarcinoma and TKI Therapy

Systemic chemotherapy is standard of care, and following the phase 3 randomized controlled trial ABC-02 trial, gemcitabine and cisplatin combination therapy has become first-line therapy for treating advanced CCA [44–46]. The trial enrolled 410 patients locally advanced or metastatic cholangiocarcinoma, gallbladder cancer, or ampullary cancer and compared gemcitabine and cisplatin combination to gemcitabine monotherapy and found a significantly higher median OS 11.7 vs. 8.1 months of the combination therapy [44–46]. Recently, more targeted therapies have been approved for treating cholangiocarcinoma. One such medication pemigatinib, an FGFR2 inhibitor, has recently been approved for advanced refractory CCA following the positive results of the FIGHT-202 trial. FIGHT-202 is a phase 2 open-label trial which enrolled 146 patients who were previously treated and had locally advanced or metastatic cholangiocarcinoma with and without FGFR2 fusions or rearrangements [47]. The primary endpoint was the proportion of patients who achieved an objective response among those with FGFR2 fusions or rearrangements [47]. 38 (35.5%) patients with FGFR2 fusions or rearrangements achieved an objective response (three complete responses and 35 partial responses) [47]. Median PFS was 6.9 months, and median overall survival was 21.1 months [47].

Cholangiocarcinoma and Immunotherapy

Immunotherapy in combination with gemcitabine and cisplatin chemotherapy has also been approved in treating CCA. The TOPAZ-1 trial, a phase 3 double-blind placebo study, showed that combining durvalumab (anti PD-L1) with gemcitabine and cisplatin significantly improved than chemotherapy in treating advanced biliary tract cancer [48]. A total of 685 patients were enrolled in the trial, and the primary objective was to assess OS [48]. 198 patients (58.1%) in the durvalumab group plus gemcitabine and cisplatin and 226 patients (65.7%) in the placebo group plus gemcitabine and cisplatin had died [48]. The estimated 24-month overall survival rate was 24.9% for durvalumab and 10.4% for placebo [48].

Pembrolizumab combined with gemcitabine and cisplatin also demonstrated significantly improved outcomes for advanced biliary tract cancer compared to chemotherapy as seen in the KEYNOTE-966 trial [49]. This was a phase 3 randomized, double-blind, placebo-controlled trial that enrolled 1069 patients [49]. The primary endpoint of overall survival was evaluated in the intention-to-treat population [49]. Median overall survival was 12.7 months in the pembrolizumab group versus 10.9 months in chemotherapy only (HR 0.85) [49]. Based on the clinically significant results from the study, the FDA approved this combination in 2023 [50].

Conclusion

HPB cancers affect millions of people each year, and they are all extremely deadly cancers as they are typically diagnosed at a later stage where curative surgery isn't feasible. Immune checkpoint inhibitors such as pembrolizumab, nivolumab, and durvalumab have been a revolutionary development in treating solid tumors in the past decade. Similarly, the benefits of these medications can be seen in the enhanced clinical outcomes including progression-free survival in advanced HCC patients and cholangiocarcinoma patients. Targeted therapy such as tyrosine kinase inhibitors including sorafenib and lenvatinib has demonstrated their superior clinical benefit when combined with TACE over TACE alone at treating advanced unresectable HCC. Another tyrosine kinase inhibitor, pemigatinib, has shown benefit in treating advanced cholangiocarcinoma. Another class of targeted therapies, KRAS inhibitors, has shown benefit in treating advanced PDAC patients with G12C mutations. Looking toward the future, new KRAS inhibitor targeting G12D mutation is currently in phase 2 trials where more PDAC patients can benefit from it as approximately 40% of PDAC patients have this mutation. In addition to KRAS inhibitors, a novel chemotherapy regimen, NALIRIFOX, has demonstrated superior clinical benefit over GEM-NABP for PDAC patients. Advances in small-molecule targeted therapy, immune checkpoint inhibitors, and novel chemotherapeutic regimens are shifting the standard of care for treating HPB cancers and improving the quality of life in these patients.

References

1. Adeniji N, Dhanasekaran R. Current and emerging tools for hepatocellular carcinoma surveillance. Hepatol Commun. 2021;5(12):1972–86. https://doi.org/10.1002/hep4.1823. Epub 2021 Sep 17. PMID: 34533885; PMCID: PMC8631096. https://pubmed.ncbi.nlm.nih.gov/34533885/
2. Zhao Y-J, Ju Q, Li G-C. Tumor markers for hepatocellular carcinoma. Mol Clin Oncol. 2013;1:593–8. https://pubmed.ncbi.nlm.nih.gov/24649215/
3. Tzartzeva K, Obi J, Rich NE, Parikh ND, Marrero JA, Yopp A, et al. Surveillance imaging and alpha fetoprotein for early detection of hepatocellular carcinoma in patients with cirrhosis: a meta-analysis. Gastroenterology. 2018;154:1706–1718.e1. https://pubmed.ncbi.nlm.nih.gov/29425931/
4. Choi J, Kim G, Han S, Lee W, Chun S, Lim Y. Longitudinal assessment of three serum biomarkers to detect very early-stage hepatocellular carcinoma. Hepatology. 2019;69:1983–94. https://pubmed.ncbi.nlm.nih.gov/30153338/
5. Kumada T, Toyoda H, Tada T, Kiriyama S, Tanikawa M, Hisanaga Y, et al. High-sensitivity Lens culinaris agglutinin-reactive alpha-fetoprotein assay predicts early detection of hepa-tocellular carcinoma. J Gastroenterol. 2014;49:555–63. https://pubmed.ncbi.nlm.nih.gov/24057163/
6. Winter K, Talar-Wojnarowska R, Dąbrowski A, Degowska M, Durlik M, Gąsiorowska A, Głuszek S, Jurkowska G, Kaczka A, Lampe P, Marek T, Nasierowska-Guttmejer A, Nowakowska-Duława E, Rydzewska G, Strzelczyk J, Śledziński Z, Małecka-Panas E. Diagnostic and therapeutic recommendations in pancreatic ductal adenocarcinoma. Recommendations of the working Group of the Polish Pancreatic Club. Prz Gastroenterol. 2019;14(1):1–18. https://doi.org/10.5114/pg.2019.83422. Epub 2019 Mar 12. PMID: 30944673; PMCID: PMC6444110. https://pmc.ncbi.nlm.nih.gov/articles/PMC6444110/
7. National Comprehensive Cancer Network. NCCN Guidelines Version 2.2018 Pancreatic Adenocarcinoma. Available at: http://www.nccn.org.
8. Mitchell RA, Stanger D, Shuster C, et al. Repeat endoscopic ultrasound-guided fine-needle aspiration in patients with suspected pancreatic cancer: diagnostic yield and associated change in access to appropriate care. Can J Gastroenterol Hepatol. 2016;2016:7678403. https://pmc.ncbi.nlm.nih.gov/articles/PMC10378084/
9. Gu YL, Lan C, Pei H, et al. Applicative value of serum CA19-9, CEA, CA125 and CA242 in diagnosis and prognosis for patients with pancreatic cancer treated by concurrent chemoradiotherapy. Asian Pac J Cancer Prev. 2015;16:6569–73. https://pubmed.ncbi.nlm.nih.gov/26434876/
10. Forner A, Vidili G, Rengo M, Bujanda L, Ponz-Sarvisé M, Lamarca A. Clinical presentation, diagnosis and staging of cholangiocarcinoma. Liver Int. 2019;39(Suppl 1):98–107. https://doi.org/10.1111/liv.14086. Epub 2019 Mar 25. PMID: 30831002. https://pubmed.ncbi.nlm.nih.gov/30831002/
11. Mar WA, Shon AM, Lu Y, et al. Imaging spectrum of cholangiocarcinoma: role in diagnosis, staging, and posttreatment evaluation. Abdom Radiol (NY). 2016;41:553–67. https://pubmed.ncbi.nlm.nih.gov/26847022/
12. Toubert C, Guiu B, Al Taweel B, Assenat E, Panaro F, Souche FR, Ursic-Bedoya J, Navarro F, Herrero A. Prolonged survival after recurrence in hcc resected patients using repeated curative therapies: never give up! Cancers (Basel). 2022;15(1):232. https://doi.org/10.3390/cancers15010232. PMID: 36612227; PMCID: PMC9818493. https://pmc.ncbi.nlm.nih.gov/articles/PMC9818493/
13. Du JS, Hsu SH, Wang SN. The current and prospective adjuvant therapies for hepatocellular carcinoma. Cancers (Basel). 2024;16(7):1422. https://doi.org/10.3390/cancers16071422. PMID: 38611100; PMCID: PMC11011082. https://pmc.ncbi.nlm.nih.gov/articles/PMC11011082/
14. Qin S, Chen M, Cheng AL, Kaseb AO, Kudo M, Lee HC, Yopp AC, Zhou J, Wang L, Wen X, Heo J, Tak WY, Nakamura S, Numata K, Uguen T, Hsiehchen D, Cha E, Hack SP, Lian Q, Ma N, Spahn JH, Wang Y, Wu C, Chow PKH, IMbrave050 investigators. Atezolizumab plus bevacizumab versus active surveillance in patients with resected or ablated high-risk hepatocellular carcinoma (IMbrave050): a randomised, open-label, multicentre, phase 3 trial. Lancet. 2023;402(10415):1835–47. https://doi.org/10.1016/S0140-6736(23)01796-8. Epub 2023 Oct 20. PMID: 37871608. https://pubmed.ncbi.nlm.nih.gov/37871608/
15. Bruix J, Takayama T, Mazzaferro V, Chau GY, Yang J, Kudo M, Cai J, Poon RT, Han KH, Tak WY, Lee HC, Song T, Roayaie S, Bolondi L, Lee KS, Makuuchi M, Souza F, Berre MA, Meinhardt G, Llovet JM, STORM investigators. Adjuvant sorafenib for hepatocellular carcinoma after resection or ablation (STORM): a phase 3, randomised, double-blind, placebo-controlled trial. Lancet Oncol. 2015;16(13):1344–54. https://doi.org/10.1016/S1470-2045(15)00198-9. Epub 2015 Sep 8. PMID: 26361969. https://pubmed.ncbi.nlm.nih.gov/26361969/
16. Chen P-J, et al. A phase III trial of muparfostat (PI-88) as adjuvant therapy in patients with hepatitis virus related hepatocellular carcinoma (HV-HCC) after resection. Ann Oncol. 28:v213. https://www.annalsofoncology.org/article/S0923-7534(20)37898-4/fulltext
17. Li SH, Mei J, Cheng Y, Li Q, Wang QX, Fang CK, Lei QC, Huang HK, Cao MR, Luo R, Deng JD, Jiang YC, Zhao RC, Lu LH, Zou JW, Deng M, Lin WP, Guan RG, Wen YH, Li JB, Zheng L, Guo ZX, Ling YH, Chen HW, Zhong C, Wei W, Guo RP. Postoperative adjuvant hepatic arterial infusion chemotherapy with FOLFOX in hepatocellular carcinoma with microvascular invasion: a multicenter, phase III, randomized study. J Clin Oncol. 2023;41(10):1898–908. https://doi.org/10.1200/JCO.22.01142. Epub 2022 Dec 16. PMID: 36525610; PMCID: PMC10082249. https://pubmed.ncbi.nlm.nih.gov/36525610/
18. Cecchini M, Salem RR, Robert M, Czerniak S, Blaha O, Zelterman D, Rajaei M, Townsend JP, Cai G, Chowdhury S, Yugawa D, Tseng R, Mejia Arbelaez C, Jiao J, Shroyer K, Thumar J, Kortmansky J, Zaheer W, Fischbach N, Persico J, Stein S, Khan SA, Cha C, Billingsley KG, Kunstman JW, Johung KL, Wiess C, Muzumdar MD, Spickard E, Aushev VN, Laliotis G, Jurdi A, Liu MC, Escobar-Hoyos L, Lacy J. Perioperative modified FOLFIRINOX for resectable pancreatic cancer: a nonrandomized controlled

trial. JAMA Oncol. 2024;10(8):1027–35. https://doi.org/10.1001/jamaoncol.2024.1575. PMID: 38900452; PMCID: PMC11190830. https://pubmed.ncbi.nlm.nih.gov/38900452/
19. Conroy T, Hammel P, Hebbar M, Ben Abdelghani M, Wei AC, Raoul JL, Choné L, Francois E, Artru P, Biagi JJ, Lecomte T, Assenat E, Faroux R, Ychou M, Volet J, Sauvanet A, Breysacher G, Di Fiore F, Cripps C, Kavan P, Texereau P, Bouhier-Leporrier K, Khemissa-Akouz F, Legoux JL, Juzyna B, Gourgou S, O'Callaghan CJ, Jouffroy-Zeller C, Rat P, Malka D, Castan F, Bachet JB, Canadian Cancer Trials Group and the Unicancer-GI–PRODIGE Group. FOLFIRINOX or gemcitabine as adjuvant therapy for pancreatic cancer. N Engl J Med. 2018;379(25):2395–406. https://doi.org/10.1056/NEJMoa1809775. PMID: 30575490. https://pubmed.ncbi.nlm.nih.gov/30575490/
20. Shroff RT, Kennedy EB, Bachini M, Bekaii-Saab T, Crane C, Edeline J, El-Khoueiry A, Feng M, Katz MHG, Primrose J, Soares HP, Valle J, Maithel SK. Adjuvant therapy for resected biliary tract cancer: ASCO clinical practice guideline. J Clin Oncol. 2019;37(12):1015–27. https://doi.org/10.1200/JCO.18.02178. Epub 2019 Mar 11. PMID: 30856044. https://pubmed.ncbi.nlm.nih.gov/30856044/
21. Primrose JN, Fox RP, Palmer DH, Malik HZ, Prasad R, Mirza D, Anthony A, Corrie P, Falk S, Finch-Jones M, Wasan H, Ross P, Wall L, Wadsley J, Evans JTR, Stocken D, Praseedom R, Ma YT, Davidson B, Neoptolemos JP, Iveson T, Raftery J, Zhu S, Cunningham D, Garden OJ, Stubbs C, Valle JW, Bridgewater J, BILCAP Study Group. Capecitabine compared with observation in resected biliary tract cancer (BILCAP): a randomised, controlled, multicentre, phase 3 study. Lancet Oncol. 2019;20(5):663–73. https://doi.org/10.1016/S1470-2045(18)30915-X. Epub 2019 Mar 25. Erratum in: Lancet Oncol. 2019;20(5):e242. doi:10.1016/S1470-2045(19)30216-5. PMID: 30922733 https://pubmed.ncbi.nlm.nih.gov/30922733/
22. Llovet JM, Kelley RK, Villanueva A, et al. Hepatocellular carcinoma. Nat Rev Dis Primers. 2021;7:6. https://doi.org/10.1038/s41572-020-00240-3.
23. Llovet JM, Ricci S, Mazzaferro V, Hilgard P, Gane E, Blanc JF, de Oliveira AC, Santoro A, Raoul JL, Forner A, Schwartz M, Porta C, Zeuzem S, Bolondi L, Greten TF, Galle PR, Seitz JF, Borbath I, Häussinger D, Giannaris T, Shan M, Moscovici M, Voliotis D, Bruix J, SHARP Investigators Study Group. Sorafenib in advanced hepatocellular carcinoma. N Engl J Med. 2008;359(4):378–90. https://doi.org/10.1056/NEJMoa0708857. PMID: 18650514. https://pubmed.ncbi.nlm.nih.gov/18650514/
24. Mulyadi R, Hasan I, Sidipratomo P, et al. Prognosis of transarterial chemoembolization-sorafenib compared to transarterial chemoembolization-alone in hepatocellular carcinoma stage C: a systematic review. J Egypt Natl Canc Inst. 2024;36:18. https://doi.org/10.1186/s43046-024-00224-4.
25. Patidar Y, Chandel K, Condati NK, Srinivasan SV, Mukund A, Sarin SK. Transarterial chemoembolization (TACE) combined with sorafenib versus TACE in patients with BCLC stage C hepatocellular carcinoma – a retrospective study. J Clin Exp Hepatol. 2022;12(3):745–54.
26. Kudo M, Finn RS, Qin S, Han KH, Ikeda K, Piscaglia F, Baron A, Park JW, Han G, Jassem J, Blanc JF, Vogel A, Komov D, Evans TRJ, Lopez C, Dutcus C, Guo M, Saito K, Kraljevic S, Tamai T, Ren M, Cheng AL. Lenvatinib versus sorafenib in first-line treatment of patients with unresectable hepatocellular carcinoma: a randomised phase 3 non-inferiority trial. Lancet. 2018;391(10126):1163–73. https://doi.org/10.1016/S0140-6736(18)30207-1. PMID: 29433850
27. Wang S, Wang Y, Yu J, Wu H, Zhou Y. Lenvatinib as first-line treatment for unresectable hepatocellular carcinoma: a systematic review and meta-analysis. Cancers (Basel). 2022;14(22):5525. https://doi.org/10.3390/cancers14225525. PMID: 36428618; PMCID: PMC9688932
28. Hu L, Zheng Y, Lin J, Shi X, Wang A. Comparison of the effects of lenvatinib and sorafenib on survival in patients with advanced hepatocellular carcinoma: a systematic review and meta-analysis. Clin Res Hepatol Gastroenterol. 2023;47(1):102061. https://doi.org/10.1016/j.clinre.2022.102061. Epub 2022 Dec 5. PMID: 36473632
29. Liu JN, Li JJ, Yan S, Zhang GN, Yi PS. Transarterial chemoembolization combined with lenvatinib versus transarterial chemoembolization combined with sorafenib for unresectable hepatocellular carcinoma: a systematic review and meta-analysis. Front Oncol. 2023;13:1074793. https://doi.org/10.3389/fonc.2023.1074793. Erratum in: Front Oncol. 2023 Jun 22;13:1233247. doi:10.3389/fonc.2023.1233247. PMID: 36910612; PMCID: PMC9995877
30. Finn RS, Qin S, Ikeda M, Galle PR, Ducreux M, Kim TY, Kudo M, Breder V, Merle P, Kaseb AO, Li D, Verret W, Xu DZ, Hernandez S, Liu J, Huang C, Mulla S, Wang Y, Lim HY, Zhu AX, Cheng AL; IMbrave150 Investigators. Atezolizumab plus Bevacizumab in Unresectable Hepatocellular Carcinoma. N Engl J Med 2020 ;382(20):1894-1905. https://doi.org/10.1056/NEJMoa1915745. PMID: 32402160.
31. https://www.targetedonc.com/view/fda-accepts-nda-for-rivoceranib-plus-camrelizumab-in-unresectable-hcc
32. Qin S, Chan SL, Gu S, Bai Y, Ren Z, Lin X, Chen Z, Jia W, Jin Y, Guo Y, Hu X, Meng Z, Liang J, Cheng Y, Xiong J, Ren H, Yang F, Li W, Chen Y, Zeng Y, Sultanbaev A, Pazgan-Simon M, Pisetska M, Melisi D, Ponomarenko D, Osypchuk Y, Sinielnikov I, Yang TS, Liang X, Chen C, Wang L, Cheng AL, Kaseb A, Vogel A, CARES-310 Study Group. Camrelizumab plus rivoceranib versus sorafenib as first-line therapy for unresectable hepatocellular carcinoma (CARES-310): a randomised, open-label, international phase 3 study. Lancet. 2023;402(10408):1133–46. https://doi.org/10.1016/S0140-6736(23)00961-3. Epub 2023 Jul 24. PMID: 37499670
33. Zhang B, Su L, Lin Y. Efficacy and safety of lenvatinib combined with PD-1/PD-L1 inhibitors in the treatment of hepatocellular carcinoma: a meta-analysis and systematic review. Oncol Lett. 2024;28(1):312. https://doi.org/10.3892/ol.2024.14445. PMID: 38803443; PMCID: PMC11129543
34. Halbrook CJ, Lyssiotis CA, Pasca di Magliano M, Maitra A. Pancreatic cancer: advances and challenges. Cell. 2023;186(8):1729–54. https://doi.org/10.1016/j.cell.2023.02.014. PMID: 37059070; PMCID: PMC10182830
35. Hosein AN, Dougan SK, Aguirre AJ, Maitra A. Translational advances in pancreatic ductal adenocarcinoma therapy. Nat Cancer. 2022;3(3):272–86. https://doi.org/10.1038/s43018-022-00349-2. Epub 2022 Mar 29. PMID: 35352061
36. Wainberg ZA, Melisi D, Macarulla T, Pazo Cid R, Chandana SR, De La Fouchardière C, Dean A, Kiss I, Lee WJ, Goetze TO, Van Cutsem E, Paulson AS, Bekaii-Saab T, Pant S, Hubner RA, Xiao Z, Chen H, Benzaghou F, O'Reilly EM. NALIRIFOX versus nab-paclitaxel and gemcitabine in treatment-naive patients with metastatic pancreatic ductal adenocarcinoma (NAPOLI 3): a randomised, open-label, phase 3 trial. Lancet. 2023;402(10409):1272-1281. https://doi.org/10.1016/S0140-6736(23)01366-1. Epub 2023 Sep 11. PMID: 37708904; PMCID: PMC11664154.
37. Nichetti F, Rota S, Ambrosini P, Pircher C, Gusmaroli E, Droz Dit Busset M, Pusceddu S, Sposito C, Coppa J, Morano F, Pietrantonio F, Di Bartolomeo M, Mariani L, Mazzaferro V, de Braud F, Niger M. NALIRIFOX, FOLFIRINOX, and gemcitabine with nab-paclitaxel as first-line chemotherapy for metastatic pancreatic cancer: a systematic review and meta-analysis. JAMA Netw Open. 2024;7(1):e2350756. https://doi.org/10.1001/jamanetworkopen.2023.50756. PMID: 38190183; PMCID: PMC10774994
38. Long SA, Amparo AM, Goodhart G, Ahmad SA, Waters AM. Evaluation of KRAS inhibitor-directed therapies for pancreatic cancer treatment. Front Oncol. 2024;14:1402128. https://

doi.org/10.3389/fonc.2024.1402128. PMID: 38800401; PMCID: PMC11116577
39. Strickler JH, Satake H, George TJ, Yaeger R, Hollebecque A, Garrido-Laguna I, Schuler M, Burns TF, Coveler AL, Falchook GS, Vincent M, Sunakawa Y, Dahan L, Bajor D, Rha SY, Lemech C, Juric D, Rehn M, Ngarmchamnanrith G, Jafarinasabian P, Tran Q, Hong DS. Sotorasib in KRAS p.G12C-mutated advanced pancreatic cancer. N Engl J Med. 2023;388(1):33–43. https://doi.org/10.1056/NEJMoa2208470. Epub 2022 Dec 21. PMID: 36546651; PMCID: PMC10506456
40. Bekaii-Saab TS, Yaeger R, Spira AI, Pelster MS, Sabari JK, Hafez N, Barve M, Velastegui K, Yan X, Shetty A, Der-Torossian H, Pant S. Adagrasib in advanced solid tumors harboring a KRASG12C mutation. J Clin Oncol. 2023;41(25):4097–106. https://doi.org/10.1200/JCO.23.00434. Epub 2023 Apr 26. PMID: 37099736; PMCID: PMC10852394
41. Kindler HL, Hammel P, Reni M, Van Cutsem E, Macarulla T, Hall MJ, Park JO, Hochhauser D, Arnold D, Oh DY, Reinacher-Schick A, Tortora G, Algül H, O'Reilly EM, Bordia S, McGuinness D, Cui K, Locker GY, Golan T. Overall survival results from the POLO trial: a phase III study of active maintenance olaparib versus placebo for germline BRCA-mutated metastatic pancreatic cancer. J Clin Oncol. 2022;40(34):3929–39. https://doi.org/10.1200/JCO.21.01604. Epub 2022 Jul 14. Erratum in: J Clin Oncol. 2024 Jun 10;42(17):2112. doi:10.1200/JCO.24.00821. PMID: 35834777; PMCID: PMC10476841
42. Moosavi F, Hassani B, Nazari S, Saso L, Firuzi O. Targeting DNA damage response in pancreatic ductal adenocarcinoma: a review of preclinical and clinical evidence. Biochim Biophys Acta Rev Cancer. 2024;1879(6):189185. https://doi.org/10.1016/j.bbcan.2024.189185. Epub 2024 Sep 24. PMID: 39326802
43. Brown TJ, Reiss KA. PARP inhibitors in pancreatic cancer. Cancer J. 2021;27(6):465–75. https://doi.org/10.1097/PPO.0000000000000554. PMID: 34904809; PMCID: PMC8682800
44. Halder R, Amaraneni A, Shroff RT. Cholangiocarcinoma: a review of the literature and future directions in therapy. Hepatobiliary Surg Nutr. 2022;11(4):555–66. https://doi.org/10.21037/hbsn-20-396. PMID: 36016753; PMCID: PMC9396092
45. Elvevi A, Laffusa A, Scaravaglio M, Rossi RE, Longarini R, Stagno AM, Cristoferi L, Ciaccio A, Cortinovis DL, Invernizzi P, Massironi S. Clinical treatment of cholangiocarcinoma: an updated comprehensive review. Ann Hepatol. 2022;27(5):100737. https://doi.org/10.1016/j.aohep.2022.100737. Epub 2022 Jul 7. PMID: 35809836
46. Valle J, Wasan H, Palmer DH, Cunningham D, Anthoney A, Maraveyas A, Madhusudan S, Iveson T, Hughes S, Pereira SP, Roughton M, Bridgewater J, ABC-02 Trial Investigators. Cisplatin plus gemcitabine versus gemcitabine for biliary tract cancer. N Engl J Med. 2010;362(14):1273–81. https://doi.org/10.1056/NEJMoa0908721. PMID: 20375404
47. Abou-Alfa GK, Sahai V, Hollebecque A, Vaccaro G, Melisi D, Al-Rajabi R, Paulson AS, Borad MJ, Gallinson D, Murphy AG, Oh DY, Dotan E, Catenacci DV, Van Cutsem E, Ji T, Lihou CF, Zhen H, Féliz L, Vogel A. Pemigatinib for previously treated, locally advanced or metastatic cholangiocarcinoma: a multicentre, open-label, phase 2 study. Lancet Oncol. 2020;21(5):671–84. https://doi.org/10.1016/S1470-2045(20)30109-1. Epub 2020 Mar 20. Erratum in: Lancet Oncol. 2024 Jan;25(1):e3. doi:10.1016/S1470-2045(23)00642-3. PMID: 32203698; PMCID: PMC8461541
48. Oh DY, Ruth He A, Qin S, Chen LT, Okusaka T, Vogel A, Kim JW, Suksombooncharoen T, Ah Lee M, Kitano M, Burris H, Bouattour M, Tanasanvimon S, McNamara MG, Zaucha R, Avallone A, Tan B, Cundom J, Lee CK, Takahashi H, Ikeda M, Chen JS, Wang J, Makowsky M, Rokutanda N, He P, Kurland JF, Cohen G, Valle JW. Durvalumab plus gemcitabine and cisplatin in advanced biliary tract cancer. NEJM Evid. 2022;1(8):EVIDoa2200015. https://doi.org/10.1056/EVIDoa2200015. Epub 2022 Jun 1. PMID: 38319896
49. Kelley RK, Ueno M, Yoo C, Finn RS, Furuse J, Ren Z, Yau T, Klümpen HJ, Chan SL, Ozaka M, Verslype C, Bouattour M, Park JO, Barajas O, Pelzer U, Valle JW, Yu L, Malhotra U, Siegel AB, Edeline J, Vogel A, KEYNOTE-966 Investigators. Pembrolizumab in combination with gemcitabine and cisplatin compared with gemcitabine and cisplatin alone for patients with advanced biliary tract cancer (KEYNOTE-966): a randomised, double-blind, placebo-controlled, phase 3 trial. Lancet. 2023;401(10391):1853–65. https://doi.org/10.1016/S0140-6736(23)00727-4. Epub 2023 Apr 16. Erratum in: Lancet. 2023 Sep 16;402(10406):964. doi:10.1016/S0140-6736(23)01904-9. Erratum in: Lancet. 2024 Mar 23;403(10432):1140. doi:10.1016/S0140-6736(24)00545-2. PMID: 37075781
50. https://www.fda.gov/drugs/resources-information-approved-drugs/fda-approves-pembrolizumab-chemotherapy-biliary-tract-cancer

20 Genitourinary Cancer: Recent Advances in Diagnosis and Treatment

Jingsong Zhang and Joseph Zimmerman

Abbreviations

AA	Abiraterone acetate
AAP	Abiraterone acetate plus prednisone
ADC	Antibody drug conjugate
ADT	Androgen deprivation therapy
ARPI	Androgen receptor signaling pathway inhibitors
BiTE	Bispecific T-cell engager
CAR T	Chimeric antigen receptor T cell
ccRCC	Clear cell renal cell carcinoma
CRS	Cytokine release syndrome
CTLA-4	Anti-cytotoxic T-lymphocyte-associated protein 4
ctDNA	Circulating tumor DNA
ddMVAC	Dose-dense methotrexate, vinblastine, doxorubicin, and cisplatin
DFS	Disease-free survival
EBRT	External beam radiation therapy
EV	Enfortumab vedotin
GU	Genitourinary cancers
HR	Hazard ratio
HRR	Homologous recombination repair
ICI	Immune checkpoint inhibitor
IMDC	International Metastatic RCC Database Consortium
KLK2	Kallikrein-related peptidase 2
KPS	Karnofsky performance score
LHRH	Luteinizing hormone-releasing hormone
LLN	Lower limit of normal
MIBC	Muscle-invasive bladder cancer
mCRPC	Metastatic castration-resistant prostate cancer
mUC	Metastatic urothelial carcinoma
MVAC	Methotrexate, vinblastine, doxorubicin, and cisplatin
NMIBC	Non-muscle-invasive bladder cancer
OS	Overall survival
PARPi	Poly ADP ribose polymerase inhibitor
PSCA	Prostate stem cell antigen
PSMA	Prostate-specific membrane antigen
Radium 223	Radium-223 dichloride
RCC	Renal cell carcinoma
rPFS	Radiographic progression-free survival
STEAP1	Six-transmembrane epithelial antigen of prostate 1
TURBT	Transurethral resection of bladder tumor
UC	Urothelial Carcinoma
ULN	Upper limit of normal
VEGF	Vascular endothelial growth factor

J. Zhang (✉)
Department of Genitourinary Oncology, Moffitt Cancer Center, Tampa, FL, USA
e-mail: jingsong.zhang@moffitt.org

J. Zimmerman
University of South Florida, Morsani College of Medicine, Tampa, FL, USA

Introduction

Genitourinary (GU) cancers include prostate cancer, renal cell carcinoma (RCC), urothelial carcinoma (UC) of the bladder, renal pelvis and ureter, cancer of the urethral, testicular cancer, and penile cancer. Prostate cancer is the second most diagnosed cancer and the fifth leading cause of cancer death globally. The newly diagnosed prostate cancer is expected to increase from 1.4 million in 2020 to 2.9 million in 2040, and the yearly death from prostate cancer is projected to be nearly doubled from *375,000* in 2020 to *700,000* in 2040 globally [1]. Bladder cancer itself is the ninth most common cancer with over 600,000 people diagnosed and more than 220,000 deaths globally in 2022. RCC has over 430,000 new cases and over 150,000 deaths per year [2]. There is an unmet need to advance the diagnosis and treatment of these lethal GU malignancies.

J. Huang, H. S.L. Jim (eds.), *Cancer Research Guidance for Clinicians and Researchers*,
https://doi.org/10.1007/978-3-032-19175-5_20

This chapter will focus on recent advances in diagnosing and treating prostate adenocarcinoma, RCC, and UC of the bladder, ureter, and renal pelvis. Data on emerging technologies and treatments will also be discussed.

Advancements in Imaging Tools to Diagnose and to Stage GU Malignancies

Prostate Cancer

Prostate MRI

In a typical presentation of newly diagnosed prostate cancer, most patients including those with bone metastases are asymptomatic. Nowadays, prostate MRIs are increasingly used after patients are referred to urology for an elevated PSA level and/or an abnormal digital rectal exam. The prostate imaging reporting and data system, also known as PI-RADS, was developed to standardize the performance and reporting of prostate MRI examinations. Prostate biopsy is indicated in PI-RADS 5, PI-RADS 4, and some PI-RADS 3 lesions. Previously, the traditional transrectal ultrasound-guided prostate biopsy could miss up to 25% of tumors. As such, transperineal US-MRI fusion-guided biopsy is now widely adopted to improve the detection rate and the accuracy of prostate biopsy [3, 4]. A systematic review and meta-analysis of 16 studies with approximately 2000 men demonstrated that US-MRI fusion-guided biopsy had a 20% higher rate of detection of significant prostate cancer and a twofold lower rate of detection of insignificant prostate cancer resulting in reduction of oversampling in patients [5].

PSMA PET Scan

After establishing the diagnosis of prostate cancer with prostate biopsy, the risk of recurrence and metastases is stratified based on PSA, Gleason sum, and clinical tumor staging (Table 20.1). Staging is accomplished with the help of PSMA, or prostate-specific membrane antigen, which is a membrane glycoprotein expressed 100 to 1000 times higher on prostate cancer cells compared to normal prostate cells. Gallium 68, Piflufolastat F 18, and flotufolastat F 18 radiolabeled PSMA PET have been shown to be superior to CT and bone scan to selectively detect metastatic prostate cancer, and these are now approved to stage unfavorable intermediate, high, or very-high-risk prostate cancer [6, 7]. In one randomized study of 302 men comparing PSMA PET to conventional CT imaging, the former demonstrated an accuracy of 92% and sensitivity of 85% compared to 65% and 38%, respectively, for CT [6]. PSMA PET is also approved to detect early metastasis when patients developed PSA progression after completing definitive local therapy [8]. In a 2022 systematic review and meta-analysis, Pozdnykaov et al. demonstrated that PSMA PET altered treatment in 56% of patients with presumed biochemical recurrence as defined by conventional CT and bone scan [9]. Another use is in castration-resistant prostate cancer in which PSMA PET detected metastatic disease in 55% of patients that had no evidence of metastasis on conventional imaging [10]. After prostate cancer has progressed to the metastatic castration-resistant stage, PSMA PET has been used to select patients for targeted radioligand therapy like lutetium Lu 177 vipivotide tetraxetan [11, 12].

Table 20.1 Prostate cancer risk groups

Risk group	Characteristics of cancers
Very-low-risk group	Small, not felt on exam, localized to a small area of the prostate, no growth outside the prostate (cT1c), grade group 1 (Gleason score 6 or less), low PSA (<10), very slow growth
Low-risk group	Larger than very-low-risk cancers (cT1 to cT2a), localized within the prostate, grade group 1 (Gleason score 6 or less), low PSA (<10), unlikely to cause symptoms or health problems
Intermediate-risk group	Can be felt on exam or seen on imaging (cT2b to cT2c), PSA between 10–20 ng/ml. Can be divided into favorable [Gleason 7 (3 + 4)/grade group 2] or unfavorable [Gleason 7 (4 + 3)/grade group 3] subcategories
High-risk group	Has one of the following features: Tumor grown outside the prostate (cT3a), grade group 4 or 5 (Gleason score 8–10), initial PSA >20. No very high-risk features
Very high-risk group	At least one of the following traits: Tumor spread to seminal vesicles (cT3b) or other structures (cT4), dominant Gleason 5 pattern, >4 cores with grade group 4 or 5, or 2–3 high-risk features

PSMA PET does not come without limitations. The expression of PSMA will be lost when prostate adenocarcinoma transforms to the aggressive neuroendocrine or small cell prostate cancer that produces no or minimal PSA. Antiandrogen therapy can modulate PSMA expression and therefore will have variable effects based on the tumor's hormone receptor expression and timing of therapeutic treatments [13]. Finally, a solitary bone lesion may be falsely interpreted as malignant when it may be a benign condition such as fibrous dysplasia [14]. It is also challenging to assess treatment response based on the maximum or mean PSMA uptakes on multiple metastatic lesions. Although the PROMISE V2 guidelines on standardizing PSMA PET reporting to assess treatment response have been proposed [15], this guideline is still at the maturing stage and has not been widely adopted in clinical practice or clinical research.

Bladder Cancer and the Use of MRI for Tumor Staging

Bladder cancer typically presents with painless hematuria which may be gross or microscopic. As up to 18 percent of adults have hematuria, it is often a benign finding that requires risk stratification to determine who needs further diagnostic evaluation. Full guidelines for this risk-based approach have been developed by the American Urological Association which include the sex, gender, smoking history, and the amount of red blood cells per high-power field on a urinalysis [16].

Initial workup for high-risk hematuria includes CT urogram or cystoscopy. If abnormal tissue is identified, this is followed by transurethral resection of bladder tumor (TURBT) to confirm the histopathologic diagnosis. Further imaging studies are performed to characterize the extent of the tumor invasion and evidence of metastasis. Although CT scan is the current study of choice, it may miss tumors <1 cm in size and may not be accurate to determine the depth of bladder-wall invasion. TUBRT is also known to frequently understage patients compared to final pathology at radical cystectomy [17]. This is suspected to be secondary to underestimation of the depth of local invasion and the presence of LN metastasis. One retrospective study of 279 patients demonstrated 48% of patients with cT1 disease were understaged with 30% higher cancer mortality due to this [18]. To improve upon this, based on MRI's high spatial resolution and soft-tissue contrast, it has been studied and shown to be better than CT to differentiate non-muscle-invasive bladder cancer (NMIBC) to MIBC [17]. Like PI-RADS in prostate cancer, VI-RADS, or Vesical Imaging Reporting and Data System, has been developed to standardize bladder MRI acquisition and interpretation [19].

Renal Cell Carcinoma and the Development of ^{89}Zr-Girentuximab PET/CT

RCC can be divided into six histology subtypes: clear cell (75%), papillary (10–15%), chromophobe (5%), collecting duct (1%), medullary (1%), and unclassified (2–3%) [20]. With the wide utilization of CT scan to work up benign conditions like abdominal pain, the incidence of small renal masses is on the rise every year. Other than RCC, a small renal mass could be a benign kidney tumor like an oncocytoma, angiomyolipoma, or metanephric adenoma. Due to the limitations of conventional CT, MRI, and FDG-PET scan to differentiate benign renal tumors from RCC, ^{89}Zr-girentuximab PET/CT is being developed to fulfill this task. Girentuxumab is a radiolabeled antibody against carbonic anhydrase IX (CAIX), a cell surface antigen that is expressed in up to 94% of clear cell RCC (ccRCC) [21]. The ^{89}Zr-girentuximab PET/CT interpretations of clinical T1 (≤ 7 cm) renal masses were compared to the histology of partial nephrectomy in the prospective, multicenter phase III ZIRCON trial. Among the 284 evaluable patients, the average sensitivity and specificity to diagnose ccRCC across different readers were 86% and 87%, respectively [22]. This impacts clinical decision-making as up to 30% of small renal masses removed by partial nephrectomy are benign [23]. Another potential application of the ^{89}Zr-girentuximab PET/CT is to assess ccRCC's response to cryoablation, as post procedure inflammation can limit the interpretation of contrast-enhanced follow-up CT or MRI.

Advancements in Perioperative Therapy of GU Cancers

The goal of perioperative therapy is to improve the cure rate or overall survival (OS) of localized cancer that is at high risk of recurrence. There are no data to support perioperative therapy in newly diagnosed high-risk prostate cancer. For high-risk prostate cancer patients electing for external beam radiation therapy (EBRT), intensification of androgen deprivation therapy (ADT) by adding 2 years of daily oral Cyp17 inhibitor and abiraterone acetate plus prednisone (AAP) to 3 years of androgen deprivation with luteinizing hormone-releasing hormone (LHRH) analog before, during, and after EBRT have been shown to prolong the OS in the phase 3 STAMPEDE trial [24]. High risk is defined as having reginal lymph node metastases (N1) or having at least 2 of the following risk factors if N0: clinical T3 or T4, Gleason 8–10, or PSA ≥40. Of note, further intensification of ADT by adding androgen receptor antagonist, enzalutamide to LHRH analog and AAP, did not add additional OS benefit compared to LHRH analog with AAP in this phase 3 STAMPEDE trial. UC and RCC will be the focus of our discussion on recent advancements in perioperative therapy of GU cancers.

Adjuvant Therapy for Clear Cell Renal Cell Carcinoma

Disease recurrence following partial or radical nephrectomy for ccRCC occurs in approximately half of the patients. Several randomized controlled phase III studies over the past decades have investigated adjuvant therapy for ccRCC to delay the disease recurrence and to improve OS. It started with adjuvant interferon-alpha, which failed to improve relapse-free survival or OS of resected pT3-4a and/or node-positive renal cell carcinoma [25]. Later, anti-VEGFR tyrosine kinase inhibitors were approved, resulting in the testing of sorafenib, sunitinib, pazopanib, and axitinib in the adjuvant setting. Except for the improvement in disease-free survival (DFS) seen with adjuvant sunitinib in the S-TARC trial [26], all the other adjuvant trials with anti-VEGFR TKIs failed to demonstrate clinical activities in delaying recurrence or prolonging survival despite their activities in metastatic RCC. Of note, adjuvant therapy with anti-VEGF monotherapy has also failed in other solid tumors like colorectal cancer.

Immune checkpoint inhibitor-based (ICI) therapy has now become a cornerstone in treating metastatic ccRCC. Adjuvant ICI therapies have been tested in multiple phase III trials for ccRCC with intermediate or high risk of recurrence after radical nephrectomy. The phase 3 KEYNOTE-564 trial was the first to demonstrate a significant improvement in DFS and OS with 1 year of pembrolizumab compared to placebo in ccRCC patients who were at intermediate or high risk for recurrence after radical nephrectomy [27]. This trial was a double-blinded, placebo-controlled trial that randomly assigned approximately 1000 patients with ccRCC with increased risk of recurrence post-surgery to receive pembrolizumab or placebo every 3 weeks for up to 17 cycles. Disease-free survival benefit, OS, and adverse events were measured within each group. After reporting a statistically significant improvement in DFS in 2021, a significant improvement in OS was reported in 2024 at the prespecified third interim analysis with a median follow-up of approximately 57 months [27]. Statistically significant improvements in DFS or OS, however, were not observed with other reported phase III adjuvant ICI trials, i.e., adjuvant atezolizumab (anti-PDL1) in Immotion 010 and adjuvant ipilimumab (anti-CTLA4) plus nivolumab (anti-PD1) in part A of CheckMate 914 [28, 29]. Of note, the inclusion criteria for intermediate and high-risk disease are slightly different among the three phase III adjuvant trials. In terms of pathological T2 staging (pT2), pT2a- (tumor measured between 7 and 10 cm) grade 4 and pT2b- (tumor is above 10 cm and limited to kidney) any grade were allowed in the CheckMate 914 trial, whereas only pathological T2-grade 4 resected clear cell dominant renal cell carcinoma were allowed in Keynote 564 and Immotion 010 trials. One year of adjuvant pembrolizumab is the current standard of care for ccRCC patients who are at intermediate or high risk for recurrence after radical nephrectomy.

Perioperative Therapy of Urothelial Carcinoma

Neoadjuvant Chemotherapy

Neoadjuvant chemotherapy has been shown to improve OS of patients with MIBC [30]. The gemcitabine-cisplatin and the MVAC (methotrexate, vinblastine, doxorubicin, and cisplatin) regimens are the two most commonly used chemotherapies in the neoadjuvant setting. The phase 3 VESPER trial randomized MIBC patients to either 6 cycles of dose-dense MVAC (ddMVAC) given at day 1 and day 2 of every 2 weeks (248 patients) versus 4 cycles of gemcitabine-cisplatin given day 1, day 8 every 3 weeks (245 patients) followed by radical cystectomy. At a recent update in 2024, the 5-year OS with ddMVAC was 66%, which was 57% with gemcitabine-cisplatin. The hazard ratio (HR) for OS was statistically significant with a value of 0.71 and 95% confidence interval of 0.52–0.97 [31].

One could argue the OS improvement seen in the VESPER trial is mainly from chemotherapy intensification and not every MIBC patient can tolerate six cycles of ddMVAC. The phase 3 Niagara trial compares four cycles of neoadjuvant gemcitabine-cisplatin with or without durvalumab given every 3 weeks followed by radical cystectomy. In the adjuvant setting, the durvalumab arm will also receive eight cycles of durvalumab versus observation in the chemotherapy only arm. When this study was reported in Sept. 2024 with a median follow-up of 42.3 months, a statistically significant improvement in event-free survival was noted [32]. Such improvement is seen regardless of PD-L1 expression level, pure urothelial carcinoma versus urothelial carcinoma with divergent histology. OS data are not yet mature, but a trend toward improved survival was noted. Adding durvalumab in the neoadjuvant setting is also well tolerated with no increase in treatment-related grade 3 or 4 adverse events.

Adjuvant Therapy in Urothelial Carcinoma

For patients who are not candidates for cisplatin due to impaired renal function, hearing loss, or poor performance status, the current standard of care is to proceed with radical cystectomy or bladder preservation with current chemoradiation therapy for selected patients. Even for patients who underwent cisplatin-based neoadjuvant chemotherapy, more than 50% of UC could have lack of pathological tumor downstaging or microscopic nodal metastases [33]. Adjuvant nivolumab is the only adjuvant therapy that is currently approved for urothelial cancer with high risk of recurrence after surgery. This approval is based on the phase 3 CheckMate 274 trial [34], which compares 1 year of adjuvant nivolumab versus placebo in patients with resected UC of the bladder or upper tract (capped at 25% of enrolled patients) that are at a high risk of recurrence. DFS was the primary endpoint, which was significantly prolonged with 1 year of adjuvant nivolumab. This DFS prolongation was more notable in UC of the bladder than UC of the ureter and renal pelvis/upper tract. The data on OS, a key secondary endpoint, are still immature. Statistically significant improvement in DFS was also reported with 1 year of adjuvant pembrolizumab versus placebo in the recently reported phase III AMBASSADOR trial [35].

Another notable area of active research in UC adjuvant therapy is to utilize circulating tumor DNA (ctDNA) as a liquid biomarker to detect minimal residual disease and to guide adjuvant therapy. Although the phase III IMvigor010 trial did not show a statistically significant improvement in DFS or OS with adjuvant atezolizumab (anti-PD-L1) compared to placebo [36], post hoc biomarker analysis revealed improvement in DFS an OS inpatients with positive ctDNA following surgery [37]. Post hoc analysis also reported that a greater reduction in ctDNA levels with atezolizumab was associated with longer OS [38]. Based on these findings, the ongoing IMvigor011 trial is selecting high-risk MIBC patients with positive ctDNA following cystectomy and randomizing them to adjuvant atezolizumab versus placebo.

Advances in Treating Metastatic GU Cancers

Metastatic Urothelial Carcinoma and Antibody Drug Conjugates as the New Corner Stone of Treatment

The biggest breakthrough in treating metastatic UC (mUC) in the past 20 years is the approval of enfortumab vedotin (EV), an antibody drug conjugate (ADC) that targets nectin-4 with a microtubule inhibitor, MMAE [39]. Nectin-4 is a cell adhesion molecule that is overexpressed in 83–87% of UC [39–41]. It is also expressed in normal skin and cornea. EV was initially approved as a monotherapy for treating cisplatin-ineligible mUC in the post ICI setting. It received FDA accelerated approval based on the 44% response rate and the 7.6 months median duration of response in the phase 2 EV-201 trial [42]. Such clinical benefits in the post platinum and or ICI setting were confirmed by the phase 3 EV-301 trial, which showed a 12.9 months median OS in the EV arm versus the 8.9 months median OS with the taxane or vinflunine chemotherapy arm [43, 44]. This was a global, open-label trial of over 600 patients with locally advanced or mUC who had already received platinum-containing chemotherapy and had disease progression during or after ICI therapy. Participants were randomized to EV or a chemotherapy with taxane or vinflunine, and the primary endpoints were OS, PFS, clinical response, and adverse events.

Much greater clinical benefits were seen when combining EV with pembrolizumab as a frontline therapy for locally advanced or mUC. The phase 3 EV-302 trial compared pembrolizumab plus EV to platinum-based chemotherapy in patients with previously untreated locally advanced or mUC [45]. At a median follow-up of 17.2 months, median PFS was 12.5 months, and median OS was 31.5 months in the EV-pembrolizumab group. Both outcomes were nearly doubled as opposed to the platinum chemotherapy arm. Furthermore, grade 3 or higher treatment-related adverse events were reduced by approximately 15% in the EV-pembrolizumab group. Of note, EV plus pembrolizumab have not been compared to EV monotherapy in the phase III setting. It is unclear how much clinical benefit pembrolizumab is adding to the highly effective EV regimen. Both treatments can cause skin toxicities, diarrhea, pneumonitis, and liver damages. Dose interruptions and reductions are not uncommon due to skin toxicities and elevated liver enzymes in real-world practice. Another common reason for dose interruption and reduction is peripheral neuropathy, which is mainly related to the MMAE payload of EV. For patients who developed grade 2 or above peripheral neuropathy, an alternative strategy would be continuing with pembrolizumab as a maintenance therapy if they achieved tumor reduction from the EV-pembrolizumab combination.

For mUC patients who are eligible for cisplatin, gemcitabine-cisplatin plus nivolumab is another frontline mUC regimen based on the phase 3 CheckMate 901 trial [46]. At a median follow-up of 33.6 months, statistically significant improvements in median OS, PFS, objective response rate, and complete response rate were reported by adding nivolumab to gemcitabine-cisplatin. Grade 3 or higher adverse events occurred at approximately a 10% higher rate in the three-drug arm compared to gemcitabine-cisplatin alone.

Trastuzumab deruxtecan is an ADC that targets HER2 with a potent topoisomerase I inhibitor. Due to the bystander effects with this ADC, it also works for HER2-low breast cancer. It received accelerated approval for adult patients with unresectable or metastatic HER2-positive (IHC3+) solid tumors who have received prior systemic treatment and have no satisfactory alternative treatment options in April 2024. This approval is based on the phase II DESTINY-Pantumor02 study. Among the 268 patients enrolled in this study, 41 patients had bladder cancer. The overall response rate was 56.3% in the 27 HER2 IHC 3+ bladder cancer patients, and the response rate was 35% in the remaining 14 patients with HER2 IHC 2+ bladder cancer [47]. Disitamab vedotin is another anti-HER2 ADC with the MMAE payload. Based on its efficacy in the early phase trials, it is being combined with pembrolizumab and compared to platinum-based chemotherapy as a frontline treatment for HER2 expressing (IHC 1–3+) locally advanced or metastatic UC.

Metastatic Renal Cell Carcinoma, Immune Checkpoint Inhibitor-Based Therapies, and Targeting Angiogenesis

In patients with locally advanced or metastatic ccRCC, systemic therapies fall under three main categories based on the mechanism of actions: ICI with either anti-PD1 (nivolumab and pembrolizumab) or anti-cytotoxic T-lymphocyte-associated protein 4 (CTLA-4) (ipilimumab); antiangiogenesis with either anti-VEGF receptor inhibitors (sunitinib, pazopanib, axitinib, Lenvatinib), or anti-VHL with belzutifan inhibitors; and targeting ccRCC survival with the mammalian (mechanistic) target of rapamycin/mTOR inhibitor such as everolimus. The selection of treatment depends on the risk stratification based on the International Metastatic RCC Database Consortium (IMDC) criteria. These criteria were developed based on patient outcomes with anti-VEGF therapy before ICI-based therapy became standard of care for metastatic RCC. The following risk factors were included in the IMDC criteria: Karnofsky performance score (KPS) less than 80%, less than 1 year from diagnosis to randomization, hemoglobin less than the lower limit of normal (LLN), corrected calcium concentration greater than the upper limit of normal (ULN), absolute neutrophil count greater than the ULN, and platelet count greater than the ULN. When the patient outcome data based on IMDC criteria were published in 2013, the median OS was 43·2 months in the favorable risk group with no risk factors, 22·5 months in the intermediate risk group with one to two risk factors, and 7·8 months in the poor risk group with three or more risk factors [48].

The IMDC criteria were then used in predefined risk stratification of all the ICI-based phase 3 randomized trials. Of note, the improved PFS and OS with frontline treatment with the ipilimumab and nivolumab combination versus sunitinib were mainly observed in the intermediate and poor risk, not good risk metastatic RCC [49]. The improved risk response rate, PFS and OS with the ICI plus anti-VEGFR therapy (pembrolizumab plus axitinib, nivolumab plus cabozantinib, and lenvatinib plus pembrolizumab) versus sunitinib as a frontline therapy for mRCC were reported in all risk categories in the phase 3 studies [50–52].

Metastatic Prostate Adenocarcinoma, Targeting Androgen Receptor and Beyond

Prior to 2010, the only life prolonging treatments for metastatic prostate cancer are LHRH analogs and docetaxel chemotherapy. Since 2010, 12 life prolonging treatments were approved. These include immunotherapy with sipuleucel-T; chemotherapy with cabazitaxel, new generation androgen receptor signaling pathway inhibitors (ARPI), abiraterone acetate (AA), enzalutamide, apalutamide, and darolutamide; radioligand therapy, radium 223, and Lutetium-177 (^{177}Lu)-PSMA-617; and poly ADP ribose polymerase inhibitor (PARPi), olaparib, rucaparib, talazaparib, and niraparib for metastatic castration-resistant prostate cancer (mCRPC) with deleterious mutation in BRCA1/2 or other genes involved in DNA homologous recombination pathways. There is an unmet need to develop new treatments for metastatic prostate cancer.

Androgen Deprivation Therapy and Second-Generation Androgen Receptor Pathway Inhibitors

Ever since Charles Higgins won the noble prize for prostate cancer androgen deprivation therapy (ADT) in 1963, ADT remains as the cornerstone for treatment of metastatic prostate adenocarcinoma with a response rate of 100% in treatment naïve patients. Blocking testosterone production by the testis with either LHRH agonist or antagonist is more preferred by the prostate cancer patients than surgical castration. 5-α reductase inhibitors are rarely used nowadays to treat prostate cancer due to its inferior activity compared to much more potent ARPIs. The new generation ARPIs include AR antagonists (enzalutamide, apalutamide, darolutamide), which blocks the action of testosterone, and the cyp17 inhibitor, AA, which blocks the production of testosterone by the cancer cells and the adrenal glands (Fig. 20.1).

One of the biggest advances in prostate cancer treatment in the past 5 years is prolongation of PFS and OS by early utilization of the new generation ARPI for combined ADT with an LHRH analog in the castration-sensitive setting. There are, however, cross resistances among the ARPIs. If patients progressed through combined ADT with an AR antagonist and LHRH analog, the response rate to AA is less

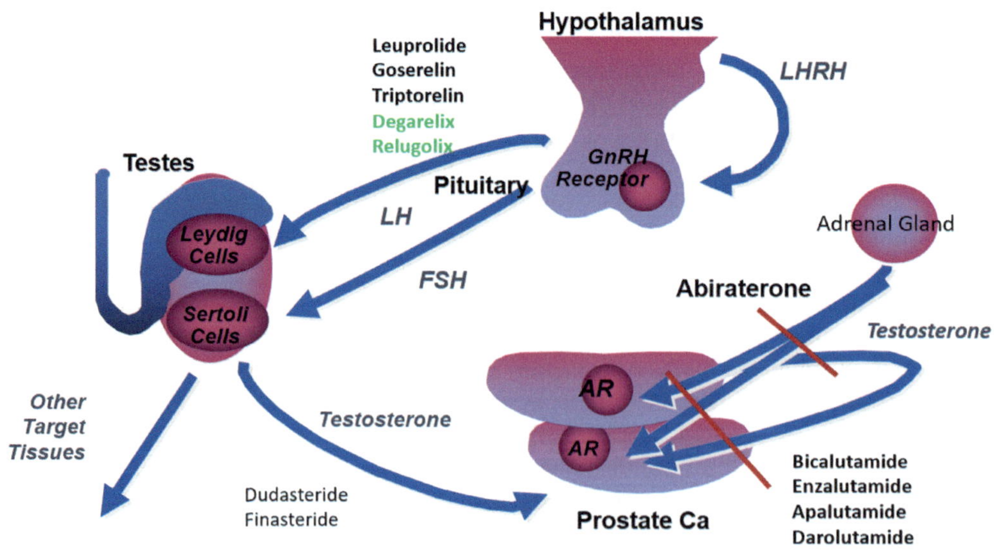

Fig. 20.1 Androgen deprivation therapy (ADT) and androgen receptor pathway inhibitors (ARPI): the cornerstones for treating advanced prostate cancer. *AR* androgen receptor, *LH* luteinizing hormone, *FSH* follicle-stimulating hormone

than 5%. Significant efforts have been spent over the past decade to develop drugs that would overcome the cross resistance. These include the failed attempts with Galeterone, which inhibits both CYP17 and AR and additionally induces AR protein degradation. Other failed attempts include CPI-1205, an EZH2 inhibitor, and EPI-7386, an AR N-terminal inhibitor, which have not been shown to provide meaningful clinical benefits either as monotherapy or added to ARPI in mCRPC after cancer progression through one line of ARPI. Currently, oral proteolysis targeting chimera degrader of AR: ARV-110/Bavdegalutamide and ARV-766 are under clinical development for mCRPC.

Immunotherapy for mCRPC

While ICIs are becoming increasingly used in UC and RCC, there has been lack of success of ICI in mCRPC either as monotherapy or in combination with docetaxel chemotherapy, enzalutamide, or PARPi. Prostate cancer is known to have reduced immunogenicity due to its immunosuppressive tumor microenvironment and low mutational burden with few tumor neoantigens [53].

Bispecific T-cell engagers (BiTEs) represent the biggest breakthrough in treating mCRPC with immunotherapy since the approval of sipuleucel-T in 2010. BiTEs are typically constructed with one antigen-binding domain to a cancer-specific tumor surface antigen while the other antigen-binding domain to a T-cell costimulatory receptor (i.e., CD3, CD28) to engage the T cell against the tumor antigen. The tumor surface antigens under clinical development include prostate-specific membrane antigen (PSMA), six-transmembrane epithelial antigen of prostate 1 (STEAP1), kallikrein-related peptidase 2 (KLK2), and prostate stem cell antigen (PSCA) [54]. Xaluritamig or AMG509 is an anti-STEAP1 xCD3 BiTE with enhanced preclinical activity based on a 2 + 1 design. Based on its promising clinical efficacy and safety data on heavily pretreated mCRPC in the phase I study [55], phase 3 trials with xaluritamig are being planned. Compared to the chimeric antigen receptor T-cell (CAR T) therapies tested in early phase trials for prostate cancer, BiTEs do not require lymphodepletion chemotherapy and immune-mediated side effects like cytokine release syndrome (CRS) tend to be less severe, occur early, and can be mitigated with step-up dosing.

PARPi and the PARPi-ARPI Combinations in Treating Metastatic Prostate Cancer

Deleterious mutations in DNA homologous recombination repair (HRR) genes are reported in about 25% of metastatic prostate cancer with BRCA2 as the most common mutated HRR genes [56]. Prostate cancers with germline mutations in BRCA2 are more likely to be diagnosed with high Gleason score, nodal or distant metastases at diagnosis compared to noncarriers [57]. With the approval of PARPi in treating mCRPC with deleterious mutations in HRR genes, it is now standard of care to screen for germline and somatic mutations in DNA repair genes after the diagnosis of metastatic prostate cancer. Based on the 2024 NCCN guidelines in prostate cancer, the germline mutation panel should include includes at least BRCA1, BRCA2, ATM, PALB2, CHEK2, HOXB13, MLH1, MSH2, MSH6, and PMS2. Although germline or somatic mutations in DNA mismatch repair genes, i.e., MLH1, MSH2, MSH6, and PMS2, represent <5% of prostate cancer, these mutations are typically associated with high tumor mutation burden and response to ICI therapy like pembrolizumab.

Olaparib and rucaparib [58, 59] are among the first two PARPi approved for mCRPC (Table 20.2). Preclinical studies indicated AR promoted DNA damage repair and the ADT upregulated PARP mediated DNA repair pathways. Three phase 3 randomized studies subsequently compared the PARPi plus ARPI combination versus ARPI as a front-line therapy for mCRPC with radiographic PFS (rPFS) as the primary endpoint and OS as a key secondary endpoint. Adding olaparib to AAP significantly prolonged rPFS versus AAP plus placebo in the unselected mCRPC population in the PROpel trial, and the rPFS and OS benefits were most notable in the BRCA1/2 mutated patients (11.8% enrolled patients) [60]. In addition to the all-comers cohort like the PROpel trial, the phase 3 TALAPRO-2 trial also included a cohort of mCRPC with known deleterious mutations in HRR genes [61]. Both cohorts met their primary endpoints of prolonging rPFS with enzalutamide plus talazoparib versus enzalutamide plus placebo. The rPFS benefits were most notable in patients with HRR mutations preselected patients based on their HRR mutation status. With 112 BRCA1/2 mutated mCRPC, MAGNITUDE trial included the largest number of BRCA-mutated patients among the three phase 3 trials. Compared to AAP plus placebo, niraparib plus AAP significantly improved rPFS in BRCA1/2 mutated mCRPC [62].

Table 20.2 *Poly(ADP-ribose) polymerase* (PARP) inhibitors and the DNA repair genes covered by each approved indication in metastatic castration resistant prostate cancer (mCRPC)

Olaparib	BRCA1, BRCA2, ATM, BRIP1, BARD1, CDK12, CHK1, CHK2, FANCL, PALB2, RAD51B, RAD51C, RDA51D, RAD51L
Rucaparib	BRCA1, BRCA2
Olaparib + abiraterone	BRCA1, BRCA2
Niraparib + abiraterone	BRCA1, BRCA2
Talazoparib + enzalutamide	BRCA1, BRCA2, ATM, ATR, CDk12, CHEK2, FANCA, MLH1, MRE11A, NBN, PALB2, RAD51C

Radioligand Therapy

The approval of Radium-223 dichloride (radium 223) in mCRPC in May 2013 represents the first approval of radioligand therapy in cancer treatment. Radium-223 is an alpha-particle-emitting calcium-mimetic radiopharmaceutical that selectively binds to areas of increased bone turnover [63]. Once bound, the alpha-particle radiation results in local cytotoxic effects in the areas of bone metastasis with reduced collateral damage to healthy tissue compared to the external beam radiation therapy. Radium 223 prolonged OS compared to placebo plus best supportive care in the phase III ALSYMPCA trial in patients with symptomatic mCRPC [64]. Of note, patients were enrolled in the ALSYMPCA trial between June 2008 and February 2011, before the new generation ARPI became widely available. The phase III PEACE-3 study enrolled asymptomatic or mildly symptomatic ARPI naïve mCRPC patients with bone metastases and randomized them 1:1 to 6 doses of radium 223 plus enzalutamide versus enzalutamide. When the preplanned interim analysis was first reported in September 2024, significant improvement in rPFS and OS was noted with the radium 223 and enzalutamide combination. No grade 3 or above treatment emerged adverse events were increased above 5% in the combination versus enzalutamide [65]. Given combined ADT with ARPI like enzalutamide is widely used nowadays in the castration-sensitive prostate cancer combined with the cross resistance among ARPIs, the clinical impacts of the PEACE-3 trial in the current treatment paradigm of mCRPC will likely be limited.

Unlike the alpha-particle radiation emitted by radium 223, lutetium Lu 177 vipivotide tetraxetan or ^{177}Lu-PSMA-617 is a radioligand with beta-particle radiation given by intravenous infusion once every 6 weeks [65]. ^{177}Lu-PSMA-617 is approved by FDA in March 2022 for mCRPC that has progressed through ARPI and at least one line of taxane-based chemotherapy. Such approval is based on the improvement in rPFS and OS in the phase III VISION trial [66]. Of note, PSMA PET scan was used to preselect patients for the VISION trial and patients with any PSMA-negative (PSMA PET uptake $\leq$ liver parenchyma) measurable metastatic lesions would be deemed ineligible for this study. As an end of line treatment option in mCRPC, best supportive care was used as the control in the VISION trial, and crossover to ^{177}Lu-PSMA-617 was not allowed at the time of progression.

The phase III PSMAfore trial subsequently evaluated ^{177}Lu-PSMA-617 versus ARPI switch in the PSMA PET-positive mCRPC that had progressed through one line of ARPI but not taxane [67]. Given chemotherapy would be preferred to ARSI switch based on the CARD trial [68], 2:1 randomization and crossover design was used for this trial. The primary endpoint on improvement of rPFS was met in both the first and the second interim analysis. No statistically significant improvement in OS, a key secondary endpoint, was observed in the second interim analysis with 82% of the patients in the ARSI switch arm had crossed over to ^{177}Lu-PSMA-617. Improvements in PSA, objective response rates, pain control, and health-related quality of life were also noted in patients treated with ^{177}Lu-PSMA-617 [69]. Other PSMA targeting radioligand therapies under late phase clinical development include 177Lu-DOTA-rosopatamab (TLX591) and177Lu-PNT2002 [54].

Conclusion

Genitourinary cancers affect millions of people per year, and as such, there are dire needs to advance the diagnosis and treatment of these cancers. The biggest diagnostic advancement in the past decade is likely the approval of PSMA PET scans for staging and treatment selection for prostate cancer. The ICI and anti-VEGF therapies have revolutionized treatment of mRCC. The clinical outcomes of mUC patients were significantly improved with EV monotherapy or in combination with pembrolizumab. The treatment paradigm for mCRPC has moved beyond targeting AR with the approval of radioligand therapies and the upcoming late phase clinical trials testing novel immunotherapies like BiTEs. In addition to developing new drugs, another important strategy to manage the incurable GU cancers would be finding better ways to use the existing drugs. As an alternative to the current treat until progression dogma, we and others have been pioneering adaptive therapy trials to integrate tumor evolutionary dynamics into the treatment of metastatic prostate cancer [70–72]. Our third-generation adaptive therapy trial in metastatic prostate cancer opened for enrollment in December 2024 with personalized modeling of PSA and testosterone kinetics (NCT06734130). Meanwhile, an adaptive therapy trial in metastatic RCC is also being planned. Overall, through a shared universal effort, we envision an improved treatment paradigm for the betterment of our patients.

References

1. Harris E. Prostate cancer cases might rise to 3 million globally by 2040. JAMA. 2024;331(20):1698.
2. Global Cancer Observatory: International Agency for Research on Cancer. World Health Organization. https://gco.iarc.fr/.
3. Pirola GM, Castellani D, Orecchia L, Giulioni C, Gubbiotti M, Rubilotta E, et al. Transperineal US-MRI fusion-guided biopsy for the detection of clinical significant prostate cancer: a systematic review and meta-analysis comparing cognitive and software-assisted technique. Cancers (Basel). 2023;15(13)
4. Watts KL, Frechette L, Muller B, Ilinksy D, Kovac E, Sankin A, et al. Systematic review and meta-analysis comparing cognitive vs. image-guided fusion prostate biopsy for the detection of prostate cancer. Urol Oncol. 2020;38(9):734.e19–25.

5. Schoots IG, Roobol MJ, Nieboer D, Bangma CH, Steyerberg EW, Hunink MG. Magnetic resonance imaging-targeted biopsy may enhance the diagnostic accuracy of significant prostate cancer detection compared to standard transrectal ultrasound-guided biopsy: a systematic review and meta-analysis. Eur Urol. 2015;68(3):438–50.
6. Hofman MS, Lawrentschuk N, Francis RJ, Tang C, Vela I, Thomas P, et al. Prostate-specific membrane antigen PET-CT in patients with high-risk prostate cancer before curative-intent surgery or radiotherapy (proPSMA): a prospective, randomised, multicentre study. Lancet. 2020;395(10231):1208–16.
7. Wondergem M, van der Zant FM, Broos WAM, Roeleveld TA, Donker R, Ten Oever D, et al. (18)F-DCFPyL PET/CT for primary staging in 160 high-risk prostate cancer patients; metastasis detection rate, influence on clinical management and preliminary results of treatment efficacy. Eur J Nucl Med Mol Imaging. 2021;48(2):521–31.
8. Hope TA, Goodman JZ, Allen IE, Calais J, Fendler WP, Carroll PR. Metaanalysis of (68)Ga-PSMA-11 PET accuracy for the detection of prostate cancer validated by histopathology. J Nucl Med. 2019;60(6):786–93.
9. Pozdnyakov A, Kulanthaivelu R, Bauman G, Ortega C, Veit-Haibach P, Metser U. The impact of PSMA PET on the treatment and outcomes of men with biochemical recurrence of prostate cancer: a systematic review and meta-analysis. Prostate Cancer Prostatic Dis. 2023;26(2):240–8.
10. Fendler WP, Weber M, Iravani A, Hofman MS, Calais J, Czernin J, et al. Prostate-specific membrane antigen ligand positron emission tomography in men with nonmetastatic castration-resistant prostate cancer. Clin Cancer Res. 2019;25(24):7448–54.
11. Hope TA, Jadvar H. Updates to appropriate use criteria for PSMA PET. J Nucl Med. 2022;63(5):14n.
12. Kratochwil C, Fendler WP, Eiber M, Hofman MS, Emmett L, Calais J, et al. Joint EANM/SNMMI procedure guideline for the use of (177)Lu-labeled PSMA-targeted radioligand-therapy ((177)Lu-PSMA-RLT). Eur J Nucl Med Mol Imaging. 2023;50(9):2830–45.
13. Emmett L, Yin C, Crumbaker M, Hruby G, Kneebone A, Epstein R, et al. Rapid modulation of PSMA expression by androgen deprivation: serial (68)Ga-PSMA-11 PET in men with hormone-sensitive and castrate-resistant prostate cancer commencing androgen blockade. J Nucl Med. 2019;60(7):950–4.
14. Phelps TE, Harmon SA, Mena E, Lindenberg L, Shih JH, Citrin DE, et al. Predicting outcomes of indeterminate bone lesions on (18)F-DCFPyL PSMA PET/CT scans in the setting of high-risk primary or recurrent prostate cancer. J Nucl Med. 2023;64(3):395–401.
15. Seifert R, Emmett L, Rowe SP, Herrmann K, Hadaschik B, Calais J, et al. Second version of the prostate cancer molecular imaging standardized evaluation framework including response evaluation for clinical trials (PROMISE V2). Eur Urol. 2023;83(5):405–12.
16. Barocas DA, Boorjian SA, Alvarez RD, Downs TM, Gross CP, Hamilton BD, et al. Microhematuria: AUA/SUFU guideline. J Urol. 2020;204(4):778–86.
17. Caglic I, Panebianco V, Vargas HA, Bura V, Woo S, Pecoraro M, et al. MRI of bladder cancer: local and nodal staging. J Magn Reson Imaging. 2020;52(3):649–67.
18. Ark JT, Keegan KA, Barocas DA, Morgan TM, Resnick MJ, You C, et al. Incidence and predictors of understaging in patients with clinical T1 urothelial carcinoma undergoing radical cystectomy. BJU Int. 2014;113(6):894–9.
19. Panebianco V, Briganti A, Boellaard TN, Catto J, Comperat E, Efstathiou J, et al. Clinical application of bladder MRI and the vesical imaging-reporting and data system. Nat Rev Urol. 2024;21(4):243–51.
20. Moch H, Cubilla AL, Humphrey PA, Reuter VE, Ulbright TM. The 2016 WHO classification of tumours of the urinary system and male genital organs – part A: renal, penile, and testicular tumours. Eur Urol. 2016;70(1):93–105.
21. Bui MH, Seligson D, Han KR, Pantuck AJ, Dorey FJ, Huang Y, et al. Carbonic anhydrase IX is an independent predictor of survival in advanced renal clear cell carcinoma: implications for prognosis and therapy. Clin Cancer Res. 2003;9(2):802–11.
22. Shuch B, Pantuck AJ, Bernhard JC, Morris MA, Master V, Scott AM, et al. [(89)Zr]Zr-girentuximab for PET-CT imaging of clear-cell renal cell carcinoma: a prospective, open-label, multicentre, phase 3 trial. Lancet Oncol. 2024;25(10):1277–87.
23. Kim JH, Li S, Khandwala Y, Chung KJ, Park HK, Chung BI. Association of Prevalence of benign pathologic findings after partial nephrectomy with preoperative imaging patterns in the United States from 2007 to 2014. JAMA Surg. 2019;154(3):225–31.
24. Attard G, Murphy L, Clarke NW, Cross W, Jones RJ, Parker CC, et al. Abiraterone acetate and prednisolone with or without enzalutamide for high-risk non-metastatic prostate cancer: a meta-analysis of primary results from two randomised controlled phase 3 trials of the STAMPEDE platform protocol. Lancet. 2022;399(10323):447–60.
25. Messing EM, Manola J, Wilding G, Propert K, Fleischmann J, Crawford ED, et al. Phase III study of interferon alfa-NL as adjuvant treatment for resectable renal cell carcinoma: an eastern cooperative oncology group/intergroup trial. J Clin Oncol. 2003;21(7):1214–22.
26. Motzer RJ, Ravaud A, Patard JJ, Pandha HS, George DJ, Patel A, et al. Adjuvant sunitinib for high-risk renal cell carcinoma after nephrectomy: subgroup analyses and updated overall survival results. Eur Urol. 2018;73(1):62–8.
27. Choueiri TK, Tomczak P, Park SH, Venugopal B, Ferguson T, Symeonides SN, et al. Overall survival with adjuvant pembrolizumab in renal-cell carcinoma. N Engl J Med. 2024;390(15):1359–71.
28. Pal SK, Uzzo R, Karam JA, Master VA, Donskov F, Suarez C, et al. Adjuvant atezolizumab versus placebo for patients with renal cell carcinoma at increased risk of recurrence following resection (IMmotion010): a multicentre, randomised, double-blind, phase 3 trial. Lancet. 2022;400(10358):1103–16.
29. Motzer RJ, Russo P, Grünwald V, Tomita Y, Zurawski B, Parikh O, et al. Adjuvant nivolumab plus ipilimumab versus placebo for localised renal cell carcinoma after nephrectomy (CheckMate 914): a double-blind, randomised, phase 3 trial. Lancet. 2023;401(10379):821–32.
30. Grossman HB, Natale RB, Tangen CM, Speights VO, Vogelzang NJ, Trump DL, et al. Neoadjuvant chemotherapy plus cystectomy compared with cystectomy alone for locally advanced bladder cancer. N Engl J Med. 2003;349(9):859–66.
31. Pfister C, Gravis G, Flechon A, Chevreau C, Mahammedi H, Laguerre B, et al. Perioperative dose-dense methotrexate, vinblastine, doxorubicin, and cisplatin in muscle-invasive bladder cancer (VESPER): survival endpoints at 5 years in an open-label, randomised, phase 3 study. Lancet Oncol. 2024;25(2):255–64.
32. Powles T, Catto JWF, Galsky MD, Al-Ahmadie H, Meeks JJ, Nishiyama H, et al. Perioperative Durvalumab with Neoadjuvant chemotherapy in operable bladder cancer. N Engl J Med. 2024;391(19):1773–86.
33. Rouprêt M, Babjuk M, Burger M, Capoun O, Cohen D, Compérat EM, et al. European association of urology guidelines on upper urinary tract urothelial carcinoma: 2020 update. Eur Urol. 2021;79(1):62–79.
34. Bajorin DF, Witjes JA, Gschwend JE, Schenker M, Valderrama BP, Tomita Y, et al. Adjuvant nivolumab versus placebo in muscle-invasive urothelial carcinoma. N Engl J Med. 2021;384(22):2102–14.

35. Apolo AB, Ballman KV, Sonpavde G, Berg S, Kim WY, Parikh R, et al. Adjuvant pembrolizumab versus observation in muscle-invasive urothelial carcinoma. N Engl J Med. 2025;392(1):45–55.
36. Bellmunt J, Hussain M, Gschwend JE, Albers P, Oudard S, Castellano D, et al. Adjuvant atezolizumab versus observation in muscle-invasive urothelial carcinoma (IMvigor010): a multicentre, open-label, randomised, phase 3 trial. Lancet Oncol. 2021;22(4):525–37.
37. Powles T, Assaf ZJ, Davarpanah N, Banchereau R, Szabados BE, Yuen KC, et al. ctDNA guiding adjuvant immunotherapy in urothelial carcinoma. Nature. 2021;595(7867):432–7.
38. Powles T, Assaf ZJ, Degaonkar V, Grivas P, Hussain M, Oudard S, et al. Updated overall survival by circulating tumor DNA status from the phase 3 IMvigor010 trial: adjuvant atezolizumab versus observation in muscle-invasive urothelial carcinoma. Eur Urol. 2024;85(2):114–22.
39. Challita-Eid PM, Satpayev D, Yang P, An Z, Morrison K, Shostak Y, et al. Enfortumab vedotin antibody-drug conjugate targeting Nectin-4 is a highly potent therapeutic agent in multiple preclinical cancer models. Cancer Res. 2016;76(10):3003–13.
40. Hoffman-Censits JH, Lombardo KA, Parimi V, Kamanda S, Choi W, Hahn NM, et al. Expression of Nectin-4 in bladder urothelial carcinoma, in morphologic variants, and nonurothelial histotypes. Appl Immunohistochem Mol Morphol. 2021;29(8):619–25.
41. Chatterjee S, Sinha S, Kundu CN. Nectin cell adhesion molecule-4 (NECTIN-4): a potential target for cancer therapy. Eur J Pharmacol. 2021;911:174516.
42. Yu EY, Petrylak DP, O'Donnell PH, Lee JL, van der Heijden MS, Loriot Y, et al. Enfortumab vedotin after PD-1 or PD-L1 inhibitors in cisplatin-ineligible patients with advanced urothelial carcinoma (EV-201): a multicentre, single-arm, phase 2 trial. Lancet Oncol. 2021;22(6):872–82.
43. Rosenberg JE, Powles T, Sonpavde GP, Loriot Y, Duran I, Lee JL, et al. EV-301 long-term outcomes: 24-month findings from the phase III trial of enfortumab vedotin versus chemotherapy in patients with previously treated advanced urothelial carcinoma. Ann Oncol. 2023;34(11):1047–54.
44. Powles T, Rosenberg JE, Sonpavde GP, Loriot Y, Durán I, Lee J-L, et al. Enfortumab vedotin in previously treated advanced urothelial carcinoma. N Engl J Med. 2021;384(12):1125–35.
45. Powles T, Valderrama BP, Gupta S, Bedke J, Kikuchi E, Hoffman-Censits J, et al. Enfortumab vedotin and pembrolizumab in untreated advanced urothelial cancer. N Engl J Med. 2024;390(10):875–88.
46. Heijden MSVD, Sonpavde G, Powles T, Necchi A, Burotto M, Schenker M, et al. Nivolumab plus gemcitabine–cisplatin in advanced urothelial carcinoma. N Engl J Med. 2023;389(19):1778–89.
47. Meric-Bernstam F, Makker V, Oaknin A, Oh DY, Banerjee S, González-Martín A, et al. Efficacy and safety of trastuzumab deruxtecan in patients with HER2-expressing solid tumors: primary results from the DESTINY-PanTumor02 phase II trial. J Clin Oncol. 2024;42(1):47–58.
48. Heng DY, Xie W, Regan MM, Harshman LC, Bjarnason GA, Vaishampayan UN, et al. External validation and comparison with other models of the international metastatic renal-cell carcinoma database consortium prognostic model: a population-based study. Lancet Oncol. 2013;14(2):141–8.
49. Motzer RJ, McDermott DF, Escudier B, Burotto M, Choueiri TK, Hammers HJ, et al. Conditional survival and long-term efficacy with nivolumab plus ipilimumab versus sunitinib in patients with advanced renal cell carcinoma. Cancer. 2022;128(11):2085–97.
50. Motzer RJ, Porta C, Eto M, Powles T, Grünwald V, Hutson TE, et al. Lenvatinib plus Pembrolizumab versus Sunitinib in first-line treatment of advanced renal cell carcinoma: final Prespecified overall survival analysis of CLEAR, a phase III study. J Clin Oncol. 2024;42(11):1222–8.
51. Rini BI, Plimack ER, Stus V, Gafanov R, Waddell T, Nosov D, et al. Pembrolizumab plus axitinib versus sunitinib as first-line therapy for advanced clear cell renal cell carcinoma: 5-year analysis of KEYNOTE-426. J Clin Oncol. 2023;41(17 suppl):LBA4501-LBA.
52. Motzer RJ, Powles T, Burotto M, Escudier B, Bourlon MT, Shah AY, et al. Nivolumab plus cabozantinib versus sunitinib in first-line treatment for advanced renal cell carcinoma (CheckMate 9ER): long-term follow-up results from an open-label, randomised, phase 3 trial. Lancet Oncol. 2022;23(7):888–98.
53. Meng L, Yang Y, Mortazavi A, Zhang J. Emerging immunotherapy approaches for treating prostate cancer. Int J Mol Sci. 2023;24(18)
54. Zhang J, Chadha JS. Developmental therapeutics in metastatic prostate cancer: new targets and new strategies. Cancers (Basel). 2024;16(17)
55. Kelly WK, Danila DC, Lin CC, Lee JL, Matsubara N, Ward PJ, et al. Xaluritamig, a STEAP1 × CD3 XmAb 2+1 immune therapy for metastatic castration-resistant prostate cancer: results from dose exploration in a first-in-human study. Cancer Discov. 2024;14(1):76–89.
56. Scott RJ, Mehta A, Macedo GS, Borisov PS, Kanesvaran R, El Metnawy W. Genetic testing for homologous recombination repair (HRR) in metastatic castration-resistant prostate cancer (mCRPC): challenges and solutions. Oncotarget. 2021;12(16):1600–14.
57. Castro E, Goh C, Olmos D, Saunders E, Leongamornlert D, Tymrakiewicz M, et al. Germline BRCA mutations are associated with higher risk of nodal involvement, distant metastasis, and poor survival outcomes in prostate cancer. J Clin Oncol. 2013;31(14):1748–57.
58. Bono J, Mateo J, Fizazi K, Saad F, Shore N, Sandhu S, et al. Olaparib for metastatic castration-resistant prostate cancer. N Engl J Med. 2020;382(22):2091–102.
59. Fizazi K, Piulats JM, Reaume MN, Ostler P, McDermott R, Gingerich JR, et al. Rucaparib or physician's choice in metastatic prostate cancer. N Engl J Med. 2023;388(8):719–32.
60. Clarke NW, Armstrong AJ, Thiery-Vuillemin A, Oya M, Shore N, Loredo E, et al. Abiraterone and Olaparib for metastatic castration-resistant prostate cancer. NEJM Evid. 2022;1(9):EVIDoa2200043.
61. Agarwal N, Azad AA, Carles J, Fay AP, Matsubara N, Heinrich D, et al. Talazoparib plus enzalutamide in men with first-line metastatic castration-resistant prostate cancer (TALAPRO-2): a randomised, placebo-controlled, phase 3 trial. Lancet. 2023;402(10398):291–303.
62. Chi KN, Rathkopf D, Smith MR, Efstathiou E, Attard G, Olmos D, et al. Niraparib and Abiraterone acetate for metastatic castration-resistant prostate cancer. J Clin Oncol. 2023;41(18):3339–51.
63. Bruland ØS, Nilsson S, Fisher DR, Larsen RH. High-linear energy transfer irradiation targeted to skeletal metastases by the alpha-emitter 223Ra: adjuvant or alternative to conventional modalities? Clin Cancer Res. 2006;12(20 Pt 2):6250s–7s.
64. Parker C, Nilsson S, Heinrich D, Helle SI, O'Sullivan JM, Fosså SD, et al. Alpha emitter Radium-223 and survival in metastatic prostate cancer. N Engl J Med. 2013;369(3):213–23.
65. Gillessen S, Choudhury A, Saad F, Gallardo E, Soares A, Loriot Y, et al. LBA1 A randomized multicenter open label phase III trial comparing enzalutamide vs a combination of Radium-223 (Ra223) and enzalutamide in asymptomatic or mildly symptomatic patients with bone metastatic castration-resistant prostate cancer (mCRPC): first results of EORTC-GUCG 1333/PEACE-3. Ann Oncol. 2024;35:S1254.
66. Sartor O, de Bono J, Chi KN, Fizazi K, Herrmann K, Rahbar K, et al. Lutetium-177-PSMA-617 for metastatic castration-resistant prostate cancer. N Engl J Med. 2021;385(12):1091–103.
67. Sartor O, Castellano Gauna DE, Herrmann K, de Bono JS, Shore ND, Chi KNN, et al. LBA13 phase III trial of [177Lu]Lu-PSMA-617 in taxane-naive patients with metastatic castration-resistant prostate cancer (PSMAfore). Ann Oncol. 2023;34:S1324–S5.

68. de Wit R, de Bono J, Sternberg CN, Fizazi K, Tombal B, Wülfing C, et al. Cabazitaxel versus Abiraterone or Enzalutamide in Metastatic Prostate Cancer. N Engl J Med. 2019;381(26):2506–18.
69. Fizazi K, Herrmann K, Krause BJ, Rahbar K, Chi KN, Morris MJ, et al. Health-related quality of life and pain outcomes with [(177)Lu]Lu-PSMA-617 plus standard of care versus standard of care in patients with metastatic castration-resistant prostate cancer (VISION): a multicentre, open-label, randomised, phase 3 trial. Lancet Oncol. 2023;24(6):597–610.
70. Zhang J, Cunningham JJ, Brown JS, Gatenby RA. Integrating evolutionary dynamics into treatment of metastatic castrate-resistant prostate cancer. Nat Commun. 2017;8(1):1816.
71. Zhang J, Cunningham J, Brown J, Gatenby R. Evolution-based mathematical models significantly prolong response to abiraterone in metastatic castrate-resistant prostate cancer and identify strategies to further improve outcomes. elife. 2022:11.
72. Zhang J, Gallaher J, Cunningham JJ, Choi JW, Ionescu F, Chatwal MS, et al. A phase 1b adaptive androgen deprivation therapy trial in metastatic castration sensitive prostate cancer. Cancers (Basel). 2022;14(21)

21 Research on GYN Cancer: Uterine, Ovarian, Vulvar

Monica Avila and Jared R. Funston

Background

Gynecologic malignancies remain one of the leading causes of death for women in the United States. The incidence of uterine, ovarian, and vulvar cancer is 28.3, 10.3, and 2.6 per 100,000 women per year. The incidence of these malignancies has been improving over the last 30 years. Unfortunately, uterine, ovarian, and vulvar cancer have a mortality rate of 5.3, 5.9, and 0.6 per 100,000 women per year [1–3]. The 5-year overall survival is largely impacted by stage at time of diagnosis. For uterine cancer, the 5-year overall survival varies from 95% for disease confined to the uterus to 19% for distant disease. For ovarian cancer, the majority of which are epithelial in origin, the 5-year overall survival varies from 93% for disease confined to the uterus to 31% for distant disease. For vulvar cancer, the 5-year overall survival varies from 86% for disease confined to the uterus to 19% for distant disease [4–6].

Prevention

Risk Factors

Uterine

The majority of uterine cancers are considered low-grade (grades 1 and 2) and stimulated by excess estrogen. Given this, many develop on a spectrum from precancer (endometrial intraepithelial neoplasia or EIN) to cancer. These are also present at an early stage and carry a good prognosis. The excess estrogen can be either produced in excess fat or taken exogenously. For example, an analysis of 14 case-control and ten cohort studies reviewing 14,000 endometrial cancer cases, the odds of developing a low-grade endometrial-type cancer based on BMI was 1.5 OR for overweight (BMI 25.0 to <30.0 kg/m^2), 2.5 OR in class 1 obesity (BMI 30.0 to <35.0 kg/m^2), 4.5 OR in class 2 obesity (BMI 35.0 to 39.9 kg/m^2), and 7.1 OR in class 3 obesity (BMI ≥40.0 kg/m^2) [7]. For high-grade (grade 3) cancers such as serous or clear cell cancers, risk factors include lower BMI, lower parity, black race, older age, and history of breast cancer.

Ovarian

The incidence of epithelial ovarian cancer increases with increasing age. In the large epidemiologic Nurses' Health Study, for women ≥50 years old, every year of life was associated with an increased risk of 11% [8]. A family history of ovarian cancer with one first- or second-degree relative can increase the risk of ovarian cancer, as well as early menarche, late menopause beyond age 52 [9, 10]. Pathogenic variants such as *BRCA1* and *BRCA2* have the greatest association with ovarian cancer. A history of nulliparity, endometriosis, and asbestos has been associated with increased risk as well [11, 12].

Vulvar

Vulvar or cervical dysplasia, history of cervical cancer, cigarette smoking, vulvar lichen sclerosus, immunodeficiency syndromes, and northern European ancestry are all risk factors for developing vulvar cancer [13, 14]. Human papillomavirus (HPV) infection can be a risk factor for dysplasia and the evolution of vulvar carcinoma. In a 92-study meta-analysis, HPV 16 was associated with approximately 40% of cases [15].

M. Avila (✉)
Department of Gynecologic Oncology, H Lee Moffitt Cancer Center, Tampa, FL, USA
e-mail: Monica.Avila@moffitt.org

J. R. Funston
Department of Surgery, AdventHealth Tampa, Tampa, FL, USA
e-mail: Jared.Funston@adventhealth.com

J. Huang, H. S.L. Jim (eds.), *Cancer Research Guidance for Clinicians and Researchers*,
https://doi.org/10.1007/978-3-032-19175-5_21

Screening

Currently, there are no standard screening options available for these malignancies. Therefore, diagnoses rely heavily on symptomatic presentation and confirmatory imaging. Patients may present with pelvic pain, vaginal bleeding, abdominal bloating, early satiety, and weight loss. Formal diagnosis for early-stage ovarian cancers is made by pathologic assessment through surgical excision to prevent spillage or seeding. For more advanced-stage ovarian cancers, diagnosis is made through diagnostic biopsies via interventional radiology or the operating room. In uterine and vulvar cancers, pre-treatment biopsies are performed via endometrial pipelle and vulvar punch biopsy. Once pathologic confirmation is obtained, these cancers are traditionally staged surgically and assisted by radiographic imaging to assess for metastatic disease.

Surgical Prevention/Vaccination

Hereditary mutations, such as BRCA, can carry an increased risk of ovarian and uterine cancers. Prophylactic surgery to remove the ovaries and/or uterus before the known age of onset can prevent the evolution of these cancers. For vulvar cancers, HPV (human papillomavirus) vaccination is the only existing primary prevention. A prospective Italian study evaluated the efficacy of HPV vaccination on the treatment of surgical pre-cancers following surgical excision. The study included 118 women, of whom 42 were vaccinated, noting a recurrence rate of 19% in the vaccinated group compared to 32% in the unvaccinated group [16]. The CDC currently recommends vaccination for females and males between ages 9 and 45 with a two- or three-dose series [17].

Treatment

Uterine

Treatment for early-stage uterine cancer is based on surgical intervention, which in some cases can be curative. Surgery consists of minimally invasive hysterectomy whenever feasible, with sentinel lymph node biopsy evaluation +/− removal of the ovaries. For those patients with high-risk factors or high-grade histologies, adjuvant chemotherapy +/− radiation therapy can be considered. Late-stage disease consists of chemotherapy plus immunotherapy plus immunotherapy maintenance. Hysterectomy can be considered based on symptoms [18]. In the last 5 years, two pivotal phase 3 randomized controlled trials have solidified the addition of immunotherapy to chemotherapy in the adjuvant frontline and advanced setting [19, 20].

Ovarian

Current treatment for early-stage ovarian cancer is rooted in surgical intervention with or without adjuvant chemotherapy. Surgical treatment involves staging with removal of the pelvic organs, including any ovarian masses, pelvic and para-aortic lymph node dissection, and omentectomy. Late-stage disease is focused on surgical debulking whenever feasible. This includes removal of the pelvic organs, omentectomy, and removal of any visible signs of cancer. This is followed by adjuvant platinum-based chemotherapy and maintenance therapy. Maintenance is given in the form of oral therapy with PARP inhibitor therapy and/or a biologic such as bevacizumab. In the setting of a recurrence, platinum-based chemotherapy is used until a patient becomes platinum-resistant, at which point the treatment algorithm shifts to non-platinum-based chemotherapy and new age therapies such as antibody-drug conjugates and immunotherapy, which are expanding on a daily basis [21].

Vulvar

For vulvar cancers, upfront treatment consists of surgical resection with or without adjuvant radiation. Surgical resection includes resection of the primary vulvar tumor and sentinel inguinal lymph node dissection. Surgical margins dictate radiation of the primary tumor site, and nodal positivity dictates radiation of the inguinal nodal beds. In advanced disease up to stage 4a, a cure can be potentially achieved with chemotherapy and radiation. For distant metastatic disease, systemic therapy has been explored with combination chemotherapy, immunotherapy, and biologics with maintenance immunotherapy [22].

Survival

Overall survival is driven by stage at time of diagnosis for gynecologic malignancies. For all epithelial ovarian cancers, the 5-year overall survival rate is 50% for all stages, with 93% for localized disease and 31% for advanced stage disease [23]. According to a 2015 NCDB, National Cancer Database, article focused on the care distribution of ovarian cancer, comprehensive community cancer programs treated 44.6% of cases, and community cancer programs accounted for another 12.3%, while academic comprehensive centers accounted for 43.1% of cases. Drivers of overall survival were based on case volume and guideline-centered care, suggesting that national efforts should focus on expanding and improving care in high-volume community care programs [24]. For uterine cancers, the 5-year overall survival rate is 81% for all stages, with 95% for localized disease and 19% for advanced stage disease [23]. For vulvar cancers, the 5-year overall survival rate is 71% for all stages, with 86% for localized disease and 19% for advanced stage disease [23].

On a national scale for the treatment of gynecologic malignancies, the National Research Group (NRG), founded in 1989, has impacted therapeutic options and survival by bringing large-scale clinical trials to communities nationwide [25]. The National Research Group (NRG) is one of five national cancer cooperative groups currently funded by the National Cancer Institute (NCI) as part of the National Clinical Trials Network (NCTN) to help advance research to improve survival for sex-specific cancers, including gynecologic, breast, and prostate malignancies. From the NRG surfaced an interconnected approach to community research, driven by both the NCI NCTN and the National Community Oncology Research Program (NCORP) [26]. NCTN and NCORP are both national networks that were launched in 2014 to advance trial access to patients in all kinds of practice settings, particularly in community settings, expediting accruals. Community sites run through the NCORP account for 33% of all patient accruals to NRG clinical trials, showing the mass benefit community research can provide [27]. To date, NRG trials have led to several practice-changing therapeutic approvals through the FDA and continue to improve survival in patients with gynecologic cancers. Below, we will focus on the strengths and limitations of research being conducted in a community setting through local, regional, and national avenues such as the NRG.

Strengths of Performing Research in a Community Setting

Regionally and locally, community research frequently arises from problems that are encountered by individual providers who receive the mass volume of upfront treatment of many gynecologic cancer patients. A recent retrospective cohort study of uterine cancer patients in a large oncology network across the United States showed that the majority of women diagnosed with uterine cancer (82.7%) received upfront treatment in a community setting [28].

Although many community locations lack resources for large trials without the help of federal funding, many real-world questions and their solutions arise from community research.

Specifically, research focused on social determinants of care, patient adherence to care, and treatment implementation can improve the delivery of care. This is largely feasible due to the concentration of cancer care within one to two providers in the community, whereas in an academic setting, this may become more piecemeal due to the availability of specialists and subspecialists. Centralizing the care within a single provider allows for closer follow-up and direct identification of patient concerns. This close connection between the provider/researcher and the patient allows for better identification of changes in the participant during the research intervention period. Community research has the benefit of a social interconnectedness to the community it serves, allowing for identification of the resources and barriers to care that may or may not be encountered during complex cancer treatment. For example, a community hospital is usually based in/near the home of the study participants, increasing the patient's chances of reaching and receiving treatment at the research site. This increases the rates of available and evaluable patients in local studies.

Community research is uniquely positioned to identify disparities in treatment and outcomes. Academic centers are largely driven by community referrals and can inherently exclude disadvantaged patients. There are fewer competing interests when working in a community setting, allowing for the community hospital to focus its resources on fewer, high-impact projects. In 2023, a prospectively collected social needs survey administered to gynecologic oncology patients showed that three factors were deemed most important in receiving their cancer care: transportation, housing insecurity, and desire to speak with a social worker. Of the patients identified by the survey, 78% were seen by a cancer care navigator and received community resources based on their needs assessment [29].

Drawbacks of Performing Research in a Community Setting

Compared to community institutions, the catchment area for a research institution is usually larger, increasing the pool of potential patients that can be enrolled in clinical research studies. This can increase the statistical power of academic research, allowing for the study of rarer conditions and novel interventions. Community providers often play the role of multiple providers given limited resources, but this is often limited. Larger institutions can offer access to multiple specialties, consolidating the patient's care into one location. A prior study of the California Cancer Registry of over 14,000 women with ovarian cancer noted that living closer to a high-quality center was associated with receiving guideline-concordant care, including fertility-preservation methods for those who qualified [30]. However, a recent cohort study evaluating whether patients with ovarian, cervical, and uterine cancers were offered fertility-sparing care in an urban vs. rural setting noted no differences between the groups [31]. This could be possible due to a growth potential over time in the community, allowing for novel fertility-sparing methods to trickle into the community after being studied and popularized in an academic setting. Academic centers also have dedicated translational researchers, allowing for the onset of preclinical foundational research. The budgets of academic research institutions have dedicated financial and personnel resources to pursue such preclinical and clinical research strategies. Therefore, the focus of studies in these communities would then be honed toward outcomes after novel practice patterns have been put into standard practice.

Strategies for High-Impact Research in a Community Setting

In order to have a significant impact in the community setting, there are several techniques that can be used to overcome the disparity with larger academic institutions. Firstly, creating a strong core research team is critical in maintaining research momentum. If the team is lacking in individuals strong in research design and implementation, then several options are available. One, the team or researcher can use independent online resources. Two, the team can collaborate with private research contractors or larger research centers. This collaboration can be pursued at various levels (national, regional, and local, if available), harnessing the brain trust of academic and community individuals. National organizations such as the NRG previously discussed and subcontractors such as the GOG can provide funding and access. This can provide direct or indirect access to clinical research, clinical resources, and professional organizations to further expand research practices. Secondly, the community researcher should establish internal support within the administration of the practice/hospital for their research. Given the positive publicity, many institutions can find monetary or personnel support for research endeavors. Community research should be tailored to the strengths of the institution, making it marketable to the administration. Gynecologic research may include debatable topics, including fertility-sparing and reproductive research practices. In such scenarios, support from local individuals or interest groups can be used to garner grassroots support for research.

Study Design and Methodology Considerations

When conducting research in a community setting, both observational and interventional studies can be initiated. Conducting single-site observational studies and quality improvement projects is a less resource-intensive first step to collect the baseline data to garner community support and necessary funding. The time and database complexity requirements are both low in this situation. The qualitative analysis of this dataset is appropriately placed into a clinical context by the practitioners. Additional quantitative data can then be referred to a freestanding statistical analysis firm or an independent consultant for low fees. Common software such as Excel(R) can be readily used to create even quite sophisticated databases for this level of information. Care must be taken in these settings to properly protect patient health information. This can normally be accomplished by de-identifying information in the database. Community health organizations, like departments of health, can provide data, insights, and even assistance in the analysis of the data from a clinic if there are additional community health implications. Once collaboration and funding are secure, these studies can then translate into larger prospective and interventional clinical trials.

Summary

Community-based research can have highly impactful and clinical applicability. The majority of gynecologic cancer patients receive their care in community settings, making it more likely that optimization of cancer care delivery in this setting is the most likely strategy to impact their survival. National networks have increased the ability of local communities to have access to current and potentially high-yield clinical trials. Community-focused research has a focus on the needs of patients in those communities and has the greatest potential to increase compliance with treatment and outcomes of care.

References

1. Uterine Cancer—Cancer Stat Facts. Accessed 9 Apr 2025. [Online]. https://seer.cancer.gov/statfacts/html/corp.html
2. Ovarian Cancer—Cancer Stat Facts. Accessed 9 Apr 2025. [Online]. Available: https://seer.cancer.gov/statfacts/html/ovary.html
3. Vulvar Cancer—Cancer Stat Facts. Accessed 9 Apr 2025. [Online]. Available: https://seer.cancer.gov/statfacts/html/vulva.html
4. SEER*Explorer Application. Accessed 31 Mar 2025. [Online]. Available: https://seer.cancer.gov/statistics-network/explorer/application.html?site=63&data_type=4&graph_type=6&compareBy=race&chk_race_1=1&chk_race_6=6&chk_race_5=5&chk_race_4=4&chk_race_8=8&chk_race_3=3&chk_race_2=2&hdn_sex=3&age_range=1&stage=101&advopt_precision=1&advopt_show_ci=on&hdn_view=0&advopt_show_apc=on&advopt_display=2#resultsRegion0
5. SEER*Explorer Application. Accessed 31 Mar 2025. [Online]. Available: https://seer.cancer.gov/statistics-network/explorer/application.html?site=61&data_type=4&graph_type=6&compareBy=race&chk_race_1=1&chk_race_6=6&chk_race_5=5&chk_race_4=4&chk_race_8=8&chk_race_3=3&chk_race_2=2&hdn_sex=3&age_range=1&stage=101&advopt_precision=1&advopt_show_ci=on&hdn_view=0&advopt_show_apc=on&advopt_display=2#resultsRegion0
6. SEER*Explorer Application. Accessed 31 Mar 2025. [Online]. Available: https://seer.cancer.gov/statistics-network/explorer/application.html?site=58&data_type=4&graph_type=6&compareBy=race&chk_race_1=1&chk_race_6=6&chk_

race_5=5&chk_race_4=4&chk_race_8=8&chk_race_3=3&chk_race_2=2&hdn_sex=3&age_range=1&stage=101&advopt_precision=1&advopt_show_ci=on&hdn_view=0&advopt_show_apc=on&advopt_display=2#resultsRegion0
7. Setiawan VW, et al. Type I and II endometrial cancers: have they different risk factors? J Clin Oncol. 2013;31(20):2607–18. https://doi.org/10.1200/JCO.2012.48.2596.
8. Gates MA, Rosner BA, Hecht JL, Tworoger SS. Risk factors for epithelial ovarian cancer by histologic subtype. Am J Epidemiol. 2010;171(1):45–53. https://doi.org/10.1093/AJE/KWP314.
9. Tsilidis KK, et al. Oral contraceptive use and reproductive factors and risk of ovarian cancer in the European prospective investigation into cancer and nutrition. Br J Cancer. 2011;105(9):1436–42. https://doi.org/10.1038/BJC.2011.371.
10. Should women with familial ovarian cancer undergo prophylactic oophorectomy?—PubMed. Accessed 17 May 2025. [Online]. Available: https://pubmed.ncbi.nlm.nih.gov/1407898/
11. Constanza Camargo M, et al. Occupational exposure to asbestos and ovarian cancer: a meta-analysis. Environ Health Perspect. 2011;119(9):1211–7. https://doi.org/10.1289/EHP.1003283.
12. Barnard ME, et al. Endometriosis typology and ovarian cancer risk. JAMA. 2024;332(6):482–9. https://doi.org/10.1001/JAMA.2024.9210.
13. Madsen BS, Jensen HL, Van Den Brule AJC, Wohlfahrt J, Frisch M. Risk factors for invasive squamous cell carcinoma of the vulva and vagina–population-based case-control study in Denmark. Int J Cancer. 2008;122(12):2827–34. https://doi.org/10.1002/IJC.23446.
14. Brinton LA, Thistle JE, Liao LM, Trabert B. Epidemiology of vulvar neoplasia in the NIH-AARP study. Gynecol Oncol. 2017;145(2):298–304. https://doi.org/10.1016/j.ygyno.2017.02.030.
15. Li Z, et al. Prevalence of human papillomavirus DNA and p16INK4a positivity in vulvar cancer and vulvar intraepithelial neoplasia: a systematic review and meta-analysis. Lancet Oncol. 2023;24(4):403–14. https://doi.org/10.1016/S1470-2045(23)00066-9.
16. Ghelardi A, et al. Surgical treatment of vulvar HSIL: adjuvant HPV vaccine reduces recurrent disease. Vaccines (Basel). 2021;9(2):1–12. https://doi.org/10.3390/VACCINES9020083.
17. HPV Vaccination Recommendations | CDC. Accessed 28 May 2025. [Online]. Available: https://www.cdc.gov/vaccines/vpd/hpv/hcp/recommendations.html
18. Uterine Neoplasms – Guidelines Detail. Accessed 26 Apr 2025. [Online]. Available: https://www.nccn.org/guidelines/guidelines-detail?category=1&id=1473
19. Eskander RN, et al. Pembrolizumab plus chemotherapy in advanced endometrial cancer. N Engl J Med. 2023;388(23):2159–70. https://doi.org/10.1056/NEJMOA2302312/SUPPL_FILE/NEJMOA2302312_DATA-SHARING.PDF.
20. Mirza MR, et al. Dostarlimab for primary advanced or recurrent endometrial cancer. N Engl J Med. 2023;388(23):2145–58. https://doi.org/10.1056/NEJMOA2216334/SUPPL_FILE/NEJMOA2216334_DATA-SHARING.PDF.
21. Ovarian Cancer/Fallopian Tube Cancer/Primary Peritoneal Cancer—Guidelines Detail. Accessed 26 Apr 2025. [Online]. Available: https://www.nccn.org/guidelines/guidelines-detail?category=1&id=1453
22. Vulvar Cancer – Guidelines Detail. Accessed 26 Apr 2025. [Online]. Available: https://www.nccn.org/guidelines/guidelines-detail?category=1&id=1476
23. Ovarian Cancer Survival Rates | Ovarian Cancer Prognosis | American Cancer Society. Accessed 29 May 2025. [Online]. Available: https://www.cancer.org/cancer/types/ovarian-cancer/detection-diagnosis-staging/survival-rates.html
24. Cliby WA, et al. Ovarian cancer in the United States: contemporary patterns of care associated with improved survival. Gynecol Oncol. 2015;136(1):11–7. https://doi.org/10.1016/j.ygyno.2014.10.023.
25. Scientific Focus. Accessed 19 Mar 2025. [Online]. Available: https://www.nrgoncology.org/About-Us/Who-We-Are-What-We-Do/Scientific-Focus
26. NRG > Committees & Programs > NRG NCORP Research Base > NCORP Resources. Accessed 26 Apr 2025. [Online]. Available: https://www.nrgoncology.org/Committees-Programs/NRG-NCORP-Research-Base/NCORP-Resources
27. Bruner D. NRG Oncology NCORP NRG NCORP Research Base PIs.
28. Monk BJ, et al. Real-world outcomes in patients with advanced endometrial cancer: a retrospective cohort study of US electronic health records. Gynecol Oncol. 2022;164(2):325–32. https://doi.org/10.1016/J.YGYNO.2021.12.008.
29. Cotangco K, Pineda E, Hingarh V, Nyakudarika NC, Cohen JG, Holschneider CH. Integrating social care into gynecologic oncology: identifying and addressing patient's social needs. Gynecol Oncol. 2023;179:138–44. https://doi.org/10.1016/J.YGYNO.2023.11.001.
30. Villanueva C, Chang J, Bartell SM, Ziogas A, Bristow R, Vieira VM. Contribution of geographic location to disparities in ovarian cancer treatment. JNCCN J Natl Compr Cancer Netw. 2019;17(11):1318–29. https://doi.org/10.6004/JNCCN.2019.7325.
31. Jorgensen K, et al. Disparities in fertility-sparing treatment and use of assisted reproductive technology after a diagnosis of cervical, ovarian, or endometrial cancer. Obstet Gynecol. 2023;141(2):341–53. https://doi.org/10.1097/AOG.0000000000005044.

Research on Soft Tissue Sarcoma

22

Leah E. Hendrick, Jae Hwan Choi, Sarah C. Tepper, Alexander Lazarides, and Rachel K. Voss

Abbreviations

STS	Soft tissue sarcoma
LFS	Li-Fraumeni syndrome
NCI	National Cancer Institute
NF1	Neurofibromatosis type 1
TARPSWG	Trans-Atlantic Retroperitoneal Sarcoma Working Group
SARC	Sarcoma Alliance for Research through Collaboration
IFS	Infantile fibrosarcoma
MRI	Magnetic resonance imaging
CT	Computed tomography
IHC	Immunohistochemistry
FISH	Fluorescence in situ hybridization
PCR	Polymerase chain reaction
DFSP	Dermatofibrosarcoma protuberans
MMP	Matrix metalloproteinase
VEGF	Vascular endothelial growth factor
LMS	Leiomyosarcoma
MAI	Mesna/adriamycin (doxorubicin)/ifosfamide
RMS	Rhabdomyosarcoma
ctDNA	Circulating tumor DNA
WDLPS	Well-differentiated liposarcoma
DDLPS	Dedifferentiated liposarcoma
SS	Synovial sarcoma
IMRT	Intensity modulated radiotherapy
SBRT	Sterotactic body radiotherapy
PFS	Progression-free survival
TCR	T-cell receptor

L. E. Hendrick (✉) · S. C. Tepper · A. Lazarides · R. K. Voss
Sarcoma Department, H. Lee Moffitt Cancer Center and Research Institute, Tampa, FL, USA
e-mail: Leah.Hendrick@moffitt.org

J. H. Choi
Department of Surgery, University of South Florida College of Medicine, Tampa, FL, USA

Introduction

Approximately 14,000 soft tissue and bone cancers were diagnosed in the United States in 2025, accounting for less than 1% of adult cancer diagnoses [1]. While even as a broad category, sarcomas meet the National Cancer Institute's (NCI) definition of rare cancers (<15 cases per 100,000 population yearly) [2], this number encompasses nearly 100 distinct sarcoma subtypes, making each individual subtype exceedingly rare. Although the etiology of most sarcomas is thought to be sporadic [3], there are known risk factors for some subtypes. Unlike most malignancies, younger age is associated with a higher risk of sarcoma diagnosis, leading to a disproportionate loss of life-years despite its rare nature. Sarcomas are currently the third leading cause of cancer death in patients under 20 years old and the fifth in patients 20–39 years old [1]. Chronic lymphedema and radiation exposure are associated with increased risk of angiosarcoma. A number of rare inherited syndromes, including Li-Fraumeni [4], neurofibromatosis type 1 (NF1) [5], Gardner syndrome [6], and Werner syndrome [7], are also associated with an increased risk of certain types of sarcomas. Certain chemical exposures, such as phenoxyacetic acid in herbicides and pesticides, as well as anthracyclines and alkylating agent exposures in children, have also been linked to the development of sarcoma.

Management of soft tissue sarcomas of the extremity and trunk involves wide surgical resection with the goal of achieving negative margins, with the addition of radiation therapy for high-grade tumors larger than 5 cm. Neoadjuvant radiation therapy is preferred for large tumors and for those likely to require flap coverage. Chemotherapy is generally reserved for select high-risk histologic subtypes such as synovial sarcoma, angiosarcoma, and high-grade undifferentiated pleomorphic sarcoma, or in the metastatic setting. For retroperitoneal sarcomas, surgery is also the primary treatment, often requiring en bloc resection of adjacent organs to achieve complete resection. The use of radiation for retro-

J. Huang, H. S.L. Jim (eds.), *Cancer Research Guidance for Clinicians and Researchers*,
https://doi.org/10.1007/978-3-032-19175-5_22

peritoneal sarcomas is more selective but may be considered preoperatively in specific histologies like liposarcoma [8]. Systemic therapy decisions are nuanced and are guided by histologic subtype, grade, and disease extent [9]. Clinical, translational, and basic science research in soft tissue sarcoma is uniquely challenging due to its marked heterogeneity combined with the rare nature of the disease. Because of this, sarcoma research relies heavily on multi-institutional and even multinational collaboration, with many of the most impactful studies coming out of groups like the Trans-Atlantic Retroperitoneal Sarcoma Working Group (TARPSWG) and the Sarcoma Alliance for Research through Collaboration (SARC) group. Despite challenges, there has been considerable progress in our understanding of the disease biology of the more common sarcoma subtypes, as well as advances in treatment and outcomes. The goal of this chapter is to summarize recent progress in clinical and translational research for the most common sarcoma subtypes.

Angiosarcoma

Angiosarcoma is a rare, aggressive malignancy of endothelial origin, representing 1–2% of all soft tissue sarcomas, and is the most common radiation-associated sarcoma subtype. It arises from blood vessels or lymphatics and may occur at any anatomic location rich in lymphovascular supply. The incidence is approximately 1.5–1.8 cases per 1,000,000 person-years, with the majority of cases involving skin, soft tissue, or visceral organs [10]. Visceral angiosarcoma is exceedingly rare [11].

Angiosarcomas can be classified either as primary or secondary; primary angiosarcomas occur de novo, whereas secondary angiosarcomas develop in association with other predisposing factors such as prior radiation, chronic lymphedema (also known as Stewart-Treves syndrome), foreign bodies such as orthopedic implants or Dacron grafts, or exposure to carcinogens such as vinyl chloride, arsenic, and thorium dioxide [12–15]. Hepatic angiosarcoma in particular is strongly associated with exposure to carcinogens such as vinyl chloride and thorium dioxide [13, 16].

Advanced-stage disease is common at presentation, which contributes to its significant clinical challenges [12, 17]. Angiosarcoma may present as nonspecific skin findings such as ecchymosis or papular rash, often leading to delayed diagnosis. For this reason, in patients with predisposing factors, such as prior therapeutic radiation, chronic lymphedema, or significant sun exposure, there should be a low threshold to pursue workup, including biopsy of the visible lesion. Visceral angiosarcomas are often detected at a more advanced stage and size, with symptoms such as pain, weight loss, or organ dysfunction [16, 17].

The mainstay of treatment for localized disease is surgical resection with negative margins, which is often challenging due to the infiltrative nature of this tumor [14, 18]. Although somewhat counterintuitive, as many angiosarcomas are associated with prior radiation exposure, they are often also treated with radiation, particularly when negative margins are not able to be achieved [19, 20]. As is the case with many sarcoma subtypes, angiosarcoma is relatively resistant to systemic therapy. The mainstay of systemic therapy is paclitaxel, which is often employed in a neoadjuvant setting or for unresectable disease [21].

Fibroblastic and Myofibroblastic Sarcomas

Fibroblastic and myofibroblastic soft tissue tumors arising from are a heterogeneous group of neoplasms with varied clinical behavior, histologic appearance, and imaging features. These lesions are stratified into benign, intermediate (locally aggressive or rarely metastasizing), and malignant categories in the most recent WHO Classification of soft tissue tumors [22]. Solitary fibrous tumor, while classified as intermediate, spans a broad biologic spectrum with some demonstrating more indolent behavior, while tumors with increased mitotic activity, necrosis, or dedifferentiation can exhibit aggressive or metastatic behavior. Solitary fibrous tumors are characterized by *NAB2-STAT6* gene fusions and have STAT6 positivity on immunohistochemistry. Desmoid-type fibromatosis is another intermediate-grade tumor, notable for its infiltrative nature and high risk of local recurrence, though it lacks metastatic potential. Management of most desmoid tumors is focused on active surveillance, with intervention reserved for symptomatic patients and those with progression. Intervention is either medical, with sorafenib, pazopanib, and nirogacestat as first-line therapies, or with cryoablation. Surgical resection is not recommended except in rare cases [23].

Malignant tumors include low-grade fibromyxoid sarcoma (LGFMS), myxofibrosarcoma, and myofibroblastic sarcoma, each with distinct molecular and histologic features. LGFMS is characterized by alternating fibrous and myxoid areas with bland spindle cells, is defined by *FUS-CREB3L2* or *CREB3L1* fusions and strong MUC4 expression, and carries a risk of late metastasis. Myxofibrosarcoma typically affects older adults, arises in the extremities, and demonstrates high-grade cytologic atypia, infiltrative margins, and a higher risk for both local recurrence and distant spread. Myofibroblastic sarcoma, though less well characterized at the molecular level, shows myofibroblastic differentiation and malignant histologic features and presents most often in the head, neck, or extremities with variable clinical aggressiveness. Imaging features such as peritumoral edema, necrosis, and poorly defined borders are associated with higher-grade lesions and aid in risk stratification. Fibrosarcoma is characterized by malignant spindle-shaped fibroblasts often arranged in a classical "herringbone" pattern. Historically, the diagnosis of fibrosarcoma has been a process of exclusion and must be distinguished from other spindle cell type tumors such as synovial sarcomas, peripheral nerve sheath tumors, angiosarcoma, leiomyosarcoma, and rhabdomyosarcoma [24]. Undifferentiated pleomorphic sarcoma (UPS), which was previously classified as malignant fibrous histiocytoma (MFH), is now categorized as a high-grade undifferentiated sarcoma and is treated similarly to other aggressive soft tissue sarcomas [25].

In recent years, there has been an increased interest in the clinical implications of fusion genes in fibroblastic and myofibroblastic sarcomas. There are a number of novel fusion genes under investigation, including COL1A1-PDGFB due to translocation t(17; 22) (q22; q13) that is frequently seen in DFSP and fibroblastoma [26], FUS-CREB3L2 in low-grade fibromyxoid sarcoma, ETV6-NTRK3 in IFS, and EWSR1-CREB3L1 in sclerosing epitheloid fibrosarcoma [27]. Multiple protein kinase inhibitors have been and are currently being studied in hopes of obtaining better clinical outcomes [28–30]. These studies included a phase I trial of flavopiridol combined with doxorubicin in 31 patients with advanced sarcomas [28], a phase II trial of anlotinib in 40 patients [29], and a phase III clinical trial involving 509 patients with advanced soft tissue sarcoma (STS) treated with doxorubicin plus olaratumab [30]. Continued research into the underlying biology of fibroblastic and myofibroblastic sarcomas and their interaction with the tumor microenvironment may prove to be pivotal for the development of future treatment options.

Leiomyosarcoma

Leiomyosarcoma (LMS) originates from smooth muscle cells, accounts for approximately 10–20% of adult soft tissue sarcomas, and carries a higher risk of metastatic recurrence compared to some other soft tissue sarcomas. It most commonly arises in the retroperitoneum, extremities, and intra-abdominal soft tissues, with a slight male predominance and peak incidence in the seventh decade [31]. While uterine cases are more frequent in women, this discussion is focused on non-uterine LMS. The pathogenesis of LMS remains incompletely understood; however, prior radiation and genetic syndromes such as Li-Fraumeni are recognized risk factors. Genomic analyses have consistently identified frequent alterations in tumor suppressor genes, including TP53, RB1, and PTEN. Clinically, LMS typically presents as a painless, enlarging mass, often diagnosed incidentally when imaging is performed for an unrelated complaint. Local recurrence rates range from 30% to 50%, predominantly within 2–3 years post-surgery, posing significant treatment challenges and morbidity. Metastatic disease, often to the lungs, liver, and peritoneum, occurs in 40–60% of high-grade LMS cases and generally confers a poor prognosis [32]. Prognosis in LMS is influenced by tumor site, grade, size, and resectability. Overall, the 5-year survival rate is approximately 55%, but outcomes are poorer for retroperitoneal and high-grade tumors [33].

Diagnosis of LMS requires a combination of imaging, biopsy, and molecular testing. Cross-sectional imaging plays a central role in the evaluation and management of these tumors. Contrast-enhanced CT is typically used for abdominal and retroperitoneal tumors, offering excellent delineation of tumor margins and detection of pulmonary or hepatic metastases. MRI is the preferred modality for extremity and pelvic LMS due to its superior soft tissue resolution and ability to evaluate involvement of neurovascular bundles and adjacent musculature. A core needle biopsy is standard for histologic confirmation, typically revealing fascicles of eosinophilic spindle cells with blunt-ended nuclei. Immunohistochemical staining for smooth muscle actin, desmin, and h-caldesmon supports the diagnosis, and molecular profiling may reveal specific gene alterations that assist in therapeutic decision-making.

Management of LMS centers on complete surgical resection with negative margins for localized disease. Surgery remains the cornerstone of curative treatment, but the development of metastatic disease is common, especially in retroperitoneal tumors. Chemotherapy is frequently used in advanced or unresectable cases, with doxorubicin alone or in combination with ifosfamide (MAI) serving as the standard first-line regimen. Recent studies have investigated alternative strategies to improve outcomes. A phase III trial, including 150 patients, demonstrated that the combination of doxorubicin and trabectedin resulted in longer progression-free survival compared to doxorubicin alone in advanced LMS [34]. The ongoing STRASS II trial will compare survival and distant metastasis rates for patients with high-risk retroperitoneal sarcomas (LMS and dedifferentiated liposarcoma) undergoing neoadjuvant doxorubicin + dacarbazine followed by surgery versus those undergoing surgery alone. This study aims to clarify the role of systemic therapy in these aggressive sarcoma subtypes and guide treatment strategies for patients who are at a higher risk of recurrence and metastasis.

Additionally, immunotherapy is an emerging area of research with some small studies demonstrating potential benefit with the addition of immunotherapy to cytotoxic chemotherapy in advanced LMS as a second-line therapy [35], though this requires more robust investigation. Enrollment in clinical trials is encouraged when available, especially in metastatic or refractory disease.

Recent studies have identified molecular markers associated with prognosis. For instance, a multi-omics study found that amplification of the CTHRC1 gene, involved in collagen remodeling, correlates with poor overall survival in uterine LMS [36]. Additionally, large-scale work is being done to better define the molecular landscape and immunogenic profile of leiomyosarcoma and other more common sarcoma histologies, with the goal of developing improved targeted therapies for these rare diseases [37]. These recurrence patterns highlight the importance of aggressive surgery and rigorous imaging surveillance. Multi-omic profiling and molecular characterization, as described by the Toronto group [38], promise to refine risk stratification, identify actionable targets, and improve systemic therapies for LMS, offering hope for better patient outcomes in this difficult-to-treat malignancy.

Rhabdomyosarcoma

Although exceedingly rare in adults, rhabdomyosarcoma (RMS) is the most common malignant soft tissue tumor of childhood, with 4.6 cases per million in patients under 20 years, and over 50% of cases diagnosed before the age of 10 [39]. Tumors are most frequently found in the head and neck, with 60% of cases in this location. Approximately 14–25% of cases occur in the genitourinary system, and 15% arise in the extremities [40]. Adult outcomes are known to be significantly worse than pediatric outcomes in this disease [41], with adult 5-year survival rates of 40–54% compared to 70% in children [42]. Like pediatric cases, adult outcomes are influenced by tumor size, resectability, site, and presence of metastatic disease [43]. There are no known environmental risk factors; however, NF1 and LFS are known risk factors for adult RMS. Several distinct histologies exist within RMS, including alveolar, embryonal, spindle cell/sclerosing, and pleomorphic. Presence of FOXO1 fusion, which is less common in adults, is associated with a worse prognosis [39].

Treatment requires a multidisciplinary approach, with multimodal therapy including surgery, chemotherapy, and radiation. Complete surgical resection is the mainstay of treatment for resectable disease. Specific chemotherapy and radiation protocols are extrapolated from pediatric management, although higher radiation doses are generally considered acceptable for adults due to less concern about long-term adverse effects compared to children [44]. First-line chemotherapy agents are vincristine, dactinomycin, and cyclophosphamide [9].

As RMS is primarily a disease of childhood, research is largely focused on the pediatric population, with findings extrapolated to adult management. Current pediatric clinical research is focused on identifying subgroups of patients with lower-risk disease who may be candidates for de-escalation of therapy and, conversely, high-risk patients who may benefit from more aggressive chemotherapy regimens. Translational work has focused on the association between detectable circulating tumor DNA (ctDNA) and survival, regardless of fusion status, and has shown promise for the use of ctDNA as a potential predictive biomarker after further validation [45, 46].

Liposarcoma

Liposarcoma, while rare, is one of the most common soft tissue sarcomas, with an annual incidence of approximately 2.5 cases per million people, accounting for 15–20% of all adult soft tissue sarcomas [1]. It is a histologically diverse tumor with four main subtypes: well-differentiated (WDLPS), dedifferentiated (DDLPS), myxoid, and pleomorphic. Accurate diagnosis requires imaging—typically CT for retroperitoneal tumors or MRI for extremity tumors—followed by core needle biopsy and molecular testing. Core needle biopsy is not necessary for well-differentiated liposarcoma, as imaging characteristics can provide a clear diagnosis. Molecular markers such as MDM2 and CDK4 amplification are key in confirming WDLPS and DDLPS, while myxoid liposarcoma typically features a FUS-DDIT3 gene fusion. These subtypes differ not only in morphology but also in prognosis, recurrence patterns, and response to therapy, making precise histologic and molecular classification essential for effective management [47].

Complete surgical resection remains the cornerstone of treatment for liposarcoma. However, local recurrence is common, particularly in retroperitoneal cases where negative margins are difficult to achieve, and long-term surveillance is required. The STRASS trial (EORTC 62092), a multicenter phase III study, including 266 patients, evaluated whether preoperative radiotherapy improves abdominal recurrence-free survival in patients with primary retroperitoneal sarcomas [8]. While the overall results were negative, a pre-specified subgroup analysis showed potential benefit in patients with WDLPS [8]. The ongoing STRASS II trial (EORTC 1809) builds on these findings, evaluating the benefit of neoadjuvant chemotherapy in high-risk retroperitoneal DDLPS and leiomyosarcoma.

Prognosis and recurrence rates in liposarcoma vary widely by subtype and anatomical location. WDLPS typically has a favorable prognosis with very low metastatic potential but high local recurrence—up to 50% in retroperitoneal tumors over 10 years, with a relatively indolent course. DDLPS, on the other hand, carries a greater risk of both local recurrence (up to 40%) and distant metastases (about 30% at 5 years). Myxoid liposarcoma has a unique metastatic pattern, often spreading to fat-rich areas such as bone and soft tissue, with high-grade tumors demonstrating a 30% metastasis rate. Five-year overall survival ranges from over 90% in WDLPS to as low as 50% in pleomorphic or high-grade DDLPS, demonstrating the varied aggressiveness of these tumors and the need for management at a high-volume center familiar with nuances of disease subtypes and the ability to provide expert multidisciplinary care [33, 48].

Emerging therapies aim to improve outcomes in advanced or recurrent disease. Immunotherapy is under active investigation, particularly following results from the SARC032 trial (143 patients), where perioperative pembrolizumab combined with radiotherapy improved disease-free survival in undifferentiated pleomorphic sarcoma and showed encouraging signals in DDLPS [49]. Targeted therapies are also being explored; MDM2 inhibitors have shown activity in early trials [50], and cell-based immunotherapies are under investigation for myxoid/round cell liposarcoma [51]. These novel strategies reflect a shift toward histology-driven, personalized medicine in the management of liposarcoma.

Synovial Sarcoma

Synovial sarcoma (SS) is a soft tissue sarcoma that accounts for 5–10% of all STS, with a predilection for adolescents and adults younger than 40 years of age [52]. It is characterized by the pathognomonic chromosomal translocation t(X;18)(p11.2;q11.2) in 90% of cases, which leads to fusion of the SS18 gene on chromosome 18 to one of the synovial sarcoma X (SSX1 or 2) genes on chromosome X, creating the SS18-SSX oncogene [53]. The type of fusion gene is clinically significant, with the SSX1 gene fusion demonstrating worse metastasis-free survival at 5 years than the SSX2 gene fusion (LADANYI 2002). Cancer testis antigen NY-ESO-1 is also expressed in 76% of SS and may help differentiate it from other spindle cell neoplasms [54]. Despite its name, synovial sarcoma does not arise from synovial tissue and is classified by WHO as a tumor of uncertain differentiation. Patients typically present with a slow-growing soft tissue mass that may have been present for years. The majority of these tumors occur in the extremities, with up to 70% located in the lower extremities, and synovial sarcoma is the most common tumor of the foot and ankle in patients 6–45 years old. These tumors typically occur near joints but are only very rarely truly intra-articular. Synovial sarcoma may also occur in various other anatomic locations such as the neck, paravertebral region, and the abdominal wall [55].

Surgical resection with negative margins remains the standard of care for resectable disease. Radiation, either adjuvant or neoadjuvant, is recommended in high-grade or larger tumors, or in cases where surgical margins are threatened [56]. Recent advances in radiation techniques have improved treatment outcomes and reduced toxicity. Intensity-modulated radiotherapy (IMRT) allows for precise dose delivery, minimizing radiation exposure and toxicity to surrounding normal tissues [57]. Proton beam therapy, though less commonly used, offers the advantage of sparing adjacent critical or radiosensitive structures [58]. Stereotactic body radiotherapy (SBRT) is also used for local control of recurrent or oligometastatic disease and is being explored as a potential perioperative therapy option [59, 60].

Cytotoxic systemic therapy is reserved for metastatic or unresectable SS and high-risk tumors and includes multi-agent chemotherapy, with ifosfamide and doxorubicin being the standard first-line regimen [61]. As compared to STS overall, SS demonstrates a better response to chemotherapy with longer progression-free and overall survival following treatment [62]. Pazopanib, a multitargeted tyrosine kinase inhibitor, has demonstrated improved progression-free survival (PFS) and has been approved for second-line use in cases with prior chemotherapy [63]. Regorafenib is another multi-kinase inhibitor which has also been shown to improve PFS when used as a second-line agent [64, 65]. Trabectedin, an alkylating agent, has similarly shown activity in many STS subtypes and is often used in SS, although substantial evidence for SS in specific cases is lacking [61, 65]. Despite improved PFS, it should be noted that no statistically significant improvement in overall survival was observed with these second-line agents. Additionally, checkpoint inhibitors, which have revolutionized treatment for other malignancies, have not seen much success in synovial sarcoma due to its relatively low tumor mutational burden and lack of immunogenicity [66].

Recent advancements in the molecular and immunologic landscape of SS have provided promising therapeutic insights. One of the most notable developments is the investigation of engineered T-cell receptor (TCR) therapy targeting cancer-testis antigens such as NY-ESO-1 and MAGE-A4. The phase II SPEARHEAD-1 trial evaluated afamitresgene autoleucel (Afami-cel), an autologous T-cell therapy targeting MAGE-A4, in patients with advanced SS with heavy pretreatment requiring a median of three lines of systemic therapy previously. The study results were promising, with an overall response rate of 39% in patients with SS [51]. This study underscores the potential for TCR-based immunotherapy for future expansion of the therapeutic arsenal against SS.

Summary

Despite the management and research challenges associated with a constellation of rare histologies like STS, survival continues to improve as we work to refine our understanding of its nuances. Future areas for advancement include further delineation of genetic and epigenetic drivers of disease and personalization of systemic therapy as we work to better understand underlying molecular drivers.

References

1. Siegel RL, Kratzer TB, Giaquinto AN, et al. Cancer statistics, 2025. CA Cancer J Clin. 2025;75(1):10–45.
2. National Cancer Institute. https://www.cancer.gov/publications/dictionaries/cancer-terms/def/rare-cancer. Accessed 29 Jan 2025.
3. Helman LJ, Meltzer P. Mechanisms of sarcoma development. Nat Rev Cancer. 2003;3(9):685–94.
4. Li FP, Fraumeni JF Jr. Rhabdomyosarcoma in children: epidemiologic study and identification of a familial cancer syndrome. J Natl Cancer Inst. 1969;43:1365–73.
5. King AA, Debaun MR, Riccardi VM, Gutmann DH. Malignant peripheral nerve sheath tumors in neurofibromatosis 1. Am J Med Genet. 2000;93:388–92.
6. Baumhoer D. Hereditäre Knochentumoren [hereditary bone tumors]. Pathologe. 2017;38(3):179–85.
7. Czarnecka AM, Synoradzki K, Firlej W, et al. Molecular biology of osteosarcoma. Cancer. 2020;12(8):2130.
8. Bonvalot S, Gronchi A, Le Péchoux C, et al. Preoperative radiotherapy plus surgery versus surgery alone for patients with primary retroperitoneal sarcoma (EORTC-62092: STRASS): a multicentre, open-label, randomised, phase 3 trial. Lancet Oncol. 2020;21(10):1366–77.
9. NCCN Clinical Practice Guidelines in Oncology (NCCN Guidelines®) for Soft Tissue Sarcoma V.1.2025. Accessed 6 June 2025.
10. Colas M, Gérazime A, Popescu D, et al. Angiosarcoma: a population-based cancer registry descriptive study of 45 consecutive cases diagnosed between 1979 and 2016. Rare Tumors. 2020;12:2036361320979216.
11. Hendrick LE, Zambetti BR, Wong DL, et al. Visceral angiosarcoma: a nationwide analysis of treatment factors and outcomes. J Surg Oncol. 2022;125(8):1231–7.
12. Gaballah AH, Jensen CT, Palmquist S, et al. Angiosarcoma: clinical and imaging features from head to toe. Br J Radiol. 2017;90(1075):20170039.
13. Rouhani P, Fletcher CDM, Devesa SS, Toro JR. Cutaneous soft tissue sarcoma incidence patterns in the U.S.: an analysis of 12,114 cases. Cancer. 2008;113(3):616–27.
14. Florou V, Wilky BA. Current management of angiosarcoma: recent advances and lessons from the past. Curr Treat Options in Oncol. 2021;22(7):61.
15. Samargandi R. Etiology, pathogenesis, and management of angiosarcoma associated with implants and foreign body: clinical cases and research updates. Medicine. 2024;103(18):e37932.
16. Zeng D, Zeng X, Duan J, Chen D, Zhu B. Clinical characteristics of primary hepatic angiosarcoma outcomes: a SEER database analysis. Transl Cancer Res. 2021;10(1):110–25.
17. Cao J, Wang J, He C, Fang M. Angiosarcoma: a review of diagnosis and current treatment. Am J Cancer Res. 2019;9(11):2303–13.
18. Yan Q, Fernandez RA, Elmi M, Gelfond J, Davies MG. Outcomes of interventions for Angiosarcoma. Front Surg. 2022;9:819099.
19. Arora TK, Terracina KP, Soong J, Idowu MO, Takabe K. Primary and secondary angiosarcoma of the breast. Gland Surg. 2014;3(1):28–34.
20. Abraham JA, Hornicek FJ, Kaufman AM, et al. Treatment and outcome of 82 patients with angiosarcoma. Ann Surg Oncol. 2007;14(6):1953–67.
21. Roy A, Gabani P, Davis EJ, et al. Concurrent paclitaxel and radiation therapy for the treatment of cutaneous angiosarcoma. Clin Transl Radiat Oncol. 2021;27:114–20.
22. WHO Classification of Tumours Editorial Board. WHO classification of tumours: soft tissue and bone tumours, vol. 3. 5th ed. Lyon: IARC Press/World Health Organization; 2020.
23. Bonvalot S, Miah A, Kasper B. Evolving concepts in the management of desmoid tumors. Hematol Oncol Clin North Am. 2025;S0889-8588(25):00047–4.
24. Haseli S, Mansoori B, Christensen D, et al. Fibroblastic and myofibroblastic soft-tissue tumors: imaging spectrum and radiologic-pathologic correlation. Radiographics. 2023;43(8):e230005.
25. Gronchi A, Miah AB, Dei Tos AP, et al. Soft tissue and visceral sarcomas: ESMO–EURACAN–GENTURIS clinical practice guidelines for diagnosis, treatment and follow-up. Ann Oncol. 2021;32(11):1348–65.
26. Simon MP, Pedeutour F, Sirvent N, et al. Deregulation of the platelet-derived growth factor B-chain gene via fusion with collagen gene COL1A1 in dermatofibrosarcoma protuberans and giant-cell fibroblastoma. Nat Genet. 1997;15(1):95–8.
27. Tang X, Hu X, Wen Y, Min L. Progressive insights into fibrosarcoma diagnosis and treatment: leveraging fusion genes for advancement. Front Cell Dev Biol. 2023;11:1284428.
28. Luke JJ, D'Adamo DR, Dickson MA, et al. The cyclin-dependent kinase inhibitor flavopiridol potentiates doxorubicin efficacy in advanced sarcomas: preclinical investigations and results of a phase I dose-escalation clinical trial. Clin Cancer Res. 2012;18(9):2638–47.
29. Li T, Dong Y, Wei Y, et al. First-line anlotinib treatment for soft-tissue sarcoma in chemotherapy-ineligible patients: an open-label, single-arm, phase 2 clinical trial. Clin Cancer Res. 2024;30(19):4310–7.
30. Tap WD, Wagner AJ, Schöffski P, ANNOUNCE Investigators, et al. Effect of doxorubicin plus olaratumab vs doxorubicin plus placebo on survival in patients with advanced soft tissue sarcomas: the announce randomized clinical trial. JAMA. 2020;323(13):1266–76.
31. Ducimetière F, Lurkin A, Ranchère-Vince D, et al. Incidence of sarcoma histotypes and molecular subtypes in a prospective epidemiological study with central pathology review and molecular testing. PLoS One. 2011;6(8):e20294.
32. Haddox CL, Papke DJ Jr, Serrano C. Leiomyosarcoma therapeutic approaches and future directions. Hematol Oncol Clin North Am. 2025;S0889-8588(25):00045-0.
33. Brennan MF, Antonescu CR, Moraco N, Singer S. Lessons learned from the study of 10,000 patients with soft tissue sarcoma. Ann Surg. 2014;260(3):416–22.
34. Pautier P, Italiano A, Piperno-Neumann S, Chevreau C, et al. Doxorubicin alone versus doxorubicin with trabectedin followed by trabectedin alone as first-line therapy for metastatic or unresectable leiomyosarcoma (LMS-04): a randomised, multicentre, open-label phase 3 trial. Lancet Oncol. 2022;23(8):1044–54. https://doi.org/10.1016/S1470-2045(22)00380-1. Epub 2022 Jul 11. PMID: 35835135
35. Kim M, Kim YJ, Suh KJ, et al. Phase 2 trial of avelumab in combination with gemcitabine in advanced leiomyosarcoma as a second-line treatment (EAGLES, Korean cancer study group UN18-09). Cancer. 2025;131(1):e35609.
36. Falcao RM, de Souza JES, Gonzalez-Molina J, et al. Deep multi-omics integration approach reveals new molecular features of uterine leiomyosarcoma. Biochim Biophys Acta Mol basis Dis. 2025;1871(3):167632.
37. Soupir A, Ospina OE, Hampton O, et al. Genomic, transcriptomic, and immunogenomic landscape of over 1300 sarcomas of diverse histology subtypes. Nat Commun. 2025;16(1):4206.
38. Anderson ND, Babichev Y, Fuligni F, et al. Lineage-defined leiomyosarcoma subtypes emerge years before diagnosis and determine patient survival. Nat Commun. 2021;12(1):4496.
39. PDQ Pediatric Treatment Editorial Board. Childhood rhabdomyosarcoma treatment (PDQ®): health professional version. 2025 Apr

11. In: PDQ cancer information summaries [internet]. Bethesda: National Cancer Institute (US); 2002.
40. Meyer WH, Spunt SL. Soft tissue sarcomas of childhood. Cancer Treat Rev. 2004;30:269–80.
41. Gerber NK, Wexler LH, Singer S, et al. Adult rhabdomyosarcoma survival improved with treatment on multimodality protocols. Int J Radiat Oncol Biol Phys. 2013;86(1):58–63.
42. Smith MA, Seibel NL, Altekruse SF, et al. Outcomes for children and adolescents with cancer: challenges for the twenty-first century. J Clin Oncol. 2010;28(15):2625–34.
43. Simon JH, Paulino AC, Ritchie JM, Mayr NA, Buatti JM. Presentation, prognostic factors and patterns of failure in adult rhabdomyosarcoma. Sarcoma. 2003;7(1):1–7.
44. Bergamaschi L, Bertulli R, Casanova M, et al. Rhabdomyosarcoma in adults: analysis of treatment modalities in a prospective single-center series. Med Oncol. 2019;36(7):59.
45. Abbou S, Klega K, Tsuji J, et al. Circulating tumor DNA is prognostic in intermediate-risk rhabdomyosarcoma: a report from the children's oncology group. J Clin Oncol. 2023;41(13):2382–93.
46. Lak NSM, van Zogchel LMJ, Zappeij-Kannegieter L, et al. Cell-free DNA as a diagnostic and prognostic biomarker in pediatric rhabdomyosarcoma. JCO Precis Oncol. 2023;7:e2200113.
47. Crago AM, Singer S. Clinical and molecular approaches to well differentiated and dedifferentiated liposarcoma. Curr Opin Oncol. 2011;23(4):373–8.
48. Gronchi A, Strauss DC, Miceli R, et al. Variability in patterns of recurrence after resection of primary retroperitoneal sarcoma (RPS): a report on 1007 patients from the multi-institutional collaborative RPS working group. Ann Surg. 2016;263(5):1002–9.
49. Mowery YM, Ballman KV, Hong AM, et al. Safety and efficacy of pembrolizumab, radiation therapy, and surgery versus radiation therapy and surgery for stage III soft tissue sarcoma of the extremity (SU2C-SARC032): an open-label, randomised clinical trial. Lancet. 2024;404(10467):2053–64.
50. Lee TY, von Mehren M. Novel pharmacotherapies for the treatment of liposarcoma: a comprehensive update. Expert Opin Pharmacother. 2024;25(17):2293–306.
51. D'Angelo SP, Druta M, Van Tine BA. Letetresgene autoleucel in advanced/metastatic myxoid/round cell liposarcoma. J Clin Oncol. 2025;43(15):1777–88.
52. Murphey MD, Gibson MS, Jennings BT, et al. Imaging of synovial sarcoma with radiologic-pathologic correlation. Radiographics. 2006;26(5):1543–65.
53. Thway K, Fisher C. Synovial sarcoma: defining features and diagnostic evolution. Ann Diagn Pathol. 2014;18(6):369–80.
54. Lai JP, Robbins PF, Raffeld M, et al. NY-ESO-1 expression in synovial sarcoma and other mesenchymal tumors: significance for NY-ESO-1-based targeted therapy and differential diagnosis. Mod Pathol. 2012;25(6):854–8.
55. Gazendam AM, Popovic S, Munir S, et al. Synovial sarcoma: a clinical review. Curr Oncol. 2021;28(3):1909–20.
56. Gingrich AA, Marrufo AS, Liu Y, et al. Radiotherapy is associated with improved survival in patients with synovial sarcoma undergoing surgery: a national cancer database analysis. J Surg Res. 2020;255:378–87.
57. Wang J, Song Y, Liu X, et al. Comparison of outcome and toxicity of postoperative intensity-modulated radiation therapy with two-dimensional radiotherapy in patients with soft tissue sarcoma of extremities and trunk. Cancer Med. 2019;8(3):902–9.
58. Laughlin BS, Golafshar MA, Ahmed S, et al. Early experience using proton beam therapy for extremity soft tissue sarcoma: a multicenter study. Int J Part Ther. 2022;9(1):1–11.
59. Kubicek GJ, Kim TW, Gutowski CJ, et al. Preoperative stereotactic body radiation therapy for soft-tissue sarcoma: results of phase 2 study. Adv Radiat Oncol. 2022;7(2):100855.
60. Feng XY, Li J, Li AM, et al. Stereotactic body radiotherapy for recurrent and oligometastatic soft tissue sarcoma. World J Surg Oncol. 2022;20(1):322.
61. Desar IME, Fleuren EDG, Van Der Graaf WTA. Systemic treatment for adults with synovial sarcoma. Curr Treat Options in Oncol. 2018;19(2):13.
62. Vlenterie M, Litière S, Rizzo E, et al. Outcome of chemotherapy in advanced synovial sarcoma patients: review of 15 clinical trials from the European Organisation for Research and Treatment of Cancer soft tissue and bone sarcoma group; setting a new landmark for studies in this entity. Eur J Cancer. 2016;58:62–72.
63. van der Graaf WTA, Blay JY, Chawla SP, et al. Pazopanib for metastatic soft-tissue sarcoma (PALETTE): a randomised, double-blind, placebo-controlled phase 3 trial. Lancet Lond Engl. 2012;379(9829):1879–86.
64. Penel N, Mir O, Wallet J, et al. A double-blind placebo-controlled randomized phase II trial assessing the activity and safety of regorafenib in non-adipocytic sarcoma patients previously treated with both chemotherapy and pazopanib. Eur J Cancer. 2020;126:45–55.
65. Carroll C, Patel N, Gunsoy NB, Stirnadel-Farrant HA, Pokras S. Meta-analysis of pazopanib and trabectedin effectiveness in previously treated metastatic synovial sarcoma (second-line setting and beyond). Future Oncol. 2022;18(32):3651–65.
66. Tawbi HA, Burgess M, Bolejack V, et al. Pembrolizumab in advanced soft-tissue sarcoma and bone sarcoma (SARC028): a multicentre, two-cohort, single-arm, open-label, phase 2 trial. Lancet Oncol. 2017;18(11):1493–501.

Research on Cutaneous Cancer

23

Anastasios T. Mitsakos, Vernon K. Sondak, and Matthew C. Perez

Introduction

Epidemiology

Cutaneous melanoma is one of the most common cancer diagnoses in the United States, with 100,640 new patients and 8290 deaths estimated in 2024 [1]. However, figures for new cases may represent a substantial underestimate, as many in situ and early-stage invasive melanomas diagnosed and managed in the community setting might not be formally reported. Incidence has been rising in the United States and worldwide, with White race, increasing age, and male gender being major non-modifiable risk factors [2]. It is estimated that in the Western population, one out of every 50 individuals will develop melanoma. Despite the rising rates of melanoma, the prognosis remains excellent for patients diagnosed with early stages of the disease [1–3]. Furthermore, prognosis and long-term survival have improved significantly for patients with more advanced stages, which is attributed to an increase in effective treatment options for recurrent and metastatic disease.

Etiology and Pathogenesis

Cutaneous melanoma originates from the melanocytes that reside in the epidermal layer of the skin. The common place of origin of all melanocytes is embryologically the neural crest, something that gives melanomas some of their characteristic immunohistochemical phenotype components [4]. Melanocytes are responsible for the production of melanin, which gives the complexion color to human skin, and at the same time, they provide a layer of protection from ultraviolet radiation [4]. Melanomas can have a wide range of pathological findings. The four most common histologic subtypes are superficial spreading melanoma, nodular melanoma, acral lentiginous melanoma, and lentigo maligna melanoma [4, 5].

Risk factors for the development of cutaneous melanoma can be divided into non-modifiable and modifiable. As mentioned earlier in this chapter, non-modifiable risk factors include White race with fair complexion, increasing age (higher risk >50 years of age), male gender, and family history. The majority of cutaneous melanomas arise as de novo lesions; only a minority of them are associated with familial syndromes. Previous melanoma or evidence of dysplastic nevi also increases the risk of a new melanoma diagnosis. The most critical modifiable factor for cutaneous melanoma is exposure to ultraviolet radiation from natural sunlight or indoor tanning, with more than 70% of cases having had such exposure in the past. Consequently, most melanoma lesions arise in the exposed areas of the trunk and extremities, with other areas of the body also affected but to a lesser extent [1, 4, 6, 7].

From a molecular pathogenesis standpoint, the Cancer Genome Atlas (TCGA) program has identified four major genomic subtypes based on DNA-, RNA-, and protein-based analyses. The BRAF-mutant subtype is the most common, with RAS-mutant and NF1-mutant subtypes coming in as second and third, while the fourth subtype is the triple wild-type (WT), which is a heterogeneous subgroup with a lack of the above mutations. BRAF-mutant, RAS-mutant, and NF1-mutant subtypes harbor an ultraviolet signature in over 90% of cases and have provided the framework for identification of potential therapeutic targets and predictive biomarkers [8, 9].

A. T. Mitsakos (✉)
Department of Cutaneous Oncology, H. Lee Moffitt Cancer Center, Tampa, FL, USA

Division of Surgical Oncology, Baxter Health, Mountain Home, AR, USA

V. K. Sondak · M. C. Perez
Department of Cutaneous Oncology, H. Lee Moffitt Cancer Center, Tampa, FL, USA

J. Huang, H. S.L. Jim (eds.), *Cancer Research Guidance for Clinicians and Researchers*,
https://doi.org/10.1007/978-3-032-19175-5_23

Diagnosis and Treatment

Diagnosis and Staging

Diagnosis of cutaneous melanoma is based on suspicious findings of skin lesions on physical exam and confirmed with a tissue biopsy. Traditionally, suspicious findings on physical exam can be summarized by the ABCDE mnemonic, which stands for asymmetry, border irregularity, color changes, diameter > 6 mm, and evolving lesion throughout time (Fig. 23.1). Even though in situ and early-stage melanoma lesions can be missed by relying completely on these clinical rules, a higher number of these examination findings have been associated with earlier recognition and diagnosis when examined by a dermatologist [10]. The American Academy of Dermatologists recommends routine total body skin evaluation (TBSE) by a medical professional, especially for patients with fair complexion, family history, and/or other established risk factors [11]. In addition, community initiatives should be implemented to promote knowledge and understanding of this disease process, since early diagnosis and treatment strongly correlate with improved survival rates [11].

Tissue biopsy is necessary for both histologic confirmation and primary tumor staging for cutaneous melanoma. While multiple biopsy methods may be performed, full-thickness biopsy and adequate sampling are the key principles when determining biopsy technique for suspicious melanocytic lesions. Excisional biopsies should be performed with narrow 1–3 mm margins and should always be oriented with a proposed definitive excision in mind. Incisional biopsies, punch biopsies, and deep scallop shave biopsies are also techniques commonly used depending on the size and location of the lesion, as long as the aforementioned key principles are taken into account [2]. In a retrospective multi-institutional study of 60 patients, Zager et al. found shave biopsy to be reliable and accurate in 97% of cases, without compromising their subsequent management [12].

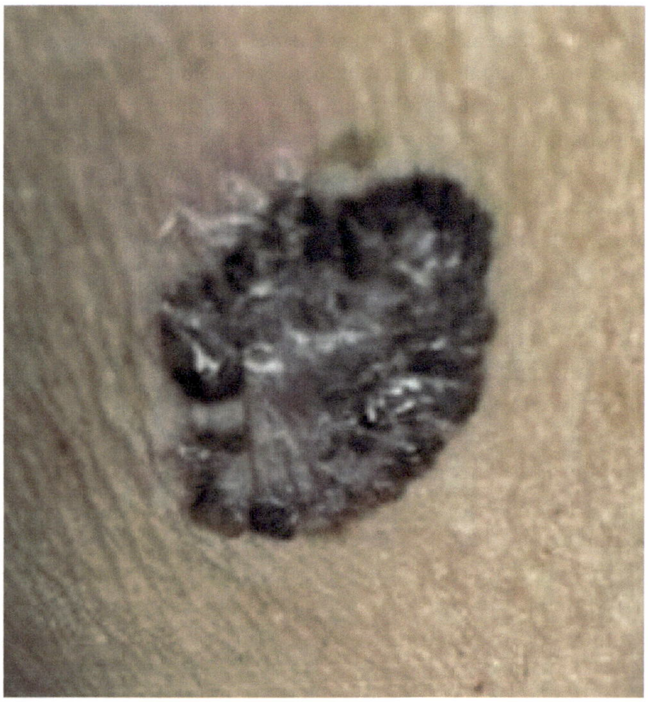

Fig. 23.1 Primary cutaneous melanoma

Histopathologic evaluation plays a key role in assessing prognostic factors and determining the staging of the disease. Breslow thickness (maximal tumor depth) and the absence/presence of ulceration are the most significant components and are therefore used in the AJCC eighth edition staging [13]. Additional factors that can aid in prognostic evaluation of the primary tumor include mitotic rate, perineural and lymphovascular invasion, neurotropism, presence of tumor-infiltrating lymphocytes, presence and extent of regression, presence of vertical growth phase, histologic subtype, and presence of microsatellite lesions. Molecular testing is especially relevant with advanced or metastatic disease when evaluating for targetable mutations to guide the use of systemic therapies [8, 14].

Staging of cutaneous melanoma is based on the TNM approach per the AJCC eighth edition. T (tumor) staging is based on Breslow thickness and presence of ulceration. N (node) staging is based on the number of tumor-involved regional lymph nodes and the presence of in-transit, satellite, or microsatellite metastases. M (metastasis) staging is based on the presence of distant metastasis and subcategorized according to anatomical site of distant metastasis and presence of elevated serum LDH [13, 15, 16].

Management of Primary Lesion

Management of cutaneous melanoma has been traditionally surgical, especially in its earlier stages, and thus, the role of the surgical oncologist as a key component in the multidisciplinary team is paramount. While many of the basic surgical principles remain unchanged, the nuances of the extent, timing, and sequencing of surgical options are an evolving field [17].

Through the 1970s, wide excision of primary melanoma with 3–5 cm radial margins was the standard of care. Five prospective randomized trials challenged the need for wide (larger than 1–2 cm) surgical margins and provided evidence for the current excision margin recommendations (Table 23.1) [18–22]. Current guidelines recommend 0.5–1 cm margins for melanoma in situ, 1 cm margins for invasive melanoma Breslow thickness ≤ 1.0 mm, 1–2 cm margins for invasive melanoma Breslow thickness > 1.0–2.0 mm, and 2 cm mar-

Table 23.1 Randomized clinical trials comparing resection margins in cutaneous melanoma

	Definition		5-year DFS		5-year OS		Local recurrence	
Study	Narrow margin (cm)	Wide margin (cm)	Narrow margin (%)	Wide margin (%)	Narrow margin (%)	Wide margin (%)	Narrow margin (%)	Wide margin (%)
French Group for Research on Malignant Melanoma ($n = 337$)	2	5	85 (10-year)	83 (10-year)	93	90	0.6	2.4
Intergroup Melanoma Surgical Trial ($n = 740$)	2	4	75	80	76	82	0.8	1.7
Swedish Melanoma Study Group ($n = 989$)	2	5	81	83	86	89	0.8	1.0
World Health Organization ($n = 612$)	1	3	82 (8-year)	84 (8-year)	90 (8-year)	90 (8-year)	1.3	0
UKMSG/BAPS/SCTN ($n = 900$)	1	3	55	48	68	70	3.3	2.9

gins where anatomic considerations allow for invasive melanomas Breslow thickness > 2.0 mm [2, 23]. Contemporary trials are underway to evaluate narrower surgical margins, especially for melanomas >2 mm in depth, in order to potentially decrease the morbidity of larger resections.

Beyond the radial margin excision, other operative considerations include the depth of excision and management of the wound defect. For primary invasive melanoma, the excision depth should routinely extend down to, but not including, the muscular fascia. While the underlying muscular fascia may be resected en bloc with the specimen if there are concerns for direct invasion through the subcutaneous fat planes, routine resection of the underlying fascia has not been shown to improve outcomes. The excision is usually performed in a fusiform or elliptical fashion along an axis to minimize tension and/or along the longitudinal axis of the involved extremity, thus facilitating primary closure. If primary closure is unable to be performed, then closure can be performed with local advancement or rotational flaps or with skin graft placement. If there are significant clinical concerns regarding potential microscopic tumor involvement of the peripheral margins of the specimen and the wound cannot be closed primarily, options include leaving the wound open until the final pathology results are obtained versus performing the margin of excision alone and leaving the central aspect of the proposed excision in vivo. Following histologic confirmation of clear margins, any additional excision needed for the tissue can then be performed, followed by definitive reconstruction of the wound.

Management of Clinically Negative Regional Lymph Nodes

Cutaneous melanoma is notorious for metastasizing to the regional lymph nodes, and a significant component of the morbidity of this disease is derived not only from the disease progression itself, but also from the different surgical and nonsurgical treatment approaches that have been used historically to control regional lymph node disease.

Sentinel lymph node biopsy (SLNB) is a surgical procedure that was developed to accurately stage the regional nodal basins in patients with primary melanoma without clinical or radiographic evidence of lymph nodal involvement. In these patients, sentinel lymph node status is a strong predictor of survival and provides improved disease-free survival, as well as provides important prognostic information to guide further treatment [24, 25].

The Multicenter Selective Lymphadenectomy Trial-I (MSLT-I) provided the background evidence for the establishment of sentinel lymph node biopsy as the standard of care for patients with intermediate and thick cutaneous melanomas. After randomizing 2001 patients with primary cutaneous melanoma to undergo wide excision with nodal observation and lymphadenectomy for nodal relapse (observation group) or wide excision with sentinel lymph node biopsy and immediate lymphadenectomy for positive sentinel lymph node (biopsy group), the study concluded that pathologic lymph node staging provides important prognostic information and identifies patients who might benefit from additional treatment. In addition, SLNB-based management was shown to prolong disease-free survival for patients with nodal metastases [26]. Current practice guidelines recommend that patients with T1b disease (Breslow thickness ≥ 0.8 mm or any Breslow thickness level with ulceration on pathological evaluation of the primary biopsy specimen) and no clinical lymphadenopathy should be considered for sentinel lymph node biopsy and carry a > 5% risk of having nodal disease [2, 23]. For patients with Breslow thickness < 0.8 mm (T1a), the risk of nodal disease is considered to be less than 5%. Thus, sentinel lymph node biopsy is not routinely performed in these patients. While it has been suggested that SLNB may be considered for T1a melanomas with high-risk features (age younger than 42 years old, head and neck location, lymphovascular invasion, high mitotic rate), this is an area of ongoing research, including prospective trials evaluating gene expression profile tests [27–29].

In the setting of primary cutaneous melanoma with negative sentinel lymph nodes on pathological evaluation, traditional management has been surveillance for disease recurrence and separate de novo skin cancers in different locations. Over the past 20 years, multiple trials have shown improved survival with systemic immunotherapy and targeted therapies for advanced melanoma, including improved recurrence-free survival in the adjuvant setting for patients with high-risk, resected stage III and IV melanoma [30, 31]. Since high-risk stage II disease (IIB and IIC) has been noted to have similar or worse disease-specific survival than stage IIIA and IIIB disease, the role of adjuvant systemic immunotherapy in high-risk stage II patients was subsequently evaluated [15, 32, 33]. The Keynote 716 trial was a multi-institutional randomized controlled trial that assessed pembrolizumab for up to 1 year as adjuvant systemic therapy for patients with stage IIB and IIC melanoma and pathologically proven negative sentinel lymph nodes. A total of 976 patients were randomized to receive adjuvant pembrolizumab or placebo. Recurrence-free survival and distant metastasis-free survival were both improved with pembolizumab when compared to placebo, and the treatment side effects were generally well tolerated and manageable [32, 34]. In a similar fashion, the CheckMate 76 K trial randomized 790 patients to receive adjuvant nivolumab or placebo and showed the efficacy and safety of adjuvant nivolumab in decreasing recurrence-free and distant metastasis-free survival in patients with stage IIB and IIC melanoma [33].

In summary, adjuvant systemic immunotherapy should be discussed in patients with stage IIB and IIC, formally weighing the risks and benefits of treatment based on their individualized risk and safety profile.

Management of Positive Sentinel Lymph Nodes

Following the identification of positive sentinel lymph nodes, patients are then staged with whole-body imaging to exclude distant metastatic disease. Historically, patients with positive sentinel nodes and no evidence of distant disease were managed with a completion lymph node dissection. However, only about 10–20% of these patients would go on to have positive non-sentinel lymph nodes, and therefore, this approach has been challenged.

The DeCOG-SLT trial randomized 483 patients with cutaneous melanoma with positive sentinel lymph node biopsy to undergo completion lymph node dissection vs. observation with serial regional nodal ultrasonography. At 3- and 6-year evaluation, completion lymph node dissection was not superior to observation in terms of distant metastasis-free survival, recurrence-free survival, and overall survival [35]. The Multicenter Selective Lymphadenectomy Trial-II (MSLT-II) also randomized 1934 patients with sentinel lymph node positive intermediate-thickness melanoma to completion lymph node dissection vs. observation with surveillance nodal ultrasonography. In this study, completion lymph node dissection did increase the rate of regional disease control and provided prognostic information. However, it did not increase melanoma-specific survival [25]. More recent retrospective studies evaluating the real-world practice of nodal observation rather than immediate completion lymph node dissection have also shown no survival benefit when reserving formal lymphadenectomy for only those patients who develop isolated regional recurrence while on surveillance [36, 37].

Current guidelines advocate for the consideration of adjuvant systemic therapy after a positive sentinel lymph node biopsy in conjunction with active surveillance of the regional nodal basin, reserving complete lymph node dissection for nodal recurrence [23, 38]. The EORTC 18071 in 2016 was the first randomized controlled trial to evaluate the role of adjuvant systemic therapy in 951 patients with stage III melanoma. In this trial, ipilimumab, a CTLA4 antibody, was given to patients with resected stage III melanoma and improved recurrence-free and overall survival at 5 years when compared to placebo [39]. However, due to significant treatment-related adverse events with ipilimumab, further adjuvant studies with anti-PD1 agents have been performed [40]. The CheckMate 238 randomized controlled trial compared adjuvant ipilimumab vs. nivolumab in 906 patients with resected stage III and IV melanoma and showed longer recurrence-free survival and a significantly lower rate of grade 3 or 4 adverse events with treatment in the nivolumab arm [41]. Lastly, pembrolizumab was also compared to placebo as adjuvant therapy in resected stage III melanoma and was associated with increased recurrence-free survival [42]. Therefore, adjuvant systemic immunotherapy with anti-PD1 blockade is currently the standard of care management for patients with resected stage III and IV melanoma over ipilimumab.

Mutational profiling via next-generation sequencing or immunohistochemistry has developed into an advanced method of identifying potential treatment targets that can assist in the management of patients with advanced melanoma (stage III or IV). The most common harboring mutation is BRAF, specifically the V600E variant. Current guidelines also advocate for combined BRAF and MEK inhibition for patients with resected stage III and IV melanoma, specifically dabrafenib and trametinib, which is associated with improved outcomes and lower incidence of adverse effects from treatment [43, 44]. Even though there has been no direct comparison between immunotherapy and BRAF/MEK-targeted therapy, it is the authors' belief that decisions on adjuvant therapy should always be made in the setting of an experienced multidisciplinary oncological team, taking both disease and patient factors into consideration.

Management of Clinically Positive Regional Lymph Nodes

Clinical examination of the regional lymph node basins is of utmost importance in localized cutaneous melanoma. All patients presenting for evaluation of a new cutaneous melanoma should be assessed for the presence of enlarged and/or firm regional lymphadenopathy. For patients with clinically evident regional nodal disease defined as detectable on either physical exam or radiographic studies, image-guided needle biopsy is the preferred approach to confirm histologic diagnosis and determine mutational status (Fig. 23.2). In addition, all patients with clinically evident stage III disease should have complete staging imaging evaluation with whole-body PET/CT and MRI brain to assess for distant metastatic disease.

Historically, the approach to clinically evident stage III disease on presentation has been mostly surgical, with resection of the primary cutaneous lesion, if not previously treated, and regional therapeutic lymph node dissection being the predominant treatment modalities. The demonstrated value of adjuvant systemic immunotherapy and targeted therapies in patients with resected stage III melanoma has been previously discussed in this chapter and should be considered in patients treated with an upfront surgical approach. However, recently published randomized trials have shifted the systemic treatment strategy in these patients toward neoadjuvant approaches [38, 45]. Advantages of neoadjuvant treatment include in vivo evaluation of the response to therapy, which may guide treatment duration, including cessation of therapy, as well as the extent of the consolidative surgical approach. Additionally, neoadjuvant treatment possesses the theoretical advantage of attacking the tumor at its initial, undisturbed immunological microenvironment and resulting in an enhanced anti-tumor immune response.

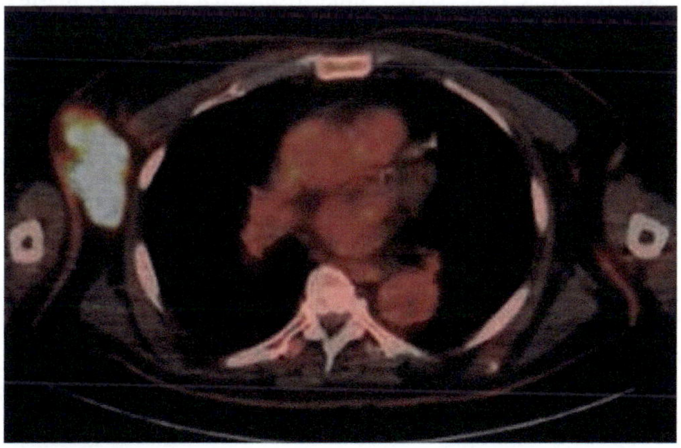

Fig. 23.2 PET-avid right axillary lymph node with metastatic melanoma

Recent randomized controlled trials have established neoadjuvant systemic immunotherapy as the new preferred standard of care in clinically evident stage III melanoma as well as resectable stage IV melanoma. The SWOG 1801 randomized controlled trial compared neoadjuvant-adjuvant pembrolizumab (three doses preoperatively and 15 doses postoperatively) with adjuvant-only pembrolizumab. A total of 313 patients were randomized in a 1:1 fashion. Event-free survival at 2 years was 72% (95% CI 0.64–0.80) in the neoadjuvant-adjuvant group and 49% (95% CI 0.41–0.59) in the adjuvant-only group ($p = 0.004$), and at the same time, no new toxic events were identified [46]. Subsequently, the NADINA trial compared neoadjuvant immunotherapy with ipilimumab and nivolumab for two cycles followed by therapeutic lymph node dissection to upfront therapeutic lymph node dissection and adjuvant nivolumab for 1 year in 423 patients with clinically evident stage III melanoma. In this trial, the adjuvant treatment of the patients in the experimental neoadjuvant arm was decided based on the pathologic response of the evaluated resected lymph nodes, with only patients with partial response (10–50% viable tumor) and nonresponse (>50% viable tumor) receiving adjuvant immunotherapy or targeted therapy. At a median follow-up of 9.9 months, the estimated 12-month event-free survival was 83.7% (99.9% CI 73.8 to 94.8) in the neoadjuvant group and 57.2% (99.9% CI 45.1 to 72.7) in the adjuvant group. The difference in restricted mean survival time was 8.00 months (99.9% CI 4.94 to 11.05; $p < 0.001$) [47].

Taking the individualized approach of patients with advanced melanoma one step further, the PRADO trial addressed the feasibility of using pathologic response after neoadjuvant ipilimumab and nivolumab as a criterion for further treatment personalization. In this extension cohort of a larger neoadjuvant trial, 99 patients with stage III melanoma received two cycles of ipilimumab and nivolumab and subsequently underwent index lymph node excision (operative excision of the index lymph node defined as the largest lymph node metastasis at baseline) with assessment of pathologic response on the specimen regarding the percentage of tumor viability. In patients achieving major pathologic response (<10% viable tumor), both therapeutic lymph node dissection and adjuvant systemic therapy were omitted. Patients with partial pathologic response (10–50% viable tumor) underwent therapeutic lymph node dissection alone without adjuvant therapy, whereas patients with pathologic nonresponse (>50% viable tumor) underwent therapeutic lymph node dissection and adjuvant immunotherapy with or without concurrent radiation therapy. The 24-month relapse-free survival and distant metastasis-free survival rates were 93% and 98% for major pathologic response, 64% and 64% for pathologic partial response, and 71% and 76% for pathologic non-response [48]. Although only 99 patients were included in this cohort, these findings have provided a rationale for consideration of surgical de-escalation with index lymph node excision rather than formal lymphadenectomy in selected patients following response to neoadjuvant therapy.

With the evolution of newer treatment strategies and molecular-based approaches, physicians who treat patients with melanoma will continue to have multiple ongoing weapons in their armamentarium. It is the responsibility of the multidisciplinary cancer treatment teams to be able to navigate through the different therapeutic pathways and to identify the best individualized approach, in coordination with the patient's comorbidities and desires, in order to achieve the best results.

Management of Metastatic and Unresectable Locoregionally Advanced Melanoma

As both the incidence of cutaneous melanoma and the survival rate of patients affected by the disease continue to increase, patients will continue to live longer with advanced metastatic disease. Melanoma is notorious for presenting with metastatic disease to multiple areas and organs of the body, from satellite and in-transit disease between the primary lesion and the regional lymph node basins to disease in the brain, gastrointestinal tract, lung, and liver.

Historically, cytotoxic chemotherapy was used for patients with advanced metastatic disease, however with low response rates and high toxicity. The role of ipilimumab immunotherapy as a CTLA4 inhibitor was established by two randomized controlled trials in 2010 and 2011, where it showed improved overall survival in 676 and 502 patients, respectively, with metastatic melanoma, both as second-line after no response to prior therapy and as first-line treatment [49, 50]. Further understanding of the immunological aspects of the disease led to the introduction of PD1 inhibitors, such as nivolumab and pembrolizumab, which have also been shown to be effective but with less toxicity [44, 51–53]. Furthermore, mutational analysis of disease specimens and identification of potential therapeutic targets have led to the development of BRAF/MEK-targeted therapies, which have improved objective response rates and progression-free survival [54, 55]. The decision for first-line treatment between immunotherapy and BRAF-targeted therapy in clinical practice should be performed by specialized providers with expertise in the management of advanced melanoma.

As survival continues to improve in patients with advanced melanoma, the importance of locoregional control has never been more critical. While surgery remains a mainstay for treatment of patients with limited, recurrent locoregional disease, specialized therapies such as intralesional talimogene laherparepvec (T-VEC) and regional infusion therapies for isolated limb disease also allow for meaningful disease control in patients with advanced locoregional disease (Fig. 23.3).

T-VEC is a novel therapeutic viral construct of the HSV1, which was approved for intralesional therapy by the FDA in 2015 after evaluation in the OPTiM trial [56, 57]. When injected intratumorally, this virus selectively targets tumor cells and causes their lytic destruction, while at the same time producing GM-CSF to recruit macrophages in the tumor microenvironment. It is generally well tolerated with limited significant adverse events, most commonly transient fatigue and pyrexia the evening of injection. In the OPTiM (Oncovex Pivotal Trial in Melanoma) phase III trial, T-VEC was compared with GM-CSF in 436 patients with advanced melanoma stage III and IV. Durable response rate and objective response rate in 6 months were significantly higher in patients receiving T-VEC, while overall survival was significantly improved in patients with stage IIIB-IVM1a melanoma [56].

Regional infusion therapy for unresectable in-transit disease isolated to an extremity has been described via two major techniques: hyperthermic isolated limb perfusion (HILP) and isolated limb infusion (ILI). Overall response rates for these procedures range from 50% to 100% in vari-

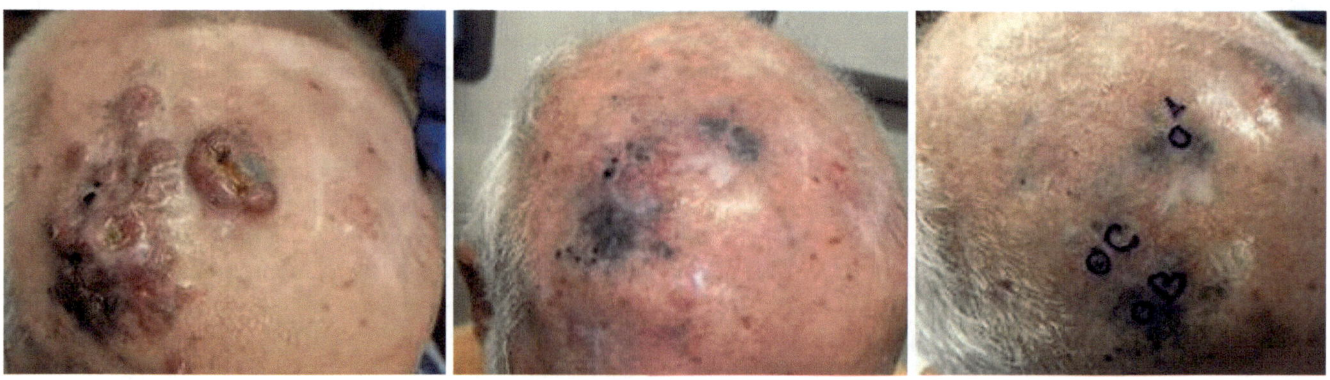

Fig. 23.3 Patient with advanced recurrent locoregional melanoma of the scalp who underwent intralesional therapy with talimogene laherparepvec. The final image shows scouting posttreatment biopsies that did not reveal any viable melanoma

ous studies, with clinical complete response rates ranging from 25% to 45%, and a myriad of patient, disease, and technique factors potentially coming into play [58, 59]. While HILP has shown higher response rates than ILI, the advantages of ILI are the less invasive percutaneous placement of catheters and therefore repeatability of the procedure [60, 61]. The acidotic and hypoxic environment created during ILI potentially contributes to the anti-tumor effects of the treatment, and the limb is washed out at the completion of the procedure, thus limiting the systemic side effects.

Uveal melanoma is a rare subtype of melanoma with a high predilection for metastatic disease, often isolated, to the liver. Additionally, systemic immune checkpoint inhibitors have been shown to not be as effective in uveal melanoma as compared to metastatic cutaneous melanoma. Percutaneous hepatic perfusion (PHP) with melphalan is a novel approach of selectively delivering regional chemotherapy to the liver intra-arterially while isolating the hepatic vasculature via veno-venous bypass. Based on a multicenter randomized controlled trial that compared PHP with best alternative care in 93 patients with uveal melanoma metastatic to the liver, hepatic progression-free survival, overall progression-free survival, and hepatic objective response were all improved with the use of PHP-melphalan [62]. Following the phase III FOCUS trial, PHP-melphalan is now FDA-approved for the treatment of metastatic uveal melanoma to the liver.

In patients with widespread metastatic melanoma, surgery should be reserved for those patients seeking palliation or with oligometastatic progression. Indications for palliation include intestinal obstruction or bleeding, as well as intractable pain. However, it is imperative that these complex patients be treated by a multidisciplinary team and highly selected. Radiation therapy may also serve as a palliative adjunct treatment option in patients with advanced, widespread metastatic melanoma.

Summary

Cutaneous melanoma represents a wide spectrum of disease intensity, which physicians in multiple practice types will encounter throughout their practice. Whether it is early-stage melanoma or advanced metastatic disease, therapeutic options and society guidelines are continuously evolving, and it is the responsibility of the practitioners to evolve along with them and stay informed to the best of their abilities. As the understanding of the immunological and mutational profile of melanoma continues to evolve, our systemic therapies and sequencing of these treatments continue to improve, which calls for the treatment of these complex patients in a multidisciplinary fashion. Furthermore, this better understanding of tumor biology, along with more "arrows in the quiver," will allow for more individualized treatment plans for these patients.

Disclosure Statement All authors have no conflict of interest and/or financial support to declare in the research presented. There are no declarations of interest.

References

1. Siegel RL, Giaquinto AN, Jemal A. Cancer statistics, 2024. CA Cancer J Clin. 2024;74(1):12–49. https://doi.org/10.3322/caac.21820. PMID: 38230766
2. National Comprehensive Cancer Network Guidelines. Melanoma: Cutaneous (Version 3.2024). https://www.nccn.org/professionals/physician_gls/pdf/cutaneous_melanoma.pdf. Accessed 24 Nov 2024.
3. Dzwierzynski WW. Melanoma risk factors and prevention. Clin Plast Surg. 2021;48(4):543–50. https://doi.org/10.1016/j.cps.2021.05.001. PMID: 34503715
4. Miller AJ, Mihm MC Jr. Melanoma. N Engl J Med. 2006;335(1):51–65. https://doi.org/10.1056/NEJMra052166. PMID: 16822996
5. Chen JY, Fernandez K, Fadadu RP, Reddy R, Kim MO, Tan J, et al. Skin cancer diagnosis by lesion, physician, and examination type: a systematic review and meta-analysis. JAMA Dermatol. 2025;161(2):135–46. https://doi.org/10.1001/jamadermatol.2024.4382. PMID: 39535756
6. Long GV, Swetter SM, Menzies AM, Gershenwald JE, Scolyer RA. Cutaneous melanoma. Lancet. 2023;402(10400):485–502. https://doi.org/10.1016/S0140-6736(23)00821-8. PMID: 37499671
7. Yeh I, Bastian BC. Melanoma pathology: new approaches and classification. Br J Dermatol. 2021;185(2):282–93. https://doi.org/10.1111/bjd.20427. PMID: 34060071
8. Tímár J, Ladányi A. Molecular pathology of skin melanoma: epidemiology, differential diagnostics, prognosis and therapy prediction. Int J Mol Sci. 2022;23(10):5384. https://doi.org/10.3390/ijms23105384. PMID: 35628196
9. Cancer Genome Atlas Network. Genomic classification of cutaneous melanoma. Cell. 2015;161(7):1681–96. https://doi.org/10.1016/j.cell.2015.05.044. PMID: 26091043
10. Duarte AF, Sousa-Pinto B, Azevedo LF, Barros AM, Puig S, Malvehy J, et al. Clinical ABCDE rule for early melanoma detection. Eur J Dermatol. 2021;31(6):771–8. https://doi.org/10.1684/ejd.2021.4171. PMID: 35107069
11. Swetter SM, Tsao H, Bichakjian CK, Curiel-Lewandrowski C, Elder DE, Gershenwald JE, et al. Guidelines of care for the management of primary cutaneous melanoma. J Am Acad Dermatol. 2019;80(1):208–50. https://doi.org/10.1016/j.jaad.2018.08.055. PMID: 30392755
12. Zager JS, Hochwald SN, Marzban SS, Francois R, Law KM, Davis AH, et al. Shave biopsy is a safe and accurate method for the initial evaluation of melanoma. J Am Coll Surg. 2011;212(4):454–60. https://doi.org/10.1016/j.jamcollsurg.2010.12.021. discussion 460-2. PMID: 21463767
13. Amin MB, Edge SB, Greene FL, editors. The American Joint Committee on Cancer (AJCC) Staging Manual, Part X: Skin. 8th ed. Cham: American College of Surgeons/Springer; 2017.
14. Scolyer RA, Rawson RV, Gershenwald JE, Ferguson PM, Prieto VG. Melanoma pathology reporting and staging. Mod Pathol. 2020;33(Suppl 1):15–24. https://doi.org/10.1038/s41379-019-0402-x. PMID: 31758078
15. Gershenwald JE, Scolyer RA, Hess KR, Sondak VK, Long GV, Ross MI, et al. Melanoma staging: evidence-based changes in the American Joint Committee on Cancer eighth edition cancer staging manual. CA Cancer J Clin. 2017;67(6):472–92. https://doi.org/10.3322/caac.21409. PMID: 29028110
16. Amin MB, Greene FL, Edge SB, Compton CC, Gershenwald JE, Brookland RK, et al. The eighth edition AJCC cancer staging

manual: continuing to build a bridge from a population-based to a more "personalized" approach to cancer staging. CA Cancer J Clin. 2017;67(2):93–9. https://doi.org/10.3322/caac.21388. PMID: 28094848
17. Sondak VK. The evolving role of surgery in melanoma. Clin Adv Hematol Oncol. 2024;22(5):227–9. PMID: 38805314
18. Khayat D, Rixe O, Martin G, Soubrane C, Banzet M, Bazex JA, et al. Surgical margins in cutaneous melanoma (2 cm vs 5 cm for lesions measuring less than 2.1-mm thick). Cancer. 2003;97(8):1941–6. https://doi.org/10.1002/cncr.11272. PMID: 12673721
19. Balch CM, Soong SJ, Smith T, Ross MI, Urist MM, Karakousis CP, et al. Long-term results of a prospective surgical trial comparing 2 cm vs. 4 cm excision margins for 740 patients with 1-4 mm melanomas. Ann Surg Oncol. 2001;8(2):101–8. https://doi.org/10.1007/s10434-001-0101-x. PMID: 11258773
20. Cohn-Cedermark G, Rutqvist LE, Andersson R, Breivald M, Ingvar C, Johansson H, et al. Long term results of a randomized study by the Swedish melanoma study group on 2-cm versus 5-cm resection margins for patients with cutaneous melanoma with a tumor thickness of 0.8-2.0 mm. Cancer. 2000;89(7):1495–501. PMID: 11013363
21. Veronesi U, Cascinelli N, Adamus J, Balch C, Bandiera D, Barchuk A, et al. Thin stage I primary cutaneous malignant melanoma. Comparison of excision with margins of 1 or 3 cm. N Engl J Med. 1988;318(18):1159–62. https://doi.org/10.1056/NEJM198805053181804. PMID: 3079582
22. Hayes AJ, Maynard L, Coombes G, Newton-Bishop J, Timmons M, Cook M, et al. Wide versus narrow excision margins for high-risk, primary cutaneous melanomas: long-term follow-up of survival in a randomised trial. Lancet Oncol. 2016;17(2):184–92. https://doi.org/10.1016/S1470-2045(15)00482-9. PMID: 26790922
23. Amaral T, Ottaviano M, Arance A, Blank C, Chiarion-Sileni V, Donia M, et al. Cutaneous melanoma: ESMO clinical practice guideline for diagnosis, treatment and follow-up. Ann Oncol. 2025;36(1):10–30. https://doi.org/10.1016/j.annonc.2024.11.006. PMID: 39550033
24. El Sharouni MA, Stodell MD, Ahmed T, Suijkerbuijk KPM, Cust AE, Witkamp AJ, et al. Sentinel node biopsy in patients with melanoma improves the accuracy of staging when added to clinicopathological features of the primary tumor. Ann Oncol. 2021;32(3):375–83. https://doi.org/10.1016/j.annonc.2020.11.015. PMID: 33253862
25. Faries MB, Thompson JF, Cochran AJ, Andtbacka RH, Mozzillo N, Zager JS, et al. Completion dissection or observation for sentinel-node metastasis in melanoma. N Engl J Med. 2017;376(23):2211–22. https://doi.org/10.1056/NEJMoa1613210. PMID: 28591523
26. Morton DL, Thompson JF, Cochran AJ, Mozzillo N, Nieweg OE, Roses DF, et al. Final trial report of sentinel-node biopsy versus nodal observation in melanoma. N Engl J Med. 2014;370(7):599–609. https://doi.org/10.1056/NEJMoa1310460. PMID: 24521106
27. Shannon AB, Sharon CE, Straker RJ 3rd, Carr MJ, Sinnamon AJ, Bogatch K, et al. Sentinel lymph node biopsy in patients with T1a cutaneous malignant melanoma: a multicenter cohort study. J Am Acad Dermatol. 2023;88(1):52–9. https://doi.org/10.1016/j.jaad.2022.09.040. PMID: 36184008
28. Bartlett EK, O'Donoghue C, Boland G, Bowles T, Delman KA, Hieken TJ, et al. Society of surgical oncology consensus statement: assessing the evidence for and utility of gene expression profiling of primary cutaneous melanoma. Ann Surg Oncol. 2025;32(3):1429–42. https://doi.org/10.1245/s10434-024-16379-2. PMID: 39470890
29. Yousaf A, Tjien-Fooh FJ, Rentroia-Pacheco B, Quattrocchi E, Kobic A, Tempel D, et al. Validation of CP-GEP (Merlin assay) for predicting sentinel lymph node metastasis in primary cutaneous melanoma patients: a U.S. cohort study. Int J Dermatol. 2021;60(7):851–6. https://doi.org/10.1111/ijd.15594. PMID: 33914348
30. Eggermont AMM, Blank CU, Mandalà M, Long GV, Atkinson VG, Dalle S, et al. Adjuvant pembrolizumab versus placebo in resected stage III melanoma (EORTC 1325-MG/KEYNOTE-054): distant metastasis-free survival results from a double-blind, randomised, controlled, phase 3 trial. Lancet Oncol. 2021;22(5):643–54. https://doi.org/10.1016/S1470-2045(21)00065-6. PMID: 33857412
31. Long GV, Hauschild A, Santinami M, Atkinson V, Mandalà M, Chiarion-Sileni V, et al. Adjuvant dabrafenib plus trametinib in stage III BRAF-mutated melanoma. N Engl J Med. 2017;377(19):1813–23. https://doi.org/10.1056/NEJMoa1708539. PMID: 28891408
32. Luke JJ, Rutkowski P, Queirolo P, Del Vecchio M, Mackiewicz J, Chiarion-Sileni V, et al. Pembrolizumab versus placebo as adjuvant therapy in completely resected stage IIB or IIC melanoma (KEYNOTE-716): a randomised, double-blind, phase 3 trial. Lancet. 2022;399(10336):1718–29. https://doi.org/10.1016/S0140-6736(22)00562-1. PMID: 35367007
33. Kirkwood JM, Del Vecchio M, Weber J, Hoeller C, Grob JJ, Mohr P, et al. Adjuvant nivolumab in resected stage IIB/C melanoma: primary results from the randomized, phase 3 CheckMate 76K trial. Nat Med. 2023;29(11):2835–43. https://doi.org/10.1038/s41591-023-02583-2. PMID: 37845511
34. Luke JJ, Ascierto PA, Khattak MA, de la Cruz Merino L, Del Vecchio M, Rutkowski P, et al. Pembrolizumab versus placebo as adjuvant therapy in resected stage IIB or IIC melanoma: final analysis of distant metastasis-free survival in the phase III KEYNOTE-716 study. J Clin Oncol. 2024;42(14):1619–24. https://doi.org/10.1200/JCO.23.02355. PMID: 38452313
35. Leiter U, Stadler R, Mauch C, Hohenberger W, Brockmeyer NH, Berking C, et al. Final analysis of DeCOG-SLT trial: no survival benefit for complete lymph node dissection in patients with melanoma with positive sentinel node. J Clin Oncol. 2019;37(32):3000–8. https://doi.org/10.1200/JCO.18.02306. PMID: 31557067
36. Broman KK, Hughes T, Dossett L, Sun J, Kirichenko D, Carr MJ, et al. Active surveillance of patients who have sentinel node positive melanoma: AN international, multi-institution evaluation of adoption and early outcomes after the Multicenter selective lymphadenectomy trial II (MSLT-II). Cancer. 2021;127(13):2251–61. https://doi.org/10.1002/cncr.33483. PMID: 33826754
37. Broman KK, Bettampadi D, Pérez-Morales J, Sun J, Kirichenko D, Carr MJ, et al. Surveillance of sentinel node-positive melanoma patients who receive adjuvant therapy without undergoing completion lymph node dissection. Ann Surg Oncol. 2021;28(12):6978–85. https://doi.org/10.1245/s10434-021-10570-5. PMID: 34363118
38. Farma JM, Olszanski AJ, Messina JL, Sondak VK. Annals of surgical oncology practice guidelines series: adjuvant and neoadjuvant therapy for melanoma. Ann Surg Oncol. 2025;32(1):3–11. https://doi.org/10.1245/s10434-024-16418-y. PMID: 39495363
39. Eggermont AMM, Chiarion-Sileni V, Grob JJ, Dummer R, Wolchok JD, Schmidt H, et al. Prolonged survival in stage III melanoma with ipilimumab adjuvant therapy. N Engl J Med. 2016;375(19):1845–55. https://doi.org/10.1056/NEJMoa1611299. PMID: 27717298
40. Tarhini AA, Lee SJ, Hodi FS, Rao UNM, Cohen GI, Hamid O, et al. Phase III study of adjuvant ipilimumab (3 or 10 mg/kg) versus high-dose interferon Alfa-2b for resected high-risk melanoma: North American intergroup E1609. J Clin Oncol. 2020;38(6):567–75. https://doi.org/10.1200/JCO.19.01381. PMID: 31880964
41. Weber J, Mandala M, Del Vecchio M, Gogas HJ, Arance AM, Cowey CL, et al. Adjuvant nivolumab versus ipilimumab in resected stage III or IV melanoma. N Engl J Med. 2017;377(19):1824–35. https://doi.org/10.1056/NEJMoa1709030. PMID: 28891423
42. Eggermont AMM, Blank CU, Mandala M, Long GV, Atkinson V, Dalle S, et al. Adjuvant pembrolizumab versus placebo in resected

stage III melanoma. N Engl J Med. 2018;378(19):1789–801. https://doi.org/10.1056/NEJMoa1802357. PMID: 29658430
43. Long GV, Stroyakovskiy D, Gogas H, Levchenko E, de Braud F, Larkin J, et al. Combined BRAF and MEK inhibition versus BRAF inhibition alone in melanoma. N Engl J Med. 2014;371(20):1877–88. https://doi.org/10.1056/NEJMoa1406037. PMID: 25265492
44. Robert C, Karaszewska B, Schachter J, Rutkowski P, Mackiewicz A, Stroiakovski D, et al. Improved overall survival in melanoma with combined dabrafenib and trametinib. N Engl J Med. 2015;372(1):30–9. https://doi.org/10.1056/NEJMoa1412690. PMID: 25399551
45. Su D, Kluger H, Olino K. Educational review: clinical application of immune checkpoint blockade for the treatment of melanoma. Ann Surg Oncol. 2024;31(3):1865–79. https://doi.org/10.1245/s10434-023-14587-w. PMID: 37989956
46. Patel SP, Othus M, Chen Y, Wright GP Jr, Yost KJ, Hyngstrom JR, et al. Neoadjuvant-adjuvant or adjuvant-only pembrolizumab in advanced melanoma. N Engl J Med. 2023;388(9):813–23. https://doi.org/10.1056/NEJMoa2211437. PMID: 36856617
47. Blank CU, Lucas MW, Scolyer RA, van de Wiel BA, Menzies AM, Lopez-Yurda M, et al. Neoadjuvant nivolumab and ipilimumab in resectable stage III melanoma. N Engl J Med. 2024;391(18):1696–708. https://doi.org/10.1056/NEJMoa2402604. PMID: 38828984
48. Reijers ILM, Menzies AM, van Akkooi ACJ, Versluis JM, van den Heuvel NMJ, Saw RPM, et al. Personalized response-directed surgery and adjuvant therapy after neoadjuvant ipilimumab and nivolumab in high-risk stage III melanoma: the PRADO trial. Nat Med. 2022;28(6):1178–88. https://doi.org/10.1038/s41591-022-01851-x. PMID: 35661157
49. Hodi FS, O'Day SJ, McDermott DF, Weber RW, Sosman JA, Haanen JB, et al. Improved survival with ipilimumab in patients with metastatic melanoma. N Engl J Med. 2010;363(8):711–23. https://doi.org/10.1056/NEJMoa1003466. PMID: 20525992
50. Robert C, Thomas L, Bondarenko I, O'Day S, Weber J, Garbe C, et al. Ipilimumab plus dacarbazine for previously untreated metastatic melanoma. N Engl J Med. 2011;364(26):2517–26. https://doi.org/10.1056/NEJMoa1104621. PMID: 21639810
51. Wolchok JD, Kluger H, Callahan MK, Postow MA, Rizvi NA, Lesokhin AM, et al. Nivolumab plus ipilimumab in advanced melanoma. N Engl J Med. 2013;369(2):122–33. https://doi.org/10.1056/NEJMoa1302369. PMID: 23724867
52. Simeone E, Grimaldi AM, Ascierto PA. Anti-PD1 and anti-PD-L1 in the treatment of metastatic melanoma. Melanoma Manag. 2015;2(1):41–50. https://doi.org/10.2217/mmt.14.30. PMID: 30190830
53. Robert C, Long GV, Brady B, Dutriaux C, Maio M, Mortier L, et al. Nivolumab in previously untreated melanoma without BRAF mutation. N Engl J Med. 2015;372(4):320–30. https://doi.org/10.1056/NEJMoa1412082. PMID: 25399552
54. Flaherty KT, Infante JR, Daud A, Gonzalez R, Kefford RF, Sosman J, et al. Combined BRAF and MEK inhibition in melanoma with BRAF V600 mutations. N Engl J Med. 2012;367(18):1694–703. https://doi.org/10.1056/NEJMoa1210093. PMID: 23020132
55. Luke JJ. Comprehensive clinical trial data summation for BRAF-MEK inhibition and checkpoint immunotherapy in metastatic melanoma. Oncologist. 2019;24(11):e1197–211. https://doi.org/10.1634/theoncologist.2018-0876. PMID: 31064886
56. Andtbacka RHI, Kaufman HL, Collichio F, Amatruda T, Senzer N, Chesney J, et al. Talimogene laherparepvec improves durable response rate in patients with advanced melanoma. J Clin Oncol. 2015;33(25):2780–8. https://doi.org/10.1200/JCO.2014.58.3377. PMID: 26014293
57. Senzer NN, Kaufman HL, Amatruda T, Nemunaitis M, Reid T, Daniels G, et al. Phase II clinical trial of a granulocyte-macrophage colony-stimulating factor-encoding, second-generation oncolytic herpesvirus in patients with unresectable metastatic melanoma. J Clin Oncol. 2009;27(34):5763–71. https://doi.org/10.1200/JCO.2009.24.3675. PMID: 19884534
58. Lidsky ME, Turley RS, Beasley GM, Sharma K, Tyler DS. Predicting disease progression after regional therapy for in-transit melanoma. JAMA Surg. 2013;148(6):493–8. https://doi.org/10.1001/jamasurg.2013.695. PMID: 23558401
59. Miura JT, Kroon HM, Beasley GM, Mullen D, Farrow NE, Mosca PJ, et al. Long-term oncologic outcomes after isolated limb infusion for locoregionally metastatic melanoma: an international multicenter analysis. Ann Surg Oncol. 2019;26(8):2486–94. https://doi.org/10.1245/s10434-019-07288-w. PMID: 30911949
60. Sharma K, Beasley G, Turley R, Raymond AK, Broadwater G, Peterson B, et al. Patterns of recurrence following complete response to regional chemotherapy for in-transit melanoma. Ann Surg Oncol. 2012;19(8):2563–71. https://doi.org/10.1245/s10434-012-2315-5. PMID: 22476748
61. Möller MG, Lewis JM, Dessureault S, Zager JS. Toxicities associated with hyperthermic isolated limb perfusion and isolated limb infusion in the treatment of melanoma and sarcoma. Int J Hyperth. 2008;24(3):275–89. https://doi.org/10.1080/02656730701805520. PMID: 18393005
62. Hughes MS, Zager J, Faries M, Alexander HR, Royal RE, Wood B, et al. Results of a randomized controlled multicenter phase III trial of percutaneous hepatic perfusion compared with best available care for patients with melanoma liver metastases. Ann Surg Oncol. 2016;23(4):1309–19. https://doi.org/10.1245/s10434-015-4968-3. PMID: 26597368

Research on Breast Cancer: From Bench to Bedside

24

Mohammed Al-Jumayli

Introduction

Breast cancer remains one of the most commonly diagnosed malignancies worldwide, accounting for approximately 11.7% of all new cancer cases globally [1]. It is a major contributor to cancer-related morbidity and mortality, particularly among women. The heterogeneity of breast cancer, which includes distinct subtypes such as hormone receptor–positive (HR+), HER2-positive, and triple-negative breast cancer (TNBC), presents significant challenges in treatment and prognosis [2]. Each subtype exhibits unique molecular characteristics that influence therapeutic response and disease progression.

Recent advancements in diagnostic tools and targeted therapies have substantially improved survival rates, particularly in early-stage breast cancer. The introduction of genomic profiling, immunotherapy, and antibody-drug conjugates (ADCs) has revolutionized breast cancer management. However, metastatic breast cancer (MBC) continues to present a poor prognosis, with limited curative options and high rates of recurrence [3]. Research efforts continue to focus on understanding the molecular mechanisms underlying tumor progression, resistance to therapy, and potential biomarkers that could further enhance personalized treatment approaches.

Several key methodologies have significantly advanced our understanding and treatment of the disease (Table 24.1).

M. Al-Jumayli (✉)
H Lee Moffitt Cancer Center and Research Institute, University of South Florida, Tampa, FL, USA
e-mail: mohammed.aljumayli@moffitt.org

J. Huang, H. S.L. Jim (eds.), *Cancer Research Guidance for Clinicians and Researchers*,
https://doi.org/10.1007/978-3-032-19175-5_24

Table 24.1 Comparison of clinical trial types

Trial type	Description	Advantages	Disadvantages
Traditional phase trials	Phase I–IV trials conducted in sequential phases to evaluate safety, efficacy, and other outcomes	Well established and widely used; clear progression from early- to late-stage trials	Time-consuming; requires separate trials for each therapy/disease combination
Platform trials	Evaluates multiple therapies simultaneously for a single disease, allowing therapies to enter/leave based on performance	Efficient use of resources; therapies can be added/removed dynamically, speeding up research	Complex design; requires detailed statistical planning and continuous monitoring
Genomic profiling	Analyzing the expression of specific genes to predict disease prognosis and treatment response	Employed in the MINDACT trial to stratify patients' risk and guide chemotherapy decisions	Genomic profiling
Basket trials	Tests one therapy across multiple diseases sharing a common molecular marker	Allows for the identification of effectiveness across different cancers sharing a molecular marker	Relies heavily on identifying relevant biomarkers across multiple diseases
Umbrella trials	Tests multiple therapies within one disease subtype, using biomarkers to guide therapy selection	Allows personalized treatment options within a single cancer subtype, optimizing patient outcomes	Requires significant biomarker stratification and complex trial design
Response adaptive trials	Adaptive phase II/III designs for oncology drug development combine phase II signal detection and phase III confirmatory trials into one adaptive study. They allow flexible decisions based on real-time data to optimize outcomes	Mitigates risk of costly phase III failures by allowing a trial to adapt based on phase II results. Efficient use of resources and time, especially in challenging fields like oncology	Requires complex statistical modeling and continuous monitoring. Relies heavily on accurate early signal detection, and if misinterpreted, could lead to suboptimal phase III outcomes
Real-world evidence (RWE) integration	Incorporating data from routine clinical practice to complement findings from controlled trials	The AURORA program collects real-world data to study metastatic breast cancer's molecular landscape	Real-world evidence (RWE) integration

Molecular and Cellular Biology

Research in molecular and cellular biology has been pivotal in identifying genetic mutations that increase susceptibility to breast cancer. Notably, mutations in the BRCA1 and BRCA2 genes have been extensively studied for their role in hereditary breast cancer [4]. Technological advancements, such as next-generation sequencing (NGS) and CRISPR-Cas9 gene editing, have facilitated the detailed exploration of these mutations and their mechanisms. NGS allows for comprehensive profiling of genetic alterations, enabling personalized treatment strategies [5]. CRISPR-Cas9, on the other hand, provides a tool for precise gene editing, offering potential therapeutic avenues to correct deleterious mutations [6]. These technologies have collectively enhanced our ability to diagnose, monitor, and develop targeted therapies for breast cancer.

In Vitro and In Vivo Models

The utilization of in vitro and in vivo models has been instrumental in studying breast cancer biology and testing therapeutic interventions. In vitro models, particularly those employing breast cancer cell lines, allow researchers to investigate tumor behavior, drug responses, and molecular pathways under controlled laboratory conditions [7]. These models are essential for high-throughput screening of potential therapeutic agents. Complementing in vitro studies, in vivo models, such as patient-derived xenografts (PDXs), involve implanting human breast cancer tissues into immunocompromised mice. PDXs closely mimic the human tumor microenvironment and heterogeneity, providing a more accurate platform for evaluating the efficacy and safety of new treatments before clinical application [8].

Omics Technologies

Advancements in omics technologies, including genomics, proteomics, and transcriptomics, have deepened our understanding of the molecular architecture of breast cancer. Genomic studies have identified numerous mutations and copy number variations associated with different breast cancer subtypes [5]. Proteomic analyses have elucidated protein expression patterns and posttranslational modifications that drive tumor progression [9]. Transcriptomic profiling has revealed gene expression signatures predictive of patient outcomes and treatment responses. Integrating data from these omics approaches facilitates the development of personalized therapies tailored to the unique molecular profile of each patient's tumor.

Tumor Microenvironment (TME)

The tumor microenvironment (TME) plays a crucial role in breast cancer development, progression, and response to therapy. The TME comprises various components, including immune cells, stromal cells, extracellular matrix, and signaling molecules, all interacting dynamically with tumor cells [10]. Understanding these interactions has led to the identification of therapeutic targets within the TME. For instance, cancer-associated fibroblasts (CAFs) contribute to tumor growth and metastasis by remodeling the extracellular matrix and secreting pro-tumorigenic factors [11]. Targeting CAFs or their signaling pathways holds potential for disrupting the supportive niche that tumors exploit. Additionally, immune cells within the TME can either suppress or promote tumor activity. Therapies aiming to enhance anti-tumor immunity, such as immune checkpoint inhibitors, have shown promise in reactivating the immune system to recognize and attack breast cancer cells [12]. Ongoing research into TME modulation continues to open new avenues for therapeutic intervention.

Collectively, these methodologies underscore the multifaceted approach required to tackle breast cancer, integrating molecular insights with translational research to inform clinical practice and improve patient outcomes.

Treatment Research in Breast Cancer

Advancements in breast cancer treatment have been shaped by rigorous clinical trials, aiming to improve survival outcomes, reduce recurrence rates, and personalize therapy based on molecular profiling.

Phase I/II Trials

Phase I and II trials focus on assessing the safety, dosage, and preliminary efficacy of novel treatments. A notable example is the DecipHER phase I trial, which explored a combination of HER2-primed dendritic cells with immune checkpoint inhibitors for treating high-risk breast cancer [13]. This trial enrolled 12 patients and demonstrated that the combination therapy was safe and elicited measurable immune responses, laying the groundwork for subsequent studies to assess its clinical efficacy. Additionally, emerging antibody-drug conjugates (ADCs), such as trastuzumab deruxtecan (T-DXd), have demonstrated promising activity in HER2 low metastatic breast cancer, as seen in the DESTINY-Breast01 and DESTINY-Breast04 trials. In the DESTINY-Breast01 trial, 184 patients with HER2-positive metastatic breast cancer received T-DXd, resulting in an objective response rate of 60.9% and a median progression-free survival of 16.4 months. Similarly, the DESTINY-Breast04 trial included 557 patients with HER2-low metastatic breast cancer, where T-DXd significantly improved progression-free survival and overall survival compared to standard chemotherapy [14].

Randomized Controlled Trials (RCTs)

Randomized controlled trials remain the gold standard for evaluating new breast cancer therapies.

- The HER2CLIMB trial demonstrated that adding tucatinib to trastuzumab and capecitabine significantly improved survival in HER2-positive metastatic breast cancer, even in patients with brain metastases. This international, randomized, placebo-controlled, double-blind trial enrolled 612 patients with metastatic HER2-positive breast cancer, including those with and without brain metastases. The addition of tucatinib reduced the risk of disease progression or death by 46% and the risk of death by 34% compared to trastuzumab and capecitabine alone [15].
- The KEYNOTE-522 trial established pembrolizumab plus chemotherapy as the standard neoadjuvant treatment for triple-negative breast cancer (TNBC), significantly increasing the pathologic complete response (pCR) rate. In this trial, 1174 patients with high-risk early-stage triple-negative breast cancer (TNBC) were enrolled. The addition of pembrolizumab to neoadjuvant chemotherapy resulted in a pathologic complete response (pCR) rate of 64.8%, compared to 51.2% with chemotherapy alone. At 36 months, the event-free survival (EFS) rate was 84.5% in the pembrolizumab-chemotherapy group versus 76.8% in the chemotherapy-alone group. At 60 months, the overall survival (OS) rate was 86.6% in the pembrolizumab-chemotherapy group, compared to 81.7% in the chemotherapy-alone group [16].
- The KATHERINE trial confirmed that switching from trastuzumab to trastuzumab emtansine (T-DM1) after residual disease post-neoadjuvant therapy reduced recurrence risk in HER2-positive early-stage breast cancer. In this trial, 1486 patients with HER2-positive early-stage breast cancer who had residual disease after neoadjuvant therapy were enrolled. The study showed that T-DM1 reduced the risk of invasive disease recurrence or death by 50%, with an invasive disease-free survival (IDFS) rate of 80.8% compared to 67.1% with trastuzumab. The overall survival (OS) rate was 89.1% in the T-DM1 group versus 84.4% in the trastuzumab group, reflecting a 34% reduction in the risk of death [17].

Real-World Evidence (RWE) Studies

Real-world evidence (RWE) complements RCTs by evaluating treatment effectiveness in diverse, everyday clinical settings.

- A real-world study by Rugo et al. (2023) evaluated the effectiveness of palbociclib plus aromatase inhibitors (AIs) in hormone receptor–positive (HR+)/HER2-negative metastatic breast cancer. The study included 270 African American patients, with 127 receiving palbociclib plus an AI and 143 receiving an AI alone. The results demonstrated that the combination therapy was associated with improved overall survival compared to AI alone [18]. Another RWE, the ASCENT trial evaluating sacituzumab govitecan in metastatic TNBC, included 132 patients and demonstrated a median PFS of 5.2 months, a median OS of 8.7 months, and an ORR of 29%, closely aligning with the ASCENT trial results [19].

Advances in Clinical Trial Designs

Innovative clinical trial designs have accelerated drug development and personalized medicine in breast cancer.

Seamless Trials

Seamless trials integrate phase I/II or II/III stages into a continuous adaptive process, reducing drug development timelines. For example, the MORPHEUS HR + BC (NCT03280563) trial, which enrolled 138 patients, employed this model for HER2-negative breast cancer therapies, improving trial efficiency [20].

Master Protocols

Master protocols, including basket and umbrella trials, have revolutionized precision oncology:

- **Basket trials** evaluate a single targeted therapy across multiple cancer subtypes sharing the same molecular alteration.
- **Umbrella trials** test multiple drugs within a single cancer subtype, tailoring treatment based on distinct molecular markers. The NeoTRIP trial, for instance, assessed different regimens for TNBC in a molecularly stratified approach. In this trial, 280 patients with high-risk or locally advanced TNBC were treated to assess atezolizumab plus chemotherapy. The pCR rate was 48.6% with atezolizumab versus 44.4% with chemotherapy alone, with no significant improvement in event-free survival (70.6% vs. 74.9%) [21].

Platform Trials

Platform trials are an innovative clinical trial design that allows for the continuous evaluation of multiple investigational therapies within a single study. Unlike traditional trials that test one treatment at a time, platform trials use real-time interim data analysis to dynamically adjust treatment arms, ensuring that the most promising therapies receive more patient allocations while ineffective treatments are discontinued. A key example is the I-SPY 2 trial, a large, multicenter adaptive trial designed to evaluate multiple therapies for high-risk, early-stage breast cancer. In I-SPY 2, patients are assigned to different investigational treatments based on their biomarker profiles and molecular characteristics, allowing for a precision medicine approach. As of November 2016, the trial had enrolled 990 patients across nine experimental drug arms, with each arm involving up to 120 patients. One of its key findings was the identification of pembrolizumab (Keytruda) as an effective therapy in triple-negative breast cancer (TNBC), which later received FDA approval. Additionally, the trial demonstrated that the combination of veliparib and carboplatin significantly increased pathologic complete response (pCR) rates in certain breast cancer subtypes. By allowing new drugs to be seamlessly added without requiring a new trial, I-SPY 2 has accelerated drug development and transformed how investigational therapies are assessed, ultimately improving treatment outcomes for breast cancer patients [22, 23].

Biomarker-Driven Research

The incorporation of biomarkers in trial design has enhanced targeted therapy selection.

- The SOLAR-1 trial, which included 341 patients with PIK3CA-mutated HR+/HER2-negative breast cancer, demonstrated that this group of breast cancer patients benefited significantly from alpelisib plus fulvestrant with improvement of median progression-free survival (PFS) to 11.0 months versus 5.7 months with placebo ($HR = 0.65$; $P = 0.001$). Median overall survival (OS) was 39.3 months with alpelisib versus 31.4 months with placebo, though not statistically significant ($P = 0.15$) [24].
- ctDNA-guided therapy trials are emerging, leveraging liquid biopsy to track minimal residual disease (MRD) and personalize treatment intensification strategies [25].

These advances in clinical trial methodology are transforming breast cancer research, enabling faster drug approval, greater treatment precision, and improved patient outcomes (Table 24.2).

Specific Landmark Studies by Breast Cancer Subtype

Breast cancer is a diverse disease with multiple subtypes classified based on hormone receptor (HR) status and HER2 expression, guiding prognosis and treatment. The claudin-low subtype, a distinct category, is characterized by molecular alterations that promote a pro-metastatic phenotype, impacting disease progression and therapy response (Fig. 24.1). Landmark clinical trials have focused on specific subtypes:

Hormone Receptor–Positive (HR+), HER2-Negative Breast Cancer

HR+/HER2− breast cancer represents the most common subtype, and clinical trials have driven key advancements in hormonal and targeted therapies.

Prevention and Diagnosis

- IBIS-II Trial [26]: A phase III randomized controlled trial (RCT) with 3864 postmenopausal women examined anastrozole for breast cancer prevention. The study found a 53% reduction in invasive HR+ breast cancer over 5 years.
- TAILORx Trial [27]: A prospective phase III trial with 10,273 patients assessed the Oncotype DX 21-gene assay to guide chemotherapy decisions. It confirmed that women with intermediate-risk scores (11–25) could safely avoid chemotherapy, significantly altering clinical practice.
- The Anthracyclines in Early Breast Cancer (ABC) Trials [28]: Six cycles of docetaxel plus cyclophosphamide (TC6) to anthracycline-taxane combinations (TaxAC) in patients with high-risk, HER2-negative early breast cancer were compared. Results showed that the 5-year invasive disease-free survival (IDFS) was 85.1% for TC6 and 86.7% for TaxAC, indicating that the noninferiority of TC6 was not demonstrated. No significant difference

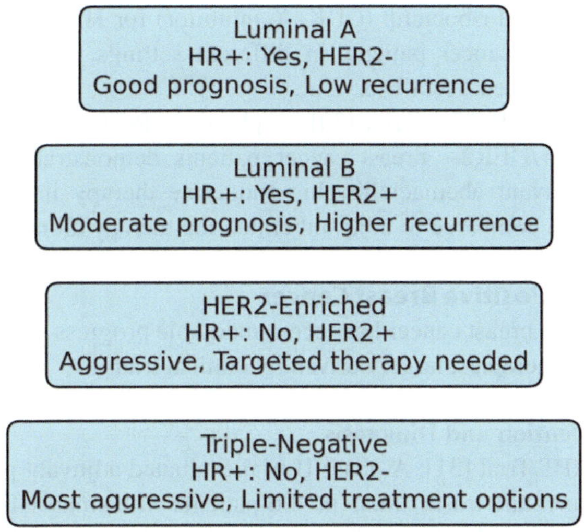

Fig. 24.1 The figure illustrates the four main breast cancer subtypes (Luminal A, Luminal B, HER2-enriched, and triple-negative) with their key characteristics, highlighting differences in hormone receptor status, HER2 expression, prognosis, and treatment options. This classification guides personalized therapy decisions, improving patient outcomes

Table 24.2 Ongoing breast cancer clinical trials

Trial name	Phase	Objective	Methodology	Key features
I-SPY 2 trial	Phase II	Evaluate the efficacy of novel agents in the neoadjuvant setting for high-risk breast cancer patients	Adaptive randomization based on biomarker profiles to match patients with promising treatments	Collaborative effort involving multiple institutions; focuses on accelerating the identification of effective therapies
MINDACT trial	Phase III	Assess the utility of the 70-gene MammaPrint assay in guiding adjuvant chemotherapy decisions	Randomized study comparing genomic risk assessment with clinical-pathological criteria	Aims to determine if genomic profiling can spare patients from unnecessary chemotherapy
AURORA program	Observational	Investigate the molecular characteristics of metastatic breast cancer to understand tumor evolution and resistance mechanisms	Comprehensive genomic and clinical data collection from patients with metastatic breast cancer	Seeks to identify actionable mutations and potential therapeutic targets
POSITIVE trial (BIG time for baby)	Phase II	Evaluate the safety of interrupting endocrine therapy to allow pregnancy in women with hormone receptor–positive breast cancer	Prospective study monitoring recurrence rates and pregnancy outcomes after temporary treatment cessation	Addresses fertility concerns, aiming to provide evidence-based guidelines for young survivors

in overall survival (OS) was observed between the groups, with 5-year OS rates of 91.8% for TC6 and 92.4% for TaxAC.

Treatment

- PALOMA-2 and PALOMA-3 Trials: Phase III trials evaluated palbociclib (CDK4/6 inhibitor) plus endocrine therapy in metastatic HR+/HER2− breast cancer. PALOMA-2 (666 patients) showed a 10-month improvement in progression-free survival (PFS) vs. letrozole alone. PALOMA-3 (521 patients) confirmed benefits in pretreated patients.
- MONALEESA-2/3/7 Trials [29]: These phase III studies assessed ribociclib (CDK4/6 inhibitor) for HR+/HER2− breast cancer patients in different settings, confirming prolonged overall survival.
- MONARCH 3 Trial [30]: A phase III RCT with 493 of HR+/HER2− breast cancer patients demonstrated that adjuvant abemaciclib plus endocrine therapy improved PFS compared to adjuvant endocrine therapy alone.

HER2-Positive Breast Cancer

HER2+ breast cancer has seen remarkable progress with targeted therapies, largely driven by clinical trials.

Prevention and Diagnosis

- APT Trial [31]: A phase II trial evaluated adjuvant paclitaxel and trastuzumab in 406 patients with small HER2+ tumors. The 7-year disease-free survival rate was 93.3%, changing treatment for low-risk patients.

Treatment

- CLEOPATRA Trial [32]: A phase III trial of 808 patients confirmed that pertuzumab, trastuzumab, and docetaxel significantly improved overall survival (56.5 vs. 40.8 months) in metastatic HER2+ breast cancer.
- KATHERINE Trial [17]: A phase III RCT evaluated 1486 patients of HER2-positive early-stage breast cancer who had residual invasive disease after neoadjuvant therapy. The result showed that switching from trastuzumab to trastuzumab emtansine (T-DM1) after neoadjuvant therapy significantly reduced recurrence.
- DESTINY-Breast01/02 Trials: The trials included HER2-positive metastatic breast cancer patients who had progressed after prior HER2 therapy [33]. With DESTINY-Breast04, Modi et al. (2022) evaluated trastuzumab deruxtecan (T-DXd) (557 patients enrolled), showing survival benefits(6.6-month improvement in median OS) in heavily pretreated HER2-low breast cancer, leading to a paradigm shift in classification [14].

Triple-Negative Breast Cancer (TNBC)

TNBC, the most aggressive subtype, has benefited from immune and chemotherapy combination trials.

Prevention and Diagnosis

- IMpassion130 Trial [34]: A phase III trial with 902 patients of metastatic triple-negative breast cancer established atezolizumab plus nab-paclitaxel as the first immune checkpoint inhibitor for PD-L1-positive metastatic TNBC, improving median overall survival (25 vs. 18 months). Although atezolizumab initially received accelerated approval, its U.S. indication was later withdrawn following confirmatory trial results.

Treatment

- KEYNOTE-522 Trial [34]: A phase III RCT with 1174 patients showed that adding pembrolizumab (PD-1 inhibitor) to chemotherapy improved pathologic complete response (pCR) in early-stage TNBC.
- ASCENT Trial [35]: A phase III RCT with 468 patients confirmed that sacituzumab govitecan, an antibody-drug conjugate, significantly improved overall survival in metastatic TNBC (12.1 vs. 6.7 months).

Summary

Advancements in breast cancer research methodologies from basic science to advanced clinical trials have significantly enhanced our understanding and treatment of the disease. Innovations such as molecular profiling, adoptive cell therapy, and real-world data integration are transforming breast cancer care, leading to more personalized treatments and improved survival rates. The ongoing evolution of targeted agents, immunotherapy, predictive biomarkers, and trial designs, including seamless and master protocols, ensures that clinical research remains at the forefront of breast cancer care, continually shaping its future.

References

1. Cao W, et al. Comparative study of cancer profiles between 2020 and 2022 using global cancer statistics (GLOBOCAN). J Natl Cancer Cent. 2024;4(2):128–34.
2. Carey LA, et al. Race, breast cancer subtypes, and survival in the Carolina breast cancer study. JAMA. 2006;295(21):2492–502.
3. Neve RM, et al. A collection of breast cancer cell lines for the study of functionally distinct cancer subtypes. Cancer Cell. 2006;10(6):515–27.
4. Miki Y, et al. A strong candidate for the breast and ovarian cancer susceptibility gene BRCA1. Science. 1994;266(5182):66–71.

5. Koboldt DC, et al. VarScan 2: somatic mutation and copy number alteration discovery in cancer by exome sequencing. Genome Res. 2012;22(3):568–76.
6. Jinek M, et al. A programmable dual-RNA–guided DNA endonuclease in adaptive bacterial immunity. Science. 2012;337(6096):816–21.
7. Holliday DL, Speirs V. Choosing the right cell line for breast cancer research. Breast Cancer Res. 2011;13(4):215.
8. DeRose YS, et al. Tumor grafts derived from women with breast cancer authentically reflect tumor pathology, growth, metastasis and disease outcomes. Nat Med. 2011;17(11):1514–20.
9. Mertins P, et al. Proteogenomics connects somatic mutations to signalling in breast cancer. Nature. 2016;534(7605):55–62.
10. Hanahan D, Lisa M. Coussens, accessories to the crime: functions of cells recruited to the tumor microenvironment. Cancer Cell. 2012;21(3):309–22.
11. Kalluri R. The biology and function of fibroblasts in cancer. Nat Rev Cancer. 2016;16(9):582–98.
12. Topalian SL, Drake CG, Pardoll DM. Immune checkpoint blockade: a common denominator approach to cancer therapy. Cancer Cell. 2015;27(4):450–61.
13. Costa RL, et al. Phase 1 dose-escalation, dose-expansion trial of intratumoral HER2 and HER3-primed dendritic cells injections for the treatment of early-stage TNBC and HR low positive breast cancer: DecipHER trial. J Clin Oncol. 2023;41(16_suppl):TPS629.
14. Modi S, et al. Trastuzumab Deruxtecan in previously treated HER2-low advanced breast cancer. N Engl J Med. 2022;387(1):9–20.
15. Murthy RK, et al. Tucatinib, Trastuzumab, and Capecitabine for HER2-positive metastatic breast cancer. N Engl J Med. 2020;382(7):597–609.
16. Schmid P, et al. Event-free survival with Pembrolizumab in early triple-negative breast cancer. N Engl J Med. 2022;386(6):556–67.
17. Minckwitz GV, et al. Trastuzumab Emtansine for residual invasive HER2-positive breast cancer. N Engl J Med. 2019;380(7):617–28.
18. Rugo HS, et al. Real-world treatment patterns for palbociclib plus an aromatase inhibitor, or an aromatase inhibitor alone, for patients with metastatic breast cancer in the flatiron database. Int J Cancer. 2024;154(4):701–11.
19. Bardia A, et al. Biomarker analyses in the phase III ASCENT study of sacituzumab govitecan versus chemotherapy in patients with metastatic triple-negative breast cancer. Ann Oncol. 2021;32(9):1148–56.
20. Zhou T, Zhang J. Types and progress of clinical trial design for breast cancer: a narrative review. Transl Breast Cancer Res. 2023;4 :20
21. Dugo M, et al. The immune-related 27-gene signature DetermaIO predicts response to Neoadjuvant Atezolizumab plus chemotherapy in triple-negative breast cancer. Clin Cancer Res. 2024;30(21):4900–9.
22. Meyer EL, et al. Why and how should we simulate platform trials? Learnings from EU-PEARL. BMC Med Res Methodol. 2025;25(1):12.
23. Wang H, Yee D. I-SPY 2: a Neoadjuvant adaptive clinical trial designed to improve outcomes in high-risk breast cancer. Curr Breast Cancer Rep. 2019;11(4):303–10.
24. André F, et al. Alpelisib for PIK3CA-mutated, hormone receptor-positive advanced breast cancer. N Engl J Med. 2019;380(20):1929–40.
25. Panet F, et al. Use of ctDNA in early breast cancer: analytical validity and clinical potential. npj Breast Cancer. 2024;10(1):50.
26. Cuzick J, et al. Tamoxifen for prevention of breast cancer: extended long-term follow-up of the IBIS-I breast cancer prevention trial. Lancet Oncol. 2015;16(1):67–75.
27. Sparano JA, et al. Adjuvant chemotherapy guided by a 21-gene expression assay in breast cancer. N Engl J Med. 2018;379(2):111–21.
28. Geyer CE, et al. Long-term follow-up of the Anthracyclines in early breast cancer trials (USOR 06-090, NSABP B-46-I/USOR 07132, and NSABP B-49 [NRG Oncology]). J Clin Oncol. 2024;42(12):1344–9.
29. Hortobagyi C, et al. Overall survival with ribociclib plus letrozole in advanced breast cancer. N Engl J Med. 2022;386:942–50.
30. Johnston S, et al. MONARCH 3 final PFS: a randomized study of abemaciclib as initial therapy for advanced breast cancer. npj Breast Cancer. 2019;5:5.
31. Tolaney SM, et al. Adjuvant paclitaxel and Trastuzumab for node-negative, HER2-positive breast cancer. N Engl J Med. 2015;372(2):134–41.
32. Swain SM, et al. Pertuzumab, trastuzumab, and docetaxel for HER2-positive metastatic breast cancer (CLEOPATRA): end-of-study results from a double-blind, randomised, placebo-controlled, phase 3 study. Lancet Oncol. 2020;21(4):519–30.
33. André F, et al. Trastuzumab deruxtecan versus treatment of physician's choice in patients with HER2-positive metastatic breast cancer (DESTINY-Breast02): a randomised, open-label, multicentre, phase 3 trial. Lancet. 2023;401(10390):1773–85.
34. Schmid P, et al. Atezolizumab and nab-paclitaxel in advanced triple-negative breast cancer. N Engl J Med. 2018;379(22):2108–21.
35. Bardia A, et al. Sacituzumab Govitecan in metastatic triple-negative breast cancer. N Engl J Med. 2021;384(16):1529–41.

Research on Malignant Hematology

25

Jiya Mulayamkuzhiyil and Julio Chavez

Introduction

Hematology is a very broad category of disease that includes classical hematology (formerly called "benign hematology") that comprises disorders of hemoglobin, coagulation factors, platelets, and white blood cells. They are not considered malignant as it does not follow malignant proliferation of cells. However, it could be associated with complicated clinical cases. Malignant hematology, per se, involves neoplasms of the various blood cells. In this regard, the most common subgroups are plasma cell neoplasms, leukemias, and lymphomas. Given the extent of the topic, we will focus on research that is practice-changing.

Lymphoma

Lymphoma is a clonal disease of blood cells and lymph nodes. It has two subtypes: Hodgkin's lymphoma (HL) and non-Hodgkin's lymphoma (NHL). In 2020, about 544,000 people were diagnosed with NHL worldwide. About 80,000 new cases of NHL are diagnosed per year, with 20,000 deaths per year. NHL consists of B-cell lymphomas, T-cell lymphomas, and NK cell lymphomas. The most common subtype is diffuse large B-cell lymphoma (DLBCL), followed by follicular lymphoma (FL), marginal zone lymphoma (MZL), mantle cell lymphoma (MCL), and T-cell NHLs and Burkitt's lymphoma (BL) [1].

J. Mulayamkuzhiyil
Department of Internal Medicine, NYU Langone Hospital, Suffolk, USA

J. Chavez (✉)
Department of Malignant Hematology, Moffitt Cancer Center, Tampa, FL, USA
e-mail: chavez.julio@mayo.edu

Etiology and Risk Factors

The etiology is heterogeneous, and there is no clear etiologic factor. Subtypes of lymphomas, such as DLBCL, BL, and HL, have been associated with Epstein-Barr virus (EBV). Other infectious agents (such as *Helicobacter pylori*) have been associated with lymphomas such as mucosa-associated lymphoid tissue (MALT) lymphomas. Environmental exposure (pesticides, burn pits, etc.) has been associated with lymphomas. Other potential risk factors are related to underlying immunosuppression, such as in patients with chronic infections (HIV and HTLV-1 cases), elderly patients, and autoimmunity.

Clinical Presentation and Staging

Symptoms of lymphoma include B symptoms such as fever, weight loss, pruritus, drenching night sweats, cytopenia including anemia leading to fatigue, thrombocytopenia leading to bleeding or petechiae, and neutropenia leading to infections. Patients can also have symptoms due to Central nervous system (CNS) or Cerebrospinal fluid (CSF) involvement, expansion of lymph nodes or spleen, and/or superior vena cava syndrome. Paraneoplastic syndromes in lymphoma include nephrotic syndrome, hemolytic anemia, and ITP. Since the introduction of rituximab, the mortality rate due to NHL has come down. The low-grade or indolent lymphomas are typically slow-growing but incurable and seen in the elderly, whereas the aggressive lymphomas are fast-growing but potentially curable and seen in all age groups. An exception to this is the mantle cell lymphoma, which is fast-growing but incurable, and the T-cell lymphoma, which is aggressive but very difficult to treat.

Standard staging is performed by imaging studies, including computed tomography (or CT scan) and FDG-PET scanning. In some cases, a bone marrow biopsy is performed. The standard staging system is the Ann Arbor staging system

J. Huang, H. S.L. Jim (eds.), *Cancer Research Guidance for Clinicians and Researchers*,
https://doi.org/10.1007/978-3-032-19175-5_25

(stages I–IV). There are also prognostic scoring systems that are specific for each lymphoma subtype. Perhaps the most used scoring system is the International Prognostic Index (IPI) score, which was mostly studied in aggressive NHLs. The IPI score is based on performance status (PS-ECOG), LDH levels, age, extranodal involvement, and stage [2]. There are scoring systems in MCL, HL, and T-cell NHLs.

Treatment

The treatment of lymphomas varies depending on the subtype, stage, and scoring system. We will discuss the treatment for DLBCL and HL, where relevant research has shown improved outcomes.

Diffuse Large B-Cell Lymphoma (DLBCL)

The standard of care for DLBCL is the CHOP regimen administered on a 21-day schedule for six cycles. R-CHOP includes rituximab 375 mg/m^2, cyclophosphamide 750 mg/m^2, doxorubicin 50 mg/m^2, and vincristine and oral prednisone 100 mg on days 1–5. Growth factor support (G-CSF) and anti-infective prophylaxis may be needed in certain patients. These regimens cure about 50–60% of patients based on the GELA study that compared R-CHOP vs. CHOP alone [3].

For years, there have been several clinical trials adding novel agents or increasing chemotherapy intensity to the R-CHOP backbone in order to improve clinical outcomes. However, they did not show improvement in outcomes. For instance, the GALGB 5303 study (524 patients) compared R-CHOP vs. DA-EPOCH-R, but there was no improvement in overall survival (OS) and progression-free survival (PFS) [4]. Adding agents such as lenalidomide and ibrutinib in different studies did not show significant survival improvements [5].

Most recently, polatuzumab vedotin, an anti-CD79b antibody-drug conjugate, in combination with R-CHP (rituximab, cyclophosphamide, doxorubicin, prednisone), a modified R-CHOP regimen, was approved for first-line therapy for patients with previously untreated DLCBL, based on the results of the POLARIX trial (double-blind, placebo-controlled, international phase 3 trial with 879 patients). The above trial demonstrated improved PFS (76.7% vs. 70.2%) in patients with age >60, high IPI, non-bulky and ABC subtype disease, and improved 2-year EFS (75.6% vs. 69.4%) in the Pola-R-CHP group compared to the R-CHOP group at 28.2 months [6].

In the relapse/refractory (R/R) setting, clinical research has shown the efficacy of novel agents, particularly with anti-CD19 chimeric antigen receptor (CAR) T-cell therapy. Three pivotal trials showed efficacy of axicabtagene ciloleucel (axi-cel, ZUMA-1), tisagenlecleucel (tisa-cel, JULIET), and lisocabtagene maraleucel (liso-cel, TRANSCEND-NHL-001) in the third-line setting. In the second-line setting, two trials have successfully challenged the treatment paradigm of salvage chemotherapy followed by autologous hematopoietic cell transplantation (auto-HCT) [7–9]. The ZUMA-7 (axi-cel) (international, phase 3 randomized trial with 180 patients) and TRANSFORM (liso-cel) (184 patients) studies showed improvement of PFS over SOC, with even OS benefit in the long-term follow-up [10, 11].

Clinical research also showed the activity of a novel generation of immunotherapy: T-cell-engaging antibodies or bispecific antibodies (BiAbs). There are two BiAbs available for R/R DLBCL in the third-line setting: epcoritamab and glofitamab. Recent trials are showing improved outcomes in earlier lines (STARGLO and SUNMO) [3].

Hodgkin's Lymphoma

Treatment is given based on risk stratification. In general, there are three groups of patients with HL: favorable early stage, unfavorable early stage, and advanced stage. The outcomes of HL have improved significantly with the introduction of multi-agent chemotherapy and radiation therapy [12].

For a favorable early stage, the standard practice consists of two cycles of ABVD (adriamycin, bleomycin, vinblastine, and dacarbazine) followed by 20 Gy involved site radiation therapy (ISRT). This regimen is based on a large randomized clinical trial (1370 patients) that used PET-based stratification and compared four groups of patients that received two to four cycles of ABVD with/without ISRT at 20–35 Gy. Given the high efficacy and low toxicity, the ABVDx2 + ISRT remains the recommended approach [12, 13].

For unfavorable early-stage HL, clinical trials showed that omission of ISRT leads to increased relapse risk. Therefore, the standard approach is consistent with four to six cycles of ABVD followed by ISRT at 30 Gy at least [14]. However, a recent PET-guided approach clinical trial (multicenter, open-label, randomized, phase 3 trial with 1100 patients) (HD17) showed that ABVD × 2 cycles + escalated (esc) BEACOPP (bleomycin, cyclophosphamide, etoposide, procarbazine, and prednisone) without radiation in PET4-negative patients (at the end of four cycles) did not impact overall outcomes raising the possibility of omitting radiation in a selected group of patients [15].

In advanced-stage HL, for years, six cycles of ABVD (or six cycles of escBEACOPP) remained the standard approach [12]. Deintensification of chemotherapy by omitting bleomycin (in RATHL trial) and switching to ABVD from BEACOP (AHL2011) (randomized, non-inferiority, phase 3 study with 823 patients) in PET2-negative patients after two initial cycles of chemotherapy showed no impact on survival outcomes and, therefore, an attractive approach to mitigate bleomycin-related toxicity [16, 17]. More recently, the CD30-targeting ADC, brentuximab, showed improved overall survival when combined with AVD (A-AVD regimen), becoming the standard of care in patients with high-risk and stage IV disease [18]. Lastly, the introduction of nivolumab (a PD-1 inhibitor) in combination with AVD (omitting bleomycin) improved the median PFS in comparison to A-AVD in the phase 3 randomized clinical trial SWOG S1826 (a phase 3, multicenter, open-label, randomized trial with 970 patients) [19]. These trials demonstrated that adding novel agents to the chemotherapy backbone in advanced-stage HL can improve survival outcomes.

Leukemias

Leukemias are a very heterogenous group of diseases that involve the malignant proliferation of different white blood cell subtypes. The clinical presentation will depend on the type of cell subtype affected. The incidence of leukemias varies depending on the subtypes, but in general, in the USA, about 14.4 per 100,000 are diagnosed with some type of leukemia. In general, the leukemias are classified as acute leukemias, such as acute myeloid leukemia (AML) and acute lymphoblastic leukemia (ALL), and chronic leukemias, such as chronic myeloid leukemia (CML) and chronic lymphocytic leukemia (CLL). Other intermediate conditions, but important to mention, are myelodysplastic syndromes. The prognosis of the leukemias is highly variable as it depends on patient characteristics, leukemia subtype, risk stratification, and associated genomic aberrations. In general, chronic leukemias have a better prognosis [20–22].

Etiology and Risk Factors

Many leukemias have been associated with specific chromosomal abnormalities. For instance, the hallmark mutation in CML is the translocation of chromosomes 9 and 21 or t (9;21) that generates the fusion protein BCR-ABL, which is targetable by tyrosine kinase inhibitors. Another important targetable mutations are FLT3-ITD (in AML) and JAK2 (in cases of myelofibrosis). Non-targetable mutations that impact the prognosis are the tumor suppressor TP53, which can impact all leukemias, particularly AML, MDS, and CLL [20–22].

Among risk factors, there are no specific factors that predispose patients with leukemias. Radiation exposure (atomic bomb survivors) had a high incidence of CML and other myeloid malignancies. Elderly patients have a higher risk of developing AML, MDS, and CLL. However, one of the best recognized risk factors is prior exposure to chemotherapy, particularly topoisomerase II inhibitors (etoposide and doxorubicin) and alkylating agents (i.e., chlorambucil) in a condition that is called secondary leukemias or therapy-related leukemias (t-AML and t-MDS) [20].

Clinical Presentation and Staging

The clinical presentation of leukemias is highly variable depending on the subtype and timing of diagnosis (with late diagnosis leading to more symptomatic disease). Patient's symptoms result from associated cytopenias and can include fatigue, pallor, increased bruising, or bleeding. Constitutional symptoms like lymphomas can also be a presenting clinical picture. Recurrent infections are also a common type of presentation. Some patients are asymptomatic at diagnosis, especially in the case of chronic leukemias. Obstructive symptoms such as abdominal pain (due to splenomegaly) or dyspnea (due to mediastinal masses) can also occur [20–22].

There are different staging systems for leukemias, and it depends on the specific subtype. For instance, the Rai staging system is commonly used for reporting in CLL trials. For instance, for AML, the most common risk stratification system is the European Leukemia Net (ELN), which was recently updated [23].

Treatment

Given the extensive list of conditions in this category, we will focus briefly on AML and CLL. However, pivotal and practice-changing clinical trials have been reported in MDS, myelofibrosis, and CML.

Acute Myeloid Leukemia

The most important goal of induction therapy in AML is to achieve CR. The standard treatment consists in induction regimen followed by post-remission therapy that could include allogeneic HCT. The choice of therapy depends on several parameters, including disease and patient factors. The backbone of intensive therapy for most fit patients remains the regimen 7 + 3 (cytarabine for 7 days and daunorubicin for 3 days) [20].

Clinical research led to important advances in the treatment of AML. One of the initial discoveries was the intensification of chemotherapy that showed benefit with a higher dose of daunorubicin (90 mg/m^2 vs. 45 mg/m^2) [24]. Targeting of FLT3-ITD in FLT3+ AML was one of the most important discoveries in recent years. The RATIFY trial (a randomized, double-blind, placebo-controlled, phase 3 trial with 3468 patients) compared standard 7 + 3 +/− midostaurin or placebo in FLT3+ AML and demonstrated PFS and OS benefit [25, 26]. Since then, several drugs targeting FLT3-ITD have emerged (quizartinib) [26]. Lastly, a phase 3 clinical trial was able to challenge the 7 + 3 regimen when CPX-351 (a liposomal formulation of daunorubicin and cytarabine in a fixed concentration ratio) showed OS benefit in secondary or t-AML, becoming a standard of care approach [27].

Several additional advances occurred in AML with the emergence of isocitrate dehydrogenase (IDH) inhibitors and menin inhibitors that may lead to further refinement of the personalized approach of AML [20].

Chronic Lymphocytic Leukemia

For years, the standard approach for CLL was chemoimmunotherapy with either the regimen FCR (fludarabine, cyclophosphamide, and rituximab) and chlorambucil and rituximab or obinutuzumab (Clb-R, Clb-O). Clinical research made a significant impact, changing the treatment landscape of CLL. The biological understanding of CLL led to the discovery of the main classes of drugs that are currently part of the standard approach for CLL: Bruton tyrosine kinase inhibitors (BTKi) and BCL2 inhibitors (venetoclax) [22].

Ibrutinib is the first in class of BTKi that was discovered over a decade ago. In a landmark study, ibrutinib was superior to chemotherapy, showing OS benefit [28]. Later studies showed that second-generation BTKi (zanubrutinib and acalabrutinib) may be at least as effective as ibrutinib but with a better safety profile [29, 30].

A landmark study (CLL14) (open-label, phase 3 trial with 432 patients) demonstrated the PFS and OS benefit of the combination of venetoclax and obinutuzumab (Ven-O) in comparison to chemoimmunotherapy (Clb-O) in elderly patients with comorbidities [31]. As a fixed duration regimen, the Ven-O option provides an advantage over BTKi that are given as indefinite therapy.

More recently, combination approaches of BTKi + BCL2i +/− anti-CD20 antibodies have become a point of interest in CLL. The FLAIR study (phase 3, multicenter, randomized, controlled, open-label study with 523 patients) showed that a combination of fixed-duration ibrutinib-venetoclax (IV) resulted in a survival benefit over standard FCR [32].

Chronic Myeloid Leukemia

Until the last century, the only treatment option that offered a cure for CML was allogeneic HCT. Treatment approaches with interferon, busulfan, or low-dose cytarabine led to short-lived responses. An important shift occurred with the discovery and development of small molecules targeting the BCR-ABL fusion protein, a key component in CML pathogenesis. The development of TKIs targeting BCR-ABL dramatically improved the survival of CML from a historical 10-year survival of 20% in the pre-imatinib era to 80–90% 10-year survival with the first-in-class TKI imatinib. Resistance mutations occur in about 10% of cases of CML, leading to disease progression, particularly the T351I mutation [21, 33, 34].

Another major advance in CML was the development of second-generation TKIs with the discovery of dasatinib, nilotinib, and bosutinib that led to deeper responses than imatinib, but it is unclear if there is a survival advantage. Therefore, all four TKIs remain as the standard initial approach for CML in chronic phase [21].

Recurrence after initial treatment with first- or second-generation TKIs remains a clinical challenge, particularly in patients who develop the T351I mutation [35]. A major advance was the development of the third-generation TKI, ponatinib, which specifically targeted the T351I mutation in CML cases. Ponatinib is currently the standard approach after first-line CML therapy. A phase 3 trial, randomized study with 405 patients discovered a novel BCR-ABL targeting approach (as oppose of kinase inhibition) by inducing conformational changes in the allosteric conformation of the BCR-ABL1. This led to the discovery of asciminib, which represents an option for patients with CML after failure of two or more TKIs [36].

Conclusions

Practice-changing innovations in malignant hematology have led to profound changes in the treatment landscape and prognosis of lymphomas and leukemias. The introduction of targeted therapies, antibody-drug conjugates, bispecific antibodies, and CAR T-cell therapy has transformed treatment algorithms, offering improved survival rates and better quality of life for patients. Genomic and molecular discoveries have enabled precise risk stratification and personalized therapy selection, evidenced by the success of targeted agents in diseases such as CML, AML, and CLL. In addition, PET-guided and risk-adapted strategies in lymphoma have optimized outcomes. Advances in clinical research, novel therapeutics, and molecular diagnostics have facilitated individualized treatment approaches, leading to improved survival and quality of life in patients with hematologic malignancies.

References

1. Siegel RL, Kratzer TB, Giaquinto AN, Sung H, Jemal A. Cancer statistics, 2025. CA Cancer J Clin. 2025;75(1):10–45.
2. International Non-Hodgkin's Lymphoma Prognostic Factors Project. A predictive model for aggressive non-Hodgkin's lymphoma. N Engl J Med. 1993;329(14):987–94.
3. Tavakkoli M, Barta SK. 2024 update: advances in the risk stratification and management of large B-cell lymphoma. Am J Hematol. 2023;98(11):1791–805.

4. Bartlett NL, Wilson WH, Jung S-H, Hsi ED, Maurer MJ, Pederson LD, et al. Dose-adjusted EPOCH-R compared with R-CHOP as frontline therapy for diffuse large B-cell lymphoma: clinical outcomes of the phase III intergroup trial alliance/CALGB 50303. J Clin Oncol. 2019;37(21):1790–9.
5. Nowakowski GS, Chiappella A, Gascoyne RD, Scott DW, Zhang Q, Jurczak W, et al. ROBUST: a phase III study of lenalidomide plus R-CHOP versus placebo plus R-CHOP in previously untreated patients with ABC-type diffuse large B-cell lymphoma. J Clin Oncol. 2021;39(12):1317–28.
6. Tilly H, Morschhauser F, Sehn LH, Friedberg JW, Trněný M, Sharman JP, et al. Polatuzumab vedotin in previously untreated diffuse large B-cell lymphoma. N Engl J Med. 2022;386(4):351–63.
7. Neelapu SS, Locke FL, Bartlett NL, Lekakis LJ, Miklos DB, Jacobson CA, et al. Axicabtagene ciloleucel CAR T-cell therapy in refractory large B-cell lymphoma. N Engl J Med. 2017;377(26):2531–44.
8. Schuster SJ, Bishop MR, Tam CS, Waller EK, Borchmann P, McGuirk JP, et al. Tisagenlecleucel in adult relapsed or refractory diffuse large B-cell lymphoma. N Engl J Med. 2019;380(1):45–56.
9. Abramson JS, Palomba ML, Gordon LI, Lunning MA, Wang M, Arnason J, et al. Lisocabtagene maraleucel for patients with relapsed or refractory large B-cell lymphomas (TRANSCEND NHL 001): a multicentre seamless design study. Lancet. 2020;396(10254):839–52.
10. Locke FL, Miklos DB, Jacobson CA, Perales M-A, Kersten M-J, Oluwole OO, et al. Axicabtagene ciloleucel as second-line therapy for large B-cell lymphoma. N Engl J Med. 2022;386(7):640–54.
11. Abramson JS, Solomon SR, Arnason J, Johnston PB, Glass B, Bachanova V, et al. Lisocabtagene maraleucel as second-line therapy for large B-cell lymphoma: primary analysis of the phase 3 TRANSFORM study. Blood. 2023;141(14):1675–84.
12. Ansell SM. Hodgkin lymphoma: 2025 update on diagnosis, risk-stratification, and management. Am J Hematol. 2024;99(12):2367–78.
13. Engert A, Plütschow A, Eich HT, Lohri A, Dörken B, Borchmann P, et al. Reduced treatment intensity in patients with early-stage Hodgkin's lymphoma. N Engl J Med. 2010;363(7):640–52.
14. Eich HT, Diehl V, Görgen H, Pabst T, Markova J, Debus J, et al. Intensified chemotherapy and dose-reduced involved-field radiotherapy in patients with early unfavorable Hodgkin's lymphoma: final analysis of the German Hodgkin study group HD11 trial. J Clin Oncol. 2010;28(27):4199–206.
15. Borchmann P, Plütschow A, Kobe C, Greil R, Meissner J, Topp MS, et al. PET-guided omission of radiotherapy in early-stage unfavourable Hodgkin lymphoma (GHSG HD17): a multicentre, open-label, randomised, phase 3 trial. Lancet Oncol. 2021;22(2):223–34.
16. Johnson P, Federico M, Kirkwood A, Fosså A, Berkahn L, Carella A, et al. Adapted treatment guided by interim PET-CT scan in advanced Hodgkin's lymphoma. N Engl J Med. 2016;374(25):2419–29.
17. Casasnovas RO, Bouabdallah R, Brice P, Lazarovici J, Ghesquieres H, Stamatoullas A, et al. PET-adapted treatment for newly diagnosed advanced Hodgkin lymphoma (AHL2011): a randomised, multicentre, non-inferiority, phase 3 study. Lancet Oncol. 2019;20(2):202–15.
18. Connors JM, Jurczak W, Straus DJ, Ansell SM, Kim WS, Gallamini A, et al. Brentuximab vedotin with chemotherapy for stage III or IV Hodgkin's lymphoma. N Engl J Med. 2018;378(4):331–44.
19. Herrera AF, LeBlanc M, Castellino SM, Li H, Rutherford SC, Evens AM, et al. Nivolumab+AVD in advanced-stage classic Hodgkin's lymphoma. N Engl J Med. 2024;391(15):1379–89.
20. Shimony S, Stahl M, Stone RM. Acute myeloid leukemia: 2025 update on diagnosis, risk-stratification, and management. Am J Hematol. 2025;100(5):860–91.
21. Jabbour E, Kantarjian H. Chronic myeloid leukemia: 2025 update on diagnosis, therapy, and monitoring. Am J Hematol. 2024;99(11):2191–212.
22. Hallek M. Chronic lymphocytic leukemia: 2025 update on the epidemiology, pathogenesis, diagnosis, and therapy. Am J Hematol. 2025;100(3):450–80.
23. Döhner H, DiNardo CD, Appelbaum FR, Craddock C, Dombret H, Ebert BL, et al. Genetic risk classification for adults with AML receiving less-intensive therapies: the 2024 ELN recommendations. Blood. 2024;144(21):2169–73.
24. Fernandez HF, Sun Z, Yao X, Litzow MR, Luger SM, Paietta EM, et al. Anthracycline dose intensification in acute myeloid leukemia. N Engl J Med. 2009;361(13):1249–59.
25. Stone RM, Mandrekar SJ, Sanford BL, Laumann K, Geyer S, Bloomfield CD, et al. Midostaurin plus chemotherapy for acute myeloid leukemia with a FLT3 mutation. N Engl J Med. 2017;377(5):454–64.
26. Erba HP, Montesinos P, Kim H-J, Patkowska E, Vrhovac R, Žák P, et al. Quizartinib plus chemotherapy in newly diagnosed patients with FLT3-internal-tandem-duplication-positive acute myeloid leukaemia (QuANTUM-first): a randomised, double-blind, placebo-controlled, phase 3 trial. Lancet. 2023;401(10388):1571–83.
27. Lancet JE, Uy GL, Newell LF, Lin TL, Ritchie EK, Stuart RK, et al. CPX-351 versus 7+3 cytarabine and daunorubicin chemotherapy in older adults with newly diagnosed high-risk or secondary acute myeloid leukaemia: 5-year results of a randomised, open-label, multicentre, phase 3 trial. Lancet Haematol. 2021;8(7):e481–e91.
28. Shanafelt TD, Wang XV, Hanson CA, Paietta EM, O'Brien S, Barrientos J, et al. Long-term outcomes for ibrutinib-rituximab and chemoimmunotherapy in CLL: updated results of the E1912 trial. Blood. 2022;140(2):112–20.
29. Brown JR, Eichhorst B, Hillmen P, Jurczak W, Kaźmierczak M, Lamanna N, et al. Zanubrutinib or ibrutinib in relapsed or refractory chronic lymphocytic leukemia. N Engl J Med. 2023;388(4):319–32.
30. Byrd JC, Hillmen P, Ghia P, Kater AP, Chanan-Khan A, Furman RR, et al. Acalabrutinib versus ibrutinib in previously treated chronic lymphocytic leukemia: results of the first randomized phase III trial. J Clin Oncol. 2021;39(31):3441–52.
31. Fischer K, Al-Sawaf O, Bahlo J, Fink A-M, Tandon M, Dixon M, et al. Venetoclax and obinutuzumab in patients with CLL and coexisting conditions. N Engl J Med. 2019;380(23):2225–36.
32. Munir T, Cairns DA, Bloor A, Allsup D, Cwynarski K, Pettitt A, et al. Chronic lymphocytic leukemia therapy guided by measurable residual disease. N Engl J Med. 2024;390(4):326–37.
33. O'Brien SG, Guilhot F, Larson RA, Gathmann I, Baccarani M, Cervantes F, et al. Imatinib compared with interferon and low dose cytarabine for newly diagnosed chronic-phase chronic myeloid leukemia. N Engl J Med. 2003;348(11):994–1004.
34. Hochhaus A, Larson RA, Guilhot F, Radich JP, Branford S, Hughes TP, et al. Long-term outcomes of imatinib treatment for chronic myeloid leukemia. N Engl J Med. 2017;376(10):917–27.
35. Cortes JE, Kim D-W, Pinilla-Ibarz J, Coutre P, Paquette R, Chuah C, et al. A Phase 2 Trial of ponatinib in Philadelphia chromosome–positive leukemias. N Engl J Med. 2013;369(19):1783–96.
36. Hochhaus A, Wang J, Kim D-W, Kim DDH, Mayer J, Goh Y-T, et al. Asciminib in newly diagnosed chronic myeloid leukemia. N Engl J Med. 2024;391(10):885–98.

Research on Pediatric Oncology

26

Jonathan Metts, Sunil S. Raikar, Krupesh Patel, Amy E. Armstrong, and Aditi Dhir

Abbreviations

AH	Aqueous humor
ALCL	Anaplastic large-cell lymphoma
ALL	Acute lymphoblastic leukemia
AML	Acute myeloid leukemia
B-LLy	B-lymphoblastic lymphoma
cfDNA	Cell-free DNA
CMMRD	Constitutional mismatch repair deficiency
CNS	Central nervous system
COG	Children's Oncology Group
DFMO	Difluromethylornithine
DNA	Deoxyribonucleic acid
EFS	Event-free survival
EpSSG	European Paediatric Soft Tissue Sarcoma Study Group
ES	Ewing sarcoma
FDG-PET	Fluorodeoxyglucose positron emission tomography
FHWT	Favorable-histology Wilms tumor
GNB	Ganglioneuroblastoma
HGG	High-grade glioma
HL	Hodgkin lymphoma
HSCT	Hematopoietic stem cell transplant
IAC	Intra-arterial chemotherapy
IDRF	Image-defined risk factor
INRG	International Neuroblastoma Risk Group
IRSS	International Retinoblastoma Staging System
LFS	Li–Fraumeni syndrome
LGG	Low-grade glioma
LOH	Loss of heterozygosity
LOI	Loss of imprinting
MEKi	MEK inhibitor
MIBG	Metaiodobenzylguanidine
MRI	Magnetic resonance imaging
NF-1	Neurofibromatosis type 1
NF-2	Neurofibromatosis type 2
NHL	Non-Hodgkin lymphoma
NK	Natural killer
OS	Overall survival
RMS	Rhabdomyosarcoma
RT	Radiation therapy
SCR	Stem cell rescue
SEGA	Subependymal giant cell astrocytoma
SMN	Secondary malignant neoplasm
TSC	Tuberous sclerosis complex
USA	United States of America
WAGR	Wilms tumor, aniridia, genitourinary abnormalities, mental retardation
WHO	World Health Organization
WT	Wilms tumor

J. Metts (✉)
Sarcoma Department, H Lee Moffitt Cancer Center and Research Institute, Tampa, FL, USA

Cancer and Blood Disorders Institute, Johns Hopkins All Children's Hospital, St Petersburg, FL, USA
e-mail: jonathan.metts@moffitt.org

S. S. Raikar
Department of Pediatrics, Emory University, Atlanta, GA, USA
e-mail: sraikar@emory.edu

K. Patel
Cancer and Blood Disorders Institute, Johns Hopkins All Children's Hospital, St Petersburg, FL, USA
e-mail: kpate128@jhmi.edu

A. E. Armstrong
Department of Pediatrics, Division of Pediatric Hematology and Oncology, Washington University in St Louis School of Medicine, St Louis, MO, USA
e-mail: armstrongae@wustl.edu

A. Dhir
Department of Pediatrics, University of Miami Miller School of Medicine, Miami, FL, USA
e-mail: aditi.dhir@med.miami.edu

J. Huang, H. S.L. Jim (eds.), *Cancer Research Guidance for Clinicians and Researchers*,
https://doi.org/10.1007/978-3-032-19175-5_26

Introduction

Cancer affects approximately 15,000 children and adolescents each year in the United States of America (USA), and most pediatric cancers meet the National Cancer Institute's definition of rare cancers (<15 cases out of 100,000 people each year) [1]. The etiology of most pediatric cancers is unknown; due to young age at diagnosis, environmental factors play a minimal role; however, identifiable cancer predispositions are thought to be present in at least 10% of pediatric cancers and are an active area of ongoing research [2]. The estimated 5-year overall survival (OS) of pediatric cancer is 85% [3]. Despite its rarity and advances in treatment, cancer remains the highest noninjury cause of death in children and adolescents in the USA [1].

Basic, translational, and clinical research in pediatric cancer presents unique challenges compared to adult cancer, including the rarity of patient samples; ethical research considerations in children, who are considered a vulnerable patient population; and relatively little investigation into therapies developed solely for pediatric cancers. Despite these challenges, considerable progress has been made in our biological understanding and treatment outcomes for pediatric cancer, due in large part to a longstanding commitment to large-scale collaborations between pediatric cancer institutions both nationally and internationally (aka cooperative groups) [4]. In this chapter, we will summarize the recent research progress for the most frequently encountered pediatric cancers.

Progress in Pediatric Cancer Research

Leukemia

The most common type of pediatric leukemia is acute lymphoblastic leukemia (ALL, 75–80% of cases), followed by acute myeloid leukemia (AML, 15–20% of cases) [5]. Other rare types include chronic myeloid leukemia, mixed phenotype acute leukemia, and juvenile myelomonocytic leukemia [5]. ALL is the most common cancer diagnosed in children less than 15 years of age, accounting for 25% of childhood cancer [6]. ALL includes two subtypes: B-cell acute lymphoblastic leukemia (B-ALL) and T-cell acute lymphoblastic leukemia (T-ALL), with B-ALL three to four times more prevalent than T-ALL [6].

Recent advances in pediatric leukemia biology center around multiomic bioinformatics. Large-scale studies utilizing whole-exome, whole-genome, and transcriptomic sequencing, as well as methylation profiling on pediatric ALL (>2500 patients) and AML (>950 patients) samples collected on St. Jude's and COG clinical trials, have characterized the genetic and molecular landscape of these leukemias [7, 8]. Single-cell multiomic analyses are underway to deeply study the biology and tumor microenvironment of leukemias and identify potential targets for therapy [9, 10].

Multi-agent chemotherapy is standard treatment for ALL and AML. In ALL, induction therapy consists of vincristine, corticosteroids, and L-asparaginase with or without daunorubicin, followed by 4–6 months of intensive chemotherapy and then a less intense maintenance chemotherapy phase for an additional 2 years [6]. Risk stratification is based on presenting WBC count, age, cytogenetics, and response to induction chemotherapy [6]. In T-ALL, a phase 3 Children's Oncology Group (COG) trial, AALL0434, which enrolled 1562 patients in a 2x2 pseudofactorial randomization, demonstrated that the addition of nelarabine improved survival in T-ALL [11]. For AML, cytarabine- and anthracycline-based intensive chemotherapy blocks are the mainstay of initial treatment, with higher-risk patients requiring allogeneic hematopoietic stem cell transplantation (HSCT) for cure. Immunotherapy (e.g., the bispecific T-cell engager blinatumomab and CD19-directed chimeric antigen receptor T-cells) is playing an increased role in the treatment of B-ALL. While the CD33-directed antibody drug conjugate gemtuzumab ozagamicin is used in AML, other immunotherapies have thus far seen limited success in AML and T-ALL [5, 12].

The OS for ALL has consistently improved over several decades, with 5-year survival now around 90% for children under 15 and 75–80% for children age 15–19 [6]. Certain low-risk subsets of B-ALL have 5-year event-free survival (EFS) rates over 95% [6]. The COG phase 3 trial AALL1731, randomizing 1440 patients, showed that the addition of blinatumomab to combination chemotherapy in standard-risk B-ALL significantly improved disease-free survival for patients with average and high risk of relapse [13]. However, a pooled retrospective analysis of 1041 patients with induction failure on cooperative group ALL trials demonstrated that these patients continue to have a poor 10-year OS of only 32% [14]. Importantly, infant ALL (<1 year at diagnosis) is a distinct entity, and a phase 3 randomized study (Interfant-06) enrolling 651 patients comparing intensive chemotherapy combinations found an extremely poor EFS of 21% for high-risk patients with a KMT2A rearrangement [15]. AML remains challenging to cure, with a 5-year EFS and OS of 46 and 64%, respectively, despite chemotherapy intensification and HSCT [5]. AML patients with low-risk disease have an OS of around 65–75%, whereas high-risk patients have an OS of 50% [5].

Lymphoma

Pediatric lymphoma is broadly categorized into two groups—Hodgkin lymphoma (HL) and non-Hodgkin lymphoma (NHL). HL is the most common malignancy among adolescents 15–19 years [16]. Pediatric NHL includes over 30 different histologies, with most cases defined within three categories—mature B-cell NHL (Burkitt lymphoma, diffuse large B-cell lymphoma, and primary mediastinal B-cell lymphoma), lymphoblastic lymphoma, and anaplastic large cell lymphoma (ALCL, Fig. 26.1) [18].

Two recent studies of 61 and 18 patients, respectively, leveraged whole-genome and single-cell RNA sequencing focused on the small portion of malignant Hodgkin and Reed-Sternberg cells present in HL tumors to study the molecular evolution and immune microenvironment of classic HL in children and adults [19, 20]. A recent comprehensive mutational and transcriptional analysis of B-lymphoblastic lymphoma (B-LLy) samples from 97 patients revealed that most molecular subtypes originally defined in B-ALL are present in B-LLy [21]. Genomic studies in various pediatric NHL subgroups continue to explore their underlying biology [22].

HL treatment includes risk-adapted chemotherapy, with or without consolidative radiation therapy (RT) [16]. Risk assignment includes staging, presence of B symptoms, and presence of bulky disease. The risk of RT-related toxicity has been greatly reduced by the use of FDG-PET to determine the need for RT. Randomized phase 3 trials enrolling >600 patients each with advanced HL have demonstrated a survival benefit to the addition of brentuximab vedotin to chemotherapy as well as nivolumab to chemotherapy [23, 24].

For mature B-cell NHL, a randomized phase 3 trial with >300 patients testing the addition of the CD20 monoclonal antibody rituximab with intensive chemotherapy greatly improved outcomes in high-risk patients [25]. B-LLy is treated with similar regimens as B-ALL. In a phase 3 randomized study enrolling >800 patients, improved EFS and OS were seen with the addition of bortezomib to chemotherapy in patients with T-LLy but not T-ALL, raising the possibility that these conditions are biologically distinct [26]. A phase 2 study in 68 children with ALCL demonstrated favorable outcomes with the combination of brentuximab vedotin and chemotherapy [27].

Patients with pediatric lymphomas have survival rates exceeding 90% for most disease subtypes. In the last two decades, a series of clinical trials through cooperative groups in North America and Europe enrolling over 5000 patients have demonstrated that long-term OS in HL regularly exceeds 95% [16, 23]. The OS of pediatric NHL has greatly improved over several decades through cooperative trials, with a survival rate of greater than 85–90% in most major subtypes [18, 22]. Hence, the focus of contemporary and future clinical trials is to reduce toxicity through the incorporation of novel targeted agents, including immunotherapy [16, 18].

Central Nervous System Tumors

Pediatric central nervous system (CNS) tumors represent 20% of childhood cancers and are the most common solid malignancies in children [28]. CNS tumors are divided into glial/glioneuronal and non-glial tumors (Fig. 26.2).

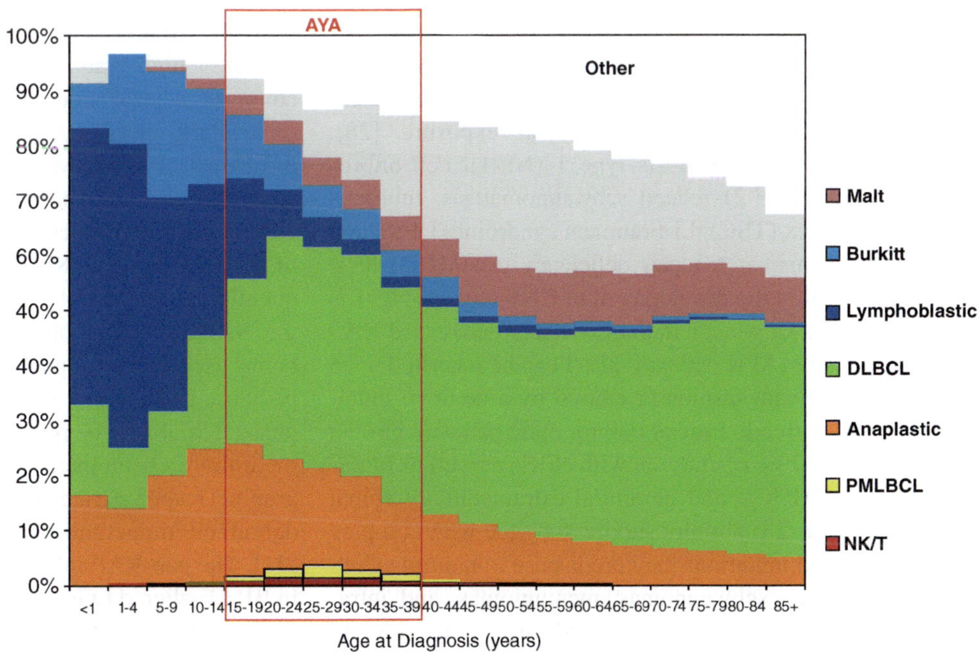

Fig. 26.1 Non-Hodgkin lymphoma histology distribution by age, United States SEER data 2000–2011. (Source: Bleyer et al. [17])

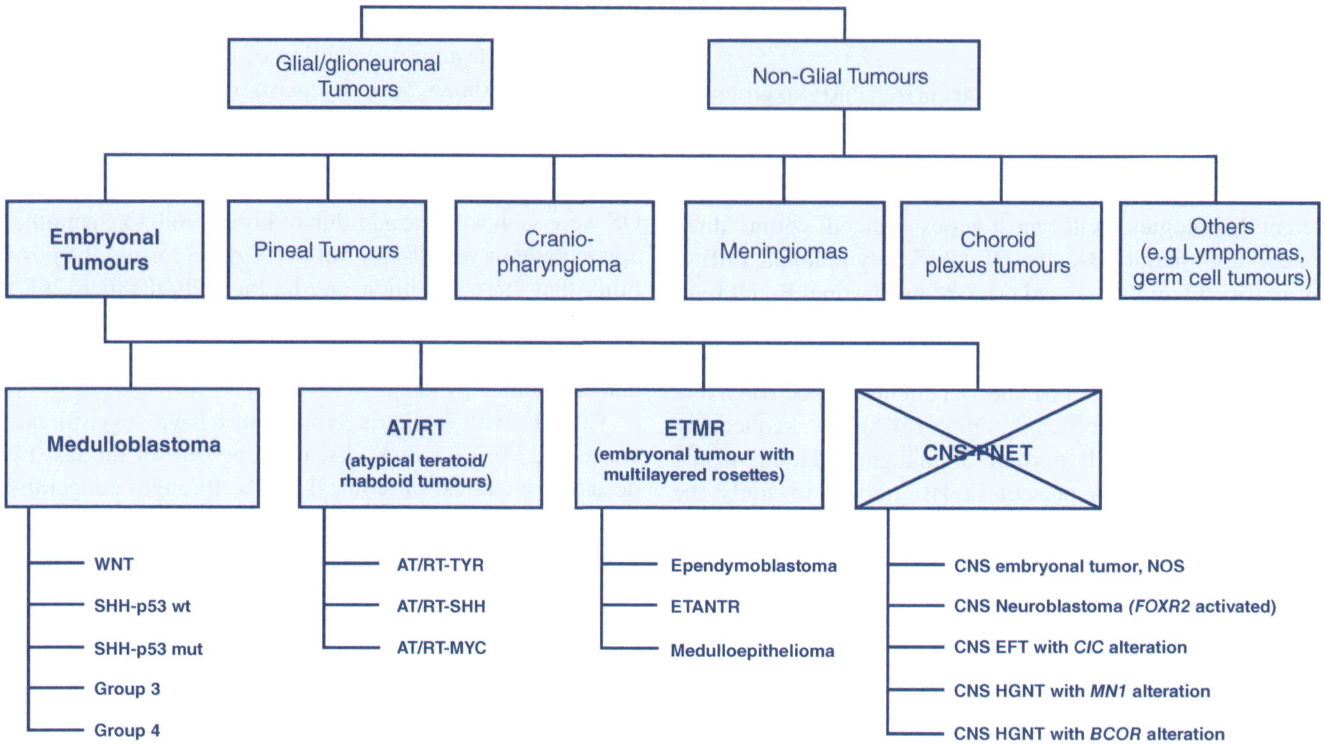

Fig. 26.2 Classification of pediatric central nervous system tumors, including newer molecularly defined classifications. (Source: Gajjar et al. [28])

Glial-based tumors can be further divided into low-grade gliomas (LGGs), high-grade gliomas (HGGs), and ependymomas. Non-glial tumors can be further divided into embryonal tumors, pineal tumors, craniopharyngiomas, meningiomas, choroid plexus tumors, and germ cell tumors [28]. In 2021, the World Health Organization (WHO) published the fifth edition of Classification of Tumors of the CNS, which heavily emphasizes molecular characterization [29].

Risk factors for developing CNS tumors include cancer predisposition syndromes (identifiable in approximately 10% of cases) and ionizing radiation exposure [28]. Specifically, neurofibromatosis type 1 (NF-1), neurofibromatosis type 2 (NF-2)–related schwannomatosis, tuberous sclerosis complex (TSC), Li-Fraumeni syndrome (LFS), and constitutional mismatch repair deficiency (CMMRD) have been implicated in the development of CNS tumors. NF-1 is a tumor suppressor gene; a mutation leads to increased RAS signaling in the MAPK pathway. NF-1 can be inherited in an autosomal dominant fashion or caused by a de novo mutation. Patients with NF-1 are at risk for optic pathway glioma (affecting up to 20% of children with NF-1) as well as brainstem gliomas, HGGs, and intradural extramedullary spinal tumors [28]. NF-2 is a tumor suppressor gene with complex interactions, and mutations may predispose to multiple CNS tumors, including schwannomas, meningiomas, and intramedullary spinal ependymomas. TSC mutations lead to mTOR hyperactivation, and CNS manifestations may include subependymal giant cell astrocytomas (SEGAs). LFS is associated with TP53 mutations and increases one's risk for CNS tumors such as HGGs, medulloblastomas, and choroid plexus carcinomas. Lastly, CMMRD is associated with mismatch repair system biallelic mutations involving MLH1, MSH2, MSH6, or PMS2. CMMRD increases the risk of LGGs, HGGs, and medulloblastomas [30].

WHO grading classifies tumors as low grade (grades 1 and 2) or high grade (grades 3 and 4). LGGs are the most common heterogenous CNS tumor group. They can be molecularly classified, including MYB or MYBL1-altered diffuse astrocytoma, MAPK-altered diffuse LGG, or MAPK-altered pilocytic astrocytoma (PA). PA is the most common LGG seen in pediatrics (~20% of all CNS tumors), and 70% of PAs harbor the KIAA1549-BRAF fusion. LGGs frequently exhibit MAPK alterations, including the fusion and the BRAFV600E mutation. MEK inhibitors (MEKis) are being used more frequently for fusion-positive patients. In pediatric LGG with a BRAFV600E mutation, a randomized phase 2 trial of 110 patients randomized to dabrafenib/trametinib vs. chemotherapy demonstrated an improved radiographic response rate and progression-free survival in the dabrafenib/trametinib arm and resulted in FDA approval [31]. The pan-RAF inhibitor tovorafenib has shown promise in BRAF-altered LGGs, including tumor responses in almost 70% of 35 patients enrolled in a phase 1b study, and an ongoing trial is comparing tovorafenib with standard chemotherapy [32]. HGGs are also heterogenous with mutations such as H3K27M seen in midline tumors and H3G34R seen in hemispheric tumors. H3K27M mutant midline gliomas have no cure; radiotherapy extends survival 3–6 months, and certain drugs such as ONC201 (selective DRD2 antagonist) have shown life prolongation in early phase trials, but not curative potential [33]. Other HGGs are generally treated with surgery, RT, and temozolomide and carry a poor prognosis. Ependymomas of the brain and spine are not chemotherapy sensitive and are treated with surgery and RT [34].

Medulloblastoma is a posterior fossa embryonal tumor and the most common malignant brain tumor in children, and 30% of patients present with mainly CNS metastatic disease. High-risk disease is based on age, postoperative residual tumor, metastases, and anaplasia/large-cell histology. Medulloblastoma is molecularly classified into WNT-activated, SHH-activated, SHH-activated with TP53-mutant, and non-WNT/non-SHH, and 70% of patients can be cured with surgery, RT, and chemotherapy. There is institutional variability in preferred systemic treatment for medulloblastoma, which may involve high-dose chemotherapy with autologous stem cell rescue (SCR) or maintenance chemotherapy. The HeadStart trials aim to spare RT with intensive therapy; the HeadStart IV trial tested three cycles of induction therapy and one cycle of high-dose chemotherapy with SCR, which showed excellent 3-year EFS and OS in localized SHH-activated medulloblastomas [35].

Neuroblastoma

Neuroblastoma is the most common extracranial pediatric solid tumor, representing 8–10% of childhood cancers but approximately 15% of childhood cancer deaths [36]. Clinical behavior ranges from localized or spontaneously regressing disease in infants to widely metastatic and aggressive presentations in slightly older children. Tumors arise from the adrenal medulla or along the sympathetic chain, and over half have metastasized at presentation. Histologic categories reflect the differentiation status of the tumor cells with a spectrum from benign ganglioneuroma (fully differentiated ganglion cells) to neuroblastoma (malignant neuroblasts). Ganglioneuroblastomas (GNBs) contain both cell types and are either nodular or intermixed; only neuroblastoma and GNB nodular are included in the current neuroblastoma risk stratification system [37].

The International Neuroblastoma Risk Group (INRG) system is widely used for risk-based treatment assignment, focusing on image-defined risk factors (IDRFs), which assess the likelihood of a successful surgical resection [38]. Specifically, locoregional tumors are classified as L1 (IDRF−) or L2 (IDRF+), and metastatic disease is stage M except in children <18 months with metastases restricted to the skin, liver, and/or limited bone marrow involvement (stage MS) [38]. Components beyond stage influencing risk assignment include *MYCN* status, age, ploidy, International Neuroblastoma Pathology Classification, and segmental chromosome aberrations [37, 39, 40].

Evaluation of patients with neuroblastoma includes the collection of urine vanillylmandelic and homovanillic acid, as catecholamine metabolites are elevated in most patients. Imaging evaluation includes an anatomical view of primary tumors to assess IDRFs, ^{123}I-metaiodobenzylguanidine (^{123}I-MIBG) for identification of primary and metastatic disease, and FDG-PET in patients with ^{123}I-MIBG non-avid tumors (<10%) [41]. A tumor biopsy is needed for histologic and molecular evaluation. However, in patients <12 months with an isolated adrenal mass (<5 cm) and elevated catecholamines or in infants with disseminated disease needing immediate intervention, an empirical diagnosis can be rendered [42]. Bilateral bone marrow samples are also required for staging.

Treatment of neuroblastoma is based on risk stratification (Fig. 26.3), ranging from observation to intense multimodal therapy including chemotherapy, surgery, high-dose chemotherapy with SCR, radiation, anti-GD2 immunotherapy, and isotretinoin for high-risk disease, which accounts for about half of patients with newly diagnosed neuroblastoma [42]. *ALK* is mutated in 10–15% of neuroblastoma and provides a potential therapeutic target; the rare familial neuroblastomas also tend to be associated with germline mutations in *ALK* [44]. Children with low- and intermediate-risk disease have a 5-year EFS >85% with recent successful reductions in therapy, but new approaches are still needed for those with high-risk presentations, in which 5-year EFS is approximately 50% [45]. Accordingly, ongoing clinical trials for high-risk neuroblastoma through COG are studying the impact of ALK inhibition and therapeutic MIBG (NCT03126916) and upfront use of immunotherapy with induction chemotherapy (NCT06172296). Additionally, eflornithine (DFMO) received FDA approval in 2023 as a maintenance therapy based on a propensity-matched analysis of >1500 patients with high-risk neuroblastoma showing improved EFS in patients receiving DFMO [46].

Wilms Tumor

Wilms tumor (WT) is the most common renal cancer in children, with approximately 500 cases annually in the USA [47]. Most WTs have favorable histology comprised of epithelial, blastemal, and/or stromal components, while a minority show anaplastic histology, which can be either focal or diffuse and carries a worse prognosis. Additionally, post-chemotherapy histologic evaluation can reveal lower-risk

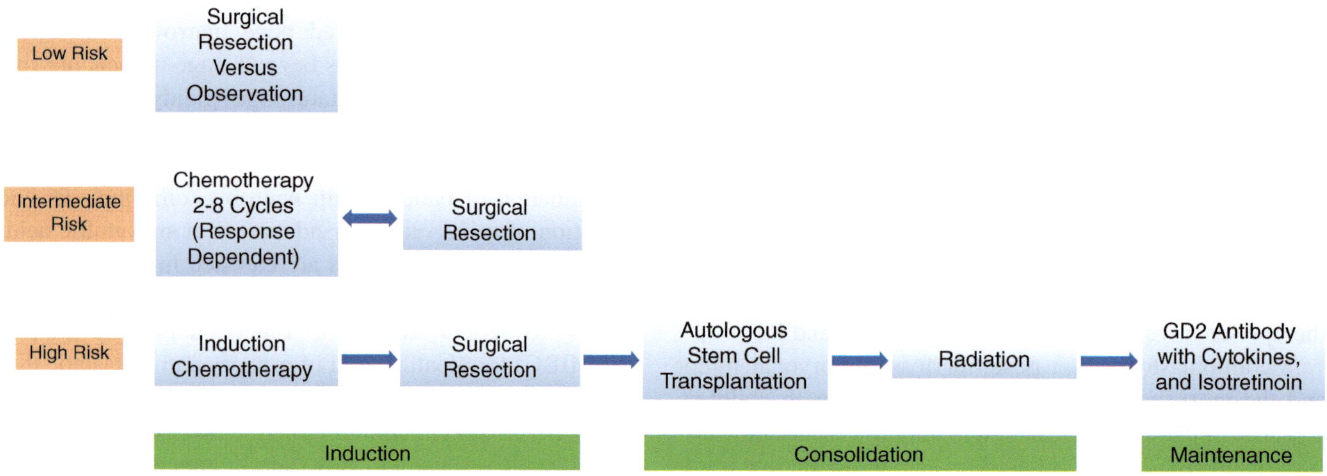

Fig. 26.3 Treatment overview for neuroblastoma by risk classification. (Source: Tolbert [43])

WT (completely necrotic) or higher-risk WT (blastemal predominant) [48]. While most WTs are sporadic, approximately 10% are associated with underlying genetic predisposition, such as WT1-related WT, Beckwith-Wiedemann, or WAGR (Wilms tumor, aniridia, genital anomalies, retardation) syndrome, and surveillance is appropriate for certain syndromes or genetic alterations [49]. Most WTs are solitary. However, 10% are multifocal in one kidney, and 5–7% have bilateral synchronous tumors at presentation. Those with unilateral multifocal or bilateral disease often have an underlying genetic predisposition [49].

Treatment of WT depends on histology and tumor stage, with slightly different approaches among cooperative groups. In the USA, upfront nephrectomy in unilateral nonsyndromic disease is preferred. The Children's Oncology Group (COG) WT staging includes stage I to stage V, where stage I–III outlines local renal tumor involvement and extension, stage IV represents metastases (most commonly to the lung), and stage V denotes bilateral renal tumors [50]. After resection, treatment may span from observation only for young patients with stage I favorable-histology WT (FHWT) to chemotherapy such as vincristine and dactinomycin, adding doxorubicin, or intensification using additional agents such as cyclophosphamide, etoposide, and carboplatin for higher-risk groups [51]. The activity of irinotecan has been found in patients with metastatic diffuse anaplasia in 14 patients treated on a phase 2 window study and retrospectively in a 14-patient cohort at relapse [52, 53]. Radiation is provided based on stage, metastatic site/response, and histology [50].

Biological factors, including karyotype abnormalities, aid in risk stratification for FHWT. Specifically, a gain of chromosome 1q is associated with worse outcomes, an increased chance of relapse, and decreased OS [54]. The combination of loss of heterozygosity (LOH) of chromosomes 1p and 16q places patients at higher risk, mitigated by augmentation of therapy as shown in 49 patients treated on the biology study ARST03B2 and the phase 3 trial ARST0532 [55]. The presence of positive lymph nodes and LOH of 1p *or* 16q is associated with worse outcomes and warrants consideration of therapy intensification [56]. In very-low-risk patients previously treated with nephrectomy only, there is an increased risk of relapse seen with LOH/LOI of 11p15 [57].

For patients with FHWT and pulmonary metastases, evaluation of response to 6 weeks of chemotherapy can guide therapy intensification and radiation use [55]. Outcomes of patients with extrapulmonary metastatic disease remain suboptimal, and there is a lack of consensus for how to control metastatic sites [58]. Patients with bilateral WT benefit from preoperative chemotherapy to facilitate nephron-sparing surgery, with further therapy guided by post-chemotherapy histology and stage [59].

Overall, risk-stratified treatment in WT has resulted in excellent 5-year survival at 90% [60].

Efforts are currently underway to improve the treatment of patients with upfront higher-risk diffuse anaplastic WT, as well as those with relapsed FHWT (NCT04322318). Furthermore, optimizing the initial approach to WT by detecting pathognomonic and prognostic features via circulating tumor DNA in liquid biopsy may help overcome tumoral heterogeneity and will be explored in future studies. A preliminary study of blood and urine samples from 50 patients on a clinical trial for WT found the ability to detect ctDNA at diagnosis in >80% of patients with a trend toward inferior EFS in those with ctDNA detected [61].

Retinoblastoma

Retinoblastoma has an age-adjusted incidence of 18.4 cases per one million children aged 1–4 years [62]. All patients should be tested for germline RB1 mutation. Dilated eye exams in children with a known RB1 genetic predisposition can lead to early retinoblastoma detection and improved outcomes. A baseline brain MRI is recommended at diagnosis to evaluate for a midline neuroblastic tumor (aka trilateral retinoblastoma). Metastatic evaluation with lumbar puncture, bone marrow evaluation, and FDG-PET should be performed in patients with suspected extraocular extension or high-risk pathology in the enucleated eye (i.e., massive choroidal invasion, involvement of the sclera, or the optic nerve extension beyond the lamina cribrosa).

Treatment requires a pediatric multidisciplinary team including ocular oncologists, hematologists/oncologists, and radiation oncologists. The International Retinoblastoma Staging System (IRSS) is the most widely used staging system. Intraocular disease is stratified to groups lettered A through F based on confinement to the retina, presence of subretinal or vitreous seeding, or diffuse/massive involvement. OS exceeds 95% for intraocular disease. However, this does not equate to "ocular survival," which is the time before enucleation is required. A conservative ocular salvage approach with local treatments, including intravitreal and intra-arterial therapy (IAC), is employed whenever possible, in conjunction with neoadjuvant chemotherapy for patients under 3 months of age and those with advanced disease [62]. The most commonly used chemotherapy agent for intra-arterial or intravitreal use is melphalan, which conveys minimal long-term side effects. Electroretinography can be used pre-IAC to assist with treatment planning, given its correlation with visual acuity [63]. Enucleation may be needed, especially for group E disease. Systemic therapy is necessary for patients with high-risk pathology in the enucleated eye, and an intensive regimen using high-dose chemotherapy and autologous SCR is often employed for patients with extraorbital disease. Radiation therapy is typically reserved for refractory disease or progression. A retrospective analysis of >2000 survivors of retinoblastoma found the most common cause of death to be secondary malignant neoplasms (SMN); it is important that these patients receive evaluations in cancer genetics and survivorship clinics [64].

An ongoing COG study, ARET2121 (NCT05504291), explores the feasibility of combining intravitreal melphalan with neoadjuvant systemic chemotherapy in patients with unilateral group D retinoblastoma with vitreous seeding or bilateral retinoblastoma with the worst eye categorized as group D and vitreous seeding. There is emerging data on the role of aqueous humor (AH) as a liquid biopsy source; a study of AH from 26 patients found the presence of ctDNA correlated with the likelihood of enucleation [65]. Salvage regimens depend on the prior treatment and nature of recurrence. A novel approach under investigation involves the use of an oncolytic adenovirus that targets *RB1* based on promising preclinical data in patient-derived retinoblastoma models [66].

Rhabdomyosarcoma

Rhabdomyosarcoma (RMS) is the most common soft tissue tumor in childhood, with an incidence of 4.6 cases per million in those under 20 years of age, with superior outcomes seen in children and adolescents vs. adults with RMS [67]. Several RMS histologies exist, including embryonal, alveolar, spindle cell/sclerosing, and pleomorphic, and risk stratification relies on the molecular classification based on the presence of *FOXO1* fusion, which portends a poor prognosis [67]. Outcomes are also influenced by age, site, tumor size, resectability, and presence of metastatic disease. While there are no known environmental risk factors, LFS, DICER1, and NF-1 are known cancer predispositions for FOXO1-negative RMS; a study of germline DNA of 580 patients with RMS found those patient with a germline cancer predisposition variant had inferior overall survival to those without [68].

A multimodal treatment approach involving surgery, chemotherapy, and radiation is often necessary, with upfront surgical resection preferred for localized disease where R0 margins are feasible. The chemotherapy backbone mostly comprises vincristine, dactinomycin, and an alkylating agent (cyclophosphamide or ifosfamide). However, duration, agents, and dosage vary by cooperative group. Clinical trials should be strongly considered whenever possible.

Current COG study ARST2032 (NCT05304585) aims to decrease therapy burden for patients with very low risk disease (stage 1 group 1, fusion negative, MYOD 1, and TP53 WT) by omission of cyclophosphamide, while COG ARST2031 (NCT04994132) aims to improve survival for high-risk patients with the introduction of vinorelbine in the upfront setting. Maintenance therapy with vinorelbine and oral cyclophosphamide has shown benefit in higher-risk nonmetastatic RMS in the EpSSG RMS 2005 trial and, therefore, is also being explored for the HR subset. In addition, a novel "evolutionary" tactic to specifically target metastatic fusion-positive RMS is also currently underway [69].

Detectable ctDNA in 124 patients with newly diagnosed intermediate-risk RMS was found to be associated with inferior survival irrespective of fusion status [70]. A European retrospective study of 57 patient samples reported poor outcomes in patients with detectable serum methylated RASSF1A [71]. The utility of these tests as predictive biomarkers necessitates further validation and is being incorporated in the ongoing prospective trials. Multiple treatment regimens have been explored in the relapse setting, including varying combinations of temsirolimus, irinotecan, temozolomide, carboplatin, and etoposide. However, treating a recurrence continues to be a challenge. Immunotherapy trials are currently underway in the relapsed-refractory setting, including using universal donor, TGFβ-imprinted expanded natural killer (NK) cells in combination with chemotherapy (NCT05634369), and pembrolizumab in PD-L1-positive tumors (NCT02332668).

Osteosarcoma

Osteosarcoma accounts for approximately 1000 cases per year in the USA and spans older childhood, adolescence, and young adulthood, with a second peak later in adulthood. The mainstays of treatment are surgical local control and intensive multiagent chemotherapy for both localized and metastatic patients. The 5-year estimated EFS is approximately 60%, with inferior survival in those with metastatic disease (approximately 30%) [72]. Cancer predisposition plays an important role in osteosarcoma, with germline cancer susceptibility variants present in almost 1/3 of patients [72].

Research in biology has focused on osteosarcoma's heterogeneity both genomically and in the immune microenvironment. Osteosarcoma has a high mutational burden compared to other pediatric solid tumors and is also characterized by complex chromosomal rearrangements and somatic copy number alterations, while the immune microenvironment is highly variable between patient samples in regard to T-cell infiltration, PD-1/PD-L1 expression, and non-T-cell immune infiltrates [73]. The osteosarcoma community has identified a lack of high-quality, clinically annotated clinical samples as an urgent need for improved understanding of osteosarcoma biology, and efforts are underway to improve sample collection and availability [74].

Clinical research efforts focus on improving prognostic stratification using new technologies such as ctDNA while improving survival outcomes in newly diagnosed and recurrent disease [72, 75]. Current clinical efforts in North America include testing the addition of the tyrosine kinase inhibitor (TKI) cabozantinib to systemic therapy in newly diagnosed osteosarcoma (NCT05691478) as well as identifying the optimal surgical approach to address lung metastases (NCT05235165).

Ewing Sarcoma

Ewing sarcoma (ES) accounts for about 300 cases per year in the USA. Localized disease has an approximately 80% 5-year EFS, while metastatic disease portends a poor prognosis (approximately 40% 3-year EFS) [72]. Standard treatment consists of interval-compressed intensive chemotherapy with surgery or radiation for local control. The interval-compressed chemotherapy strategy was shown recently on a long-term analysis of >500 patients from a randomized phase 3 trial AEWS0031 to have particularly increased efficacy in patients with large tumor size. The highest-reported survival outcomes in localized ES were seen in a recent phase 3 randomized trial of >600 patients using 17 cycles of compressed therapy [76]. A recent phase 3 randomized study testing the addition of ganitumab to chemotherapy in >200 patients with metastatic Ewing sarcoma did not find a survival benefit in those treated with ganitumab [77].

ES is a translocation-driven sarcoma defined by the fusion of FET and ETS family genes, with the most common fusion being EWS::FLI1 [78]. Recent biology studies have elucidated the function of the fusion in oncogenesis as well as ES fusion dependence, identifying the great potential of fusion-targeting therapies in the future [79]. Similar to osteosarcoma, acquisition and curation of high-quality patient samples will be indispensable for further advances [74]. Recent and ongoing studies and clinical trials test the utility of ctDNA as a prognostic biomarker in ES, the safety and efficacy of fusion targeting therapies (either directly or indirectly), and the incorporation of novel agents into frontline therapy to improve outcomes for metastatic ES [72].

Summary

Despite the rarity, great heterogeneity, and logistical challenges of research in pediatric cancer, our understanding of these cancers and survival outcomes has improved dramatically. Future challenges for the pediatric oncology community include studying ever-more-rare subtypes of disease that are molecularly defined, developing pharmacologic interventions tailored to pediatric cancers, and reducing the burden of treatment-related toxicities in patients with a long life expectancy following cancer treatment.

References

1. Siegel DA, King JB, Lupo PJ, Durbin EB, Tai E, Mills K, et al. Counts, incidence rates, and trends of pediatric cancer in the United States, 2003–2019. J Natl Cancer Inst. 2023;115(11):1337–54.
2. Roganovic J. Genetic predisposition to childhood cancer. World J Clin Pediatr. 2024;13(3):95010.
3. Siegel DA, Richardson LC, Henley SJ, Wilson RJ, Dowling NF, Weir HK, et al. Pediatric cancer mortality and survival in the United States, 2001–2016. Cancer. 2020;126(19):4379–89.
4. Ehrlich PF. The impact of cooperative group studies on childhood cancer: improving outcomes and quality and international collaboration. Semin Pediatr Surg. 2019;28(6):150857.
5. Cooper TM, Alonzo TA, Tasian SK, Kutny MA, Hitzler J, Pollard JA, et al. Children's Oncology Group's 2023 blueprint for research: myeloid neoplasms. Pediatr Blood Cancer. 2023;70(Suppl 6):e30584.

6. Raetz EA, Bhojwani D, Devidas M, Gore L, Rabin KR, Tasian SK, et al. Children's oncology group blueprint for research: acute lymphoblastic leukemia. Pediatr Blood Cancer. 2023;70(Suppl 6):e30585.
7. Brady SW, Roberts KG, Gu Z, Shi L, Pounds S, Pei D, et al. The genomic landscape of pediatric acute lymphoblastic leukemia. Nat Genet. 2022;54(9):1376–89.
8. Bolouri H, Farrar JE, Triche TJ, Ries RE, Lim EL, Alonzo TA, et al. The molecular landscape of pediatric acute myeloid leukemia reveals recurrent structural alterations and age-specific mutational interactions. Nat Med. 2018;24(1):103–12.
9. Mumme H, Thomas BE, Bhasin SS, Krishnan U, Dwivedi B, Perumalla P, et al. Single-cell analysis reveals altered tumor microenvironments of relapse and remission-associated pediatric acute myeloid leukemia. Nat Commun. 2023;14(1):6209.
10. Xu J, Chen C, Sussman JH, Yoshimura S, Vincent T, Polonen P, et al. A multiomic atlas identifies a treatment-resistant, bone marrow progenitor-like cell population in T cell acute lymphoblastic leukemia. Nat Cancer. 2024;6(1):102–22.
11. Dunsmore KP, Winter SS, Devidas M, Wood BL, Esiashvili N, Chen Z, et al. Children's Oncology Group AALL0434: a phase III randomized clinical trial testing nelarabine in newly diagnosed T-cell acute lymphoblastic leukemia. J Clin Oncol. 2020;38(28):3282–93.
12. Fleischer LC, Spencer HT, Raikar SS. Targeting T cell malignancies using CAR-based immunotherapy: challenges and potential solutions. J Hematol Oncol. 2019;12(1):141.
13. Gupta S, Rau RE, Kairalla JA, Rabin KR, Wang C, Angiolillo AL, et al. Blinatumomab in standard-risk B-cell acute lymphoblastic leukemia in children. N Engl J Med. 2024;392(9):875–91.
14. Schrappe M, Hunger SP, Pui C, Saha V, Gaynon PS, Baruchel A, et al. Outcomes after induction failure in childhood acute lymphoblastic leukemia. N Engl J Med. 2012;366(15):1371–81.
15. Pieters R, De Lorenzo P, Ancliffe P, Aversa LA, Brethon B, Biondi A, et al. Outcome of infants younger than 1 year with acute lymphoblastic leukemia treated with the Interfant-06 protocol: results from an international phase III randomized study. J Clin Oncol. 2019;37(25):2246–56.
16. Castellino SM, Giulino-Roth L, Harker-Murray P, Kahn JM, Forlenza C, Cho S, et al. Children's Oncology Group's 2023 blueprint for research: Hodgkin lymphoma. Pediatr Blood Cancer. 2023;70(Suppl 6):e30580.
17. Bleyer WA, et al. Cancer in adolescents and young adults. 2nd ed. Springer International Publishing; 2017.
18. El-Mallawany NK, Alexander S, Fluchel M, Hayashi RJ, Lowe EJ, Giulino-Roth L, et al. Children's Oncology Group's 2023 blueprint for research: Non-Hodgkin lymphoma. Pediatr Blood Cancer. 2023;70(Suppl 6):e30565.
19. Maura F, Ziccheddu B, Xiang JZ, Bhinder B, Rosiene J, Abascal F, et al. Molecular evolution of classic Hodgkin lymphoma revealed through whole-genome sequencing of Hodgkin and Reed Sternberg cells. Blood Cancer Discov. 2023;4(3):208–27.
20. de Kanter JK, Steemers AS, Gonzalez DM, van Ineveld RL, Blijleven C, Groenen N, et al. Single-cell RNA sequencing of pediatric Hodgkin lymphoma to study the inhibition of T cell subtypes. Hemasphere. 2024;8(9):e149.
21. Kroeze E, Iaccarino I, Kleisman MM, Mondal M, Beder T, Khouja M, et al. Mutational and transcriptional landscape of pediatric B-cell precursor lymphoblastic lymphoma. Blood. 2024;144(1):74–83.
22. Cairo MS. "The state of the science" of childhood, adolescent and young adult Non Hodgkin Lymphoma (NHL). Best Pract Res Clin Haematol. 2023;36(2):101482.
23. Castellino SM, Pei Q, Parsons SK, Hodgson D, McCarten K, Horton T, et al. Brentuximab vedotin with chemotherapy in pediatric high-risk Hodgkin's Lymphoma. N Engl J Med. 2022;387(18):1649–60.
24. Herrera AF, LeBlanc M, Castellino SM, Li H, Rutherford SC, Evens AM, et al. Nivolumab+AVD in advanced-stage classic Hodgkin's Lymphoma. N Engl J Med. 2024;391(15):1379–89.
25. Minard-Colin V, Auperin A, Pillon M, Burke GAA, Barkauskas DA, Wheatley K, et al. Rituximab for high-risk, mature B-Cell Non-Hodgkin's Lymphoma in Children. N Engl J Med. 2020;382(23):2207–19.
26. Teachey DT, Devidas M, Wood BL, Chen Z, Hayashi RJ, Hermiston ML, et al. Children's Oncology Group Trial AALL1231: a phase III clinical trial testing bortezomib in newly diagnosed T-Cell acute lymphoblastic leukemia and lymphoma. J Clin Oncol. 2022;40(19):2106–18.
27. Lowe EJ, Reilly AF, Lim MS, Gross TG, Saguilig L, Barkauskas DA, et al. Brentuximab vedotin in combination with chemotherapy for pediatric patients with ALK+ ALCL: results of COG trial ANHL12P1. Blood. 2021;137(26):3595–603.
28. Gajjar A, Reaman G, Racadio J, Smith F. Brain Tumors in Children. Springer Nature; 2018.
29. d'Amati A, Bargiacchi L, Rossi S, Carai A, Bertero L, Barresi V, et al. Pediatric CNS tumors and 2021 WHO classification: what do oncologists need from pathologists? Front Mol Neurosci. 2024;13(17):1268038.
30. Durno C, Ercan AB, Bianchi V, Edwards M, Aronson M, Galati M, et al. Survival benefit for individuals with constitutional mismatch repair deficiency undergoing surveillance. J Clin Oncol. 2021;39(25):2779–90.
31. Bouffet E, Hansford JR, Garre ML, Hara J, Plant-Fox A, Aerts I, et al. Dabrafenib plus trametinib in pediatric glioma with BRAF V600 mutations. N Engl J Med. 2023;389(12):1108–20.
32. van Tilburg CM, Kilburn LB, Perreault S, Schmidt R, Azizi AA, Cruz-Martinez O, et al. LOGGIC/FIREFLY-2: a phase 3, randomized trial of tovorafenib vs. chemotherapy in pediatric and young adult patients with newly diagnosed low-grade glioma harboring an activating RAF alteration. BMC Cancer. 2024;24(1):147–x.
33. Gardner SL, Tarapore RS, Allen J, McGovern SL, Zaky W, Odia Y, et al. Phase I dose escalation and expansion trial of single agent ONC201 in pediatric diffuse midline gliomas following radiotherapy. Neurooncol Adv. 2022;4(1):vdac143.
34. Smith A, Lensing S, Onar-Thomas A, Leary S, Fouladi M, Foreman N, et al. Is the outcome of supratentorial ependymoma with ZFTA fusion really poor? Neuro Oncol. 2024;26(Suppl 4):154–155.
35. Dhall G, Stanek J, Blue M, Patel P, Thomas D, Pierson C, Tamrazi B, Mahadeo K, Fleming J, Bell E, K MI, Grischow O, Liszkay T, Owen S, Hastings C, Tsui K, Mazewski C, Friedman G, Moertel C, Hanson D, Koschman C, Brock G, Asgharzadeh S, Chakravarti A, Wong K, Nelson M, Bouc D, Biegel J, Mardis E, Finlay J. Outcomes of infants and young children with newly diagnosed SHH Medulloblastoma treated on The NEXT Consortium "Head Start 4" protocol. Neuro Oncol. 2024;26(Suppl 4)
36. Park JR, Eggert A, Caron H. Neuroblastoma: biology, prognosis, and treatment. Hematol Oncol Clin North Am. 2010;24(1):65–86.
37. Shimada H, Ambros IM, Dehner LP, Hata J, Joshi VV, Roald B, et al. The International Neuroblastoma Pathology Classification (the Shimada system). Cancer. 1999;86(2):364–72.
38. Irwin MS, Naranjo A, Zhang FF, Cohn SL, London WB, Gastier-Foster JM, et al. Revised neuroblastoma risk classification system: a report from the Children's Oncology Group. J Clin Oncol. 2021;39(29):3229–41.
39. Brisse HJ, McCarville MB, Granata C, Krug KB, Wootton-Gorges SL, Kanegawa K, et al. Guidelines for imaging and staging of neuroblastic tumors: consensus report from the International Neuroblastoma Risk Group Project. Radiology. 2011;261(1):243–57.
40. Irwin MS, Goldsmith KC. Current and emerging biomarkers: impact on risk stratification for neuroblastoma. J Natl Compr Canc Netw. 2024;22(6):e247051. https://doi.org/10.6004/jnccn.2024.7051.
41. Matthay KK, Shulkin B, Ladenstein R, Michon J, Giammarile F, Lewington V, et al. Criteria for evaluation of disease extent by (123) I-metaiodobenzylguanidine scans in neuroblastoma: a report for the

International Neuroblastoma Risk Group (INRG) Task Force. Br J Cancer. 2010;102(9):1319–26.
42. Qiu B, Matthay KK. Advancing therapy for neuroblastoma. Nat Rev. Clin Oncol. 2022;19(8):515–33.
43. Tolbert V. Neuroblastoma: clinical and biological approach to risk stratification and treatment. Cell Tissue Res. 2018;372(2):195–209. PubMed ID 29572647
44. Matthay KK, Maris JM, Schleiermacher G, Nakagawara A, Mackall CL, Diller L, et al. Neuroblastoma. Nat Rev. Dis Primers. 2016;10(2):16078.
45. DuBois SG, Macy ME, Henderson TO. High-Risk and relapsed neuroblastoma: toward more cures and better outcomes. Am Soc Clin Oncol Educ Book. 2022;42:1–13.
46. Oesterheld J, Ferguson W, Kraveka JM, Bergendahl G, Clinch T, Lorenzi E, et al. Eflornithine as postimmunotherapy maintenance in high-risk neuroblastoma: externally controlled, propensity score-matched survival outcome comparisons. J Clin Oncol. 2024;42(1):90–102.
47. Bernstein L, Linet M, Smith M, Olshan A, Tumors R. In: Gloeckler L, Smith M, Gurney J, Linet M, Tamra T, Young J, et al., editors. Cancer Incidence and Survival Among Children and Adolescents: United States SEER Program 1975-1995. National Cancer Institute; 1999. p. 79–90.
48. Parsons LN. Wilms Tumor: challenges and newcomers in prognosis. Surg Pathol Clin. 2020;13(4):683–93.
49. Turner J, Brzezinski J, Dome J. Wilms Tumor Predisposition. In: Adam M, Feldman J, Mirzaa G, Pagon R, Wallace S, Amemiya A, editors. Gene Reviews. Seattle: University of Washington; 2003. p. 1993–2024.
50. Pater L, Melchior P, Rube C, Cooper BT, McAleer MF, Kalapurakal JA, et al. Wilms tumor. Pediatr Blood Cancer. 2021;68(Suppl 2):e28257.
51. Balis F, Green DM, Anderson C, Cook S, Dhillon J, Gow K, et al. Wilms tumor (nephroblastoma), version 2.2021, NCCN clinical practice guidelines in oncology. J Natl Compr Canc Netw. 2021;19(8):945–77.
52. Daw NC, Chi Y, Kalapurakal JA, Kim Y, Hoffer FA, Geller JI, et al. Activity of vincristine and irinotecan in diffuse anaplastic Wilms tumor and therapy outcomes of stage II to IV disease: results of the children's oncology group AREN0321 study. J Clin Oncol. 2020;38(14):1558–68.
53. Hol JA, van den Heuvel-Eibrink MM, Graf N, Pritchard-Jones K, Brok J, van Tinteren H, et al. Irinotecan for relapsed Wilms tumor in pediatric patients: SIOP experience and review of the literature-a report from the SIOP renal tumor study group. Pediatr Blood Cancer. 2018;65(2):26849. Epub 2017 Oct 27
54. Gratias EJ, Dome JS, Jennings LJ, Chi Y, Tian J, Anderson J, et al. Association of chromosome 1q gain with inferior survival in favorable-histology Wilms tumor: a report from the children's oncology group. J Clin Oncol. 2016;34(26):3189–94.
55. Dix DB, Fernandez CV, Chi Y, Mullen EA, Geller JI, Gratias EJ, et al. Augmentation of therapy for combined loss of heterozygosity 1p and 16q in favorable histology Wilms tumor: a children's oncology group AREN0532 and AREN0533 study report. J Clin Oncol. 2019;37(30):2769–77.
56. Evageliou N, Renfro LA, Geller J, Perlman E, Kalapurakal J, Paulino A, et al. Prognostic impact of lymph node involvement and loss of heterozygosity of 1p or 16q in stage III favorable histology Wilms tumor: a report from children's oncology group studies AREN03B2 and AREN0532. Cancer. 2024;130(5):792–802.
57. Fernandez CV, Perlman EJ, Mullen EA, Chi Y, Hamilton TE, Gow KW, et al. Clinical outcome and biological predictors of relapse after nephrectomy only for very low-risk Wilms tumor: a report from children's oncology group AREN0532. Ann Surg. 2017;265(4):835–40.
58. Benedetti DJ, Varela CR, Renfro LA, Tornwall B, Dix DB, Ehrlich PF, et al. Treatment of children with favorable histology Wilms tumor with extrapulmonary metastases: a report from the COG studies AREN0533 and AREN03B2 and NWTSG study NWTS-5. Cancer. 2024;130(6):947–61.
59. Ehrlich P, Chi YY, Chintagumpala MM, Hoffer FA, Perlman EJ, Kalapurakal JA, et al. Results of the first prospective multi-institutional treatment study in children with bilateral Wilms tumor (AREN0534): a report from the children's oncology group. Ann Surg. 2017;266(3):470–8.
60. Nelson MV, van den Heuvel-Eibrink MM, Graf N, Dome JS. New approaches to risk stratification for Wilms tumor. Curr Opin Pediatr. 2021;33(1):40–8.
61. Madanat-Harjuoja LM, Renfro LA, Klega K, Tornwall B, Thorner AR, Nag A, et al. Circulating tumor DNA as a biomarker in patients with stage III and IV Wilms tumor: analysis from a children's oncology group trial, AREN0533. J Clin Oncol. 2022;40(26):3047–56.
62. PDQ Pediatric Treatment Editorial Board. Retinoblastoma treatment (PDQ(R)): health professional version. In: PDQ cancer information summaries, Bethesda (MD); 2002.
63. Levin AM, Francis JH, McFadden M, Brodie S, Gobin YP, Abramson DH. Association of electroretinography with visual outcomes after ophthalmic artery chemosurgery for retinoblastoma in ICRb D and E eyes. PLoS One. 2019;14(1):e0210647.
64. Kleinerman RA, Tucker MA, Sigel BS, Abramson DH, Seddon JM, Morton LM. Patterns of cause-specific mortality among 2053 survivors of retinoblastoma, 1914-2016. J Natl Cancer Inst. 2019;111(9):961–9.
65. Berry JL, Xu L, Kooi I, Murphree AL, Prabakar RK, Reid M, et al. Genomic cfDNA analysis of aqueous humor in retinoblastoma predicts eye salvage: the surrogate tumor biopsy for retinoblastoma. Mol Cancer Res. 2018;16(11):1701–12.
66. Pascual-Pasto G, Bazan-Peregrino M, Olaciregui NG, Restrepo-Perdomo CA, Mato-Berciano A, Ottaviani D, et al. Therapeutic targeting of the RB1 pathway in retinoblastoma with the oncolytic adenovirus VCN-01. Sci Transl Med. 2019;11(476):eaat9321. https://doi.org/10.1126/scitranslmed.aat9321.
67. PDQ Pediatric Treatment Editorial Board. Childhood rhabdomyosarcoma treatment (PDQ(R)): health professional version. In: PDQ cancer information summaries, Bethesda (MD); 2002.
68. Martin-Giacalone BA, Li H, Scheurer ME, Casey DL, Dugan-Perez S, Marquez-Do DA, et al. Germline genetic testing and survival outcomes among children with rhabdomyosarcoma: a report from the children's oncology group. JAMA Netw Open. 2024;7(3):e244170.
69. Reed DR, Metts J, Pressley M, Fridley BL, Hayashi M, Isakoff MS, et al. An evolutionary framework for treating pediatric sarcomas. Cancer. 2020;126(11):2577–87.
70. Abbou S, Klega K, Tsuji J, Tanhaemami M, Hall D, Barkauskas DA, et al. Circulating tumor DNA is prognostic in intermediate-risk rhabdomyosarcoma: a report from the children's oncology group. J Clin Oncol. 2023;41(13):2382–93.
71. Lak NSM, van Zogchel LMJ, Zappeij-Kannegieter L, Javadi A, van Paemel R, Vandeputte C, et al. Cell-free DNA as a diagnostic and prognostic biomarker in pediatric rhabdomyosarcoma. JCO Precis Oncol. 2023;7:e2200113.
72. Reed DR, Grohar P, Rubin E, Binitie O, Krailo M, Davis J, et al. Children's oncology group's 2023 blueprint for research: bone tumors. Pediatr Blood Cancer. 2023;70(Suppl 6):e30583.
73. Wu C, Livingston JA. Genomics and the immune landscape of osteosarcoma. Adv Exp Med Biol. 2020;1258:21–36.
74. Green D, van Ewijk R, Tirtei E, Andreou D, Baecklund F, Baumhoer D, et al. Biological sample collection to advance research and treatment: a fight osteosarcoma through European research and Euro Ewing Consortium statement. Clin Cancer Res. 2024;30(16):3395–406.

75. Shulman DS, Klega K, Imamovic-Tuco A, Clapp A, Nag A, Thorner AR, et al. Detection of circulating tumour DNA is associated with inferior outcomes in Ewing sarcoma and osteosarcoma: a report from the children's oncology group. Br J Cancer. 2018;119(5):615–21.
76. Leavey PJ, Laack NN, Krailo MD, Buxton A, Randall RL, DuBois SG, et al. Phase III trial adding vincristine-topotecan-cyclophosphamide to the initial treatment of patients with non metastatic Ewing sarcoma: a children's oncology group report. J Clin Oncol. 2021;39(36):4029–38.
77. DuBois SG, Krailo MD, Glade-Bender J, Buxton A, Laack N, Randall RL, et al. Randomized phase III trial of ganitumab with interval-compressed chemotherapy for patients with newly diagnosed metastatic Ewing sarcoma: a report from the children's oncology group. J Clin Oncol. 2023;41(11):2098–107.
78. Apfelbaum AA, Wrenn ED, Lawlor ER. The importance of fusion protein activity in Ewing sarcoma and the cell intrinsic and extrinsic factors that regulate it: a review. Front Oncol. 2022;24(12):1044707.
79. Flores G, Grohar PJ. One oncogene, several vulnerabilities: EWS/FLI targeted therapies for Ewing sarcoma. J Bone Oncol. 2021;01(31):100404.

Pathology and Cancer Research

27

Xu Hongzhi, Jasreman Dhillon, Aram Vosoughi,
and Vaibhav Chumbalkar

The Role of Pathology in Enhancing Cancer Care in the Modern Era

Pathology, the indispensable cornerstone of diagnostic medicine, has played a pivotal role in the evolution of cancer care. As the medical specialty dedicated to the study of disease through the examination of tissues, cells, and molecular markers, pathology is central to enhancing cancer diagnosis, prognostication, and the development of targeted therapies. In an era of increasingly complex cancer management, advanced pathology services are more critical than ever. This section elucidates the multifaceted contributions of modern pathology to cancer care, underscoring key advancements and their implications for clinical practice in the community hospital setting.

The Central Role of Pathology in Cancer Diagnosis

Accurate diagnosis is the bedrock of effective cancer management, and pathology remains central to this process. Histopathological examination, employing hematoxylin and eosin (H&E) staining, continues to be the gold standard. H&E staining allows for the assessment of tumor morphology and architecture, which remains fundamental to diagnostic pathology. Refinements in tissue processing, staining techniques, and microscopic analysis have significantly improved diagnostic precision [1].

The advent of immunohistochemistry (IHC) in the 1980s marked a significant milestone. IHC allows for the identification of specific antigens in cells, aiding in tumor classification, determining the tissue of origin in metastatic cancers, and predicting therapeutic responses. This technique has provided invaluable diagnostic precision, especially in distinguishing between morphologically similar tumor types. Additionally, IHC plays a crucial role in assessing therapeutic targets, such as PD-L1 in non-small-cell lung cancer, which guides immunotherapy decisions. The assessment of hormone receptor status (estrogen and progesterone receptors) and HER2 in breast cancer via IHC has been integral in guiding targeted therapies, leading to significant improvements in patient outcomes [2].

Advancements in Molecular Pathology

The emergence of molecular pathology has revolutionized cancer diagnostics and therapeutics. Techniques such as polymerase chain reaction (PCR), fluorescence in situ hybridization (FISH), and next-generation sequencing (NGS) have enabled the detection of genetic mutations, chromosomal alterations, and gene expression profiles with unprecedented accuracy [3]. NGS, in particular, allows for the simultaneous detection of multiple mutations, saving time and tissue. This information directly impacts treatment decisions, allowing us to select the most effective targeted therapy for each patient, based on the specific molecular profile of their tumors. Nowadays, molecular testing has become essential in the management of various cancers. For example, in non-small-cell lung cancer (NSCLC), identifying mutations in EGFR, ALK rearrangements, and ROS1 fusions has transformed treatment paradigms, allowing for personalized therapy with tyrosine kinase inhibitors [4]. Similarly, the discovery of BRAF mutations in melanoma has led to the development of targeted therapies, significantly improving patient outcomes. The increasing role of liquid biopsies should also be noted, allowing for less invasive molecular testing.

X. Hongzhi (✉) · J. Dhillon · A. Vosoughi · V. Chumbalkar
Department of pathology, H. Lee Moffitt Cancer Center and Research Institute, Tampa, FL, USA
e-mail: hongzhi.xu@moffitt.org; jasreman.dhillon@moffitt.org; aram.vosoughi@moffitt.org; vaibhav.chumbalkar@moffitt.org

J. Huang, H. S.L. Jim (eds.), *Cancer Research Guidance for Clinicians and Researchers*,
https://doi.org/10.1007/978-3-032-19175-5_27

Pathology and the Evolution of Cancer Classification

Pathologists have been instrumental in the continuous refinement of cancer classification systems, which are critical for accurate diagnosis, treatment planning, and prognostication. The World Health Organization (WHO) classifications, regularly updated based on pathological, immunophenotypic, and molecular findings, provide standardized diagnostic criteria that facilitate uniformity in diagnosis and research globally [5].

Historically, cancer classification was primarily based on morphological features observed under the microscope. However, the integration of IHC and molecular data into traditional histopathological classification has led to more precise tumor subtyping. For example, the classification of gliomas now incorporates isocitrate dehydrogenase (IDH) mutation status and 1p/19q co-deletion, which are critical for prognosis and therapeutic decisions. Similarly, breast cancer classification has evolved from histological types to molecular subtypes, driven by the expression of hormone receptors and HER2 status, influencing treatment strategies [6].

Contribution to Prognostication and Predictive Biomarkers

Pathology not only aids in diagnosis but also in prognostication and prediction of therapeutic responses. The identification of prognostic markers, such as the Ki-67 proliferation index, has provided insights into tumor aggressiveness. Predictive biomarkers identified through pathological techniques have guided the use of targeted therapies and immunotherapies [7]. The assessment of PD-L1 expression in tumors, for example, has become a standard practice to determine eligibility for immune checkpoint inhibitors in cancers such as NSCLC and urothelial carcinoma.

The Role of Digital Pathology and Artificial Intelligence

The digital revolution has ushered in new possibilities for pathology. Digital pathology, involving the scanning and analysis of whole-slide images, has enhanced diagnostic workflows and supported educational endeavors. Artificial intelligence (AI) and machine learning algorithms are increasingly being integrated into pathology practice. These technologies assist in pattern recognition, quantification of biomarkers, and prediction of patient outcomes, augmenting the diagnostic capabilities of pathologists [8].

Pathology's Role in Cancer Research and Clinical Trials

Pathologists play a critical role in cancer research, contributing to the understanding of tumor biology, the development of new therapies, and the advancement of precision oncology. One of the key contributions of pathology to cancer research is the establishment and management of tissue biobanks and biorepositories. These resources provide high-quality, well-annotated specimens that are essential for molecular studies, biomarker discovery, and the development of targeted therapies. Pathologists oversee the procurement, processing, and preservation of these samples, ensuring their integrity for downstream analyses.

In clinical trials, pathologists are indispensable for several critical functions. They provide histopathological confirmation of cancer diagnoses, a prerequisite for patient enrollment in most oncology trials. Additionally, pathologists assess therapeutic responses through standardized criteria, such as the RECIST (Response Evaluation Criteria in Solid Tumors) guidelines [9], and evaluate treatment-related histological changes, which are crucial for understanding drug efficacy and mechanisms of action.

Conclusion

Throughout the last several decades, pathology has evolved from traditional histological examination to a dynamic specialty integrating molecular diagnostics, digital technologies, and AI. Its contributions have been fundamental in enhancing cancer diagnosis, guiding personalized therapies, and advancing cancer research. As oncology continues to progress, pathology will remain at the forefront, driving innovations that improve patient care and outcomes.

For community physicians interested in conducting clinical research, collaboration with pathologists is essential. By leveraging pathology-driven biomarker studies, utilizing biorepositories, and incorporating molecular diagnostics into research initiatives, community hospitals can contribute significantly to cancer research. Understanding and applying pathology principles in clinical research will enable more effective patient stratification, foster the development of novel therapeutic strategies, and enhance the overall quality of cancer care.

Basic Science Research in Pathology

Pathology is a vital field of medical science that examines disease causes and effects at the molecular, cellular, and tissue levels. It serves as a bridge between basic research and clinical practice, driving advancements in diagnostics, therapeutics, and precision medicine. The integration of technologies such as artificial intelligence (AI), next-generation sequencing (NGS), and organoid models has transformed pathology, enabling breakthroughs in disease detection and management [10].

The Role of Basic Science in Pathology

Basic science research in pathology investigates the underlying biological processes that contribute to disease. This includes exploring genetic mutations, cellular responses to injury, immune system interactions, and biomarker identification. These fundamental studies are essential for elucidating disease mechanisms and developing novel diagnostic and therapeutic strategies [11].

Key Areas of Research

Molecular Pathology

- Examines genetic and molecular alterations in diseases
- Employs techniques such as polymerase chain reaction (PCR), NGS, and fluorescence in situ hybridization (FISH) to detect genetic abnormalities
- Studies gene expression patterns and epigenetic modifications to understand disease progression
- Investigates the role of noncoding RNAs and microRNAs in regulating gene expression in pathological conditions [12]

Cellular Pathology

- Studies cellular responses to injury, infection, and genetic changes
- Investigates apoptosis, necrosis, and autophagy to understand disease progression
- Analyzes how cellular stress responses influence cancer development and resistance to treatments
- Explores how organelle dysfunction, such as mitochondrial abnormalities, contributes to disease pathogenesis [13]

Immunopathology

- Explores immune system dysregulation in autoimmune disorders, infections, and cancer [14]
- Examines cytokine signaling, antigen presentation, and immune cell interactions
- Investigates novel immunotherapies, such as checkpoint inhibitors and chimeric antigen receptor (CAR)-T-cell therapies [15]
- Studies the impact of the gut microbiome on immune function and its potential in modulating disease responses

Histopathology

- Analyzes tissue morphology using microscopic techniques
- Utilizes immunohistochemistry (IHC) and special stains to identify disease-specific markers
- Advances in digital pathology and image analysis enhance diagnostic precision
- Investigates the potential of multiplex imaging techniques to provide comprehensive insights into tissue architecture and disease progression [16]

Microbial Pathogenesis

- Investigates pathogen-host interactions
- Studies antimicrobial resistance and vaccine development [17]
- Develops novel strategies for combating multidrug-resistant pathogens through innovative antimicrobial agents and therapies

Basic Science Research in Community Hospital Settings

Community hospitals play a growing role in pathology research by leveraging their access to diverse patient populations and real-world clinical data. Conducting research in these settings can lead to meaningful contributions to medical knowledge and improve patient care. Key aspects include

- Establishing collaborative networks with academic institutions and research organizations to access advanced technologies and expertise
- Implementing biobanking initiatives to collect and store tissue samples for translational research
- Utilizing electronic medical records (EMRs) for retrospective studies and real-world data analysis
- Conducting investigator-initiated studies on local disease trends, treatment responses, and biomarker validation
- Engaging in clinical trials to evaluate new diagnostic tools and therapeutic interventions

Technological Advancements in Basic Science Research in Pathology

Basic science research in pathology has dramatically benefited from technological innovations, including the following:

- *Omics Technologies*: Genomics, proteomics, and metabolomics enable comprehensive disease profiling, facilitating personalized medicine approaches [18].
- *Artificial Intelligence (AI) and Machine Learning*: Enhance diagnostic accuracy, predictive modeling, and large-scale data analysis in pathology [19].
- *CRISPR and Gene Editing*: Enable functional studies of genetic mutations, potential gene therapies, and the development of disease models [20].
- *Organoids and 3D Cell Cultures*: Provide more physiologically relevant models for studying disease progression and drug responses [21].
- *Nanotechnology in Pathology*: Advances in nanomedicine offer improved diagnostic and therapeutic techniques, enabling early disease detection at the molecular level [22].
- *Liquid Biopsy and Noninvasive Testing*: Emerging technologies allow for early cancer detection, disease progression monitoring, and real-time assessment of treatment efficacy without invasive procedures [23].

Impact on Clinical Medicine

Findings from basic pathology research directly influence clinical practice by

- Improving diagnostic precision through biomarker discovery and advanced imaging techniques [24]
- Enhancing treatment strategies via targeted therapies, immunotherapies, and personalized medicine approaches
- Informing preventive measures based on genetic predisposition and lifestyle factors
- Refining disease classification, enabling early detection, and improving patient stratification for tailored therapies
- Facilitating the development of minimally invasive diagnostic tools that improve patient compliance and reduce healthcare costs

Future Directions of Basic Science Research in Pathology

The future of pathology research lies in integrating multi-omics data, computational pathology, and innovative biotechnologies. Advancements in single-cell sequencing, spatial transcriptomics, and AI will continue to revolutionize disease diagnostics and therapeutic decision-making [25]. Furthermore, fostering interdisciplinary collaborations between pathologists, bioinformaticians, and biomedical engineers will drive the next wave of disease understanding and treatment breakthroughs. Additionally, regenerative medicine and stem cell research hold promise for tissue repair and the development of novel treatment modalities.

In summary, basic science research in pathology is fundamental to understanding disease mechanisms and translating discoveries into medical advancements. Continued investment in research, interdisciplinary collaboration, and technological integration will drive the future of pathology, ultimately improving patient outcomes and shaping the future of medicine. As new discoveries emerge, pathology will continue to evolve, refining diagnostic techniques, therapeutic interventions, and disease prevention strategies for years to come.

Clinical Research in Pathology for Cancer Prevention

Cancer remains one of the leading causes of morbidity and mortality worldwide. Clinical research in cancer prevention is a crucial aspect of oncology, particularly in pathology, where early detection and risk assessment play vital roles. Pathologists contribute significantly through the following approaches such as (1) *histopathological screening*—routine histological evaluation of tissues aids in detecting precancerous lesions, such as dysplasia, which may progress to malignancy if left untreated; (2) *molecular biomarkers*—identification of molecular alterations, including genetic and epigenetic changes, facilitates early diagnosis and targeted interventions; and (3) *risk stratification*—pathology enables categorization of individuals based on their risk levels, supporting personalized prevention strategies.

For community physicians, integrating clinical research into daily practice can be challenging due to limited resources and infrastructure. However, leveraging pathology-driven studies can enhance cancer prevention efforts in community hospital settings. This section explores various clinical research interests aimed at preventing cancer, emphasizing pathological approaches for community physicians.

Key Areas of Clinical Research in Cancer Prevention

Biomarker Discovery and Validation

Biomarkers are essential for detecting cancer at its earliest stages. Currently, clinical research focuses on identifying novel biomarkers that can predict cancer susceptibility, including

- DNA mutations and methylation patterns
- RNA expression profiles
- Protein signatures in blood and tissue samples
- Circulating tumor cells and extracellular vesicles

One of the notable clinical trials focusing on DNA methylation patterns as biomarkers is the study on clinical validation of peripheral blood mononuclear cell DNA methylation for diagnosis of early-stage hepatocellular carcinoma conducted by Cheishvili D. et al., published in *Communications Medicine* in 2024 [26]. This study utilized a cohort of 402 participants, including healthy controls, chronic hepatitis patients, and HCC patients from Bangladesh, to evaluate DNA methylation signatures in peripheral blood mononuclear cells (PBMC). The authors performed targeted next-generation sequencing on selected genes previously identified to assess their methylation dynamics. The development of M8 and M4 scores was based on these dynamics, using receiver operating characteristic (ROC) analysis to determine their effectiveness in detecting early-stage HCC alongside existing markers such as epiLiver and alpha-fetoprotein (AFP). In this study, they found that integration of M8 and M4 scores with epiLiver and AFP significantly enhances diagnostic sensitivity for early-stage HCC. The M4+epiLiver score achieves a sensitivity of 79.4% in Stage A HCC, while combining M4 with AFP increases sensitivity to 88.2–95.7% across all stages, indicating a superior diagnostic performance compared to each marker used alone. This study confirms that combining gene methylation profiles with established diagnostic markers substantially improves the sensitivity of detecting early-stage HCC. The research underscores the potential of epigenetic modifications as biomarkers in cancer detection, offering an avenue for innovative screening methods. Community physicians can collaborate with pathology departments to collect, analyze, and interpret biomarker data, ultimately facilitating early intervention and improving patient outcomes. Furthermore, implementing these findings into routine clinical practice can enhance early detection strategies in community healthcare settings, bridging the gap between research advancements and real-world application.

Screening and Early Detection Programs

Population-based screening programs, supported by pathology, play a pivotal role in reducing cancer incidence. A notable clinical study is the Canadian Cervical Cancer Screening Trial (CCCaST) [27]. This randomized controlled trial was designed to determine whether testing the DNA of oncogenic HPV is superior to the Papanicolaou (Pap) test for cervical cancer screening. The authors compared HPV testing, using an assay approved by the Food and Drug Administration, with conventional Pap testing as a screening method to identify high-grade cervical intraepithelial neoplasia in women ages 30 to 69 years in Montreal and St. John's, Canada. Women with abnormal Pap test results or a positive HPV test (at least 1 pg of high-risk HPV DNA per milliliter) underwent colposcopy and biopsy, as did a random sample of women with negative tests. A total of 10,154 women were randomly assigned to testing. Both tests were performed on all women in a randomly assigned sequence at the same session. The sensitivity of HPV testing for cervical intraepithelial neoplasia of grade 2 or 3 was 94.6% (95% confidence interval [CI], 84.2 to 100), whereas the sensitivity of Pap testing was 55.4% (95% CI, 33.6 to 77.2; $P = 0.01$). The specificity was 94.1% (95% CI, 93.4 to 94.8) for HPV testing and 96.8% (95% CI, 96.3 to 97.3; $P < 0.001$) for Pap testing. Performance was unaffected by the sequence of the tests. The sensitivity of both tests used together was 100%, and the specificity was 92.5%. Triage procedures for Pap or HPV testing resulted in fewer referrals for colposcopy than did either test alone but were less sensitive. Based on these results, the authors concluded that HPV testing has greater sensitivity for the detection of cervical intraepithelial neoplasia, as compared with Pap testing.

Several additional important screening efforts include (1) *mammography and breast biopsy analysis* for early breast cancer detection; (2) *serum PSA testing and prostate biopsy*, where PSA testing serves as a common screening tool for prostate cancer, with elevated levels prompting biopsy for confirmation; (3) *colonoscopy with histopathological examination* for colorectal cancer screening; and (4) *liquid biopsy technologies* for noninvasive detection of early-stage malignancies [3]. Community physicians can contribute to these programs by promoting patient participation, ensuring adherence to screening guidelines, and working closely with pathologists to interpret results.

Chemoprevention Studies

Chemoprevention involves the use of natural or synthetic agents to prevent cancer progression. For instance, some clinical trials investigate the effectiveness of aspirin and NSAIDs in colorectal cancer prevention [28], the role of selective estrogen receptor modulators (SERMs) in breast cancer prevention, or the impact of dietary phytochemicals, such as curcumin and resveratrol, on cancer risk reduction.

The Selenium and Vitamin E Cancer Prevention Trial (SELECT) is one of the significant clinical trials investigating the role of natural agents in cancer chemoprevention [29]. This large-scale, randomized, placebo-controlled study aimed to determine whether selenium and vitamin E supplements could reduce the risk of prostate cancer. The trial enrolled 35,533 men from 427 participating sites in the United States, Canada, and Puerto Rico, randomly assigned to four groups (selenium, vitamin E, selenium + vitamin E, and placebo) in a double-blind fashion between August 22, 2001, and June 24, 2004. Baseline eligibility included age 50 years or older (African American men) or 55 years or older (all other men), a serum prostate-specific antigen level of 4 ng/mL or less, and a digital rectal examination not suspicious for prostate cancer. Participants were followed for an average of 5.5 years to monitor the development of prostate cancer. They found that the hazard ratios (99% confidence intervals [CIs]) for prostate cancer were 1.13 (99% CI, 0.95–1.35; $n = 473$) for vitamin E, 1.04 (99% CI, 0.87–1.24; $n = 432$) for selenium, and 1.05 (99% CI, 0.88–1.25; $n = 437$) for selenium + vitamin E vs. 1.00 ($n = 416$) for placebo. There were no significant differences (all $P > 0.15$) in any other prespecified cancer end points. There were statistically nonsignificant increased risks of prostate cancer in the vitamin E group ($P = 0.06$) and type 2 diabetes mellitus in the selenium group (relative risk, 1.07; 99% CI, 0.94–1.22; $P = 0.16$) but not in the selenium + vitamin E group. The trial concluded that neither selenium nor vitamin E, alone or in combination, reduced the risk of prostate cancer. The SELECT trial provided robust evidence that supplementation with selenium and vitamin E does not confer a protective effect against prostate cancer in healthy men. These findings underscore the necessity of rigorous clinical trials to evaluate the efficacy and safety of dietary supplements for cancer prevention. Community physicians can participate in chemoprevention research by identifying eligible patients, educating them about preventive interventions, monitoring their adherence to prescribed regimens, assessing treatment responses, and systematically reporting outcomes to contribute to broader clinical research efforts.

Immunoprevention Research

Immunoprevention utilizes vaccines and immune-modulating agents to prevent cancer. Research in this domain includes

- HPV vaccination to prevent cervical and oropharyngeal cancers
- Hepatitis B vaccination to lower hepatocellular carcinoma risk
- Checkpoint inhibitors in high-risk populations to prevent malignant transformation

A landmark clinical study evaluating the efficacy of human papillomavirus (HPV) vaccination is the Costa Rica HPV Vaccine Trial (CVT) [30]. This randomized, double-blind, controlled trial aimed to assess the effectiveness of the bivalent HPV vaccine, Cervarix, in preventing HPV infections and related cervical lesions. The trial enrolled 7466 healthy women aged 18 to 25 years in Costa Rica. The participants were divided into 1) vaccine group—participants received three doses of the bivalent HPV-16/18 vaccine, Cervarix—and 2) control group—participants received a control vaccine against hepatitis A. Participants were monitored over a period of 4 years, with regular cervical cytology and HPV DNA testing to detect incident infections and cervical lesions. According-to-protocol (ATP) cohorts included compliant HPV-negative women; intention-to-treat (ITT) cohorts included all randomized women. ATP VE was 90.9% (95% CI, 82.0–95.9) against HPV-16/18 infections, 44.5% against HPV-31/33/45 (95% CI, 17.5–63.1), and 12.4% (95% CI, −3.2 to 25.6) against any oncogenic infection. Overall, ITT VE against HPV-16/18 infections was 49.0%, but ATP and ITT VE almost reached 100% in year 4 of follow-up. ATP efficacy against HPV-16/18 was similar by age, but ITT VE was greatest among the youngest women (68.9% among those 18–19 years of age; 21.8% among those 24–25 years of age) and 79.8% among virgins. The CVT provided robust evidence supporting the use of the bivalent HPV vaccine in preventing HPV-16 and HPV-18 infections and associated cervical precancerous lesions. These findings have been instrumental in shaping global HPV vaccination programs aimed at reducing the incidence of cervical cancer. This study exemplifies the critical role of immunoprevention strategies, such as HPV vaccination, in reducing the burden of cervical cancer worldwide. Community physicians can engage in immunoprevention research by participating in post-marketing surveillance studies, monitoring vaccine efficacy in real-world settings, and contributing to population-based studies assessing long-term immunization outcomes. Collaborating with pathology departments and research institutions can further enhance their role in advancing immunoprevention strategies, ensuring evidence-based interventions reach broader patient populations.

Genomic and Epigenetic Studies

Understanding genetic predisposition and epigenetic modifications aids in designing personalized prevention strategies. Clinical research of interest includes

- Familial cancer syndromes such as BRCA mutations in breast and ovarian cancer
- Epigenetic modifiers, including DNA methylation inhibitors, for cancer prevention
- CRISPR-based gene editing for correcting oncogenic mutations

Published in the *British Journal of Cancer* in 2018, Hitchins et al. conducted a significant clinical study exploring the genetic and epigenetic foundations of Lynch syndrome, titled "Primary constitutional MLH1 epimutations: a focal epigenetic event" [31]. This research delves into the role of primary constitutional epimutations in the MLH1 gene, a critical component of the DNA mismatch repair system, and their contribution to Lynch syndrome. Twelve

MLH1 epimutation carriers, 61 Lynch syndrome patients, and 41 healthy controls were analyzed by the Infinium 450 K array. Targeted molecular techniques were used to characterize the MLH1 epimutation carriers and their inheritance pattern. This study found that no nucleotide or structural variants were identified *in cis* on the epimutated allele in ten carriers, in which inter-generational methylation erasure was demonstrated in two, suggesting a primary type of epimutation. CNVs outside the *MLH1* locus were found in two cases. *EPM2AIP1-MLH1* CpG island was identified as the sole differentially methylated region in *MLH1* epimutation carriers compared to controls. This research demonstrated that primary constitutional *MLH1* epimutations arise as a focal epigenetic event at the *EPM2AIP1-MLH1* CpG island in the absence of *cis*-acting genetic variants. It underscores the importance of considering epigenetic mechanisms, such as primary constitutional MLH1 epimutations, in the diagnostic evaluation of Lynch syndrome. Recognizing these epigenetic alterations can enhance the accuracy of diagnoses and inform personalized prevention strategies for individuals predisposed to Lynch syndrome–associated cancers.

Future Directions

Advancements in artificial intelligence (AI) and digital pathology promise to revolutionize cancer prevention research. AI-driven histopathological analysis enhances early detection accuracy, while integrative multi-omics approaches provide deeper insights into cancer susceptibility. Additionally, precision medicine continues to evolve, tailoring prevention strategies based on an individual's genetic and molecular profile [32].

Conducting Clinical Research in Community Hospital Settings

Community physicians can engage in clinical research by integrating cancer prevention studies into their practice. Key strategies include

- *Establishing Collaborative Networks*: Partnering with academic centers, pathology laboratories, and research organizations enhances access to expertise and resources.
- *Utilizing Existing Patient Data*: Retrospective analyses of pathology reports and screening outcomes provide valuable insights into cancer prevention.
- *Participating in Clinical Trials*: Community hospitals can serve as recruitment sites for larger multicenter studies, contributing to cancer prevention research.
- *Leveraging Digital Pathology and AI*: Digital pathology platforms and AI tools can assist in data interpretation, improving research efficiency and accuracy.
- *Seeking Research Funding and Support*: Physicians can apply for grants from organizations such as the National Cancer Institute (NCI) or collaborate with industry partners.

Conclusion

Clinical research in pathology is instrumental in advancing cancer prevention efforts. Community physicians play a vital role in translating research findings into practice by promoting early detection, participating in screening programs, and collaborating with pathologists in biomarker studies. By actively engaging in clinical research, community hospitals can contribute to reducing the global cancer burden and improving patient outcomes. Continued innovation, interdisciplinary collaboration, and support for research infrastructure in community settings will be crucial in making cancer prevention efforts more effective and accessible.

Clinical Research in Pathology for Cancer Treatment

The role of pathologists in cancer treatment is crucial, encompassing multiple aspects such as diagnosis, subclassification, grading, staging, biomarker testing, molecular profiling, and other characterizations of cancer cells and their surrounding environment. Information derived from these activities informs treatment decisions throughout the patient's journey. In community hospital settings, pathologists are increasingly involved in clinical research efforts, leveraging real-world patient data and collaborating with oncologists to refine cancer diagnostics and treatment approaches.

Study of Histological Features of Cancer

Histological features are identified using hematoxylin and eosin (H&E) staining, special chemical stains, immunohistochemical (IHC) stains, and in situ hybridization (ISH) tests. Despite being one of the oldest diagnostic methods, histological analysis remains invaluable in research and development.

One of the recent significant examples includes the diagnosis of noninvasive follicular thyroid neoplasm with papillary-like nuclear features (NIFTP) [33]. This landmark study reclassified a subset of thyroid tumors that were previously diagnosed as encapsulated follicular variant of papillary thyroid carcinoma (EFVPTC) into a new entity, NIFTP, to reduce overtreatment of indolent lesions. In this retrospective study, patients with thyroid nodules diagnosed as EFVPTC, including 109 patients with noninvasive EFVPTC, were observed for 10 to 26 years, and 101 patients with invasive EFVPTC were observed for 1 to 18 years. Digitized histologic slides collected at 13 sites in five countries were reviewed by 24 thyroid pathologists from seven countries. The investigators found that all 109 patients with noninvasive EFVPTC (67 treated with only lobectomy, none received radioactive iodine ablation) were alive with no evidence of disease at final follow-up (median [range], 13 [10–26] years). An adverse event was seen in 12 of 101 (12%) of the cases of invasive EFVPTC, including five patients developing distant metastases, two of whom died of disease. Based on the outcome information for noninvasive EFVPTC, the name "noninvasive follicular thyroid neoplasm with papillary-like nuclear features" (NIFTP) was adopted. This study redefined the diagnostic criteria for NIFTP, promoting a shift toward less aggressive treatment for patients with these tumors. The reclassification has significantly impacted clinical practice, leading to reduced overtreatment, improved risk stratification, and better patient outcomes.

Other noteworthy examples include

1. Redefining prostate cancer grading into grade groups, significantly altering prognostic understanding and standard care [34]
2. The development of predictive markers, such as ER, PR, and HER2 in breast cancer [35] and HER2 expression for trastuzumab deruxtecan in various cancers [36]

In community hospitals, histological research extends to retrospective studies using stored biopsy samples, where pathologists analyze morphological patterns that correlate with treatment outcomes. Digital pathology tools are increasingly employed to facilitate large-scale histological studies, allowing for automated quantification of features such as tumor-infiltrating lymphocytes, which are predictive of immunotherapy responses.

Molecular Profiling

Technological advancements have cemented molecular profiling as part of standard care, significantly impacting patient outcomes. It is integral to precision oncology and can be performed through various methods, such as

1. *Next-Generation Sequencing (NGS)*: Analyzes hundreds of genes from minimal tissue samples, detecting mutations and gene fusions with increasing sensitivity and coverage [37].
2. *RNA Sequencing*: Identifies gene fusions, copy number alterations, and gene expression levels. It aids in tumor classification (e.g., medulloblastomas) and guides treatment [38].
3. *Epigenetic Analysis*: Examines methylation status, such as MGMT methylation in brain tumors. Genome-wide methylation arrays have become standard in neuro-oncology diagnostics [39].

In a study [37] aiming to evaluate the role of next-generation sequencing (NGS) in identifying genomic alterations in advanced prostate cancer to guide targeted therapy, Robinson et al. conducted integrative clinical genomic analysis using NGS to uncover actionable mutations that could influence treatment strategies. They established a multi-institutional clinical sequencing infrastructure to conduct prospective whole-exome and transcriptome sequencing of bone or soft tissue tumor biopsies from a cohort of 150 castration-resistant prostate cancer (mCRPC) patients. The researchers found that aberrations of AR, ETS genes, TP53, and PTEN were frequent (40–60% of cases), with TP53 and AR alterations enriched in mCRPC compared to primary prostate cancer. They identified new genomic alterations in PIK3CA/B, R-spondin, BRAF/RAF1, APC, β-catenin, and ZBTB16/PLZF. Moreover, aberrations of BRCA2, BRCA1, and ATM were observed at substantially higher frequencies (19.3% overall) compared to those in primary prostate cancers. A total of 89% of patients harbored a clinically actionable aberration, including 62.7% with aberrations in AR, 65% in other cancer-related genes, and 8% with actionable pathogenic germline alterations. This milestone study highlighted the utility of NGS in precision oncology, paving the way for genetically guided treatments in advanced prostate cancer. The results have been instrumental in developing targeted therapies and clinical guidelines for prostate cancer management.

In community hospital settings, molecular profiling is being integrated into routine pathology workflows, enabling clinicians to access real-time genomic data for treatment decisions. Local research efforts often involve testing cost-effective, rapid sequencing methodologies to improve accessibility to advanced diagnostics for cancer patients in nonacademic centers.

Digital Pathology and Artificial Intelligence (AI)

Digital pathology tools enhance workflow efficiency and enable remote diagnostics. Research focuses on developing advanced scanners and software tools for image analysis, improving biomarker assessment accuracy, such as Ki-67 expression [40]. AI is revolutionizing cancer pathology. AI tools assist in image analysis, aiding diagnosis and grading, as seen in prostate biopsies [41]. Moreover, AI integrates pathologic, radiologic, and clinical data to optimize treatment strategies.

Cancers of unknown primary (CUPs) are challenging to treat due to the lack of an identified tissue origin, leading to delays in targeted therapy selection. A study by Lu et al. [42] investigated whether artificial intelligence (AI)–driven digital pathology analysis could accurately predict the tissue of origin for CUP cases, enhancing treatment selection and outcomes. The authors developed a deep learning–based algorithm—Tumor Origin Assessment via Deep Learning (TOAD)—that provides a differential diagnosis for the origin of the primary tumor using routinely acquired histology slides. Their model predictions resulted in concordance for 61% of cases and a top-three agreement of 82%. This study demonstrated that AI-powered digital pathology could aid in CUP diagnosis, enabling personalized cancer treatment when conventional diagnostics are inconclusive.

Development of New Methods

Innovative methods, such as mass spectrometry and Raman spectroscopy [43], offer rapid, nondestructive tissue analysis, providing valuable real-time diagnostic insights during intraoperative consultations. These techniques enable the identification of biochemical and molecular characteristics of tissues, aiding in the differentiation of malignant and benign lesions without the need for extensive tissue processing. In community hospital settings, research is focused on refining these techniques to make them more accessible and practical for routine clinical use.

In summary, clinical research in pathology continues to play a fundamental role in cancer treatment, driving advancements in diagnostic accuracy, biomarker discovery, and personalized medicine. Histological evaluation, molecular profiling, digital pathology, artificial intelligence, and multiplex technologies are transforming the field, allowing for more precise and effective treatment strategies. Emerging technologies, including mass spectrometry and Raman spectroscopy, provide novel avenues for rapid intraoperative decision-making. As pathology integrates more sophisticated methodologies, its contributions to oncology will remain indispensable, ensuring improved patient outcomes and continued innovations in cancer care.

Clinical Research in Pathology for Cancer Survival

The rising incidence and improved treatment of cancer have increased the number of survivors. Cancer survival rates are key indicators of healthcare effectiveness, with pathologists playing a pivotal role in survival prediction and intervention. Beyond their traditional diagnostic roles, pathologists contribute significantly to understanding the biological behavior of cancers, which directly informs survival outcomes and long-term patient management. The following are some important clinical research areas in pathology focusing on cancer survival:

1. Predictive Biomarkers for Treatment Response

   One of the key challenges in oncology is predicting which patients will respond to specific treatments. As treatment modalities such as immunotherapy and targeted therapies advance, predictive biomarkers are essential for optimizing patient outcomes and improving cancer survival. Some key research areas include

   (a) Minimal Residual Disease (MRD) Detection for Monitoring Recurrence—MRD detection helps identify small numbers of cancer cells remaining after treatment, guiding decisions on the need for additional therapy to prevent relapse [44].

   (b) PD-L1 Expression and Tumor Mutational Burden (TMB)—PD-L1 expression and TMB are critical biomarkers in immunotherapy, as they help predict responses to immune checkpoint inhibitors, improving treatment selection [45].

   (c) Molecular Subtyping and Targeted Therapy Selection—Molecular profiling enables classification of cancers into subtypes, allowing for precise therapeutic targeting and the development of personalized treatment regimens to enhance patient outcomes [46].

A landmark clinical trial, "Impact of Conditioning Intensity of Allogeneic Transplantation for Acute Myeloid Leukemia with Genomic Evidence of Residual Disease," published in the *Journal of Clinical Oncology* in April 2020 [47], explored the role of minimal residual disease (MRD) detection in guiding treatment decisions for acute myeloid leukemia (AML) patients undergoing allogeneic hematopoietic stem cell transplantation (HSCT). Led by Dr. Christopher S. Hourigan and colleagues, the study investigated whether the intensity of pretransplant conditioning influenced survival outcomes in patients with MRD-positive disease. The trial followed 99 AML patients who had detectable genomic MRD before undergoing HSCT. To assess the impact of conditioning intensity, the participants were divided into two groups: 1) 70 patients received myeloablative conditioning (MAC), a high-intensity regimen designed to eradicate as many cancer cells as possible before transplant, and 2) 29 patients received reduced-intensity conditioning (RIC), a milder approach used for patients who may not tolerate aggressive treatment. MRD detection was performed using genomic sequencing techniques, identifying even the smallest traces of remaining leukemia cells before transplant. Researchers then tracked overall survival (OS) and relapse rates over three years. The results were striking. Patients who underwent the more intensive MAC regimen had a significantly higher three-year overall survival rate of 63%, compared to only 32% in the RIC group. Furthermore, the cumulative incidence of relapse was dramatically lower in the MAC group at 23%, while those in the RIC group faced a much higher relapse rate of 59%. This study provided compelling evidence that AML patients with MRD-positive disease benefit from a more aggressive pretransplant regimen. The findings suggest that for these patients, myeloablative conditioning (MAC) offers a significant survival advantage, reducing the risk of relapse and improving long-term outcomes. By reinforcing the clinical significance of MRD detection, this study underscores its value in guiding treatment intensity and personalizing transplant strategies. For AML patients facing high relapse risk, MRD testing is proving to be a crucial tool in shaping therapeutic decisions and improving survival in the battle against leukemia.

2. Tumor Microenvironment and Cancer Progression

   The tumor microenvironment (TME) plays a crucial role in cancer progression, treatment resistance, and survival. Understanding immune infiltration, fibrosis, and cellular heterogeneity in the TME can improve prognostic stratification and guide treatment decisions. Some key research areas include

   (a) Immune Infiltration Profiles as Survival Predictors: The presence of tumor-infiltrating lymphocytes (TILs) in cancers like breast and lung cancer has been correlated with improved survival and response to immunotherapy [48].
   (b) Role of Fibrosis and Hypoxia in Tumor Aggressiveness: Desmoplastic reaction and stromal fibrosis are linked to worse outcomes in pancreatic and colorectal cancers [49].
   (c) Spatial Transcriptomics and Cellular Heterogeneity: Spatial transcriptomics enables mapping of gene expression in relation to tumor architecture, helping understand how cellular heterogeneity affects survival [50].

A notable clinical study titled "Prediction of Survival in Follicular Lymphoma Based on Molecular Features of Tumor-Infiltrating Immune Cells" was published in the *New England Journal of Medicine* in 2004 [51]. This research aimed to develop a molecular predictor of survival length in patients with follicular lymphoma by analyzing gene expression profiles of tumor-biopsy specimens obtained at diagnosis. In this study, gene expression profiling was performed on 191 biopsy specimens obtained from patients with untreated follicular lymphoma. Supervised methods were used to discover expression patterns associated with the length of survival in a training set of 95 specimens. A molecular predictor of survival was constructed from these genes and validated in an independent test set of 96 specimens. They found that individual genes that predicted the length of survival were grouped into gene expression signatures on the basis of their expression in the training set, and two such signatures were used to construct a survival predictor. The two signatures allowed patients with specimens in the test set to be divided into four quartiles with widely disparate median lengths of survival (13.6, 11.1, 10.8, and 3.9 years), independently of clinical prognostic variables. Flow cytometry showed that these signatures reflected gene expression by nonmalignant tumor-infiltrating cells. This pioneering study demonstrated that the molecular characteristics of tumor-infiltrating immune cells are critical determinants of survival in follicular lymphoma patients. The findings suggest that assessing the immune landscape within tumors can provide valuable prognostic information and potentially guide therapeutic strategies.

AI and Digital Pathology in Cancer Survival Prediction

Artificial intelligence (AI) is transforming pathology by enhancing diagnostic accuracy and prognostic assessment. AI-powered tools can assist pathologists in identifying high-risk patients, predicting survival, and improving workflow efficiency, which is particularly beneficial for community hospitals with limited resources. Some key research areas include

- AI-Based Image Analysis for Tumor Grading and Prognosis: AI-driven analysis of histopathological slides can standardize tumor grading and provide survival predictions [52].

- Deep Learning for Automated Survival Prediction: Machine learning models trained on digital pathology images can correlate tumor morphology with survival outcomes [53].
- Digital Pathology and Electronic Health Record (EHR) Integration: Digital pathology allows for automated slide scanning and AI-assisted reporting, improving efficiency in remote or understaffed hospitals [54].

A notable clinical study on deep learning for fully automated prediction of overall survival was led by Dr. Nai-Ming Cheng and colleagues, who developed a deep learning–based, fully automated tool named DeepPET-OPSCC to predict overall survival in patients with oropharyngeal squamous cell carcinoma (OPSCC) using [^{18}F]fluorodeoxyglucose (FDG) positron emission tomography (PET) imaging [55]. In this study, the DeepPET-OPSCC prediction model was built and tested internally on a discovery cohort ($n = 268$) by integrating five convolutional neural network models for volumetric segmentation and ten models for OS prognostication. Two external test cohorts were enrolled—the first based on the Cancer Imaging Archive (TCIA) database ($n = 353$) and the second being a clinical deployment cohort ($n = 31$)—to assess the DeepPET-OPSCC performance and goodness of fit. After adjustment for potential confounders, DeepPET-OPSCC was found to be an independent predictor of OS in both discovery and TCIA test cohorts [HR = 2.07; 95% confidence interval (CI), 1.31–3.28 and HR = 2.39; 95% CI, 1.38–4.16; both $P = 0.002$]. The tool also revealed good predictive performance, with a c-index of 0.707 (95% CI, 0.658–0.757) in the discovery cohort, 0.689 (95% CI, 0.621–0.757) in the TCIA test cohort, and 0.787 (95% CI, 0.675–0.899) in the clinical deployment test cohort; the average time taken was 2 min for calculation per exam. The integrated nomogram of DeepPET-OPSCC and clinical risk factors significantly outperformed the clinical model [AUC at 5 years: 0.801 (95% CI, 0.727–0.874) vs. 0.749 (95% CI, 0.649–0.842); $P = 0.031$] in the TCIA test cohort. These data show that the DeepPET-OPSCC model demonstrated a significant capability to predict overall survival, effectively distinguishing between high-risk and low-risk patients. This study highlights the potential of deep learning algorithms in processing complex medical imaging data to provide accurate survival predictions. The DeepPET-OPSCC model exemplifies how artificial intelligence can enhance prognostic evaluations in oncology, leading to more tailored and effective treatment strategies.

Conclusion

Advancements in pathology-driven clinical research are revolutionizing cancer survival predictions and personalized treatment approaches. Predictive biomarkers such as MRD detection, PD-L1 expression, and molecular subtyping are refining therapeutic decisions, improving patient outcomes, and reducing recurrence rates. Research on the tumor microenvironment, particularly immune infiltration profiles, is uncovering critical survival determinants, while AI-driven digital pathology is enhancing prognostic accuracy and workflow efficiency. These innovations collectively strengthen the role of pathology in precision oncology, enabling more targeted interventions and improved long-term survival for cancer patients. Continued research in these areas will be instrumental in optimizing cancer care and guiding future therapeutic strategies.

References

1. Rosai J. Rosai and Ackerman's surgical pathology. 10th ed. Mosby; 2011.
2. Allison KH, Hammond ME, Dowsett M, et al. Estrogen and progesterone receptor testing in breast cancer: ASCO/CAP guideline update. J Clin Oncol. 2020;38(12):1346–66.
3. Chan HT, Chin YMD, Nakamura Y, Low SK. Clonal hematopoiesis in liquid biopsy: from biological noise to valuable clinical implications. Cancers. 2020;12(8):2277.
4. Lindeman NI, Cagle PT, Aisner DL, et al. Updated molecular testing guideline for the selection of lung cancer patients for treatment with targeted tyrosine kinase inhibitors. J Mol Diagn. 2018;20(2):129–59.
5. WHO Classification of Tumours Editorial Board. WHO classification of tumours. 5th ed. Lyon: IARC; 2020.
6. Louis DN, Perry A, Reifenberger G, et al. The 2016 WHO classification of tumors of the central nervous system: a summary. Acta Neuropathol. 2016;131(6):803–20.
7. Topalian SL, Hodi FS, Brahmer JR, et al. Safety, activity, and immune correlates of anti-PD-1 antibody in cancer. N Engl J Med. 2012;366(26):2443–54.
8. Pantanowitz L, Sharma A, Carter AB, Kurc T, Sussman A, Saltz J. Twenty years of digital pathology: an overview of the road traveled, challenges, and the future. J Pathol Inform. 2020;11(1):1–14.
9. Eisenhauer EA, Therasse P, Bogaerts J, et al. New response evaluation criteria in solid tumours: revised RECIST guideline (version 1.1). Eur J Cancer. 2009;45(2):228–47.
10. Siegel RL, Miller KD, Fuchs HE, Jemal A. Cancer statistics, 2021. CA: A Cancer J Clin. 2021;71(1):7–33.
11. Hanahan D, Weinberg RA. Hallmarks of cancer: the next generation. Cell. 2011;144(5):646–74.
12. Koboldt DC, Steinberg KM, Larson DE, Wilson RK, Mardis ER. The next-generation sequencing revolution and its impact on genomics. Cell. 2013;155(1):27–38.
13. Green DR, Galluzzi L, Kroemer G. Cell biology. Metabolic control of cell death. Science. 2014;345(6203):1250256.
14. Murphy KM, Weaver CT. Janeway's immunobiology. 9th ed. Garland Science; 2016.
15. Ribas A, Wolchok JD. Cancer immunotherapy using checkpoint blockade. Science. 2018;359(6382):1350–5.
16. van der Laak J, Litjens G, Ciompi F. Deep learning in histopathology: the path to the clinic. Nat Med. 2021;27(5):775–84.
17. Laxminarayan R, Matsoso P, Pant S, Brower C, Røttingen JA, Klugman K, Davies S. Access to effective antimicrobials: a worldwide challenge. Lancet. 2016;387(10014):168–75.

18. Hasin Y, Seldin M, Lusis A. Multi-omics approaches to disease. Genome Biol. 2017;18(1):83.
19. Bera K, Schalper KA, Rimm DL, Velcheti V, Madabhushi A. Artificial intelligence in digital pathology—new tools for diagnosis and precision oncology. Nat Rev Clin Oncol. 2019;16(11):703–15.
20. Doudna JA, Charpentier E. The new frontier of genome engineering with CRISPR-Cas9. Science. 2014;346(6213):1258096.
21. Lancaster MA, Knoblich JA. Organogenesis in a dish: modeling development and disease using organoid technologies. Science. 2014;345(6194):1247125.
22. Wicki A, Witzigmann D, Balasubramanian V, Huwyler J. Nanomedicine in cancer therapy: challenges, opportunities, and clinical applications. J Control Release. 2015;200:138–57.
23. Wan JCM, Massie C, Garcia-Corbacho J, et al. Liquid biopsies come of age: towards implementation of circulating tumour DNA. Nat Rev Cancer. 2017;17(4):223–38.
24. Yadav VK, De S. An overview of biomarkers in cancer detection and diagnosis. Adv Clin Chem. 2021;103:1–32.
25. Stuart T, Satija R. Integrative single-cell analysis. Nat Rev Genet. 2019;20(5):257–72.
26. Cheishvili D, et al. Clinical validation of peripheral blood mononuclear cell DNA methylation for diagnosis of early-stage hepatocellular carcinoma. Commun Med. 2024;4(1):220.
27. Mayrand MH, et al. Canadian Cervical Cancer Screening Trial (CCCaST): human papillomavirus DNA versus Papanicolaou screening test. N Engl J Med. 2007;357(16):1579–88.
28. Etzioni R, et al. The case for early detection. Nat Rev Cancer. 2003;3(4):243–52.
29. Lippman SM, et al. Effect of selenium and vitamin E on risk of prostate cancer and other cancers: the Selenium and Vitamin E Cancer Prevention Trial (SELECT). JAMA. 2009;301(1):39–51.
30. Herrero R, et al. Costa Rica HPV vaccine trial (cvt): Rationale, design, and methods. Vaccine. 2008;26(51):6708–14.
31. Hitchins MP, et al. Primary constitutional MLH1 epimutations: a focal epigenetic event. Br J Cancer. 2018;119(2):208–21.
32. Haffner MC, et al. AI in pathology: Opportunities and challenges. Nat Rev Cancer. 2022;22(4):235–46.
33. Nikiforov YE, Seethala RR, Tallini G, et al. Nomenclature revision for encapsulated follicular variant of papillary thyroid carcinoma: a paradigm shift to reduce overtreatment of indolent tumors. JAMA Oncol. 2016;2(8):1023–9.
34. Pierorazio PM, Walsh PC, Partin AW, Epstein JI. Prognostic Gleason grade grouping: data-based modeling to identify a clinically relevant classification system for prostate cancer. J Clin Oncol. 2013;31(6):871–6.
35. Onitilo AA, Engel JM, Greenlee RT, Mukesh BN. Breast cancer subtypes based on ER/PR and HER2 expression: comparison of clinicopathologic features and survival. Clin Med Res. 2009;7(1–2):4–13.
36. U.S. Food and Drug Administration. FDA approves trastuzumab deruxtecan for HER2-low breast cancer. Published 2025. Accessed 12 Feb 2025.
37. Robinson DR, Wu YM, Lonigro RJ, et al. Integrative clinical genomics of advanced prostate cancer. Cell. 2015;161(5):1215–28.
38. Ahmed Z, Javed A, Riaz N, et al. RNA sequencing in precision oncology: applications and emerging trends. Cancer Res. 2024;84(3):245–60.
39. Pratt D, Salomon MP, Wu HT, et al. Genome-wide methylation profiling in neuro-oncology diagnostics. Neuro Oncol. 2021;23(5):778–91.
40. Omar N, Smith AE, Jones B, et al. Digital pathology and machine learning in Ki-67 assessment: improving accuracy and reproducibility. Mod Pathol. 2024;37(2):210–25.
41. Shafi AA, Parwani AV. The role of artificial intelligence in prostate cancer pathology. Am J Pathol. 2023;193(7):947–60.
42. Lu MY, Chen TY, Williamson DF, et al. AI-based pathology predicts origins for cancers of unknown primary. Nature. 2021;594(7861):106–10.
43. Huang P, Liu Y, Xu C, et al. Rapid and non-destructive tumor tissue analysis using Raman spectroscopy. Sci Transl Med. 2023;15(676):eabc1234.
44. Paietta E. Minimal residual disease in acute lymphoblastic leukemia: hematology. Am Soc Hematol Educ Program. 2012;2012(1):35–42.
45. Topalian SL, Taube JM, Pardoll DM. Mechanism-driven biomarkers to guide immune checkpoint blockade in cancer therapy. Nat Rev Cancer. 2016;16(5):275–87.
46. Perou CM, Sorlie T, Eisen MB, et al. Molecular portraits of human breast tumours. Nature. 2000;406(6797):747–52.
47. Hourigan CS, Dillon R, O'Brien MM, et al. Impact of conditioning intensity of allogeneic transplantation for acute myeloid leukemia with genomic evidence of residual disease. J Clin Oncol. 2020;38(15):1273–83.
48. Denkert C, Loibl S, Noske A, et al. Tumor-infiltrating lymphocytes and prognosis in different subtypes of breast cancer: a pooled analysis of 3771 patients treated with neoadjuvant therapy. Lancet Oncol. 2018;19(1):40–50.
49. Neesse A, Algül H, Tuveson DA, et al. Stromal biology and therapy in pancreatic cancer: a changing paradigm. Gut. 2015;64(9):1476–84.
50. Stahl PL, Salmen F, Vickovic S, et al. Visualization and analysis of gene expression in tissue sections by spatial transcriptomics. Science. 2016;353(6294):78–82.
51. Dave SS, Wright G, Tan B, et al. Prediction of survival in follicular lymphoma based on molecular features of tumor-infiltrating immune cells. N Engl J Med. 2004;351(21):2159–69.
52. Campanella G, Hanna MG, Geneslaw L, et al. Clinical-grade computational pathology using weakly supervised deep learning on whole slide images. Nat Med. 2019;25(8):1301–9.
53. Lu MY, Chen TY, Williamson DFK, et al. AI-based pathology predicts origins for cancers of unknown primary. Nature. 2021;594(7861):106–10.
54. Pantanowitz L, Sharma A, Carter AB, et al. Twenty years of digital pathology: an overview of the road travelled, challenges, and the future. J Pathol Inform. 2018;9:40.
55. Cheng NM, Yao J, Cai J, et al. Deep learning for fully automated prediction of overall survival in patients with oropharyngeal cancer using FDG-PET imaging. Clin Cancer Res. 2021;27(14):3948–59.

Anesthesia and Cancer Research

28

Raha West and Daqing Ma

Introduction

Cancer is a leading cause of death worldwide, with approximately 1.9 million new cases reported in the United States in 2021 and nearly 39% of individuals facing a cancer diagnosis in their lifetime [1]. Globally, cancer cases reached 18 million in 2020, with projections estimating an increase to 28 million by 2040 [2]. More than 80% of cancer patients undergo at least one surgery for their cancer management, making surgery and its related care a central part of oncology treatment [3].

Traditionally, anesthesia was viewed as a neutral factor in cancer surgery—simply a means to keep patients anesthetized, comfortable, and safe during operations. However, emerging evidence suggests that anesthesia techniques, anesthetic drugs, and pain management strategies may influence long-term cancer outcomes, including recurrence and survival [4]. The possibility that anesthetic and analgesic choices may affect tumor biology and metastatic risk has led to a new line of investigation often referred to as "onco-anesthesia" research [5].

The onco-anesthesia field looks at various perioperative factors that might influence cancer outcomes, including the surgical stress response, inflammation, immune function, general anesthesia, regional anesthesia, opioids, beta-blockers, anti-inflammatory drugs, and local anesthetics (LAs) used during and/or after surgery [6]. The idea is that certain anesthetic and analgesic approaches may help preserve the body's ability to fight any residual tumor cells after surgery [7].

While the exact mechanisms remain partly understood, the surgery procedure itself may spread cancer cells into the circulation as circulating tumor cells (CTCs) [8]. Immunosuppression due to stress hormone release and a heightened inflammatory microenvironment can facilitate the implantation and proliferation of CTCs at distant sites [9]. Cancer long-term outcomes following surgery may be improved by choosing anesthetics and analgesics that reduce stress, maintain stronger immune function, and minimize pro-tumor signaling.

Surgical Stress, Immune System, and Tumor Microenvironment

Surgical Stress Response

Major surgical interventions elicit a complex stress response comprising both neuroendocrine and cytokine-inflammatory elements [10]. Elevated levels of cortisol, catecholamines, and proinflammatory mediators (including various interleukins) collectively diminish the function of critical immune effectors—particularly natural killer (NK) cells and cytotoxic T cells—which play a crucial role in identifying and eliminating residual malignant cells [11].

Surgical stress may shift the immune response from a tumoricidal Th1 orientation toward a more immunosuppressive Th2 phenotype [12]. Prostaglandin and stress hormone transiently compromise NK cell cytotoxicity, coinciding with the critical window during which CTCs seek to establish metastatic foci [13]. Consequently, mitigating this perioperative stress response may help reduce recurrence.

R. West
Division of Anaesthetics, Pain Medicine & Intensive Care, Department of Surgery & Cancer, Faculty of Medicine, Imperial College London, Chelsea & Westminster Hospital, London, UK
e-mail: r.west21@imperial.ac.uk

D. Ma (✉)
Division of Anaesthetics, Pain Medicine & Intensive Care, Department of Surgery & Cancer, Faculty of Medicine, Imperial College London, Chelsea & Westminster Hospital, London, UK

Perioperative and Systems Medicine Laboratory and Department of Anesthesiology, Children's hospital, Zhejiang University School of Medicine, National Clinical Research Center for Child Health, Hangzhou, China
e-mail: d.ma@imperial.ac.uk

J. Huang, H. S.L. Jim (eds.), *Cancer Research Guidance for Clinicians and Researchers*,
https://doi.org/10.1007/978-3-032-19175-5_28

Inflammation and Tumor Progression

Surgical tissue injury induces an inflammatory cascade, which, although necessary for wound healing, can inadvertently support malignant cell survival and dissemination [14]. High cytokines such as IL-6 and TNF-α, coupled with enhanced COX-2 activity and increased VEGF production, collectively foster tumor growth and neovascularization [6]. Furthermore, neutrophils may promote cancer progression by generating neutrophil extracellular traps (NETs), allowing malignant cells to evade immune-mediated destruction [11]. Modulating this inflammatory milieu and immune cell function could mitigate metastatic potential.

Circulating Tumor Cells and Metastatic Spread

During oncologic surgery, direct manipulation of the primary tumor often dislodges malignant cells locally or into the circulation, increasing the burden of CTCs [15]. Under normal conditions, the host immune system can eliminate a significant fraction of these cells.

However, the perioperative period frequently coincides with a state of immunosuppression and heightened inflammation, both enabling CTC survival and eventual colonization of distant sites [16, 17]. Elevated levels of catecholamines, cortisol, and proinflammatory cytokines (e.g., IL-6, TNF-α) can impair NK and T-cell function, reduce cytokine production that supports anti-tumor immunity, and promote endothelial adhesion and vascular permeability, facilitating extravasation of CTCs [18].

Moreover, the production of angiogenic factors such as VEGF and the recruitment of immunosuppressive cell populations can create a permissive microenvironment at potential metastatic niches [19]. This environment allows CTCs to adhere to the endothelium, pass through the vessel wall, and eventually thrive as micrometastases. In addition, perioperative factors such as opioid administration, volatile anesthetics, or beta-adrenergic stimulation may indirectly support CTC survival and integration into distant tissues [20].

Minimizing perioperative immunosuppression and inflammation might help reduce these events. Strategies such as optimizing anesthetic choice, e.g., propofol-based total intravenous anesthesia (TIVA), employing regional anesthesia to limit opioid use, and using targeted anti-inflammatory or immunomodulatory drugs help maintain immune competence and reduce metastatic foci [21, 22]. Ongoing large-scale randomized controlled trials (RCTs), including those examining the effects of different anesthetic regimens and perioperative interventions on long-term cancer outcomes, aim to clarify which measures better preserve immune surveillance and hinder CTC-mediated metastasis.

Anesthetic and Analgesic Techniques: Potential Pathways Affecting Cancer

Multiple perioperative interventions may influence the interaction between surgical stress, immune function, and tumor cell behavior:

- *Regional anesthesia*: By attenuating the neuroendocrine stress response and reducing opioid requirements, regional anesthetic techniques may limit immunosuppression and inflammatory signaling, thereby potentially constraining metastatic processes [23].
- *Propofol-based TIVA*: Propofol's immunomodulatory and anti-inflammatory properties, observed in laboratory studies, suggest it may better preserve NK cell function and overall immune competence compared to volatile anesthetics in certain contexts [24].
- *Volatile anesthetics*: The effects of inhalational agents on cancer progression remain complex and tumor-specific [25]. Some evidence indicates volatile anesthetics can promote immunosuppression and aid tumor cell survival, and other studies note neutral or even inhibitory effects on particular cancer subtypes [26, 27].
- *Opioids*: Opioids remain central to pain management, but their potential to suppress cellular immunity and possibly support tumor cell survival remains controversial [28]. Their ultimate effect may depend on specific tumor genetics and the expression of opioid receptors within the tumor microenvironment [22, 29].
- *Nonsteroidal anti-inflammatory drugs (NSAIDs) and COX-2 inhibitors*: By reducing prostaglandin synthesis and dampening inflammation, these agents may disrupt pathways that support tumor proliferation, angiogenesis, and metastasis [30, 31].
- *LAs, for example, lidocaine*: Preclinical data suggest that lidocaine not only mitigates perioperative stress and inflammation but may also exert direct antiproliferative and pro-apoptotic effects on malignant cells [32, 33].
- *Beta-blockers*: These agents may blunt the catecholamine surge associated with surgery and stress, inhibiting pathways that facilitate tumor cell adhesion, extravasation, and metastasis [30].
- *Dexmedetomidine*: While promising for its stress-attenuating and anti-inflammatory attributes, definitive evidence of dexmedetomidine's role in improving oncologic outcomes remains inconclusive and requires further investigation [34, 35].
- *Ketamine*: With multifaceted immunological effects, ketamine's ultimate influence on cancer progression is unclear [36]. Some reports indicate immunosuppression and enhanced metastasis, whereas others show neutral or context-dependent results, warranting additional study.

Common Cancers and Anesthesia

Breast Cancer

Initial investigations in breast cancer surgery posited that integrating regional anesthesia techniques (e.g., paravertebral blocks) with propofol-based TIVA might reduce recurrence rates [37]. While early observational studies showed promising indications, subsequent RCTs did not demonstrate a significant difference in recurrence when compared to volatile anesthesia and opioid-based regimens [21, 38, 39]. An important exception is peritumoral lidocaine infiltration before breast cancer excision, shown in one large trial to significantly improve both disease-free and overall survival [40].

Colorectal Cancer

In colorectal cancer, early observational and pilot studies indicated that epidural anesthesia and intravenous lidocaine infusions might offer oncologic benefits [32, 33]. Nonetheless, RCTs are still ongoing. Although propofol-based TIVA may be advantageous, large registry analyses remain conflicting [38].

Lung Cancer

Lung cancer surgery is intrinsically high-risk, involving extensive tissue manipulation and intense postoperative pain. While TIVA or agents such as dexmedetomidine might reduce inflammation and preserve immune surveillance, early trials have not shown meaningful improvements in long-term outcomes with epidural anesthesia [41]. Data remain inconclusive for TIVA or dexmedetomidine on recurrence or survival [42].

Ovarian Cancer

Ovarian cancer surgeries, often involving techniques such as hyperthermic intraperitoneal chemotherapy (HIPEC), present complex scenarios [43]. Encouraged by findings in breast cancer, some hypothesize that peritumoral local anesthetic approaches might confer benefits in ovarian malignancies, but sparse data remain heterogeneous [40, 44].

Basic Science and Clinical Research

Basic Science Findings

A growing body of preclinical evidence shows that anesthetics and perioperative drugs can affect cancer cell behavior and host immune responses through complex mechanisms [6, 16, 45, 46]. The perioperative period, characterized by the surgical stress response and tissue injury, could tip the balance in favor of tumor cell survival, proliferation, angiogenesis, and metastasis [11, 16].

Volatile Anesthetics vs. Propofol

Laboratory studies suggest volatile anesthetics may enhance metastatic potential and tumor cell proliferation by impairing immune effectors and favoring tumor-supportive microenvironments [7, 16, 17]. In contrast, propofol-based TIVA demonstrates antitumor properties in numerous models, inhibiting proliferation and migration of various cancer cell lines and promoting apoptosis [24, 47]. Serum samples from patients receiving propofol combined with regional anesthesia have shown reduced tumor cell proliferation and invasion in vitro compared to those from patients receiving volatile anesthesia [48].

Opioids

Opioids can suppress NK cell cytotoxicity and T-cell function and upregulate pathways associated with tumor angiogenesis and metastasis [28, 49]. However, animal studies show mixed results, reflecting differences in tumor types, specific opioids, and genetic factors [50, 51].

Local Anesthetics (e.g., Lidocaine)

LAs, including lidocaine, emerged as potential antitumor agents in laboratory settings [52]. Lidocaine reduced proinflammatory cytokines such as IL-1 and TNF-α, blocked voltage-gated sodium channels in tumor cells, and lowered angiogenic and metastatic signaling [52]. Animal studies showed that intravenous lidocaine infusions counteract the pro-metastatic influence of volatile anesthesia and enhance the efficacy of chemotherapy [32]. Preclinical models of breast cancer indicated that lidocaine decreased the number of pulmonary metastases and improved survival in mouse models [32].

α_2-Adrenergic Agonist (Dexmedetomidine)

Experimental research on α2-adrenoceptor agonists reveals that dexmedetomidine might increase tumor cell survival and angiogenesis through HIF-1α, survivin, and STAT3 signaling [53, 54].

NSAIDs and Other Agents

In vitro and translational studies suggest that NSAIDs may reduce immunosuppression, angiogenesis, and regulatory T-cell infiltration, thereby diminishing metastatic potential [55]. Glucocorticoids show mixed effects in experimental models, potentially promoting or suppressing tumor progression [56]. Ketamine and thiopental raise concerns by inhibiting NK cell activity and promoting metastasis in some animal studies [57]. Nitrous oxide appears to have neutral or inconclusive effects [58].

Overall, preclinical data offer insights into how anesthetics may shape the tumor microenvironment, immune function, and metastatic pathways. However, human tumors are genetically diverse, and patients present unique immunological states not fully mirrored in laboratory conditions [59]. Well-designed clinical trials remain necessary.

Observational Clinical Studies

Table 28.1 summarizes selected observational studies (2018 onward) examining how anesthetic techniques may influence cancer outcomes.

Propofol TIVA vs. Volatile Agents

Initial mechanistic research indicated that propofol-based TIVA could yield immunological or anti-inflammatory advantages over volatile inhalation agents. Yet a meta-analysis of 23 retrospective observational studies ($n = 1611$) did not detect differences in perioperative inflammatory biomarkers (IL-6, IL-10, TNF-α, and CRP) between patients receiving propofol TIVA and those given volatile anesthesia [73].

A landmark retrospective propensity-matched study of 6428 cancer patients undergoing elective surgery (2010–2013) compared volatile inhalational anesthesia and TIVA. After matching ($n = 2607$ per group), mortality was significantly higher with volatile anesthesia (22.8% vs. 15.6%), with an adjusted hazard ratio (HR) of 1.46 (95% confidence interval [CI] 1.29–1.66), suggesting a survival benefit for TIVA [74]. This was the first large-scale clinical evidence linking anesthetic technique to cancer survival, prompting further meta-analyses and controlled trials.

Despite the lack of biochemical marker differences, specific observational data pointed toward improved oncologic outcomes with propofol TIVA. A systematic review and meta-analysis of 19 retrospective observational studies found that patients receiving propofol-based TIVA during cancer surgery demonstrated significantly better overall survival compared to those receiving volatile anesthesia (HR = 0.79, 95% CI 0.66–0.94, $P = 0.008$) [27]. However, recurrence-free survival showed no statistically significant difference between the two anesthetic approaches (HR = 0.81, 95% CI 0.61–1.07, $P = 0.137$). Subgroup analyses indicated that propofol TIVA was associated with improved overall survival compared to desflurane (HR = 0.54, 95% CI 0.36–0.80, $P = 0.003$), though no survival advantage was observed when compared to sevoflurane (HR = 0.92, 95% CI 0.74–1.14, $P = 0.439$) [27]. Another meta-analysis including over 18,000 patients highlighted that propofol TIVA was associated with improved overall survival (HR = 0.76, 95% CI 0.63–0.92, $P < 0.01$) and recurrence-free survival (HR = 0.78, 95% CI 0.65–0.94, $P < 0.01$) across a variety of cancer types [45].

However, large-scale registry data did not confirm these findings uniformly. A retrospective propensity score-matched study conducted in Sweden analyzed more than 4600 breast cancer patients undergoing surgery and compared survival outcomes between patients receiving propofol-based TIVA and those receiving volatile anesthesia. The measurements focused on survival at a median follow-up of 1 year, and the study found no significant difference in survival outcomes between the two anesthetic modalities, providing no conclusive evidence favoring one approach [26]. In Denmark, a registry-based retrospective propensity-matched study investigated the effect of inhalation anesthesia on recurrence risk in colorectal cancer patients. This study included data from national registries, examining recurrence patterns and calculating hazard ratios. They found that volatile anesthesia was associated with an increased recurrence risk, with a hazard ratio (HR) of 1.12 (95% CI 1.02–1.23), suggesting that volatile anesthesia might negatively impact oncological outcomes [38]. These findings from retrospective studies emphasize the need for further RCTs to determine whether anesthetic modality influences cancer outcomes definitively.

Table 28.1 Selected observational studies (2018–present) on anesthetic techniques and cancer outcomes after surgery

Authors (publication year)	Cancer site	Study design	Sample size, n =	Intervention	Comparator	Key results	Conclusions
Enlund et al. (2022) [26]	Breast	Retrospective national registry cohort	18,674 total → 4658 matched pairs	Propofol TIVA	Volatile anesthesia	Unmatched data favored propofol, but after propensity matching, there was no significant survival difference (HR ~0.98, $P = 0.756$)	No association was found between anesthesia type (propofol vs. volatile) and overall survival in matched patients undergoing breast surgery
Zhang et al. (2021) [37]	Breast	Retrospective, propensity-matched cohort	2760	Propofol TIVA with RA	Volatile anesthesia	In multivariate analysis, TIVA-RA significantly reduced the risk of local-regional recurrence compared to volatile anesthesia (HR 0.67). Higher tumor grade (II/III), advanced stage (clinical/pT/pN), and HER2 positivity increased recurrence, while adjuvant radiotherapy lowered it	TIVA-RA may be beneficial for reducing local-regional recurrence in women with breast cancer who undergo surgery compared to volatile anesthesia
Enlund et al. (2020) [60]	Breast	Retrospective, multicenter database analysis	6305	Propofol TIVA	Volatile anesthesia	The 5-year survival rates were 91.0% (propofol) vs. 81.8% (sevoflurane), but different statistical adjustments yielded varying significance. At best, there was a 9.2% survival difference favoring propofol	Propofol may confer a survival advantage over sevoflurane in breast cancer, though the retrospective design poses inherent limitations
Yoo et al. (2019) [61]	Breast	Retrospective cohort study	5331 (1766 pairs after matching)	Propofol TIVA	Volatile anesthesia	No significant difference in 5-year recurrence-free or overall survival (93.2% vs. 93.8%)	No association between anesthesia type and long-term prognosis in breast cancer; no clear basis to prefer TIVA or volatile anesthesia
Huang et al. (2019) [62]	Breast	Retrospective cohort study	976 total (632 vs. 344) →after matching: 592 vs. 296	Propofol TIVA	Volatile anesthesia	No significant difference in 5-year overall mortality (both 4%) or locoregional recurrence; adjusted HR 1.13 (95% CI 0.67–1.92)	Neither propofol nor desflurane significantly impacted breast cancer prognosis or survival in this retrospective analysis
Kim et al. (2019) [63]	Breast	Retrospective cohort, propensity matched	2628 (236 received dexamethasone)	Single perioperative dexamethasone dose	No dexamethasone	No significant increase in recurrence (HR 1.44, $P = 0.071$) or mortality (HR 1.26, $P = 0.361$). Propensity matching yielded similar findings	A single perioperative dose of dexamethasone was not associated with higher recurrence or mortality in breast cancer surgery

(continued)

Table 28.1 (continued)

Authors (publication year)	Cancer site	Study design	Sample size, n =	Intervention	Comparator	Key results	Conclusions
Hasselager et al. (2022) [38]	Colorectal	Retrospective registry-based cohort	11,618 total (3496 epidural vs. 8122 no epidural)	Epidural analgesia	No epidural analgesia	No significant difference in colorectal cancer recurrence (HR ≈ 0.91) or mortality (HR ≈ 1.01) after propensity	Epidural analgesia was not associated with reduced recurrence or improved survival in colorectal cancer surgery
Wu et al. (2018) [64]	Colon	Retrospective cohort study	1363 total → after matching: 579 in each group	Propofol TIVA	Volatile anesthesia	The propofol group showed significantly better survival (HR range ~ 0.22 to 0.42) across different TNM stages; fewer deaths compared to desflurane (15.0% vs. 32.6%)	Propofol anesthesia was associated with improved survival in colon cancer surgery, regardless of tumor stage
Makito et al. (2020) [65]	Digestive tract	Retrospective cohort study	196,303 (volatile group: 166,966; TIVA group: 29,337)	Propofol TIVA	Volatile anesthesia	No significant difference in overall or recurrence-free survival (HR ~1.0). Instrumental variable analysis suggested a minor advantage for TIVA in recurrence-free survival (HR = 0.92), but subgroup analyses were negative	Overall and recurrence-free survival were similar, so anesthetic choice should be guided by other factors
Lai et al. (2019) [66]	Hepatocellular carcinoma (HCC)	Retrospective single-center cohort	944 total → 335 matched pairs	Propofol TIVA	Volatile anesthesia	After matching, propofol TIVA was linked to a significantly lower HR for mortality (HR ~0.47). Subgroup analyses also favored propofol, especially when distant metastasis or local recurrence was absent	Propofol TIVA was associated with improved survival after hepatectomy for HCC, warranting prospective confirmation
Zheng et al. (2018) [67]	Gastric	Retrospective cohort study	2856 total (after matching: 897 TIVA vs. 897 volatile)	Propofol TIVA	Volatile anesthesia	The TIVA group showed better survival (HR ~0.65 in multivariate analysis), with a lower risk of death compared to volatile anesthesia. Cancer stage and tumor differentiation also influenced outcomes	TIVA might be linked to improved survival in gastric cancer patients undergoing surgical resection
Zhang et al. (2020) [68]	Pancreatic	Retrospective cohort (propensity matched)	2239	Intraoperative IV lidocaine (bolus + continuous infusion)	No lidocaine	Lower intraoperative opioid requirement and lower postoperative analgesic use with lidocaine; no DFS difference, but improved overall survival (HR ≈ 0.62)	IV lidocaine infusion was linked to better overall survival after pancreatectomy, warranting further investigation
Du et al. (2018) [69]	Esophageal adenocarcinoma & squamous cell carcinoma (SCC)	Retrospective analysis	725	Higher-dose intraoperative opioids	Lower-dose intraoperative opioids	In squamous cell carcinoma, higher intraoperative opioid doses were linked to better RFS and OS; no clear association in adenocarcinoma	High opioid dosing correlated with improved survival in SCC but not adenocarcinoma, though further validation is needed

Huang et al. (2018) [70]	Non-small-cell lung	Retrospective cohort study	588	Various perioperative factors (including dexamethasone, flurbiprofen)	Not receiving dexamethasone/ flurbiprofen	In multivariable analysis, dexamethasone alone and in combination with flurbiprofen were associated with improved overall survival; limited resection and larger tumors were linked to worse outcomes	Certain perioperative factors (dexamethasone ± flurbiprofen) may enhance long-term survival after lung surgery, but findings need validation by prospective trials
Oh et al. (2018) [71]	Non-small-cell lung (NSCLC)	Retrospective cohort study	943 total → 196 matched pairs	Propofol TIVA	Volatile anesthesia	No significant difference in recurrence-free ($P = 0.233$) or overall survival ($P = 0.551$) between TIVA and inhalation groups	Propofol TIVA did not provide a survival advantage over inhalation anesthesia for NSCLC surgery in this retrospective analysis
Connolly et al. (2021) [29]	Lung adenocarcinoma	Retrospective database review	740	Intraoperative opioid exposure; adjunct ketamine or dexmedetomidine	Varying intraoperative opioid doses/no adjunct	Higher opioid doses were linked to worse overall survival; ketamine was associated with improved recurrence-specific survival. Certain tumor genomic changes modified these effects	Intraoperative opioids may worsen overall survival, whereas ketamine may help recurrence-free survival in lung adenocarcinoma
Mao et al. (2020) [72]	Bladder (urothelial carcinoma)	Retrospective single-center study	185	Perioperative glucocorticoids	No glucocorticoids	Kaplan-Meier analysis showed that the glucocorticoids group had a higher distant metastasis rate; multivariable analysis was nonsignificant after adjusting for transfusions	Perioperative glucocorticoids may be linked to increased risk of distant metastasis, especially in patients not receiving transfusions. Further research needed

TIVA total intravenous anesthesia, *HR* hazard ratio, *RA* regional anesthesia, *DFS* disease-free survival, *RFS* recurrence-free survival, *OS* overall survival

Regional Anesthesia

Regional anesthesia, such as paravertebral blocks for breast cancer surgery, was among the earliest techniques investigated for potential long-term oncologic benefits. The initial rationale was that controlling postoperative pain and mitigating the surgical stress response could help prevent the proliferation of residual cancer cells. This interest extended to epidural anesthesia, which has been hypothesized to preserve immune function and reduce the risk of metastasis. However, large retrospective datasets have often yielded inconsistent outcomes. A Danish retrospective cohort study, using the Danish Colorectal Cancer Group Database and the Danish Anesthesia Database, analyzed data from 11,618 patients who underwent colorectal cancer surgery between 2004 and 2018. Among these, 3496 patients (30.1%) received epidural analgesia before surgery. The propensity score-matched analysis included 2980 patients in each group with balanced baseline covariates. The primary outcome was cancer recurrence, and the secondary outcome was mortality, with a median follow-up of 58 months (IQR 29–86). Cancer recurrence occurred in 19.0% of patients who received epidural analgesia compared to 20.5% of those who did not. The study found no statistically significant association between epidural analgesia and cancer recurrence (HR 0.91, 95% CI 0.82–1.02) or mortality (HR 1.01, 95% CI 0.92–1.10). These findings suggest that epidural analgesia does not significantly influence long-term oncologic outcomes in colorectal cancer surgery [38].

Amide Local Anesthetics (e.g., Lidocaine)

Amide LAs, particularly lidocaine, have drawn attention for their potential inhibitory effects on cancer progression, as demonstrated in preclinical studies. Observational clinical studies, however, have presented mixed results. For example, a retrospective analysis involving 2239 pancreatic cancer patients examined the effect of perioperative lidocaine infusion (bolus 1.5 mg/kg at induction followed by 2 mg/kg/h) on survival outcomes. The study measured overall survival and disease-free survival as primary and secondary endpoints, respectively. It reported a significant association between lidocaine infusion and improved overall survival at 3 years (hazard ratio [HR] 0.62, 95% confidence interval [CI] 0.29–0.78), but no improvement in disease-free survival [68]. Despite this initial retrospective suggestion, subsequent prospective trials failed to replicate these survival benefits, indicating that observational findings alone cannot confirm a causal advantage.

Opioids

The role of opioids in cancer outcomes has been extensively studied due to preclinical evidence suggesting potential links to immunosuppression, angiogenesis, and tumor progression. However, clinical findings from observational studies remain inconclusive. A large prospective cohort study involving 34,188 early-stage breast cancer patients investigated the relationship between postsurgical opioid prescriptions and cancer recurrence. Using detailed prescription and follow-up data, the study assessed opioid type, dose, and duration while adjusting for confounders. No significant association was found between opioid use and cancer recurrence (HR = 1.0, 95% CI 0.92–1.1), regardless of the opioid type or duration. These findings suggest that opioids used for postsurgical pain management in breast cancer patients may not adversely affect long-term outcomes [75]. Additional retrospective studies examining perioperative opioid use during cancer surgery have yielded mixed results. In non-small-cell lung cancer (NSCLC) patients, a study of over 900 individuals reported that high intraoperative fentanyl doses were associated with reduced overall survival in patients with stage 1 disease (HR = 1.12, 95% CI 0.99–1.27, P = 0.053) [76]. However, this association was not observed in patients with more advanced stages (stages 2 and 3). Similarly, conflicting findings were reported in esophageal cancer studies, where one analysis associated high-dose opioid treatment with increased disease recurrence [77], while another found improved survival outcomes [69]. Meanwhile, a retrospective study involving over 1600 colorectal cancer patients found no association between intraoperative opioid administration and recurrence-free or overall survival [78].

NSAIDs/COX-2 Inhibitors and Beta-Blockers

Laboratory studies have indicated that inhibiting prostaglandin synthesis through NSAIDs or blocking adrenergic signaling via beta-blockers may reduce metastatic risk. However, clinical evidence from observational studies remains inconclusive. A prospective cohort study in Denmark examined 34,188 stage I–III breast cancer patients diagnosed between 1996 and 2008, assessing the association between post-diagnostic use of aspirin, NSAIDs, and selective COX-2 inhibitors with breast cancer recurrence. The study found no significant association between the use of these medications and recurrence rates, with adjusted hazard ratios of 1.0 (95% CI 0.90–1.1) for aspirin, 0.99 (95% CI 0.92–1.1) for NSAIDs, and 1.1 (95% CI 0.98–1.2) for selective COX-2 inhibitors. Interestingly, pre-diagnostic use of these drugs was associated with a reduced recurrence rate, suggesting potential benefits warranting further investigation [79].

Regarding beta-blockers, a retrospective cohort study involving 1413 patients with stage I–III breast cancer found that 102 patients (7%) used beta-blockers. The study reported a decreased risk of relapse among beta-blocker users, with a relative risk of 0.52 (95% CI 0.31–0.88). This association was particularly pronounced in patients with triple-negative breast cancer, where the relative risk of relapse was 0.30 (95% CI 0.10–0.87). These findings suggest a potential benefit of beta-blocker use in reducing breast cancer recurrence, especially in certain subtypes [80].

In contrast, a study examining the concurrent use of NSAIDs, beta-blockers, and metformin found no significant association with clinical benefits in cancer patients [81]. The research indicated that the effect of these medications might vary across different cancer types and patient populations, highlighting the need for further studies to clarify their roles in cancer therapy [81].

Overall, while preclinical data suggest potential anticancer effects of NSAIDs and beta-blockers, observational studies have produced mixed results.

Dexamethasone, Dexmedetomidine, and Ketamine

Observational studies investigating the perioperative use of dexamethasone, dexmedetomidine, and ketamine in cancer patients have produced inconsistent findings. A retrospective cohort study involving 2628 breast cancer patients assessed the effects of a single intraoperative dose of dexamethasone on cancer recurrence and mortality. Among the 8.5% of patients who received dexamethasone, there was no significant increase in the risk of recurrence (hazard ratio [HR] 1.389; 95% confidence interval [CI], 0.904–2.132; $P = 0.133$) or mortality (HR 1.506; 95% CI 0.886–2.561; $P = 0.130$) [63]. In contrast, a retrospective study of 185 bladder cancer patients undergoing radical resection found that those who received glucocorticoids had a shortened metastasis-free survival time (HR 1.790; $P = 0.030$), indicating a potential adverse effect on cancer progression [72]. A separate retrospective cohort study of 588 non-small-cell lung cancer (NSCLC) patients found that perioperative dexamethasone use was associated with improved long-term survival (HR 0.70; 95% CI 0.54–0.90; $P = 0.006$). Additionally, combined administration of dexamethasone and flurbiprofen axetil was linked to even longer survival (HR 0.57; 95% CI 0.38–0.84; $P = 0.005$) [70]. Evidence from preclinical studies suggests that dexmedetomidine may promote cancer cell survival via HIF-1α upregulation and enhance metastasis through MMPs. However, there is currently no robust clinical data to confirm its impact on cancer outcomes [82]. Similarly, while ketamine has demonstrated antitumor effects in preclinical models, no clinical evidence supports its perioperative use for improving cancer outcomes [83].

Randomized Controlled Trials (RCTs)

Table 28.2 provides an overview of selected RCTs (2018 onward) that investigate the effect of anesthetic approaches on long-term oncologic outcomes.

Propofol TIVA vs. Volatile Anesthesia

Several RCTs have investigated whether propofol-based TIVA offers superior long-term oncologic outcomes compared to volatile anesthetics. A double-blind RCT involving 210 primary breast cancer patients compared sevoflurane anesthesia to propofol TIVA, measuring circulating tumor cell counts at 0, 48, and 72 h postoperatively. The study found no significant differences between the two groups, suggesting that neither anesthetic approach had a distinct impact on this surrogate marker of metastasis [39]. In another pilot, RCTs, a single-blind trial, 40 patients from the Breast Cancer Recurrence and Anesthesia trial were evaluated for NETosis markers, which are implicated in cancer progression and metastasis. Markers were measured before and 24 h after surgery, and no significant differences were identified between volatile-opioid or regional and propofol-based TIVA techniques [84].

Another RCT examined 153 colorectal cancer patients randomized to receive either propofol TIVA or sevoflurane anesthesia. The study measured immune profiles, specifically NK cell activity and T-cell fractions. It found no significant differences in immune cell subsets between the two anesthetic approaches [85]. Another secondary analysis of an RCT in breast cancer patients examined the neutrophil-to-lymphocyte ratio (NLR), a marker of inflammation linked to adverse cancer outcomes. Patients randomized to propofol-paravertebral anesthesia had a lower postoperative NLR compared to those receiving volatile-opioid anesthesia (3.0 [2.4–4.2] vs. 4.0 [2.9–5.4], $P = 0.001$) [90]. However, this immunological finding did not translate into improved long-term oncologic outcomes in subsequent trials [41].

The largest RCT to date, involving 1228 Chinese patients aged 65–90 undergoing major cancer surgeries, randomized participants to sevoflurane or propofol TIVA. The primary endpoint was overall survival, with secondary endpoints of recurrence-free and event-free survival. After a median follow-up of 43 months, there were no significant differences in overall survival (adjusted HR 1.02, 95% CI 0.83–1.26; $P = 0.834$), recurrence-free survival (HR 1.07, 95% CI 0.89–1.30; $P = 0.465$), or event-free survival (HR 1.09, 95% CI 0.93–1.29; $P = 0.298$) [41, 89].

Table 28.2 Selected randomized controlled trials (2018–present) on anesthetic techniques and cancer outcomes

Authors (publication year)	Cancer site	Study design	Sample size, n =	Intervention	Comparator	Key results	Conclusions
Badwe et al. (2023) [40]	Early breast	RCT	1583 (796 lidocaine vs. 804 control)	Peritumoral lidocaine injection before surgery	No lidocaine injection (standard care)	At ~5-year follow-up, DFS was 86.6% (lidocaine) vs. 82.6% (control) (HR = 0.74), and OS was 90.1% vs. 86.4% (HR = 0.71). Lidocaine also reduced distant recurrences	Presurgical peritumoral lidocaine significantly improved disease-free and overall survival in early breast cancer, suggesting a preventive effect on metastasis
Aghamelu et al. (2021) [84]	Breast	Pilot RCT	40	Propofol TIVA with RA	Propofol TIVA	No difference in postoperative NETosis (neutrophil extracellular traps) markers (MPO, citrullinated histone H3) between groups; recurrence was low overall	Anaesthetic technique (volatile vs. propofol-paravertebral) did not alter NETosis expression in breast cancer surgery patients
Coombes et al. (2021) [31]	Breast (HER2–)	RCT	2639	Celecoxib (400 mg daily, 2 yrs)	Placebo	At ~5-year follow-up, no significant difference in disease-free survival (84% vs. 83%, HR = 0.97)	Two-year celecoxib adjuvant therapy did not improve disease-free survival in patients with HER2-negative breast cancer
Hovaguimian et al. (2020) [39]	Breast	RCT (two-center)	210 (sevoflurane $n = 107$, propofol $n = 103$)	Propofol TIVA	Volatile anesthesia	CTC counts over 72 h did not differ between groups, although a secondary analysis suggested higher maximal counts with sevoflurane	No overall difference in perioperative CTC levels between sevoflurane and propofol, implying no clear advantage for either
Sessler et al. (2019) [21]	Breast	RCT (multicentre)	2132 (1043 vs. 1065)	Propofol TIVA with RA	Volatile anesthesia + opioids	No significant difference in breast cancer recurrence (10% vs. 10%, HR 0.97) or persistent incisional pain at 6–12 months	Regional anesthesia-analgesia with propofol did not reduce recurrence or chronic pain compared to volatile anesthesia with opioids
Xu et al. (2021) [41]	Lung	RCT	400 total (200 epidural + GA vs. 200 GA)	Epidural + GA	GA + opioids	No difference in recurrence-free survival (27% vs. 24% events; adjusted HR ~0.90, $P = 0.608$) or overall and cancer-specific survival between groups. The epidural group had more intraoperative hypotension	Epidural anesthesia-analgesia did not enhance survival outcomes after lung cancer surgery compared with general anesthesia alone
Rangel et al. (2021) [22]	Prostate	RCT	146	Opioid-free anesthesia	Opioid-based anesthesia	No difference in biochemical recurrence-free survival (17 vs. 14 events); Cox analysis identified obesity, high risk, laparoscopic surgery, and positive margins as significant risk factors	Intraoperative opioid use did not affect biochemical recurrence rates or recurrence-free survival in intermediate/high-risk prostate cancer surgery
Oh et al. (2022) [85]	Colorectal	RCT	153	Propofol TIVA	Volatile anesthesia	No significant differences in fractions of NK cells, helper T cells, cytotoxic T cells, or NLR between propofol and sevoflurane groups up to 24 h postoperatively	Propofol was not superior to volatile anesthesia in preserving immune cell populations during colorectal cancer surgery

Falk et al. (2021) [86]	Colorectal	RCT	221	Thoracic epidural analgesia (TEA)	Patient-controlled IV morphine analgesia (PCA)	Five-year disease-free survival: 76% (TEA) vs. 69% (PCA) (HR ~1.19, $P = 0.61$). Pain relief was slightly better in the TEA group for the first 24 h only	TEA did not significantly improve 5-year disease-free survival vs. IV PCA, though it provided better early postoperative analgesia
Cho et al. (2021) [87]	Colorectal	RCT	100	Low-dose ketamine (bolus + infusion)	Normal saline (placebo)	No significant difference in postoperative NK cell activity or inflammatory markers (IL-6, TNF-α, CRP), and the 2-year recurrence rate was similar (10% vs. 8%)	Subanesthetic ketamine did not provide immunological or recurrence-free survival benefits in colorectal cancer surgery patients
Haldar et al. (2020) [30]	Colorectal	RCT	34	Propranolol (β-blocker) + Etodolac (COX2 inhibitor)	Placebo	Improved tumor biomarkers (less EMT, enhanced immune cell infiltration) and a trend toward lower 3-year recurrence in protocol-compliant patients	Perioperative blockade of β-adrenergic and COX2 pathways may favorably influence metastasis-related biomarkers and potentially reduce recurrence
Zhang et al. (2022) [88]	Pancreatic	RCT	563	Intraoperative IV lidocaine (bolus + continuous infusion)	Saline placebo	No difference in 3-yr overall (HR = 0.98) or disease-free survival (HR = 0.91). Lidocaine reduced intraoperative opioid use and circulating NETs, but not tumor-associated NETs	Lidocaine infusion did not improve survival in pancreatic cancer resection, despite some opioid-sparing and transient NET reduction
Cho et al. (2021) [34]	Uterine	RCT	100	Perioperative dexmedetomidine infusion	Standard care	No significant benefit in NK cell activity or long-term outcomes; dexmedetomidine increased interferon-γ, lowered early pain scores, and reduced opioid use	Dexmedetomidine did not enhance immune function or survival but offered better pain control and reduced opioid consumption in uterine cancer surgery
Hayden et al. (2020) [43]	Ovarian (advanced)	RCT	40	Intraperitoneal ropivacaine during/after cytoreductive surgery (72 h infusion)	Placebo (saline)	Time to chemotherapy initiation was shorter with ropivacaine (median 21 vs. 29 days; $P = 0.021$), with no difference in pain or complication rates	Intraperitoneal ropivacaine appeared safe and may allow earlier start of postoperative chemotherapy in advanced ovarian cancer
Cao et al. (2023) [89]	Various cancers	Multicentre RCT (14 hospitals)	1195	Propofol TIVA	Volatile anesthesia	After a median 43-mo follow-up, no significant difference in overall (31% vs. 29% deaths) or recurrence-free survival between propofol and sevoflurane (adjusted HR ≈ 1.0)	Propofol TIVA did not improve long-term survival or recurrence-free outcomes compared to sevoflurane in older patients having major cancer surgery

TIVA total intravenous anesthesia, *HR* hazard ratio, *RA* regional anesthesia, *DFS* disease-free survival, *RFS* recurrence-free survival, *OS* overall survival, *CTC* circulating tumor cell, *EMT* epithelial-to-mesenchymal transition, *NETs* neutrophil extracellular traps

Although retrospective studies have previously suggested that propofol may prolong disease-free or overall survival compared to volatile agents, available RCTs do not support this hypothesis. Future trials, such as the ongoing VAPOR-C trial, are expected to provide more definitive answers by focusing on specific tumor types, such as colorectal cancer and non-small-cell lung cancer (NSCLC), to avoid the heterogeneity that has confounded prior analyses [91].

Regional Anesthesia

Early enthusiasm for the potential oncologic benefits of regional anesthesia, particularly paravertebral blocks for breast cancer surgery, led to RCTs. The largest multicenter RCT to date, involving 2108 breast cancer patients, compared paravertebral block combined with propofol TIVA against general anesthesia with sevoflurane and opioid analgesia. The primary endpoint was cancer recurrence at a median follow-up of 36 months. The study reported no significant difference in recurrence rates between the two groups (10% in both arms, HR 0.97, 95% CI 0.74–1.28), indicating no oncologic advantage for paravertebral anesthesia [21].

Similarly, smaller RCTs evaluating regional anesthesia in colorectal cancer patients have yielded comparable results. One trial examined epidural anesthesia versus systemic opioid use in 211 patients undergoing colorectal cancer surgery. The primary outcome, 5-year disease-free survival, was 76% for epidural and 69% for opioid (HR 1.31, 95% CI 0.74–2.32; $P = 0.35$). Epidural provided better pain relief in the first 24 h, but there were no significant differences in complications, hospital stay, or return to oncologic therapy [86]. Another RCT investigated the effect of perioperative epidural analgesia on recurrence-free survival in patients undergoing major abdominal cancer surgery. The study included 503 patients randomized to receive either general anesthesia with epidural analgesia or general anesthesia alone. After a median follow-up of 2.8 years, the results showed no significant difference in recurrence-free survival between the two groups (hazard ratio [HR] 0.95, 95% confidence interval [CI] 0.76–1.17; $P = 0.61$) [92]. Additionally, an RCT of 400 lung cancer patients compared combined epidural-general anesthesia with general anesthesia alone. At a median follow-up of 32 months, no significant differences were found in recurrence-free survival (27% vs. 24%, HR 0.90, 95% CI 0.60–1.35, $P = 0.608$), overall survival, or cancer-specific survival [41].

Taken collectively, these trials suggest that while regional anesthesia provides effective pain relief and may have short-term benefits, it does not consistently lead to improved cancer-related survival or reduced recurrence.

Amide Local Anesthetics (Lidocaine)

Promising retrospective associations on systemic lidocaine use have not held up in RCTs. Following the initial observational suggestion in pancreatic resection patients, a large RCT ($n = 563$) comparing intravenous lidocaine to placebo found no difference in overall (HR 0.98, 95% CI 0.8–1.2) or disease-free survival (HR 0.9, 95% CI 0.7–1.2) [88]. However, a notable exception emerged from an Indian RCT involving nearly 1600 women undergoing breast cancer surgery. Peritumoral infiltration of lidocaine (0.5 mg/kg up to 4.5 mg/kg) given 7–10 minutes before resection improved both 5-year disease-free survival (87% vs. 83%; HR 0.74, 95% CI 0.58–0.95; $P = 0.017$) and overall survival (90% vs. 86%; HR 0.71, 95% CI 0.53–0.94; $P = 0.019$), with no reported adverse effects [40]. This outlier suggests that specific administration routes and timing may matter.

Opioids, NSAIDs/COX-2 Inhibitors, Beta-Blockers, Dexamethasone, Dexmedetomidine, and Ketamine

RCTs investigating these perioperative agents in cancer surgery have largely yielded neutral or inconclusive results. A small Brazilian RCT ($n = 146$) compared opioid-free anesthesia with opioid-based anesthesia in prostatectomy patients, measuring biochemical recurrence through prostate-specific antigen levels. The trial reported no significant differences between groups (17 vs. 14 recurrences, $P = 0.54$), suggesting that opioids do not influence recurrence in this context, though the study was underpowered [22]. Similarly, RCTs on celecoxib and NSAID/COX-2 inhibitors have not shown improvements in disease-free survival [31, 93].

Beta-blockers combined with NSAIDs were evaluated in a small colorectal cancer RCT ($n = 34$). While some biomarker changes were noted, no definitive recurrence benefits were observed [30]. A small RCT ($n = 100$) comparing dexmedetomidine infusion versus placebo in uterine cancer surgery found no significant differences in 2-year recurrence (16.3% vs. 8.7%, $P = 0.227$) or mortality (6.7% vs. 2.2%, $P = 0.318$), likely due to limited statistical power [34]. However, a follow-up analysis of a larger RCT ($n = 620$) suggested that dexmedetomidine might improve recurrence-free survival (22% vs. 32%, HR 0.67, 95% CI 0.49–0.92, $P = 0.012$) and event-free survival (39% vs. 47%, HR 0.78, 95% CI 0.61–1.00), although overall survival was unaffected [35]. RCT on ketamine in colorectal cancer patients ($n = 100$) reported no differences in postoperative immune markers, recurrence, or metastasis rates within 2 years, but these studies remain underpowered to assess oncologic outcomes [87].

Summary of Current Evidence

Over a decade of research into the impact of anesthesia and analgesia on cancer outcomes has yielded largely inconclusive results.

- *Regional Anesthesia*: Despite initial promise, large RCTs (e.g., paravertebral blocks in breast cancer, epidural anesthesia in colorectal and lung cancer) consistently show no improvements in recurrence-free or overall survival, suggesting limited oncologic benefits.
- *Propofol TIVA vs. Volatile Anesthesia*: Retrospective and meta-analyses suggested potential survival advantages for propofol TIVA, but large RCTs have not substantiated these findings. Ongoing studies, such as the VAPOR-C trial, aim to clarify its role in specific cancers.
- *Opioids*: Concerns from laboratory studies about opioids promoting tumor growth have not been confirmed clinically, with current evidence showing neutral or mixed effects based on tumor type and genomic profiles.
- *NSAIDs/COX-2 Inhibitors*: While preclinical studies showed reduced metastasis, clinical trials failed to demonstrate consistent survival benefits.
- *Lidocaine*: Systemic lidocaine infusions showed mixed results, but a large RCT demonstrated significant survival benefits with peritumoral lidocaine infiltration in breast cancer, highlighting the importance of administration route and timing.
- *Dexmedetomidine*: Preliminary evidence from RCTs suggests potential benefits for recurrence-free survival, but these findings require confirmation in dedicated trials.

The evidence emphasizes that individual patient biology, tumor genetics, and stage of disease influence outcomes more than any single anesthetic approach. Personalization and multidisciplinary collaboration are key moving forward.

Future Directions

1. *Personalized Onco-Anesthesia*: Biomarker-driven strategies identifying tumor and immune profiles may guide anesthetic selection, such as when propofol TIVA or lidocaine might provide benefits.
2. *Multimodal Strategies*: Combining regional techniques, systemic anesthetics, and adjuncts (e.g., NSAIDs, dexmedetomidine) could maximize potential benefits through synergistic mechanisms.
3. *Large-Scale RCTs*: Trials like VAPOR-C, which target specific cancers (e.g., colorectal, NSCLC), aim to provide clearer answers by addressing heterogeneity in prior studies.
4. *Integrated Care Models*: Anesthesiologists should collaborate closely with oncologists and surgeons to ensure perioperative interventions align with broader cancer treatment goals.
5. *Mechanistic Studies*: Understanding how anesthetics modulate tumor biology, immune responses, and microenvironments will refine future trials and patient selection.

Conclusion

While most RCTs have failed to confirm consistent survival or recurrence benefits for specific anesthetic techniques, emerging evidence, such as that from the lidocaine RCT, suggests the potential for targeted interventions under specific conditions. Future onco-anesthesia research must prioritize individualized care, integrate multidisciplinary efforts, and focus on biomarker-driven strategies to optimize cancer outcomes.

References

1. Siegel RL, Miller KD, Fuchs HE, Jemal A. Cancer statistics, 2021. CA Cancer J Clin. 2021;71(1):7–33.
2. Ward ZJ, Scott AM, Hricak H, Abdel-Wahab M, Paez D, Lette MM, et al. Estimating the impact of treatment and imaging modalities on 5-year net survival of 11 cancers in 200 countries: a simulation-based analysis. Lancet Oncol. 2020;21(8):1077–88.
3. Meara JG, Leather AJM, Hagander L, Alkire BC, Alonso N, Ameh EA, et al. Global surgery 2030: evidence and solutions for achieving health, welfare, and economic development. Lancet. 2015;386(9993):569–624.
4. Ramly MS, Buggy DJ. Anesthetic techniques and cancer outcomes: what is the current evidence? Anesth Analg. 2025 Apr 1; 140(4):768–777
5. Guo R, Yang WW, Zhong ML, Rao PG, Luo X, Liao BZ, et al. The relationship between anesthesia, surgery and postoperative immune function in cancer patients: a review. Front Immunol. 2024;15:1441020.
6. Murphy O, Forget P, Ma D, Buggy DJ. Tumour excisional surgery, anaesthetic-analgesic techniques, and oncologic outcomes: a narrative review. Br J Anaesth. 2023;131(6):989–1001.
7. Choi H, Hwang W. Anesthetic approaches and their impact on cancer recurrence and metastasis: a comprehensive review. Cancer. 2024;16(24):4269.
8. Raskov H, Orhan A, Salanti A, Gögenur I. Premetastatic niches, exosomes and circulating tumor cells: early mechanisms of tumor dissemination and the relation to surgery. Int J Cancer. 2020;146(12):3244–55.
9. Cheng X, Zhang H, Hamad A, Huang H, Tsung A. Surgery-mediated tumor-promoting effects on the immune microenvironment. Semin Cancer Biol. 2022;86(Pt 3):408–19.
10. Cusack B, Buggy DJ. Anaesthesia, analgesia, and the surgical stress response. BJA Educ. 2020;20(9):321–8.

11. Onuma AE, Zhang H, Gil L, Huang H, Tsung A. Surgical stress promotes tumor progression: a focus on the impact of the immune response. J Clin Med. 2020;9(12):4096.
12. Decker D, Schöndorf M, Bidlingmaier F, Hirner A, von Ruecker AA. Surgical stress induces a shift in the type-1/type-2 T-helper cell balance, suggesting down-regulation of cell-mediated and up-regulation of antibody-mediated immunity commensurate to the trauma. Surgery. 1996;119(3):316–25.
13. Angka L, Khan ST, Kilgour MK, Xu R, Kennedy MA, Auer RC. Dysfunctional natural killer cells in the aftermath of cancer surgery. Int J Mol Sci. 2017;18(8):1787.
14. Tang F, Tie Y, Tu C, Wei X. Surgical trauma-induced immunosuppression in cancer: recent advances and the potential therapies. Clin Transl Med. 2020;10(1):199–223.
15. Weitz J, Kienle P, Lacroix J, Willeke F, Benner A, Lehnert T, et al. Dissemination of tumor cells in patients undergoing surgery for colorectal cancer. Clin Cancer Res. 1998;4(2):343–8.
16. Xia SH, Zhou D, Ge F, Sun M, Chen X, Zhang H, et al. Influence of perioperative anesthesia on cancer recurrence: from basic science to clinical practice. Curr Oncol Rep. 2023;25(2):63–81.
17. Brogi E, Forfori F. Anesthesia and cancer recurrence: an overview. J Anesth Analg Crit Care. 2022;2(1):33.
18. Gottschalk A, Sharma S, Ford J, Durieux ME, Tiouririne M. Review article: the role of the perioperative period in recurrence after cancer surgery. Anesth Analg. 2010;110(6):1636–43.
19. Coffey JC, Wang JH, Smith MJF, Bouchier-Hayes D, Cotter TG, Redmond HP. Excisional surgery for cancer cure: therapy at a cost. Lancet Oncol. 2003;4(12):760–8.
20. Cata JP, Ramirez MF, Velasquez JF, Di AI, Popat KU, Gottumukkala V, et al. Lidocaine stimulates the function of natural killer cells in different experimental settings. Anticancer Res. 2017;37(9):4727–32.
21. Sessler DI, Pei L, Huang Y, Fleischmann E, Marhofer P, Kurz A, et al. Recurrence of breast cancer after regional or general anaesthesia: a randomised controlled trial. Lancet. 2019;394(10211):1807–15.
22. Rangel FP, JOC A, MJC C, Cordeiro MD, Nahas WC, Coelho RF, et al. Opioids and premature biochemical recurrence of prostate cancer: a randomised prospective clinical trial. Br J Anaesth. 2021;126(5):931–9.
23. Dockrell L, Buggy DJ. The role of regional anaesthesia in the emerging subspecialty of onco-anaesthesia: a state-of-the-art review. Anaesthesia. 2021;76(S1):148–59.
24. Jansen L, Dubois BFH, Hollmann MW. The effect of propofol versus inhalation anesthetics on survival after oncological surgery. J Clin Med. 2022;11(22):6741.
25. Welch DR, Hurst DR. Defining the hallmarks of metastasis. Cancer Res. 2019;79(12):3011–27.
26. Enlund M, Berglund A, Enlund A, Bergkvist L. Volatile versus Propofol general anesthesia and long-term survival after breast cancer surgery: a National Registry Retrospective Cohort Study. Anesthesiology. 2022;137(3):315–26.
27. Chang CY, Wu MY, Chien YJ, Su IM, Wang SC, Kao MC. Anesthesia and long-term oncological outcomes: a systematic review and meta-analysis. Anesth Analg. 2021;132(3):623–34.
28. Smith L, Cata JP, Forget P. Immunological insights into opioid-free Anaesthesia in oncological surgery: a scoping review. Curr Oncol Rep. 2022;24(10):1327–36.
29. Connolly JG, Tan KS, Mastrogiacomo B, Dycoco J, Caso R, Jones GD, et al. Intraoperative opioid exposure, tumour genomic alterations, and survival differences in people with lung adenocarcinoma. Br J Anaesth. 2021;127(1):75–84.
30. Haldar R, Ricon-Becker I, Radin A, Gutman M, Cole SW, Zmora O, et al. Perioperative COX2 and β-adrenergic blockade improves biomarkers of tumor metastasis, immunity, and inflammation in colorectal cancer: a randomized controlled trial. Cancer. 2020;126(17):3991–4001.
31. Coombes RC, Tovey H, Kilburn L, Mansi J, Palmieri C, Bartlett J, et al. Effect of celecoxib vs placebo as adjuvant therapy on disease-free survival among patients with breast cancer: the REACT randomized clinical trial. JAMA Oncol. 2021;7(9):1291–301.
32. Wall TP, Buggy DJ. Perioperative intravenous lidocaine and metastatic cancer recurrence – a narrative review. Front Oncol. 2021 Aug 2;11:688896
33. Johnson MZ, Crowley PD, Foley AG, Xue C, Connolly C, Gallagher HC, et al. Effect of perioperative lidocaine on metastasis after sevoflurane or ketamine-xylazine anaesthesia for breast tumour resection in a murine model. Br J Anaesth. 2018;121(1):76–85.
34. Cho JS, Seon K, Kim MY, Kim SW, Yoo YC. Effects of perioperative Dexmedetomidine on immunomodulation in uterine cancer surgery: a randomized, controlled trial. Front Oncol. Nov 16;11:749003
35. Zhang D-F, Su X, Meng Z-T, Li H-L, Wang D-X, Li X-Y, et al. Impact of Dexmedetomidine on long-term outcomes after noncardiac surgery in elderly: 3-year follow-up of a randomized controlled trial. Ann Surg. 2019;270(2):356–63.
36. Hou M, Zhou N, Li H, Wang B, Wang X, Wang X, et al. Morphine and ketamine treatment suppress the differentiation of T helper cells of patients with colorectal cancer in vitro. Exp Ther Med. 2019;17(1):935–42.
37. Zhang J, Chang CL, Lu CY, Chen HM, Wu SY. Paravertebral block in regional anesthesia with propofol sedation reduces locoregional recurrence in patients with breast cancer receiving breast conservative surgery compared with volatile inhalational without propofol in general anesthesia. Biomed Pharmacother. 2021;142:111991.
38. Hasselager RP, Hallas J, Gögenur I. Epidural analgesia and recurrence after colorectal cancer surgery: a Danish retrospective registry-based cohort study. Anesthesiology. 2022;136(3):459–71.
39. Hovaguimian F, Braun J, Z'graggen BR, Schläpfer M, Dumrese C, Ewald C, et al. Anesthesia and circulating tumor cells in primary breast cancer patients: a randomized controlled trial. Anesthesiology. 2020;133(3):548–58.
40. Badwe RA, Parmar V, Nair N, Joshi S, Hawaldar R, Pawar S, et al. Effect of Peritumoral infiltration of local anesthetic before surgery on survival in early breast cancer. J Clin Oncol. 2023;41(18):3318–28.
41. Xu ZZ, Li HJ, Li MH, Huang SM, Li X, Liu QH, et al. Epidural anesthesia-analgesia and recurrence-free survival after lung cancer surgery: a randomized trial. Anesthesiology. 2021;135(3):419–32.
42. Wall T, Sherwin A, Ma D, Buggy DJ. Influence of perioperative anaesthetic and analgesic interventions on oncological outcomes: a narrative review. Br J Anaesth. 2019;123(2):135–50.
43. Hayden JM, Oras J, Block L, Thörn S-E, Palmqvist C, Salehi S, et al. Intraperitoneal ropivacaine reduces time interval to initiation of chemotherapy after surgery for advanced ovarian cancer: randomised controlled double-blind pilot study. Br J Anaesth. 2020;124(5):562–70.
44. Tang Y, Tang L, Yao Y, Huang H, Chen B. Effects of anesthesia on long-term survival in cancer surgery: a systematic review and meta-analysis. Heliyon. 2024;10(3):e24791.
45. Yap A, Lopez-Olivo MA, Dubowitz J, Hiller J, Riedel B, Riedel B, et al. Anesthetic technique and cancer outcomes: a meta-analysis of total intravenous versus volatile anesthesia. Can J Anesth/J Can Anesth. 2019;66(5):546–61.
46. Alam A, Rampes S, Patel S, Hana Z, Ma D. Anesthetics or anesthetic techniques and cancer surgical outcomes: a possible link. Korean J Anesthesiol. 2021;74(3):191–203.
47. Sun P, Huang H, Ma J-C, Feng B, Zhang Y, Qin G, et al. Repurposing propofol for breast cancer therapy through promoting apoptosis and arresting cell cycle. Oncol Rep. 2024;52(5):155.
48. Jaura AI, Flood G, Gallagher HC, Buggy DJ. Differential effects of serum from patients administered distinct anaesthetic techniques on

apoptosis in breast cancer cells in vitro: a pilot study. Br J Anaesth. 2014;113(Suppl 1):i63–7.
49. Wang R, Li S, Wang B, Wang G, Zheng H. Impact of opioids and mu-opioid receptors on oncologic metastasis. Am J Cancer Res. 2024;14(9):4236–47.
50. Zhang HW, Wang F, Zhou YQ, Xu SP, Yu SY, Zhang ZG. Morphine suppresses liver cancer cell tumor properties in vitro and in vivo. Front Oncol. 2021;11:666446.
51. Belltall A, Mazzinari G, Garrido-Cano I, Giner F, Marí AM, Eroles P, et al. Opioid receptor expression in colorectal cancer: a nested matched case-control study. Front Oncol. Apr 6;12:801714
52. Ahn HJ. Anesthesia and cancer recurrence: a narrative review. APM. 2024;19(2):94–108.
53. Carnet Le Provost K, Kepp O, Kroemer G, Bezu L. Trial watch: dexmedetomidine in cancer therapy. Onco Targets Ther. 2024;13(1):2327143.
54. Lavon H, Matzner P, Benbenishty A, Sorski L, Rossene E, Haldar R, et al. Dexmedetomidine promotes metastasis in rodent models of breast, lung, and colon cancers. Br J Anaesth. 2018;120(1):188–96.
55. Yin T, Wang G, Ye T, Wang Y. Sulindac, a non-steroidal anti-inflammatory drug, mediates breast cancer inhibition as an immune modulator. Sci Rep. 2016;6(1):19534.
56. Khadka S, Druffner SR, Duncan BC, Busada JT. Glucocorticoid regulation of cancer development and progression. Front Endocrinol (Lausanne). 2023;14:1161768.
57. Melamed R, Bar-Yosef S, Shakhar G, Shakhar K, Ben-Eliyahu S. Suppression of natural killer cell activity and promotion of tumor metastasis by ketamine, thiopental, and halothane, but not by propofol: mediating mechanisms and prophylactic measures. Anesth Analg. 2003;97(5):1331–9.
58. Mintz J, Vedenko A, Rosete O, Shah K, Goldstein G, Hare JM, et al. Current advances of nitric oxide in cancer and anticancer therapeutics. Vaccines (Basel). 2021 Jan 27;9(2):94
59. Kim R. Effects of surgery and anesthetic choice on immunosuppression and cancer recurrence. J Transl Med. 2018;16(1):8.
60. Enlund M, Berglund A, Ahlstrand R, Walldén J, Lundberg J, Wärnberg F, et al. Survival after primary breast cancer surgery following propofol or sevoflurane general anesthesia-a retrospective, multicenter, database analysis of 6305 Swedish patients. Acta Anaesthesiol Scand. 2020;64(8):1048–54.
61. Yoo S, Lee H-B, Han W, Noh D-Y, Park S K, Kim WH, et al. Total intravenous anesthesia versus inhalation anesthesia for breast cancer surgery: a retrospective cohort study. Anesthesiology. 2019;130(1):31–40.
62. Huang YH, Lee MS, Lou YS, Lai HC, Yu JC, Lu CH, et al. Propofol-based total intravenous anesthesia did not improve survival compared to desflurane anesthesia in breast cancer surgery. PLoS One. 2019;14(11):e0224728.
63. Kim MH, Kim DW, Park S, Kim JH, Lee KY, Hwang J, et al. Single dose of dexamethasone is not associated with postoperative recurrence and mortality in breast cancer patients: a propensity-matched cohort study. BMC Cancer. 2019;19(1):251.
64. Wu ZF, Lee MS, Wong CS, Lu CH, Huang YS, Lin KT, et al. Propofol-based total intravenous anesthesia is associated with better survival than desflurane anesthesia in colon cancer surgery. Anesthesiology. 2018;129(5):932–41.
65. Makito K, Matsui H, Fushimi K, Yasunaga H. Volatile versus Total intravenous anesthesia for cancer prognosis in patients having digestive cancer surgery: a Nationwide retrospective cohort study. Anesthesiology. 2020;133(4):764–73.
66. Lai HC, Lee MS, Lin C, Lin KT, Huang YH, Wong CS, et al. Propofol-based total intravenous anaesthesia is associated with better survival than desflurane anaesthesia in hepatectomy for hepatocellular carcinoma: a retrospective cohort study. Br J Anaesth. 2019;123(2):151–60.
67. Zheng X, Wang Y, Dong L, Zhao S, Wang L, Chen H, et al. Effects of propofol-based total intravenous anesthesia on gastric cancer: a retrospective study. Onco Targets Ther. 2018;11:1141–8.
68. Zhang H, Yang L, Zhu X, Zhu M, Sun Z, Cata JP, et al. Association between intraoperative intravenous lidocaine infusion and survival in patients undergoing pancreatectomy for pancreatic cancer: a retrospective study. Br J Anaesth. 2020;125(2):141–8.
69. Du KN, Feng L, Newhouse A, Mehta J, Lasala J, Mena GE, et al. Effects of intraoperative opioid use on recurrence-free and overall survival in patients with esophageal adenocarcinoma and squamous cell carcinoma. Anesth Analg. 2018;127(1):210–6.
70. Huang WW, Zhu WZ, Mu DL, Ji XQ, Nie XL, Li XY, et al. Perioperative management may improve long-term survival in patients after lung cancer surgery: a retrospective cohort study. Anesth Analg. 2018;126(5):1666–74.
71. Oh TK, Kim K, Jheon S, Lee J, Do SH, Hwang JW, et al. Long-term oncologic outcomes for patients undergoing volatile versus intravenous anesthesia for non-small cell lung cancer surgery: a retrospective propensity matching analysis. Cancer Control. 2018;25(1):1073274818775360.
72. Mao S, Wu Y, Wang R, Guo Y, Yuan J, Zhang W, et al. Association between perioperative glucocorticoids and cancer metastasis and survival in patients undergoing radical cystectomy for urothelial carcinoma of the bladder: a single-center retrospective study. Investig Clin Urol. 2020;61(4):382–9.
73. O'Bryan LJ, Atkins KJ, Lipszyc A, Scott DA, Silbert BS, Evered LA. Inflammatory biomarker levels after propofol or sevoflurane anesthesia: a meta-analysis. Anesth Analg. 2022;134(1):69–81.
74. Wigmore TJ, Mohammed K, Jhanji S. Long-term survival for patients undergoing volatile versus IV anesthesia for cancer surgery: a retrospective analysis. Anesthesiology. 2016;124(1):69–79.
75. Cronin-Fenton DP, Heide-Jørgensen U, Ahern TP, Lash TL, Christiansen PM, Ejlertsen B, et al. Opioids and breast cancer recurrence: a Danish population-based cohort study. Cancer. 2015;121(19):3507–14.
76. Cata JP, Keerty V, Keerty D, Feng L, Norman PH, Gottumukkala V, et al. A retrospective analysis of the effect of intraoperative opioid dose on cancer recurrence after non-small cell lung cancer resection. Cancer Med. 2014;3(4):900–8.
77. Oh TK, Jeon JH, Lee JM, Kim MS, Kim JH, Lim H, et al. Association of high-dose postoperative opioids with recurrence risk in esophageal squamous cell carcinoma: reinterpreting ERAS protocols for long-term oncologic surgery outcomes. Dis Esophagus. 2017;30(10):1–8.
78. Tai Y-H, Wu H-L, Chang W-K, Tsou M-Y, Chen H-H, Chang K-Y. Intraoperative fentanyl consumption does not impact cancer recurrence or overall survival after curative colorectal cancer resection. Sci Rep. 2017;7(1):10816.
79. Cronin-Fenton DP, Heide-Jørgensen U, Ahern TP, Lash TL, Christiansen P, Ejlertsen B, et al. Low-dose aspirin, nonsteroidal anti-inflammatory drugs, selective COX-2 inhibitors and breast cancer recurrence. Epidemiology. 2016;27(4):586–93.
80. Melhem-Bertrandt A, Chavez-Macgregor M, Lei X, Brown EN, Lee RT, Meric-Bernstam F, et al. Beta-blocker use is associated with improved relapse-free survival in patients with triple-negative breast cancer. J Clin Oncol. 2011;29(19):2645–52.
81. Zhang Y, Chen H, Chen S, Li Z, Chen J, Li W. The effect of concomitant use of statins, NSAIDs, low-dose aspirin, metformin and beta-blockers on outcomes in patients receiving immune checkpoint inhibitors: a systematic review and meta-analysis. Onco Targets Ther. 2021;10(1):1957605.
82. Huh J, Hwang W. The role of anesthetic management in lung cancer recurrence and metastasis: a comprehensive review. J Clin Med. 2024 Nov 7;13(22):6681

83. Rodriguez Arango JA, Zec T, Khalife M. Perioperative ketamine and cancer recurrence: a comprehensive review. J Clin Med. 2024 Mar 26;13(7):1920.
84. Aghamelu O, Buggy P, Smith G, Inzitari R, Wall T, Buggy DJ. Serum NETosis expression and recurrence risk after regional or volatile anaesthesia during breast cancer surgery: a pilot, prospective, randomised single-blind clinical trial. Acta Anaesthesiol Scand. 2021;65(3):313–9.
85. Oh CS, Park HJ, Piao L, Sohn KM, Koh SE, Hwang DY, et al. Expression profiles of immune cells after propofol or sevoflurane anesthesia for colorectal cancer surgery: a prospective double-blind randomized trial. Anesthesiology. 2022;136(3):448–58.
86. Falk W, Magnuson A, Eintrei C, Henningsson R, Myrelid P, Matthiessen P, et al. Comparison between epidural and intravenous analgesia effects on disease-free survival after colorectal cancer surgery: a randomised multicentre controlled trial. Br J Anaesth. 2021;127(1):65–74.
87. Cho JS, Kim NY, Shim J-K, Jun JH, Lee S, Kwak Y-L. The immunomodulatory effect of ketamine in colorectal cancer surgery: a randomized-controlled trial. Can J Anesth/J Can Anesth. 2021;68(5):683–92.
88. Zhang H, Qu M, Guo K, Wang Y, Gu J, Wu H, et al. Intraoperative lidocaine infusion in patients undergoing pancreatectomy for pancreatic cancer: a mechanistic, multicentre randomised clinical trial. Br J Anaesth. 2022;129(2):244–53.
89. Cao S-J, Zhang Y, Zhang Y-X, Zhao W, Pan L-H, Sun X-D, et al. Long-term survival in older patients given propofol or sevoflurane anaesthesia for major cancer surgery: follow-up of a multicentre randomised trial. Br J Anaesth. 2023;131(2):266–75.
90. A NE, Burns D, Riedel B, Sessler DI, Buggy DJ. The effect of anaesthetic technique during primary breast cancer surgery on neutrophil-lymphocyte ratio, platelet-lymphocyte ratio and return to intended oncological therapy. Anaesthesia. 2018;73(5):603–11.
91. Dubowitz JA, Cata JP, De Silva AP, Braat S, Shan D, Yee K, et al. Volatile anaesthesia and peri-operative outcomes related to cancer: a feasibility and pilot study for a large randomised control trial. Anaesthesia. 2021;76(9):1198–206.
92. Myles PS, Peyton P, Silbert B, Hunt J, Rigg JRA, Sessler DI. Perioperative epidural analgesia for major abdominal surgery for cancer and recurrence-free survival: randomised trial. BMJ. 2011;342:d1491.
93. Meyerhardt JA, Shi Q, Fuchs CS, Meyer J, Niedzwiecki D, Zemla T, et al. Effect of celecoxib vs placebo added to standard adjuvant therapy on disease-free survival among patients with stage III colon cancer: the CALGB/SWOG 80702 (Alliance) randomized clinical trial. JAMA. 2021;325(13):1277–86.

Radiology in Cancer Research

29

Erez Klein, Ghassan El-Haddad, Vaiva Gustainyte, Hakob Kocharyan, and Altan Ahmed

Introduction

Radiology serves an essential role in cancer research, acting as a cornerstone for the detection, diagnosis, monitoring, and treatment of cancer. The integration of advanced imaging techniques such as computed tomography (CT), magnetic resonance imaging (MRI), positron emission tomography (PET), and ultrasound has revolutionized oncology by providing detailed insights into tumor morphology, metabolism, and molecular characteristics. Imaging facilitates early detection of malignancies, often before they become symptomatic, thereby allowing for timely intervention and significantly improving patient outcomes. Imaging is indispensable for accurate staging of cancer, which is critical for selecting appropriate therapeutic strategies, assessing prognosis, guiding invasive procedures, and delivering targeted therapies. Innovations such as functional imaging and radiomics are pushing the boundaries even further, offering the potential to visualize the biological behavior of tumors and personalize treatment plans based on individual tumor profiles. The synergy between medical imaging and cancer research is fundamental, driving advancements that continuously improve the understanding and management of cancer, ultimately aiming for improved survival rates and quality of life for patients.

E. Klein (✉) · G. El-Haddad · V. Gustainyte · H. Kocharyan · A. Ahmed
Department of Diagnostic Imaging and Interventional Radiology, Moffitt Cancer Center, Tampa, FL, USA
e-mail: Erez.Klein@moffitt.org; Ghassan.Elhaddad@moffitt.org; Vaiva.Gustainyte@moffitt.org; Hakob.Kocharyan@moffitt.org; Altan.Ahmed@moffitt.org

Fundamental Elements of Radiology in Oncologic Clinical Care and Research

1. **Screening and Early Cancer Detection**

Imaging technologies like CT, MRI, PET, radiography, and ultrasound are being researched for improving early cancer detection. Early detection through screening is key for maximizing treatment options and reducing the risk of regional or widespread metastatic disease, which can develop through mechanisms such as clonal expansion and diversification of cancer cell populations [1].

In breast cancer, technologies such as contrast-enhanced mammography (CEM) demonstrate enhanced sensitivity and specificity in the detection of breast cancer compared to digital mammography alone, particularly in the setting of dense breast tissue [2–4]. Similarly, MRI is being investigated for screening beyond select populations, histologic subtyping, treatment decision-making, and response assessment [5–10].

CT colonography is another example of a minimally invasive screening technique. While limited by the inability to obtain a tissue for histologic diagnosis and by its lack of therapeutic potential, the sensitivity and specificity for the detection of cancer approach that of optical colonoscopy. A prospective multicenter randomized controlled trial compared colonoscopy (n = 1072) to CT colonography (n = 538) and found similar sensitivity for the detection of colorectal cancer. Further research is needed on the utility of CT colonography as a first-line screening tool and the long-term clinical impact of extra-colonic findings identified during screening [11–15].

2. **Tumor Characterization and Staging**

Understanding the impact of tumor characteristics, such as vascularity, metabolism, and heterogeneity, and the impact of these characteristics on prognosis and response to therapy

J. Huang, H. S.L. Jim (eds.), *Cancer Research Guidance for Clinicians and Researchers*,
https://doi.org/10.1007/978-3-032-19175-5_29

is an evolving component of oncologic radiology research. Radiomics combines additional features such as texture, shape, and enhancement intensity to aid with these assessments. Techniques like dynamic contrast-enhanced MRI (DCE-MRI), diffusion-weighted MRI (DW-MRI), and MR spectroscopy are being developed to provide more accurate characterization of tumors [7]. In renal cell carcinoma, low T1 signal and cystic features on MRI are associated with less aggressive histologic features and improved clinical prognosis [16]. MRI evidence of extramural venous invasion or tumor deposits has been shown to correlate with distant recurrence in rectal cancer, whereas the traditional TNM (tumor and nodal components) system has not [17].

Dual-energy CT (DECT) or spectral CT acquires images at different energy spectra to enhance material characterization and differentiation [18]. Retrospective studies in patients with papillary thyroid cancer have shown that arterial phase iodine concentration (IC), effective atomic number (Z_{eff}), and the spectral Hounsfield unit curve (λ_{HU}) are higher in metastatic lymph nodes as compared to benign lymph nodes [19, 20]. Similar findings have been presented in thoracic oncology, where malignant pulmonary nodules tend to demonstrate higher IC and normalized iodine concentration compared with benign nodules [21]. DECT may also provide additional insight into lymphovascular invasion and Ki-67 expression in both gastric and colorectal cancers [22–25].

3. **Image-Guided Therapy**

Image-guided interventions, such as intra-arterial therapy, percutaneous ablation, radiation therapy, and minimally invasive surgery, rely on a variety of imaging modalities for guidance and response assessment techniques. Areas of research include dose reduction in ionizing imaging modalities, robotic-assisted guidance technologies, increasing the conformality of locoregional therapies, predicting response, and radiation dosimetry.

Percutaneous ablation involves the introduction of a thermal (e.g., microwave, radiofrequency, cryogenic) or nonthermal (e.g., irreversible electroporation) energy into tumors to destroy tissue in situ. Ablation zone prediction and confirmation are among the challenges in percutaneous image-guided ablation procedures, as it directly affects treatment efficacy. Accurately determining the extent and location of the ablation zone is essential to ensure complete tumor destruction. Multiple retrospective analyses with cohorts ranging from 68 to 113 patients have demonstrated that intraprocedural minimum ablation margin (MAM) assessment via three-dimensional volumetric analysis correlates with risk of local tumor progression across multiple tumor types [26–30]. Physiologic and histologic assessments utilizing methods including ^{18}F-FDG PET/CT, ammonia perfusion PET, and immunofluorescence viability analysis offer a more detailed assessment of the ablation zone and MAM but require further investigation before incorporation into practice [31–33].

4. **Personalized Treatment Planning**

Advances in imaging are enabling more precise therapy planning and delivery, thereby minimizing injury to surrounding tissues and increasing tumor control. Functional imaging, which includes techniques like PET-CT/MRI, provides both functional and anatomic information to further guide therapy.

Somatostatin receptor–based imaging agents such as ^{68}Ga-DOTATATE PET/CT have demonstrated significant advantages compared with traditional imaging methods and planar scintigraphy [34]. A study of 97 consecutive patients, 78 of whom had both ^{68}Ga-DOTATATE PET/CT and ^{111}In-pentetreotide imaging, found that ^{68}Ga-DOTATATE imaging changed the care plan in 36% of patients and had lower patient radiation exposure [35]. Apart from initial staging, these analogs provide an additional tool for localizing the primary site of tumors, for which it is otherwise unknown, which may facilitate treatment. Patients with tumors that demonstrate somatostatin receptor positivity and appropriate disease distribution may be candidates for peptide receptor radionuclide therapy [35, 36]. Response can also be monitored utilizing the same imaging techniques [37]. The identification of additional theragnostic agents, discussed in more detail below, is a major need across cancers of many types.

Radioembolization is a locoregional therapy for the treatment of many primary and secondary hepatic malignancies. Radiologic-pathologic correlation studies have demonstrated a clear dose-response relationship. This is best demonstrated in the treatment of hepatocellular carcinoma, where two retrospective studies have shown increased rates of complete pathologic necrosis following radioembolization utilizing ablative dosimetry [38–40]. For Yttrium-90 radioembolization, utilization of ^{99m}Tc-macroaggregated albumin (^{99m}Tc-MAA) as ^{90}Y surrogate has allowed for more accurate dosimetry and prediction of tumor response when multi-compartment personalized dosimetry models are utilized [41–43]. There is an ongoing need for accurate methods to predict distribution, tumor dose, and parenchymal dose. Future research may involve the identification of alternative surrogates and imaging methodologies to facilitate optimal treatment planning.

5. **Prognostics and Treatment Response**

Monitoring treatment response and assessing tumor recurrence is a core element of imaging in oncology. Cross-sectional imaging modalities are regularly used to track the size and characteristics of tumors during and after treatment. PET-CT/MRI adds a physiologic assessment to conventional imaging and may provide additional insights into response and detect recurrence earlier. Advanced imaging techniques such as iodine mapping with DECT are being investigated to assess response to systemic and locoregional therapies [44]. A retrospective study of 25 patients with pancreatic cancer demonstrated a correlation between extracellular volume fraction, derived from iodine maps, and treatment response [45].

Molecular imaging is an area of rapid innovation in oncologic radiology. Noninvasive methods of assessing therapeutic targets could enhance tumor identification, treatment selection, patient stratification, and response to therapy. Preclinical studies have investigated methods to assess therapeutic targets, including PD-1, PD-L1, and CTLA-4 [46–50].

RECIST: Response Evaluation Criteria in Solid Tumors

RECIST is a set of standardized criteria used to measure the response of solid tumors to treatment in clinical trials and practice [51].

Clinical Relevance

RECIST criteria are fundamental in oncology for determining the efficacy of treatments in clinical trials, guiding therapy decisions, and facilitating communication among healthcare providers. The criteria help in making informed decisions about continuing, changing, or stopping treatments based on the objective response of tumors [52].

Key Features of RECIST [51, 53]

1. **Measurement Categories**

   - **Complete Response (CR)**: Disappearance of all target lesions, with any pathological lymph nodes reduced to less than 10 mm in short-axis measurement.
   - **Partial Response (PR)**: At least a 30% decrease in the sum of the diameters of target lesions, compared to the baseline sum.
   - **Stable Disease (SD)**: Neither sufficient shrinkage to qualify for PR nor sufficient increase to qualify for progressive disease.
   - **Progressive Disease (PD)**: At least a 20% increase in the sum of diameters of target lesions, taking as reference the smallest sum on study (including baseline if that is the smallest). An absolute increase of at least 5 mm is also required, or the appearance of one or more new lesions.

2. **Lesion Types**

   - **Target Lesions**: These are chosen based on being measurable and representative of the tumor burden. Up to five lesions in total, with a maximum of two per organ, can be selected.
   - **Nontarget Lesions**: These include all other lesions or sites of disease, such as small lesions or those not easily measurable. Their presence or absence contributes to the overall assessment.

3. **Special Considerations**

   - **Coalescing Lesions**: When lesions merge into a single mass, the longest diameter of the merged lesion is measured.
   - **Fragmented Lesions**: If a lesion splits into smaller lesions, the sum of the longest diameters of the individual parts is used.
   - **New Lesions**: The appearance of new lesions is a strong indicator of progressive disease.

4. **Updates and Versions**

   - **RECIST 1.1**: The most current version, updated to refine the measurement criteria and improve clarity. It includes guidance on lymph node measurement and new lesion assessment [53].
   - **iRECIST**: A modified version designed to address the unique responses seen with immunotherapy [54].

Radiomics in Cancer Research

Radiomics is an emerging field within medical imaging and oncology that involves the extraction and analysis of quantitative features from medical images using data-characterization algorithms [55]. The goal of radiomics is to improve diagnostic, prognostic, and predictive accuracy by providing more detailed objective data from imaging studies than what is available through traditional qualitative assessments [56]. Some of the key aspects and components of radiomics are as follows.

Key Concepts [56–59]

1. **Image Acquisition**: Radiomics begins with the acquisition of high-quality medical images. These can include various imaging modalities such as CT, MRI, and PET.
2. **Segmentation**: This step involves delineating the region of interest (ROI) within the images. Segmentation can be manual, semiautomatic, or fully automatic. Accurate segmentation is crucial as it directly influences the subsequent feature extraction process.
3. **Feature Extraction**: Once the ROI is identified, a large number of quantitative features are extracted. These features can be broadly categorized into

   - **Shape-Based Features**: Describe the geometry of the ROI, such as volume, surface area, and sphericity.
   - **Intensity-Based Features**: Quantify the distribution of voxel intensities within the ROI, including first-order statistics like mean, median, and standard deviation.
   - **Texture-Based Features**: Capture the spatial arrangement of voxel intensities, providing information about the texture of the tissue. These include gray-level co-occurrence matrix (GLCM) features and gray-level run-length matrix (GLRLM) features.
   - **Wavelet Features**: Decompose the image into different frequency components to extract additional texture information.

4. **Data Preprocessing**: This involves normalizing and standardizing the extracted features to reduce variability and improve the robustness of the analysis.
5. **Feature Selection**: Given the high dimensionality of radiomic data, feature selection techniques are employed to identify the most relevant features that contribute to the clinical outcome of interest. Methods can include statistical tests, machine learning algorithms, and dimensionality reduction techniques like PCA (principal component analysis).
6. **Model Building**: The selected features are then used to build predictive models using machine learning algorithms. Commonly used algorithms include logistic regression, support vector machines (SVM), random forests, and neural networks.
7. **Validation**: Models are validated using independent datasets to assess their performance and generalizability. Validation techniques include cross-validation, bootstrapping, and external validation with separate cohorts.

Applications of Radiomics [60–63]

1. **Cancer Diagnosis and Characterization**: Radiomics can help differentiate between benign and malignant lesions, characterize tumor subtypes, and identify molecular and genetic profiles of tumors.
2. **Prognosis and Outcome Prediction**: By analyzing radiomic features, it is possible to predict patient outcomes such as overall survival, disease-free survival, and recurrence.
3. **Treatment Response Assessment**: Radiomics can be used to evaluate how well a patient is responding to treatment, allowing for adjustments in therapy if needed.
4. **Personalized Medicine**: By integrating radiomic data with other clinical and genomic information, personalized treatment plans can be developed to optimize patient care.

Challenges and Considerations [64–66]

1. **Reproducibility**: Ensuring the reproducibility of radiomic features across different imaging protocols and institutions is a major challenge.
2. **Standardization**: Developing standardized methods for image acquisition, feature extraction, and analysis is crucial for the widespread adoption of radiomics.
3. **Data Integration**: Integrating radiomic data with other types of clinical and biological data requires advanced data integration techniques and robust computational frameworks.
4. **Regulatory and Ethical Issues**: The clinical implementation of radiomics involves regulatory and ethical considerations, including patient privacy, data security, and the clinical validation of radiomic biomarkers.

Theragnostics

Theragnostics, also known as theranostics, is a combination of "therapy" and "diagnostics." It refers to a field of medicine that combines diagnostic imaging and targeted therapy [67].

Key Concepts [68, 69]

1. **Personalized Medicine**: Theragnostics aims to tailor medical treatment to the individual characteristics of each patient. By using diagnostic tools to identify specific biomarkers or molecular targets, therapies can be customized to the patient's unique disease profile.
2. **Targeted Therapy**: This approach involves using treatments that specifically target the molecular and cellular mechanisms of a disease. Targeted therapies can include monoclonal antibodies, small-molecule inhibitors, and radiopharmaceuticals.
3. **Diagnostic Imaging**: Advanced imaging techniques such as PET, SPECT (single-photon emission computed tomography), MRI, and CT are used to visualize disease processes in the body. These imaging modalities can identify the location, extent, and molecular characteristics of a disease.
4. **Radiopharmaceuticals**: These are radioactive compounds used in both diagnostic imaging and therapy. Radiopharmaceuticals can be designed to target specific cells or receptors, allowing for precise imaging and treatment of diseases.

Applications of Theragnostics [70]

- **Cancer Diagnosis**: Theragnostic approaches can identify specific cancer biomarkers, aiding in the diagnosis and staging of cancer.
- **Treatment Planning**: By visualizing tumor biology, clinicians can select the most appropriate targeted therapies.
- **Monitoring Treatment Response**: Imaging can be used to monitor how well a patient is responding to therapy, allowing for adjustments in treatment if necessary.

Techniques and Technologies [67–69, 71]

1. **Molecular Imaging**: Uses molecular probes to visualize and quantify biological processes at the molecular and cellular levels in living organisms.
2. **Radioligands**: These are radioactively labeled substances that bind to specific proteins or receptors in the body. Radioligands are used in both diagnostic imaging and targeted therapy.
3. **Biomarker Identification**: Identifying specific biomarkers is crucial for theragnostics. Biomarkers can be proteins, genes, or other molecules that indicate the presence or progression of a disease.
4. **Nanotechnology**: Nanoparticles can be used to deliver drugs directly to diseased cells, enhancing the efficacy of the therapy and reducing side effects [72].

Advantages of Theragnostics [67, 68]

1. **Precision**: Provides highly targeted treatments that reduce damage to healthy tissues and improve patient outcomes.
2. **Personalization**: Tailors treatments to individual patient profiles, improving efficacy and minimizing side effects.
3. **Improved Monitoring**: Allows for real-time monitoring of treatment responses, enabling timely adjustments to therapy.
4. **Cost-Effectiveness**: By improving the accuracy and efficacy of treatments, theragnostics may reduce the overall cost of care by decreasing the need for multiple treatment attempts.

Challenges and Considerations [73, 74]

1. **Complexity**: The integration of diagnostics and therapy requires sophisticated technology along with integrated workflows and expertise.
2. **Regulation**: Ensuring the safety and efficacy of theragnostic agents involves rigorous regulatory processes.
3. **Cost**: The development and implementation of theragnostic approaches can be expensive.
4. **Ethical Issues**: The use of personalized data in theragnostics raises ethical concerns regarding patient privacy and data security.

Examples of Theragnostic Agents [69, 71]

1. **Iodine-131**: Used in the treatment and imaging of thyroid cancer
2. **Lutetium-177**: Used in the treatment of neuroendocrine tumors (Fig. 29.1) and prostate cancer
3. **Gallium-68**: Used for PET imaging to diagnose neuroendocrine tumors

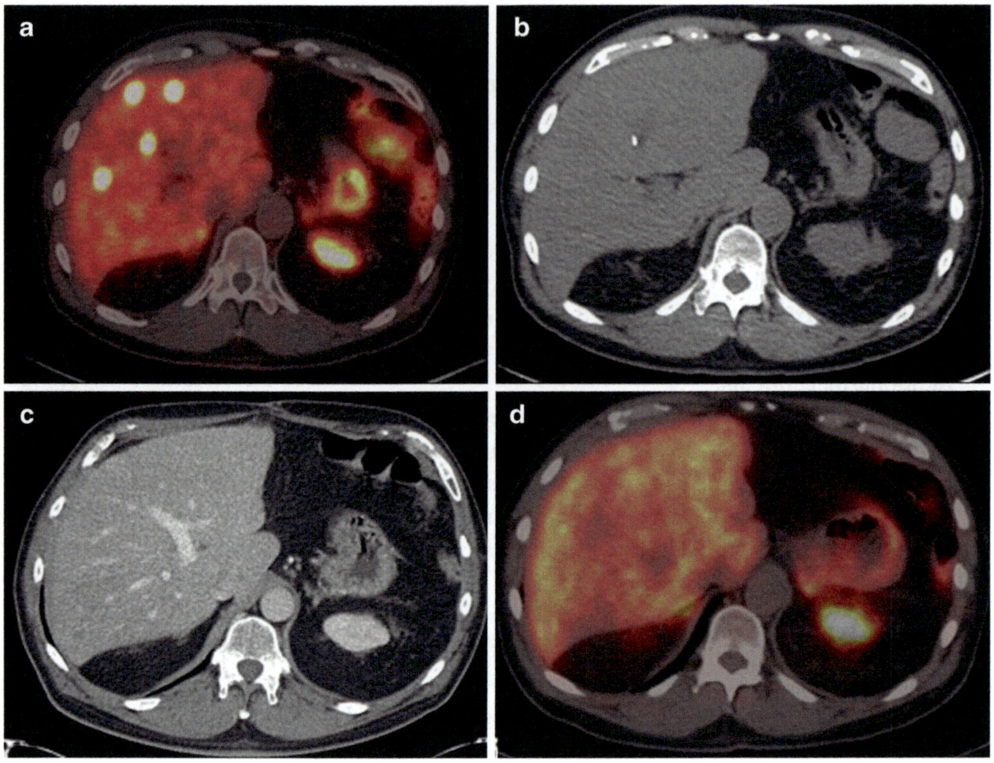

Fig. 29.1 A patient with hepatic metastatic neuroendocrine tumor underwent 68Ga-DOTATATE PET/CT (**a**) demonstrating multiple somatostatin receptor-positive metastases. These are not readily identified on the source non-contrast-enhanced CT (**b**) or same-day contrast-enhanced CT (**c**). 68Ga-DOTATATE PET/CT after completion of peptide receptor radionuclide therapy (**d**) demonstrates treatment response

Future Directions [67, 68, 70]

1. **Integration with Genomics**: Combining theragnostics with genomic data to further personalize treatments
2. **Artificial Intelligence**: Using AI to analyze imaging data and predict treatment responses
3. **Advanced Imaging Techniques**: Developing new imaging modalities to improve the precision and accuracy of theragnostic approaches
4. **Broader Applications**: Expanding the use of theragnostics beyond oncology to other fields such as infectious diseases and chronic conditions

Theragnostics represents a significant advancement in the field of medicine, providing a more integrated and personalized approach to disease management.

Artificial Intelligence (AI) in Oncologic Radiology

AI offers the potential to enhance diagnostic accuracy, improve workflow efficiency, and support decision-making processes. Research into AI in radiology focuses on the development of machine learning (ML) algorithms, particularly deep learning models, to analyze medical images with greater speed and precision than traditional methods. AI has demonstrated significant promise in various areas, such as early detection of cancer [59, 75–78].

ML algorithms, trained on vast datasets of medical images, can identify subtle patterns and anomalies that may be indicative of malignancy. For example, AI models have been shown to improve breast cancer detection in mammography by increasing sensitivity and reducing false positives [79, 80]. In lung cancer screening, AI-assisted CT scans are effective in identifying small nodules that may be missed by human radiologists [81]. However, challenges remain in integrating AI into clinical practice, such as ensuring the generalizability of models across diverse populations and reducing the risk of bias in algorithmic decision-making. Furthermore, the interpretability of AI models remains an area of active investigation, as understanding the rationale behind AI-generated recommendations is essential for clinical trust and regulatory approval [75]. Ongoing research is focused on improving the accuracy, transparency, and usability of AI tools to complement radiologists' expertise and enhance patient outcomes [77].

Summary

Radiology is fundamental in cancer research, playing a critical role in screening, diagnosis, prognostication, treatment, and clinical trials. Advanced imaging techniques are essential for accurately diagnosing cancer; assessing tumor size, location, and extent; and providing crucial information for treatment planning. In cancer clinical trials, imaging is vital for monitoring disease progression, evaluating treatment efficacy, and ensuring patient eligibility and safety. As the field advances, imaging is set to become even more integral to personalized medicine, with innovations like AI-enhanced imaging and molecular imaging enabling highly targeted and individualized treatment plans. These developments promise to improve diagnostic precision, patient outcomes, and the overall management of cancer.

References

1. Greaves M, Maley CC. Clonal evolution in cancer. Nature. 2012;481:306–13. https://doi.org/10.1038/nature10762.
2. Cheung Y-C, Lin Y-C, Wan Y-L, et al. Diagnostic performance of dual-energy contrast-enhanced subtracted mammography in dense breasts compared to mammography alone: interobserver blind-reading analysis. Eur Radiol. 2014;24:2394–403. https://doi.org/10.1007/s00330-014-3271-1.
3. Fallenberg EM, Dromain C, Diekmann F, et al. Contrast-enhanced spectral mammography versus MRI: initial results in the detection of breast cancer and assessment of tumour size. Eur Radiol. 2014;24:256–64. https://doi.org/10.1007/s00330-013-3007-7.
4. Jochelson MS, Lobbes MBI. Contrast-enhanced mammography: state of the art. Radiology. 2021;299:36–48. https://doi.org/10.1148/radiol.2021201948.
5. Kuhl CK. Abbreviated magnetic resonance imaging (MRI) for breast cancer screening: rationale, concept, and transfer to clinical practice. Annu Rev Med. 2019;70:501–19. https://doi.org/10.1146/annurev-med-121417-100403.
6. Bakker MF, de Lange SV, Pijnappel RM, et al. Supplemental MRI screening for women with extremely dense breast tissue. N Engl J Med. 2019;381:2091–102. https://doi.org/10.1056/NEJMoa1903986.
7. Huang Y, Wang X, Cao Y, et al. Multiparametric MRI model to predict molecular subtypes of breast cancer using Shapley additive explanations interpretability analysis. Diagn Interv Imaging. 2024;105:191–205. https://doi.org/10.1016/j.diii.2024.01.004.
8. Mann GB, Skandarajah AR, Zdenkowski N, et al. Postoperative radiotherapy omission in selected patients with early breast cancer following preoperative breast MRI (PROSPECT): primary results of a prospective two-arm study. Lancet. 2024;403:261–70. https://doi.org/10.1016/S0140-6736(23)02476-5.
9. Partridge SC, Gibbs JE, Lu Y, et al. Accuracy of MR imaging for revealing residual breast cancer in patients who have undergone neoadjuvant chemotherapy. AJR Am J Roentgenol. 2002;179:1193–9. https://doi.org/10.2214/ajr.179.5.1791193.
10. Esserman L, Kaplan E, Partridge S, et al. MRI phenotype is associated with response to doxorubicin and cyclophosphamide Neoadjuvant chemotherapy in stage III breast cancer. Ann Surg Oncol. 2001;8:549–59. https://doi.org/10.1007/s10434-001-0549-8.
11. Johnson CD, Chen M-H, Toledano AY, et al. Accuracy of CT Colonography for detection of large adenomas and cancers. N Engl J Med. 2008;359:1207–17. https://doi.org/10.1056/NEJMoa0800996.
12. Atkin W, Dadswell E, Wooldrage K, et al. Computed tomographic colonography versus colonoscopy for investigation of patients with symptoms suggestive of colorectal cancer (SIGGAR): a multicentre randomised trial. Lancet. 2013;381:1194–202. https://doi.org/10.1016/S0140-6736(12)62186-2.
13. Cash BD, Riddle MS, Bhattacharya I, et al. CT Colonography of a Medicare-aged population: outcomes observed in an analysis of more than 1400 patients. Am J Roentgenol. 2012;199:W27–34. https://doi.org/10.2214/AJR.11.7729.
14. Pickhardt PJ, Kim DH, Meiners RJ, et al. Colorectal and Extracolonic cancers detected at screening CT Colonography in 10 286 asymptomatic adults. Radiology. 2010;255:83–8. https://doi.org/10.1148/radiol.09090939.
15. Kim DH, Pickhardt PJ, Taylor AJ, et al. CT Colonography versus colonoscopy for the detection of advanced neoplasia. N Engl J Med. 2007;357:1403–12. https://doi.org/10.1056/NEJMoa070543.
16. Doshi AM, Huang WC, Donin NM, Chandarana H. MRI features of renal cell carcinoma that predict favorable Clinicopathologic outcomes. Am J Roentgenol. 2015;204:798–803. https://doi.org/10.2214/AJR.14.13227.
17. Lord AC, D'Souza N, Shaw A, et al. MRI-diagnosed tumor deposits and EMVI status have superior prognostic accuracy to current clinical TNM staging in rectal cancer. Ann Surg. 2022;276:334–44. https://doi.org/10.1097/SLA.0000000000004499.
18. Wang X, Shen H, Zhang J, et al. Dual-energy CT: a new frontier in oncology imaging. Meta-Radiology. 2023;1:100044. https://doi.org/10.1016/j.metrad.2023.100044.
19. Wu Y, Wei C, Wang C, et al. Preoperative prediction of cervical nodal metastasis in papillary thyroid carcinoma: value of quantitative dual-energy CT parameters and qualitative morphologic features. Am J Roentgenol. 2021;216:1335–43. https://doi.org/10.2214/AJR.20.23516.
20. Zou Y, Sun S, Liu Q, et al. A new prediction model for lateral cervical lymph node metastasis in patients with papillary thyroid carcinoma: based on dual-energy CT. Eur J Radiol. 2021;145:110060. https://doi.org/10.1016/j.ejrad.2021.110060.
21. Zegadło A, Żabicka M, Kania-Pudło M, et al. Assessment of solitary pulmonary nodules based on virtual monochrome images and iodine-dependent images using a single-source dual-energy CT with fast kVp switching. J Clin Med. 2020;9(8):2514. https://doi.org/10.3390/jcm9082514.
22. Li J, Wang Y, Wang R, et al. Spectral CT for preoperative prediction of lymphovascular invasion in resectable gastric cancer: with external prospective validation. Front Oncol. 2022;12:942425. https://doi.org/10.3389/fonc.2022.942425.
23. Cheng S-M, Ling W, Zhu J, et al. Dual energy spectral CT imaging in the assessment of gastric cancer and cell proliferation: a preliminary study. Sci Rep. 2018;8:17619. https://doi.org/10.1038/s41598-018-35712-w
24. Gao W, Zhang Y, Dou Y, et al. Association between extramural vascular invasion and iodine quantification using dual-energy computed tomography of rectal cancer: a preliminary study. Eur J Radiol. 2023;158:110618. https://doi.org/10.1016/j.ejrad.2022.110618.
25. Wang Y-L, Zhang H-W, Mo Y-Q, et al. Application of dual-layer spectral detector computed tomography to evaluate the expression of Ki-67 in colorectal cancer. J Chin Med Assoc. 2022;85(5):610–6. https://doi.org/10.1097/JCMA.0000000000000706.
26. Laimer G, Schullian P, Jaschke N, et al. Minimal ablative margin (MAM) assessment with image fusion: an independent predictor for local tumor progression in hepatocellular carcinoma after stereotactic radiofrequency ablation. Eur Radiol. 2020;30:2463–72. https://doi.org/10.1007/s00330-019-06609-7.
27. Laimer G, Verdonschot KHM, Kopf L, et al. Multicenter and inter-software evaluation of ablative margins after thermal ablation of colorectal liver metastases. Eur Radiol. 2025;35:1046–56. https://doi.org/10.1007/s00330-024-10956-5.
28. Lin Y-M, Paolucci I, Albuquerque Marques Silva J, et al. Ablative margin quantification using deformable versus rigid image registration in colorectal liver metastasis thermal ablation: a retrospective single-center study. Eur Radiol. 2024;34:5541–50. https://doi.org/10.1007/s00330-024-10632-8.

29. Lin Y-M, Paolucci I, Albuquerque Marques Silva J, et al. Intraprocedural versus initial follow-up minimal ablative margin assessment after colorectal liver metastasis thermal ablation: which one better predicts local outcomes? Investig Radiol. 2024;59:314–9. https://doi.org/10.1097/RLI.0000000000001023.
30. Kaye EA, Cornelis FH, Petre EN, et al. Volumetric 3D assessment of ablation zones after thermal ablation of colorectal liver metastases to improve prediction of local tumor progression. Eur Radiol. 2019;29:2698–705. https://doi.org/10.1007/s00330-018-5809-0.
31. Shyn PB, Casadaban LC, Sainani NI, et al. Intraprocedural ablation margin assessment by using ammonia perfusion PET during FDG PET/CT-guided liver tumor ablation: a pilot study. Radiology. 2018;288:138–45. https://doi.org/10.1148/radiol.2018172108.
32. Vasiniotis Kamarinos N, Vakiani E, Fujisawa S, et al. Immunofluorescence assay of ablated colorectal liver metastases: the frozen section of image-guided tumor ablation? J Vasc Interv Radiol. 2022;33:308–315.e1. https://doi.org/10.1016/j.jvir.2021.11.008.
33. Cornelis FH, Petre EN, Vakiani E, et al. Immediate Postablation 18F-FDG injection and corresponding SUV are surrogate biomarkers of local tumor progression after thermal ablation of colorectal carcinoma liver metastases. J Nucl Med. 2018;59:1360–5. https://doi.org/10.2967/jnumed.117.194506.
34. Galgano SJ, Iravani A, Bodei L, et al. Imaging of neuroendocrine neoplasms: monitoring treatment response— AJR expert panel narrative review. Am J Roentgenol. 2022;218:767–80. https://doi.org/10.2214/AJR.21.27159.
35. Deppen SA, Liu E, Blume JD, et al. Safety and efficacy of 68Ga-DOTATATE PET/CT for diagnosis, staging, and treatment Management of Neuroendocrine Tumors. J Nucl Med. 2016;57:708–14. https://doi.org/10.2967/jnumed.115.163865.
36. Qian ZR, Li T, Ter-Minassian M, et al. Association between somatostatin receptor expression and clinical outcomes in neuroendocrine tumors. Pancreas. 2016;45:1386–93. https://doi.org/10.1097/MPA.0000000000000700.
37. Sanli Y, Garg I, Kandathil A, et al. Neuroendocrine tumor diagnosis and management: 68 Ga-DOTATATE PET/CT. Am J Roentgenol. 2018;211:267–77. https://doi.org/10.2214/AJR.18.19881.
38. Montazeri SA, De la Garza-Ramos C, Silver C, et al. Achieving complete pathologic necrosis in hepatocellular carcinoma treated with radiation Segmentectomy before liver transplantation: a comprehensive glass microsphere analysis. Eur J Nucl Med Mol Imaging. 2025;52(9):3145–50. https://doi.org/10.1007/s00259-025-07179-1.
39. Montazeri SA, De la Garza-Ramos C, Lewis AR, et al. Hepatocellular carcinoma radiation segmentectomy treatment intensification prior to liver transplantation increases rates of complete pathologic necrosis: an explant analysis of 75 tumors. Eur J Nucl Med Mol Imaging. 2022;49:3892–7. https://doi.org/10.1007/s00259-022-05776-y.
40. Gabr A, Riaz A, Johnson GE, et al. Correlation of Y90-absorbed radiation dose to pathological necrosis in hepatocellular carcinoma: confirmatory multicenter analysis in 45 explants. Eur J Nucl Med Mol Imaging. 2021;48:580–3. https://doi.org/10.1007/s00259-020-04976-8.
41. Garin E, Lenoir L, Rolland Y, et al. Dosimetry based on 99mTc-macroaggregated albumin SPECT/CT accurately predicts tumor response and survival in hepatocellular carcinoma patients treated with 90Y-loaded glass microspheres: preliminary results. J Nucl Med. 2012;53:255–63. https://doi.org/10.2967/jnumed.111.094235.
42. Garin E, Tselikas L, Guiu B, et al. Personalised versus standard dosimetry approach of selective internal radiation therapy in patients with locally advanced hepatocellular carcinoma (DOSISPHERE-01): a randomised, multicentre, open-label phase 2 trial. Lancet Gastroenterol Hepatol. 2021;6:17–29. https://doi.org/10.1016/S2468-1253(20)30290-9.
43. Garin E, Rolland Y, Pracht M, et al. High impact of macroaggregated albumin-based tumour dose on response and overall survival in hepatocellular carcinoma patients treated with 90 Y-loaded glass microsphere radioembolization. Liver Int. 2017;37:101–10. https://doi.org/10.1111/liv.13220.
44. Park SY, Kim CK, Park BK. Dual-energy CT in assessing therapeutic response to radiofrequency ablation of renal cell carcinomas. Eur J Radiol. 2014;83:e73–9. https://doi.org/10.1016/j.ejrad.2013.11.022.
45. Noid G, Godfrey G, Hall W, et al. Predicting treatment response from extracellular volume fraction for Chemoradiation therapy of pancreatic cancer. Int J Radiat Oncol Biol Phys. 2023;115:803–8. https://doi.org/10.1016/j.ijrobp.2022.09.084.
46. Hettich M, Braun F, Bartholomä MD, et al. High-resolution PET imaging with therapeutic antibody-based PD-1/PD-L1 checkpoint tracers. Theranostics. 2016;6:1629–40. https://doi.org/10.7150/thno.15253.
47. Natarajan A, Mayer AT, Xu L, et al. Novel radiotracer for Immuno PET imaging of PD-1 checkpoint expression on tumor infiltrating lymphocytes. Bioconjug Chem. 2015;26:2062–9. https://doi.org/10.1021/acs.bioconjchem.5b00318.
48. Higashikawa K, Yagi K, Watanabe K, et al. 64Cu-DOTA-anti-CTLA-4 mAb enabled PET visualization of CTLA-4 on the T-cell infiltrating tumor tissues. PLoS One. 2014;9:e109866. https://doi.org/10.1371/journal.pone.0109866.
49. Chatterjee S, Lesniak WG, Gabrielson M, et al. A humanized antibody for imaging immune checkpoint ligand PD-L1 expression in tumors. Oncotarget. 2016;7:10215–27. https://doi.org/10.18632/oncotarget.7143.
50. Heskamp S, Hobo W, Molkenboer-Kuenen JDM, et al. Noninvasive imaging of tumor PD-L1 expression using radiolabeled anti-PD-L1 antibodies. Cancer Res. 2015;75:2928–36. https://doi.org/10.1158/0008-5472.CAN-14-3477.
51. Therasse P, Arbuck SG, Eisenhauer EA, et al. New guidelines to evaluate the response to treatment in solid tumors. European Organization for Research and Treatment of cancer, National Cancer Institute of the United States, National Cancer Institute of Canada. J Natl Cancer Inst. 2000;92:205–16. https://doi.org/10.1093/jnci/92.3.205.
52. Morse B, Jeong D, Ihnat G, Silva AC. Pearls and pitfalls of response evaluation criteria in solid tumors (RECIST) v1.1 non-target lesion assessment. Abdom Radiol. 2019;44:766–74. https://doi.org/10.1007/s00261-018-1752-4.
53. Eisenhauer EA, Therasse P, Bogaerts J, et al. New response evaluation criteria in solid tumours: revised RECIST guideline (version 1.1). Eur J Cancer. 2009;45:228–47. https://doi.org/10.1016/j.ejca.2008.10.026.
54. Seymour L, Bogaerts J, Perrone A, et al. iRECIST: guidelines for response criteria for use in trials testing immunotherapeutics. Lancet Oncol. 2017;18:e143–52. https://doi.org/10.1016/S1470-2045(17)30074-8.
55. Lambin P, Leijenaar RTH, Deist TM, et al. Radiomics: the bridge between medical imaging and personalized medicine. Nat Rev Clin Oncol. 2017;14:749–62. https://doi.org/10.1038/nrclinonc.2017.141.
56. Mendes Serrão E, Klug M, Moloney BM, et al. Current status of cancer genomics and imaging phenotypes: what radiologists need to know. Radiol Imaging Cancer. 2023;5:e220153. https://doi.org/10.1148/rycan.220153.
57. Lo Gullo R, Daimiel I, Morris EA, Pinker K. Combining molecular and imaging metrics in cancer: radiogenomics. Insights Imaging. 2020;11:1. https://doi.org/10.1186/s13244-019-0795-6.
58. Kummar S, Lu R. Using Radiomics in cancer management. JCO Precis Oncol. 2024;8:e2400155. https://doi.org/10.1200/PO.24.00155.

59. Horvat N, Papanikolaou N, Koh D-M. Radiomics beyond the hype: a critical evaluation toward oncologic clinical use. Radiol Artif Intell. 2024;6:e230437. https://doi.org/10.1148/ryai.230437.
60. Qi Y-J, Su G-H, You C, et al. Radiomics in breast cancer: current advances and future directions. Cell Rep Med. 2024;5:101719. https://doi.org/10.1016/j.xcrm.2024.101719.
61. Miranda J, Horvat N, Araujo-Filho JAB, et al. The role of Radiomics in rectal cancer. J Gastrointest Cancer. 2023;54:1158–80. https://doi.org/10.1007/s12029-022-00909-w.
62. Ye J-Y, Fang P, Peng Z-P, et al. A radiomics-based interpretable model to predict the pathological grade of pancreatic neuroendocrine tumors. Eur Radiol. 2024;34:1994–2005. https://doi.org/10.1007/s00330-023-10186-1.
63. Fusco R, Granata V, Setola SV, et al. The application of radiomics in cancer imaging with a focus on lung cancer, renal cell carcinoma, gastrointestinal cancer, and head and neck cancer: a systematic review. Phys Med. 2025;130:104891. https://doi.org/10.1016/j.ejmp.2025.104891.
64. Verma V, Simone CB, Krishnan S, et al. The rise of Radiomics and implications for oncologic management. J Natl Cancer Inst. 2017;109 https://doi.org/10.1093/jnci/djx055.
65. Liu Z, Wang S, Dong D, et al. The applications of Radiomics in precision diagnosis and treatment of oncology: opportunities and challenges. Theranostics. 2019;9:1303–22. https://doi.org/10.7150/thno.30309.
66. Fusco R, Granata V, Simonetti I, et al. An informative review of Radiomics studies on cancer imaging: the Main findings, challenges and limitations of the methodologies. Curr Oncol. 2024;31:403–24. https://doi.org/10.3390/curroncol31010027.
67. Burkett BJ, Bartlett DJ, McGarrah PW, et al. A review of Theranostics: perspectives on emerging approaches and clinical advancements. Radiol Imag Cancer. 2023;5:e220157. https://doi.org/10.1148/rycan.220157.
68. Turner JH. An introduction to the clinical practice of theranostics in oncology. Br J Radiol. 2018;91:20180440. https://doi.org/10.1259/bjr.20180440.
69. Aboagye EO, Barwick TD, Haberkorn U. Radiotheranostics in oncology: making precision medicine possible. CA Cancer J Clin. 2023;73:255–74. https://doi.org/10.3322/caac.21768.
70. Pascual TNB, Paez D, Iagaru A, et al. Guiding principles on the education and practice of theranostics. Eur J Nucl Med Mol Imaging. 2024;51:2320–31. https://doi.org/10.1007/s00259-024-06657-2.
71. Jadvar H, Chen X, Cai W, Mahmood U. Radiotheranostics in cancer diagnosis and management. Radiology. 2018;286:388–400. https://doi.org/10.1148/radiol.2017170346.
72. Duan H, Iagaru A, Aparici CM. Radiotheranostics-precision medicine in nuclear medicine and molecular imaging. Nano. 2022;6:103–17. https://doi.org/10.7150/ntno.64141.
73. Giammarile F, Paez D, Zimmermann R, et al. Production and regulatory issues for theranostics. Lancet Oncol. 2024;25:e260–9. https://doi.org/10.1016/S1470-2045(24)00041-X.
74. Bodei L, Herrmann K, Schöder H, et al. Radiotheranostics in oncology: current challenges and emerging opportunities. Nat Rev Clin Oncol. 2022;19:534–50. https://doi.org/10.1038/s41571-022-00652-y.
75. Perez-Lopez R, Ghaffari Laleh N, Mahmood F, Kather JN. A guide to artificial intelligence for cancer researchers. Nat Rev Cancer. 2024;24:427–41. https://doi.org/10.1038/s41568-024-00694-7.
76. Hosny A, Parmar C, Quackenbush J, et al. Artificial intelligence in radiology. Nat Rev Cancer. 2018;18:500–10. https://doi.org/10.1038/s41568-018-0016-5.
77. Bi WL, Hosny A, Schabath MB, et al. Artificial intelligence in cancer imaging: clinical challenges and applications. CA Cancer J Clin. 2019;69:127–57. https://doi.org/10.3322/caac.21552.
78. Bera K, Braman N, Gupta A, et al. Predicting cancer outcomes with radiomics and artificial intelligence in radiology. Nat Rev Clin Oncol. 2022;19:132–46. https://doi.org/10.1038/s41571-021-00560-7.
79. Taylor CR, Monga N, Johnson C, et al. Artificial intelligence applications in breast imaging: current status and future directions. Diagnostics (Basel). 2023;13(12):2041. https://doi.org/10.3390/diagnostics13122041.
80. Zhang J, Wu J, Zhou XS, et al. Recent advancements in artificial intelligence for breast cancer: image augmentation, segmentation, diagnosis, and prognosis approaches. Semin Cancer Biol. 2023;96:11–25. https://doi.org/10.1016/j.semcancer.2023.09.001.
81. de Margerie-Mellon C, Chassagnon G. Artificial intelligence: a critical review of applications for lung nodule and lung cancer. Diagn Interv Imaging. 2023;104:11–7. https://doi.org/10.1016/j.diii.2022.11.007.

Palliative Care and Cancer Research

30

Samuel Harris, Lora M. A. Thompson, and Sahana Rajasekhara

Introduction

There were an estimated 2,000,000 new cancer diagnoses and 600,000 cancer-related deaths in the United States in 2024 [1]. Globally, one in five individuals is expected to be diagnosed with cancer in their lifetime, with the incidence projected to continue to rise [2, 3]. This, combined with advancements in anticancer therapy that have led to improved survival, has resulted in a growing population of patients living with advanced cancer [4]. Facing a cancer diagnosis can be physically and emotionally overwhelming for patients, their families, and caregivers. Patients with advanced cancer may experience distressing symptoms such as pain and fatigue [5]. Palliative care (PC), also known as supportive care, aims to enhance patients' quality of life throughout the cancer continuum by effectively managing disease-related symptoms and treatment-associated side effects. The National Comprehensive Cancer Network (NCCN) defines PC as "an approach to patient-/family-/caregiver-centered health care that focuses on optimal management of distressing symptoms, while incorporating psychosocial, spiritual support according to patient/family/caregiver needs, values, beliefs, and cultures" [6]. This chapter provides an overview of the existing PC research in oncology, focusing on the integration of palliative and oncologic care, associated outcomes, advanced care planning, models of care delivery, quality of life, and symptom management.

S. Harris
Hospice and Palliative Medicine Fellowship Program, University of South Florida, Tampa, FL, USA

L. M. A. Thompson · S. Rajasekhara (✉)
Department of Supportive Care Medicine, Moffitt Cancer Center, Tampa, FL, USA

Department of Oncologic Sciences, University of South Florida, Tampa, FL, USA
e-mail: lora.thompson@moffitt.org; sahana.rajasekhara@moffitt.org

History of Palliative Care Research: Methodologies and Challenges

The principles of PC have existed for decades; however, as a formal medical specialty, they are relatively recent. Consequently, the body of research remains limited compared to the vast number of oncology studies, although it is growing. Over the past three decades, the scope of PC research has evolved significantly in terms of its quantity, methodology, and focus. A 1996 review of publicly available abstracts identified 384 PC research studies, the majority of which focused on defining the patient population and specialty, as expected in an emerging field [7]. The review also found a lack of a cohesive research methodology, with only 5% of these studies being randomized controlled trials (RCTs). A subsequent analysis of PC research published between 1997 and 2006 found that only 14% of the 215 identified studies were quantitative, with only one RCT [8].

PC research faces numerous challenges due to the complex nature of end-of-life care and the vulnerability of patients. One of the primary challenges faced by PC researchers is the lack of a universally agreed upon and replicated definition of what constitutes delivery of palliative care, including where it should occur, who should be involved, how frequently, or when it should begin [9]. Consequently, there was heterogeneity across studies, including participant selection and intervention type. For example, participants may be selected based on prognosis or disease stage and have varying life expectancies, cancer types, or symptom burdens. These differences can lead to difficulties replicating studies between institutions and provider groups.

A multitude of ethical concerns can arise when the study population comprises patients at the end of their lives. The

J. Huang, H. S.L. Jim (eds.), *Cancer Research Guidance for Clinicians and Researchers*,
https://doi.org/10.1007/978-3-032-19175-5_30

measured outcomes are complex as they may encompass physical, spiritual, and emotional aspects. Blinding of study participants is difficult, if not impractical. Patients may hold a negative perspective regarding PC as associated with end-of-life care, potentially affecting participation and follow-up. Additionally, there is a relative lack of funding for PC research in oncology [10]. Although many of these methodological challenges persist, the quality of evidence has improved, and a significantly greater number of quantitative studies, including RCTs and mixed-method studies, have been published since 2006. This is evidenced by a nearly fivefold increase in the number of articles on PC published worldwide from 2002 to 2020 [11].

Key Areas of Research in Palliative Care and Oncology

Integration of Palliative Care in Oncology Practice and Outcomes

PC was first introduced in the 1950s by Dr. Cicely Saunders, who presented a model that was most consistent with modern hospice care. It was not until the 1970s that PC, as a holistic approach occurring throughout the cancer continuum, was introduced and advocated by the surgical oncologist Dr. Balfour Mount [12]. It took many years before the evidence of the benefits caught up to the recommendations of Dr. Mount in 1974. In 2003, the NCCN issued its first recommendation for routine PC. Since then, other professional organizations have issued similar recommendations, including the American Society of Clinical Oncology (ASCO), American College of Surgeons, and European Society for Medical Oncology (ESMO) [13, 14]. These guidelines reflect one of the key research areas in oncologic integration of PC.

Much of the early research efforts centered on proving the validity and benefits of the field. A systematic review of 22 RCTs conducted between 1984 and 2007 with patients with advanced illness concluded that the existing research had widespread limitations [15]. A landmark parallel-group RCT study by Temel et al. in 2010 provided the strongest evidence supporting the benefits of integrating early PC with standard cancer care [16]. A total of 151 patients with newly diagnosed metastatic non-small-cell lung cancer who were randomized into an integrated PC intervention showed statistically significant improvements in quality of life and depression, longer survival, and decreased aggressive care at the end-of-life compared to those receiving standard oncologic care. This well-designed study paved the way for many other RCTs to assess the effects of integration. See Table 30.1 for a summary of eight systematic reviews and meta-analyses [17–24]. Based on these analyses, it is difficult to conclude with certainty that integrated palliative care improves symptom management and mood disorders, as the pooled data are inconclusive and at times conflicting. Similarly, the survival benefits of integrated PC are inconclusive, with only two of six meta-analyses supporting survival benefits [20, 21]. However, some evidence for survival benefits has been shown in a large cohort study, which included 23,154 patients with stage IIIB or IV advanced lung cancer and a randomized trial that included 207 patients with advanced cancer [25, 26]. A positive finding is that integrated PC is not associated with a decrease in survival [17–19, 23]. The most consistent finding across these systematic reviews and meta-analyses was that the integration of PC improves patients' quality of life.

Advance Care Planning

A key aspect of PC is facilitating early advance care planning and goals of care discussions. The significance of these conversations lies in facilitating communication that enables patients to actively engage in healthcare decisions aligned with their values, needs, and preferences, thereby promoting goal-concordant care. The intended outcome is the reduction of futile interventions at the end of life, while preserving patient dignity and decreasing healthcare costs during this period.

Research has focused on the utilization of structured communication tools to increase the frequency of these goals of care discussions, completion of advance directives, and provision of goal-concordant care [27]. To date, no single communication tool has proven to be more effective than others, highlighting a potential area for future research [28]. The need for improvement in this domain was emphasized in a 2011 RCT involving 151 patients, which found that 69% of patients with metastatic non-small-cell lung cancer endorsed "getting rid of all of the cancer" as one of their goals of care in their baseline survey [29]. Patients who received early PC intervention were 23% more likely than those who received standard oncologic care to attain an accurate prognostic understanding and five times less likely to receive chemotherapy within the last 60 days of life. Multiple RCTs and cohort studies have consistently demonstrated that early PC, irrespective of disease trajectory, is associated with reduced hospital utilization, less aggressive end-of-life care, and increased use of hospice services [30–34]. Furthermore, engaging in end-of-life conversations is not associated with heightened worry or depression among patients [35]. Consistent with the observed reduction in health care utilization and less aggressive treatment, PC has also been associated with lower healthcare costs. This cost-effectiveness has been demonstrated in large cohort studies of cancer patients [36] and in mixed PC patients, including those with cancer [37].

Table 30.1 Summary of systematic reviews and meta-analyses of PC interventions

Publication	Total number of studies	Total number of patients	Population	Outcomes: statistically significant	Outcomes: no difference	Notes
Kavalieratos et al. [17]	43 RCTs	12,731	Cancer and non-cancer	Quality of life (1–3 months) and symptom burden	Quality of life (4–6 months) and survival	Narrative review of a subset of studies suggests mixed results for improved advanced care planning, patient/caregiver satisfaction, and lower health care utilization
Gaertner et al. [18]	10 RCTs	2454	Cancer and non-cancer	Quality of life	Pain, survival, mood, and healthcare cost	Quality of life benefit amplified in cancer patients with early palliative care involvement
Haun et al. [19]	7 RCTs	1614	Cancer	Quality of life and symptom burden	Survival and depression	Evidence certainty was rated as low confidence in the outcomes
Kassianos et al. [24]	11 (6 RCTs, 5 pre/poststudies)	2939	Cancer	Quality of life		Narrative review suggested a possible benefit in symptom burden, including mood
Fulton et al. [20]	10 RCTs	2385	Cancer	Quality of life, symptom burden, and survival	Mood	Qualitative analysis results: trend toward less aggressive end-of-life care; inconclusive for health care utilization
Hoerger et al. [21]	8 RCTs	2092	Cancer	1-year survival and quality of life		Significant results from studies with high methodological quality
Oluyase et al. [23]	42 RCTs	7779	Cancer and non-cancer	Quality of life, symptom burden, patient satisfaction, and depression	Pain, anxiety, survival	Studies with qualitative analyses (N = 10) suggest perceived benefits in communication, shared decision-making, and quality of care
Xu et al. [22]	12 RCTs	2356	Cancer	Quality of life at 12–18 weeks, depression	Overall quality of life and anxiety	Palliative intervention categorized as inpatient, outpatient, and mixed settings

Models of Palliative Care Delivery

PC for cancer patients is delivered through various models: outpatient clinics, inpatient consultation teams, acute palliative care units, community-based PC, and hospices, each addressing specific care needs along the disease continuum [38].

Outpatient clinics, either free-standing or embedded, have demonstrated the highest efficacy in RCTs for improving patient outcomes [39]. Despite the lack of standardized interventions, RCTs examining community-based PC have shown improved symptom control and patient satisfaction, with home-based PC increasing the rate of death at home [38]. Although evidence of benefit remains limited, telehealth for PC delivery has also been well received by patients and providers [39].

Variability in outcomes across PC studies may be attributed to different models that vary by intervention type, care location, team composition, and care recipient. This lack of standardization affects both research replicability and the standardization of clinical care. Evidence suggests that physician-led interdisciplinary teams achieve superior outcomes compared to individual providers or nurse-led initiatives [40, 41]. However, the optimal composition and level of each member's involvement remain unclear.

Another component of enhancing care delivery is determining the most effective referral process, which identifies patients who would benefit the most from PC, while minimizing unnecessary referrals. Universal referral is impractical due to resource scarcity. Relying on the classical model of oncologists' best judgment can overlook patients with unmet needs. Emerging evidence supports the use of trigger-based models that can effectively identify patients who would benefit from PC, based on prognosis, risk factors, and patient-reported symptom assessments, leading to earlier and more systematic integration across different clinical settings [39, 40, 42–44]. This is an area of ongoing research with potential, given advancements in large data sets, improvements in electronic medical record functionalities, compatibility with research platforms, automation, and artificial intelligence.

Symptom Management

Expert symptom management is the cornerstone of PC, addressing common symptoms such as pain, dyspnea, fatigue, nausea, and cachexia. Reduced symptom burden is associated with improved quality of life, greater adherence to cancer treatment, and increased survival in some cases [5]. While symptom management research has explored novel applications of existing medications, progress in the development of new pharmacological agents remains limited.

Cancer pain management is one of the most extensively studied symptoms, with multiple evidence-based guidelines supporting a stepwise approach [45]. Current research emphasizes a multimodal approach, integrating both pharmacologic and non-pharmacologic interventions. Opioids remain the mainstay of treatment for moderate to severe cancer-related pain [46]. There is no single best opioid, and the selection should be based on factors such as bioavailability, half-life, neurotoxicity, and cost [47]. Evidence from a large systematic review showed that 95% of patients with moderate to severe cancer pain can achieve mild pain or complete pain relief within two weeks [48]. Non-opioid analgesics, such as acetaminophen, NSAIDs, corticosteroids, anticonvulsants, and antidepressants, all have evidence to support their use in certain cases. Additionally, integrative therapies such as acupuncture, hypnosis, and massage have shown some benefits [49].

Pharmacologic and non-pharmacologic approaches are used to manage dyspnea in advanced cancer patients. Opioid therapy is the only pharmacological intervention with proven benefits after optimization of underlying conditions [50]. Evidence extends beyond ASCO guidelines, with multiple systematic reviews and meta-analyses demonstrating efficacy and safety. A systematic review by Luo et al. found that opioids had a small but significant positive effect on cancer-related dyspnea [51]. Yamaguchi et al.'s real-world observational study, which included 402 patients, showed that systemic opioids provided significant relief within 72 h, with somnolence (~10%) being the most common adverse event [52]. Non-pharmacologic interventions, such as fan therapy, where air is directed toward the patient's face, have supporting evidence and remain an important adjunct to pharmacologic treatment [53].

The primary objective in managing cancer-related fatigue (CRF), a prevalent and debilitating symptom, is to identify and address reversible contributing factors. The ASCO guidelines recommend a combination of exercise and psychological interventions such as cognitive-behavioral therapy (CBT) and mind-body practices (e.g., mindfulness, tai chi) for managing CRF [54]. These recommendations are based on clinical trials that included patients across all cancer types and stages, with approximately 13% of studies focusing on advanced cancer and/or those at the end of life. The exercise analysis included 17 trials (N = 2606), along with three RCTs (N = 480) that assessed CBT, five RCTs (N = 498)—two assessing tai chi, two qigong, and one both—and three RCTs (n = 404) on mindfulness-based programs. Substantial evidence supports exercise interventions, including both aerobic and resistance training, in reducing CRF [54, 55]. Pharmacotherapies, such as methylphenidate and modafinil, have been utilized in clinical practice for many years. However, evidence regarding their effectiveness remains inconclusive, and their use is not widely endorsed. There is insufficient evidence to determine the benefits and harms of corticosteroids in CRF [56]. Further research is warranted to substantiate the comparative effectiveness of various interventions.

Evidence-based management of nausea and vomiting in advanced cancer requires a multifaceted approach addressing both treatment-related and nontreatment-related etiologies. 5-HT3 receptor antagonists combined with corticosteroids constitute standard antiemetic therapy for chemotherapy-induced nausea and vomiting (CINV) [57]. Olanzapine's efficacy in CINV prophylaxis and treatment is supported by multiple clinical trials and systematic reviews [58, 59]. A randomized pilot trial including a total of 30 patients, with a mean (range) age of 63 (39–79) years, demonstrated that olanzapine significantly reduced chronic nausea unrelated to chemotherapy and improved the quality of life in advanced cancer patients [60]. A review of integrative and non-pharmacological interventions recommended acupuncture, dietary counseling, and progressive muscle relaxation alone or with guided imagery as adjuncts to standard antiemetic therapy while emphasizing the need for higher-quality trials [61]. Compared to other causes, CINV has been extensively studied, and several evidence-based guidelines are available [62].

Cancer-associated cachexia (CC), characterized by unintentional weight loss, muscle atrophy, fatigue, and metabolic changes, is associated with poor clinical outcomes, reduced therapeutic response, diminished quality of life, and decreased survival [63]. In 2020, ASCO published evidence-based guidance on nutritional, pharmacological, and other interventions, drawing from 20 systematic reviews and 13 RCTs [64]. Based on limited evidence, dietary counseling for patients and caregivers has been reported to promote weight gain; routine use of enteral feeding tubes or parenteral nutrition has been discouraged [64, 65]. Currently, there is no FDA-approved drug for CC, and until recently, insufficient evidence prevented the recommendation of a specific pharmacological intervention as the standard of care [64]. The publication of a 2023 RCT prompted ASCO to issue a recommendation update, noting that low-dose olanzapine significantly improved appetite and weight gain compared to placebo and was well tolerated by patients with minimal side effects [66, 67]. Pharmacological interventions, such as progesterone analogs and short-term corticosteroids, may be considered; however, both medications have significant side effects [64]. Despite advancements, there is no single, consistently effective pharmacotherapy for CC, and a multimodal approach incorporating exercise and nutrition remains crucial [64, 68]. Recent updates have highlighted promising targeted therapies, including ghrelin receptor agonists such as anamorelin, that improve lean body mass, weight, and appetite-related quality of life [68]. Other investigational drugs, such as the nonselective β-blockers espindolol, thalidomide, and cannabinoids, are under investigation for their potential therapeutic effects [68].

Advancements in symptom management have not progressed at the same pace as in cancer therapy. With the increasing availability of genetic information for both patients and their diseases, there is a significant opportunity for future research on personalized symptom management. This approach has the potential to enhance patient care, reduce healthcare burdens, and minimize time-consuming trial-and-error processes in symptom management.

Conclusion

Palliative care research in oncology has made significant progress despite the methodological limitations of existing studies. It is well established that the integration of PC in oncology offers considerable benefits, including improvements in symptom management, quality of life, and end-of-life care for both the patient and the medical system. Early PC interventions are widely recognized as being advantageous. However, further research is needed to define the optimal timing, communication tools, patient population, referral process, and models of care delivery to maximize the benefits while minimizing the burdens on the healthcare system. With advancements in artificial intelligence and access to large data sets, there is a potential for rapid progress. Additionally, genetic research holds promise for breakthroughs in individualized treatment, personalized to the genetic profiles of patients and their diseases. The field of PC and cancer research is rapidly advancing with a growing body of evidence supporting its effectiveness, with a benefit for patients and the future of oncology care.

References

1. Cancer Stat Facts: Cancer of Any Site [Internet]. National Cancer Institute: Surveillance, Epidemiology, and End Results Program; 2024. Available from: https://seer.cancer.gov/statfacts/html/all.html.
2. Bray F, Laversanne M, Sung H, Ferlay J, Siegel RL, Soerjomataram I, et al. Global cancer statistics 2022: GLOBOCAN estimates of incidence and mortality worldwide for 36 cancers in 185 countries. CA Cancer J Clin. 2024;74(3):229–63. https://doi.org/10.3322/caac.21834.
3. Bizuayehu HM, Ahmed KY, Kibret GD, Dadi AF, Belachew SA, Bagade T, et al. Global disparities of cancer and its projected burden in 2050. JAMA Netw Open. 2024;7(11):e2443198-e. https://doi.org/10.1001/jamanetworkopen.2024.43198.
4. Devasia TP, Howlader N, Dewar RA, Stevens JL, Mittu K, Mariotto AB. Increase in the life expectancy of patients with cancer in the United States. Cancer Epidemiol Biomarkers Prev. 2024;33(2):196–205. https://doi.org/10.1158/1055-9965.Epi-23-1006.
5. Henson LA, Maddocks M, Evans C, Davidson M, Hicks S, Higginson IJ. Palliative care and the Management of Common Distressing Symptoms in advanced cancer: pain, breathlessness, nausea and vomiting, and fatigue. J Clin Oncol. 2020;38(9):905–14. https://doi.org/10.1200/jco.19.00470.
6. Walling AM, Campbell T, Agarwal R, Bauer A, Beck AC, Carey EC, et al. Palliative Care: National Comprehensive Cancer Network; 2024. Available from: https://www.nccn.org/professionals/physician_gls/pdf/palliative.pdf.
7. Corner J. Is there a research paradigm for palliative care? Palliat Med. 1996;10(3):201–8. https://doi.org/10.1177/026921639601000304.
8. Payne SA, Turner JM. Research methodologies in palliative care: a bibliometric analysis. Palliat Med. 2008;22(4):336–42. https://doi.org/10.1177/0269216308090072.
9. van der Steen JT, Bloomer MJ, Martins PS. The importance of methodology to palliative care research: A new article type for palliative medicine. Palliat Med. 2022;36(1):4–6. https://doi.org/10.1177/02692163211069566.
10. Reyna YZ, Bennett MI, Bruera E. Ethical and practical issues in designing and conducting clinical trials in palliative care. In: Addington-Hall JM, Bruera E, Higginson IJ, Payne S, editors. Research methods in palliative care. Oxford University Press; 2007. p. 27–42.
11. Abu-Odah H, Molassiotis A, Liu JYW. Global palliative care research (2002-2020): bibliometric review and mapping analysis. BMJ Support Palliat Care. 2022;12(4):376–87. https://doi.org/10.1136/bmjspcare-2021-002982.
12. Loscalzo MJ. Palliative care: an historical perspective. Hematology. 2008;2008(1):465. https://doi.org/10.1182/asheducation-2008.1.465.
13. Fahy BN. Current guidelines for integration of palliative Care in Oncology. Surg Oncol Clin N Am. 2021;30(3):431–47. https://doi.org/10.1016/j.soc.2021.02.002.
14. Jordan K, Aapro M, Kaasa S, Ripamonti CI, Scotté F, Strasser F, et al. European Society for Medical Oncology (ESMO) position paper on supportive and palliative care. Ann Oncol. 2018;29(1):36–43. https://doi.org/10.1093/annonc/mdx757.
15. Zimmermann C, Riechelmann R, Krzyzanowska M, Rodin G, Tannock I. Effectiveness of specialized palliative care: A systematic review. JAMA. 2008;299(14):1698–709. https://doi.org/10.1001/jama.299.14.1698.
16. Temel JS, Greer JA, Muzikansky A, Gallagher ER, Admane S, Jackson VA, et al. Early palliative care for patients with metastatic non-small-cell lung cancer. N Engl J Med. 2010;363(8):733–42. https://doi.org/10.1056/NEJMoa1000678.
17. Kavalieratos D, Corbelli J, Zhang D, Dionne-Odom JN, Ernecoff NC, Hanmer J, et al. Association between palliative care and patient and caregiver outcomes: A systematic review and meta-analysis. JAMA. 2016;316(20):2104–14. https://doi.org/10.1001/jama.2016.16840.
18. Gaertner J, Siemens W, Meerpohl JJ, Antes G, Meffert C, Xander C, et al. Effect of specialist palliative care services on quality of life in adults with advanced incurable illness in hospital, hospice, or community settings: systematic review and meta-analysis. BMJ. 2017;357:j2925. https://doi.org/10.1136/bmj.j2925.
19. Haun MW, Estel S, Rücker G, Friederich HC, Villalobos M, Thomas M, et al. Early palliative care for adults with advanced cancer. Cochrane Database Syst Rev. 2017;6(6):Cd011129. https://doi.org/10.1002/14651858.CD011129.pub2.
20. Fulton JJ, LeBlanc TW, Cutson TM, Porter Starr KN, Kamal A, Ramos K, et al. Integrated outpatient palliative care for patients with advanced cancer: A systematic review and meta-analysis. Palliat Med. 2019;33(2):123–34. https://doi.org/10.1177/0269216318812633.
21. Hoerger M, Wayser GR, Schwing G, Suzuki A, Perry LM. Impact of interdisciplinary outpatient specialty palliative care on survival and quality of life in adults with advanced cancer: A meta-analysis of

randomized controlled trials. Ann Behav Med. 2019;53(7):674–85. https://doi.org/10.1093/abm/kay077.
22. Xu S, Wang X, Wang R. The effects of integrated palliative care on quality of life and psychological distress in patients with advanced cancer: a systematic review and meta-analysis. Ann Palliat Med. 2022;11(8):2586–99. https://doi.org/10.21037/apm-22-162.
23. Oluyase AO, Higginson IJ, Yi D, Gao W, Evans CJ, Grande G, et al. Hospital-based specialist palliative care compared with usual care for adults with advanced illness and their caregivers: a systematic review. NIHR J Library. 2021; https://doi.org/10.3310/hsdr09120.
24. Kassianos AP, Ioannou M, Koutsantoni M, Charalambous H. The impact of specialized palliative care on cancer patients' health-related quality of life: a systematic review and meta-analysis. Support Care Cancer. 2018;26(1):61–79. https://doi.org/10.1007/s00520-017-3895-1.
25. Sullivan DR, Chan B, Lapidus JA, Ganzini L, Hansen L, Carney PA, et al. Association of Early Palliative Care use with Survival and Place of death among patients with advanced lung cancer receiving Care in the Veterans Health Administration. JAMA Oncol. 2019;5(12):1702–9. https://doi.org/10.1001/jamaoncol.2019.3105.
26. Bakitas MA, Tosteson TD, Li Z, Lyons KD, Hull JG, Li Z, et al. Early versus delayed initiation of concurrent palliative oncology care: patient outcomes in the ENABLE III randomized controlled trial. J Clin Oncol. 2015;33(13):1438–45. https://doi.org/10.1200/jco.2014.58.6362.
27. Oczkowski SJ, Chung HO, Hanvey L, Mbuagbaw L, You JJ. Communication tools for end-of-life decision-making in ambulatory care settings: A systematic review and meta-analysis. PLoS One. 2016;11(4):e0150671. https://doi.org/10.1371/journal.pone.0150671.
28. Myers J, Cosby R, Gzik D, Harle I, Harrold D, Incardona N, et al. Provider tools for advance care planning and goals of care discussions: A systematic review. Am J Hosp Palliat Care. 2018;35(8):1123–32. https://doi.org/10.1177/1049909118760303.
29. Temel JS, Greer JA, Admane S, Gallagher ER, Jackson VA, Lynch TJ, et al. Longitudinal perceptions of prognosis and goals of therapy in patients with metastatic non-small-cell lung cancer: results of a randomized study of early palliative care. J Clin Oncol. 2011;29(17):2319–26. https://doi.org/10.1200/jco.2010.32.4459.
30. Greer JA, Moy B, El-Jawahri A, Jackson VA, Kamdar M, Jacobsen J, et al. Randomized trial of a palliative care intervention to improve end-of-life care discussions in patients with metastatic breast cancer. J Natl Compr Cancer Netw. 2022;20(2):136–43. https://doi.org/10.6004/jnccn.2021.7040.
31. Seow H, Sutradhar R, Burge F, McGrail K, Guthrie DM, Lawson B, et al. End-of-life outcomes with or without early palliative care: a propensity score matched, population-based cancer cohort study. BMJ Open. 2021;11(2):e041432. https://doi.org/10.1136/bmjopen-2020-041432.
32. Maltoni M, Scarpi E, Dall'Agata M, Schiavon S, Biasini C, Codecà C, et al. Systematic versus on-demand early palliative care: A randomised clinical trial assessing quality of care and treatment aggressiveness near the end of life. Eur J Cancer. 2016;69:110–8. https://doi.org/10.1016/j.ejca.2016.10.004.
33. Iupati S, Stanley J, Egan R, MacLeod R, Davies C, Spence H, et al. Systematic review of models of effective community specialist palliative Care Services for Evidence of improved patient-related outcomes, equity, integration, and health service utilization. J Palliat Med. 2023;26(11):1562–77. https://doi.org/10.1089/jpm.2022.0461.
34. Michael N, Beale G, O'Callaghan C, Melia A, DeSilva W, Costa D, et al. Timing of palliative care referral and aggressive cancer care toward the end-of-life in pancreatic cancer: a retrospective, single-center observational study. BMC Palliat Care. 2019;18(1):13. https://doi.org/10.1186/s12904-019-0399-4.
35. Wright AA, Zhang B, Ray A, Mack JW, Trice E, Balboni T, et al. Associations between end-of-life discussions, patient mental health, medical care near death, and caregiver bereavement adjustment. JAMA. 2008;300(14):1665–73. https://doi.org/10.1001/jama.300.14.1665.
36. Seow H, Barbera LC, McGrail K, Burge F, Guthrie DM, Lawson B, et al. Effect of early palliative care on end-of-life health care costs: A population-based, propensity score-matched cohort study. JCO Oncol Pract. 2022;18(1):e183–e92. https://doi.org/10.1200/op.21.00299.
37. Morrison RS, Penrod JD, Cassel JB, Caust-Ellenbogen M, Litke A, Spragens L, et al. Cost savings associated with US hospital palliative care consultation programs. Arch Intern Med. 2008;168(16):1783–90. https://doi.org/10.1001/archinte.168.16.1783.
38. Hui D, Bruera E. Models of palliative care delivery for patients with cancer. J Clin Oncol. 2020;38(9):852–65. https://doi.org/10.1200/jco.18.02123.
39. Mathews J, Hannon B, Zimmermann C. Models of integration of specialized palliative care with oncology. Curr Treat Options in Oncol. 2021;22(5):44. https://doi.org/10.1007/s11864-021-00836-1.
40. Hui D, Hannon BL, Zimmermann C, Bruera E. Improving patient and caregiver outcomes in oncology: team-based, timely, and targeted palliative care. CA Cancer J Clin. 2018;68(5):356–76. https://doi.org/10.3322/caac.21490.
41. Ferrell B, Sun V, Hurria A, Cristea M, Raz DJ, Kim JY, et al. Interdisciplinary palliative Care for Patients with Lung Cancer. J Pain Symptom Manag. 2015;50(6):758–67. https://doi.org/10.1016/j.jpainsymman.2015.07.005.
42. Rodin R, Swami N, Pope A, Hui D, Hannon B, Le LW, et al. Impact of early palliative care according to baseline symptom severity: secondary analysis of a cluster-randomized controlled trial in patients with advanced cancer. Cancer Med. 2022;11(8):1869–78. https://doi.org/10.1002/cam4.4565.
43. Zimmermann C, Pope A, Hannon B, Krzyzanowska MK, Rodin G, Li M, et al. Phase II trial of symptom screening with targeted early palliative Care for Patients with Advanced Cancer. J Natl Compr Cancer Netw. 2021;20(4):361–70.e3. https://doi.org/10.6004/jnccn.2020.7803.
44. Adelson K, Paris J, Horton JR, Hernandez-Tellez L, Ricks D, Morrison RS, et al. Standardized criteria for palliative care consultation on a solid tumor oncology service reduces downstream health care use. J Oncol Pract. 2017;13(5):e431–e40. https://doi.org/10.1200/jop.2016.016808.
45. Robert S, Youngwerth J, Agne J, et al. NCCN Guidelines Adult Cancer Pain; 2024. Available from: https://www.nccn.org/professionals/physician_gls/pdf/pain.pdf.
46. Paice JA, Bohlke K, Barton D, Craig DS, El-Jawahri A, Hershman DL, et al. Use of opioids for adults with pain from cancer or cancer treatment: ASCO guideline. J Clin Oncol. 2023;41(4):914–30. https://doi.org/10.1200/jco.22.02198.
47. DiGiulio S. ASCO issues opioid use guidelines for adult cancer patients with pain. Oncol Times. 2023;45(8):1–8. https://doi.org/10.1097/01.COT.0000931968.62670.eb.
48. Wiffen PJ, Wee B, Derry S, Bell RF, Moore RA. Opioids for cancer pain - an overview of Cochrane reviews. Cochrane Database Syst Rev. 2017;7(7):Cd012592. https://doi.org/10.1002/14651858.CD012592.pub2.
49. Mao JJ, Ismaila N, Bao T, Barton D, Ben-Arye E, Garland EL, et al. Integrative medicine for pain Management in Oncology: Society for Integrative Oncology–ASCO guideline. J Clin Oncol. 2022;40(34):3998–4024. https://doi.org/10.1200/jco.22.01357.
50. Mori M, Miwa S, Ikari T, Kako J, Hasegawa T, Matsunuma R, et al. Current management options for dyspnea in cancer patients. Curr Treat Options in Oncol. 2023;24(6):565–79. https://doi.org/10.1007/s11864-023-01081-4.

51. Luo N, Tan S, Li X, Singh S, Liu S, Chen C, et al. Efficacy and safety of opioids in treating cancer-related dyspnea: A systematic review and meta-analysis based on randomized controlled trials. J Pain Symptom Manag. 2021;61(1):198–210.e1. https://doi.org/10.1016/j.jpainsymman.2020.07.021.
52. Yamaguchi T, Matsunuma R, Matsuda Y, Tasaki J, Ikari T, Miwa S, et al. Systemic opioids for dyspnea in cancer patients: A real-world observational study. J Pain Symptom Manag. 2023;65(5):400–8. https://doi.org/10.1016/j.jpainsymman.2022.12.146.
53. Gupta A, Sedhom R, Sharma R, Zhang A, Waldfogel JM, Feliciano JL, et al. Nonpharmacological interventions for managing breathlessness in patients with advanced cancer: A systematic review. JAMA Oncol. 2021;7(2):290–8. https://doi.org/10.1001/jamaoncol.2020.5184.
54. Bower JE, Lacchetti C, Alici Y, Barton DL, Bruner D, Canin BE, et al. Management of Fatigue in adult survivors of cancer: ASCO–Society for integrative oncology guideline update. J Clin Oncol. 2024;42(20):2456–87. https://doi.org/10.1200/jco.24.00541.
55. Cramp F, Byron-Daniel J. Exercise for the management of cancer-related fatigue in adults. Cochrane Database Syst Rev. 2012;11(11):Cd006145. https://doi.org/10.1002/14651858.CD006145.pub3.
56. Sandford A, Haywood A, Rickett K, Good P, Khan S, Foster K, et al. Corticosteroids for the management of cancer-related fatigue in adults with advanced cancer. Cochrane Database Syst Rev. 2023;1(1):Cd013782. https://doi.org/10.1002/14651858.CD013782.pub2.
57. Schnell FM. Chemotherapy-induced nausea and vomiting: the importance of acute antiemetic control. Oncologist. 2003;8(2):187–98. https://doi.org/10.1634/theoncologist.8-2-187.
58. Berger MJ, Ettinger DS, Aston J, Barbour S, Bergsbaken J, Bierman PJ, et al. NCCN Guidelines Insights: Antiemesis, Version 2.2017. J Natl Compr Cancer Netw. 2017;15(7):883–93. https://doi.org/10.6004/jnccn.2017.0117.
59. Navari RM, Qin R, Ruddy KJ, Liu H, Powell SF, Bajaj M, et al. Olanzapine for the prevention of chemotherapy-induced nausea and vomiting. N Engl J Med. 2016;375(2):134–42. https://doi.org/10.1056/NEJMoa1515725.
60. Navari RM, Pywell CM, Le-Rademacher JG, White P, Dodge AB, Albany C, et al. Olanzapine for the treatment of advanced cancer-related chronic nausea and/or vomiting: A randomized pilot trial. JAMA Oncol. 2020;6(6):895–9. https://doi.org/10.1001/jamaoncol.2020.1052.
61. Molassiotis A, Affronti ML, Fleury M, Olver I, Giusti R, Scotte F. 2023 MASCC/ESMO consensus antiemetic guidelines related to integrative and non-pharmacological therapies. Support Care Cancer. 2023;32(1):30. https://doi.org/10.1007/s00520-023-08225-0.
62. Kennedy SKF, Goodall S, Lee SF, DeAngelis C, Jocko A, Charbonneau F, et al. 2020 ASCO, 2023 NCCN, 2023 MASCC/ESMO, and 2019 CCO: a comparison of antiemetic guidelines for the treatment of chemotherapy-induced nausea and vomiting in cancer patients. Support Care Cancer. 2024;32(5):280. https://doi.org/10.1007/s00520-024-08462-x.
63. Ni J, Zhang L. Cancer cachexia: definition, staging, and emerging treatments. Cancer Manag Res. 2020;12:5597–605. https://doi.org/10.2147/cmar.S261585.
64. Roeland EJ, Bohlke K, Baracos VE, Bruera E, Del Fabbro E, Dixon S, et al. Management of Cancer Cachexia: ASCO guideline. J Clin Oncol. 2020;38(21):2438–53. https://doi.org/10.1200/jco.20.00611.
65. de van der MAE S, Laviano A, Blanchard H, Jourdan M, Arends J, Baracos VE. Systematic review and meta-analysis of the evidence for oral nutritional intervention on nutritional and clinical outcomes during chemo(radio)therapy: current evidence and guidance for design of future trials. Ann Oncol. 2018;29(5):1141–53. https://doi.org/10.1093/annonc/mdy114.
66. Sandhya L, Devi Sreenivasan N, Goenka L, Dubashi B, Kayal S, Solaiappan M, et al. Randomized double-blind placebo-controlled study of olanzapine for chemotherapy-related anorexia in patients with locally advanced or metastatic gastric, Hepatopancreaticobiliary, and lung cancer. J Clin Oncol. 2023;41(14):2617–27. https://doi.org/10.1200/jco.22.01997.
67. Roeland EJ, Bohlke K, Baracos VE, Smith TJ, Loprinzi CL. Cancer cachexia: ASCO guideline rapid recommendation update. J Clin Oncol. 2023;41(25):4178–9. https://doi.org/10.1200/jco.23.01280.
68. Pandey S, Bradley L, Del Fabbro E. Updates in cancer cachexia: clinical management and pharmacologic interventions. Cancers (Basel). 2024;16(9) https://doi.org/10.3390/cancers16091696.

Hospice and Cancer Research

31

John F. Shuler, Joanna Veazey Brooks, and Christian T. Sinclair

Abbreviations

PCHs	Patients with cancer in hospice
CoPCHs	Caregivers of patients with cancer in hospice
EOL	End of life
RCT	Randomized controlled trial
CRP	Cancer-related pain
IDT	Interdisciplinary team

Overview

About half of Medicare beneficiaries who died in 2022 utilized hospice care, with a wide variation of use in different states, ranging from 21 to 60%. In 2021, cancer accounted for 23% of hospice cases with an average length of stay of 52 days. Half of the people who die with cancer receive hospice care [1]. In the United States, hospice is a care model focused on symptom control, patient, and caregiver support when patients forego further life-prolonging treatments. In cancer care, hospice is usually initiated after chemotherapy, immunotherapy, radiation, surgeries, and transfusions are no longer pursued. The prognosis of advanced disease is the key element to determine eligibility for the Medicare Hospice Benefit in the United States. A physician must certify "that the individual's prognosis is for a life expectancy of 6 months or less if the terminal illness runs its normal course" [2]. Coverage guidelines for demonstrating a 6-month prognosis for adults with a cancer diagnosis include evidence of a "disease with metastases at presentation or progression from an earlier stage of disease to metastatic disease with either: A continued decline in spite of therapy; or patient declines further disease directed therapy" [3]. Compared to eligibility criteria for modern cancer research, hospice guidelines are considerably more vague and open to interpretation. A 2016 systematic review of 42 studies on clinician prognostication showed evidence that clinicians are frequently inaccurate [4]. Many studies have devised and validated prognostic tools of varying complexity, but their application in general practice is minimal and without ongoing published research to demonstrate effective use. There have been calls for more standardized outcome reporting and measurements in prognosis science, which could be helpful to the intersection of hospice and cancer research [5].

Research in the hospice setting has typically taken the form of observational or retrospective studies, with clinical trials being rare. This is despite 45% of hospice patients being interested in therapeutic intervention research [6].

Hospice Utilization

Longer hospice admissions are associated with better patient quality of life, lower caregiver depression scores, and lower rates of complicated grief. Despite this, only about 50% of patients utilize hospice at EOL, and about a third of hospice admissions are less than 7 days in duration [1]. Shorter hospice admissions are associated with poor outcomes like worse pain, higher incidence of depression, and lower quality of EOL care as perceived by caregivers. Many factors can help explain the suboptimal hospice utilization rates, including patient awareness and perception of hospice during advanced care planning. El-Jawarhi et al. [7] conducted an RCT looking at the effect of a 6-min video depicting hospice care versus a verbal description alone on 150 hospitalized

J. F. Shuler (✉) · C. T. Sinclair
Division of Palliative Medicine, University of Kansas Medical Center, Kansas City, KS, USA
e-mail: jshuler@kumc.edu; csinclair@kumc.edu

J. V. Brooks
Department of Population Health and Division of Palliative Medicine, University of Kansas Medical Center, Kansas City, KS, USA
e-mail: jbrooks6@kumc.edu

J. Huang, H. S.L. Jim (eds.), *Cancer Research Guidance for Clinicians and Researchers*,
https://doi.org/10.1007/978-3-032-19175-5_31

advanced cancer patients' preferences for hospice. Patients and caregivers who viewed the video were more informed about hospice and had a more favorable perception of hospice. Patients who reviewed the video were more likely to use hospice and have a longer length of stay.

Research has shown several disparities in hospice enrollment and use for patients with cancer. Abbas et al. [8] found that among patients undergoing cancer surgery, individuals living in counties with a high social vulnerability index were less likely to be enrolled in hospice. In addition, minority patients were less likely to utilize hospice, and this disparity by race increased as social vulnerability increased. Barragan-Carillo et al. [9] argued that the Hispanic/Latinx population is understudied when it comes to EOL care and that this population disproportionately underutilizes EOL care compared to the general population. Increased barriers are faced by patients with limited English proficiency due to a lack of interpreters, inconsistent translation, and interpreter style around EOL communication, including hospice [10]. Finally, patients in rural communities receive hospice care at a lower rate than their urban counterparts [11], which is likely due to a number of factors, including the availability of hospice staff [12].

A range of factors and reasons underlie the disparities in hospice utilization. For some patients on complex and costly treatments like chemotherapy or parenteral nutrition, specific hospice enrollment policies may create barriers to hospice access. Historically marginalized and underrepresented populations face increased rates of social vulnerability, discrimination, or social determinants of health that create barriers to accessing hospice [8, 13]. For the Hispanic/Latinx population, research indicates that a combination of "socio-cultural, financial, and health system-related" barriers is in play [9]. Other researchers argue that strong sociocultural values around fighting cancer constrain hospice utilization [14].

Hematological malignancies are a cancer subgroup that presents with a difficult dichotomy between death and cure, given advances in stem cell transplants. Combined with other factors, these patients are twice as likely to die in an inpatient setting compared to other cancers in one meta-analysis of studies from 1966 to 2010 [15]. A barrier to hospice in the United States is that patients with hematologic malignancies are often transfusion-dependent, which often delays enrollment in hospice. Transfusion-dependent patients with leukemia have a median hospice length of stay of 6 days compared to 11 days when those patients are not transfusion-dependent (i.e., requiring two or more transfusions in 30 days before death or hospice enrollment) [16].

Some describe the decision between hospice care and ongoing cancer-directed treatment as a "terrible choice." Concurrent hospice care is a novel approach that allows patients to receive the comfort-focused treatments of hospice while continuing to receive life-prolonging treatments, such as cancer-directed treatment. In the USA, currently, only children and veterans are eligible for this type of care. The Veterans Health Administration (VHA) has been allowing concurrent care since 2005, and since that time, veterans' hospice enrollment has tripled [17]. In 2010, the Affordable Care Act allowed pediatric Medicaid beneficiaries to receive concurrent care. CMS has begun studying the viability of this type of care in the broader Medicare population. The Medicare Care Choices Model (MCCM) is a pilot program that began in 2016 and utilized hospice agencies to provide supportive care for patients nearing the end of life (i.e., 6 months or less to live) without requiring them to forego treatments directed at their terminal diagnosis, as is required when someone signs onto hospice. They analyzed Medicare claims data for patients enrolled in MCCM (n = 4575) compared to similar patients not enrolled ($n = 13{,}575$) and calculated the regression-adjusted differences in outcome measures for the two groups. They found that Medicare expenditures were $7254 (14%) lower in the MCCM group. This was primarily driven by a decrease in inpatient expenditures (−39%) as well as skilled nursing facility expenditures (−22%). It also reduced the overall number of hospital/clinic visits (inpatient admissions −26%, hospital readmissions −28%, emergency department visits −14%, and ambulatory visits −14%). MCCM participants had lower rates of aggressive treatment in the 30 days prior to death. This effect was seen most significantly in patients with cancer and chronic obstructive pulmonary disease. Racial minority patients and dually eligible (i.e., Medicare and Medicaid) patients had less favorable outcomes, which require further exploration [18].

Symptom Management

There is a high prevalence of bothersome symptoms for patients at the EOL, in hospice, and even more so for PCH [19]. One observational cohort study in Ontario, Canada, monitored Edmonton Symptom Assessment System (ESAS) scores routinely for cancer patients ($n = 10{,}752$) and looked at these scores over the last 6 months of life. They found that levels of pain, nausea, anxiety, and depression remained relatively stable over the last 6 months, compared with dyspnea, fatigue, and lack of appetite, which increased in severity over that time, especially in the last month of life. Over one-third of patients had moderate to severe scores for the majority of symptoms in the last month of life [20].

Pain

Pain related to cancer is common and can be difficult to treat. It often requires alternative strategies to standard analgesics. About two-thirds of patients with advanced cancer experience pain, increasing to 80% in the terminal stage, and it is often undertreated or refractory [21, 22]. The mainstay of

CRP treatment, and especially in the end stages, is opioids. While often effective, standard opioid therapy is associated with common troublesome side effects (i.e., constipation, nausea, sedation) as well as issues with misuse and diversion. Much of the recent research on CRP in PCH revolves around nonstandard, nonopioid modalities.

One nonopioid option for treating cancer-related pain is parenteral lidocaine. A review of seven articles (one retrospective chart review, three practice guidelines, two case series, and one case study) looked at a total of 73 patients receiving parenteral lidocaine (i.e., intravenous or subcutaneous), who had treatment started in the hospital and continued at home. They all showed positive outcomes in pain management with no severe adverse effects [22]. An RCT by Hawley et al. [23] looked at the viability of doing home lidocaine infusions. It analyzed the effect of a 10 mg/kg infusion of subcutaneous lidocaine over 5.5 h on chronic cancer-related pain. The study excluded patients with a prognosis of less than 3 months. It was a small study with only 25 patients receiving the lidocaine infusion. No significant analgesic response was seen in 23 of the 25 patients. However, blood levels of lidocaine did not reach a therapeutic level in most patients, suggesting possible inadequate dosing.

Another nonopioid approach to pain management involves interventional pain techniques (e.g., neuraxial analgesia, vertebral procedures, sympathetic neurolysis, peripheral nerve blocks, neuromodulation, and neurosurgical procedures). Catheter-based continuous peripheral nerve blocks (i.e., non-neuraxial) are frequently utilized in postsurgical pain management but have not been widely used to treat CRP. One review showed that a majority of 25 studies, all of which were small and non-RCT, showed a reduction in pain with very few adverse events, most often migration, which was remedied by tunneling. The longest duration of continuous catheter usage was 217 days and was usually monotherapy with bupivacaine or ropivacaine. The authors of the study proposed that this intervention has the potential to bridge the gap between single-shot injections and more invasive procedures for CRP [24]. The feasibility of this type of treatment for PCH still needs to be studied.

Some hospice agencies utilize massage therapy as part of a pain and symptom management plan. An RCT by Kutner et al. [25] looked at the effect of six 30-min massages over the course of 2 weeks ($n = 151$) versus simple touch ($n = 147$) on moderate to severe CRP. Most of the patients were enrolled in hospice. Both groups had improvements in pain and mood ratings, with massage being superior for both. There was no difference in the amount of time in pain, quality of life, symptom distress, or analgesic medication use. The authors suggest that massage may have immediate beneficial effects on pain and mood, but these were not sustained. The ability to do frequent massage visits on hospice is limited by cost and staffing. Moosvi et al. [26] conducted a pretest/posttest feasibility study in which caregivers ($n = 39$) provided four daily massages to hospice patients. They found that this intervention was not overly burdensome for caregivers and seemed to foster connection with the patient (e.g., laughter, story sharing, closure activities). Further prospective studies are needed to determine symptom benefit for patients.

Dyspnea

Dyspnea is another common symptom experienced by people with terminal cancer. It tends to worsen in the last days to weeks of life and can be difficult to manage during that time. Uncontrolled dyspnea can be incredibly distressing for patients and their caregivers. Along with delirium, it is the most common reason for utilizing palliative sedation. Treatment of dyspnea during the last days of life is rarely studied. A review by Mori et al. provides a nice summary of the evidence [27]. Morphine is the most studied opioid for dyspnea in cancer patients, but studies typically focus on single-dose administration in cognitively intact patients. Aabom et al. [28] performed a randomized, double-blind crossover trial ($n = 12$) comparing liquid morphine with ethanol (aka red morphine drops, commonly used in Denmark) and without for the relief of dyspnea. They found that in the first 3 minutes after receiving a dose, the formulation with ethanol was superior. They postulate that ethanol may facilitate morphine absorption in the mouth. Very limited studies have suggested that hydromorphone and oxycodone can be effective for terminal dyspnea, but the effect of fentanyl is unknown [27].

There is clearly an association between dyspnea and anxiety in patients with terminal cancer. Benzodiazepines are commonly used for refractory dyspnea. However, no studies have clarified whether benzodiazepines can treat dyspnea independently from opioids or if they are better used as an adjunct for dyspnea that is difficult to control. An RCT by Navigante et al. looked at the role of midazolam as an adjunct to morphine for the treatment of dyspnea in terminally ill cancer patients. Patients were randomized to receive around-the-clock morphine with midazolam rescue doses in case of breakthrough dyspnea ($n = 35$), around-the-clock midazolam with morphine rescues ($n = 33$), or around-the-clock morphine plus midazolam with morphine rescue doses ($n = 33$). Their findings suggested that adding around-the-clock midazolam to around-the-clock morphine reduced levels of dyspnea in the last days of life [29].

Corticosteroids are sometimes used for terminal breathlessness in cancer patients, but no studies support their broad use. Rather, clinical guidelines recommend utilizing corticosteroids for specific complications of cancer, such as lymphangitic carcinomatosis, superior vena cava syndrome, and airway obstruction. The psychoactive side effects of corticosteroids in patients nearing the end of life should be considered in risk–benefit assessments [27].

Nonpharmacological interventions for terminal breathlessness have also been studied, with fan therapy showing the most promise. Kako et al. conducted an RCT which showed the benefit of a fan blowing across the face ($n = 20$) relative to a fan blowing over the legs ($n = 20$) [30]. The use of supplemental oxygen in the absence of hypoxia is not supported by evidence but can be used if it provides subjective relief for patients and is not causing burdensome side effects (i.e., extra tubing, mask hindering communication, drying effects on nasal mucosa, which can cause bleeding) [27].

Delirium

Delirium in terminal cancer patients can be quite distressing, especially for caregivers. Delirium is managed with behavioral interventions and medications, with antipsychotics being the most common class. Van Der Vorst et al. [31] conducted a multicenter RCT to compare the efficacy and tolerability of olanzapine ($n = 49$) versus haloperidol ($n = 49$) for the treatment of delirium in hospitalized patients with advanced cancer. There was no statistically significant difference between the two with regard to efficacy or safety. Agar et al. [32] compared risperidone, haloperidol, and placebo for the treatment of delirium in advanced cancer patients. They conducted a double-blind RCT of 249 patients at 11 Australian inpatient hospice or hospital palliative care services. Delirium scores were higher in the haloperidol and risperidone arms compared to placebo. Extrapyramidal symptoms were more common in the treatment arms. Overall survival was higher in the placebo arm compared to haloperidol. One exclusion criterion was a clinician-predicted survival of 7 days or less, which limits this study's application to "terminal delirium." All groups received supportive care and attempts to address reversible contributors to delirium. The authors suggest that effective delirium management relies on effective screening, addressing underlying causes, and providing support.

Terminal Secretions

Audible upper airway secretions (AKA "the death rattle") are common in the final hours to days of life. Guidance routinely given to caregivers is that the secretions are not bothersome to the patient but can be difficult for those caring for the patient to witness. Repositioning (i.e., lateral recumbent, raising the head of the bed) and reassurance are considered first-line interventions followed by anticholinergic medications. A secondary analysis of a cluster randomized trial of clinically assisted hydration in cancer patients found that 55% of cancer patients developed audible upper airway secretions during the final days of life, but only 35% of patients had them at the time of death. Their prevalence increased closer to the time of death, more significantly during the last 12 to 16 h of life. The natural history of audible secretions is variable, with some patients having multiple episodes and others having none [33]. An RCT by van Esch et al. [34] examined the effect of prophylactic subcutaneous scopolamine ($n = 79$) four times daily versus placebo ($n = 78$). Most patients had cancer (~85%). They found that audible secretions occurred on 13% of the scopolamine group compared to 27% in the placebo group. Differences in restlessness, dry mouth, and urinary retention were not statistically significant. Patients were excluded if they were not able to give written consent. Of the ones who could, 50% chose to participate in the study. The authors commented on the challenges of performing a clinical trial on hospice patients. They suggest that the process can be facilitated by using advanced consent, having the hospice physician as a local researcher, and using a structured template to monitor patient care in the dying phase. They suggest their study could be a model for future trials in this patient population.

Caregiver Experience

Caregivers take an active role in monitoring and managing symptoms for PCH. The act of caregiving can take a psychological and physical toll. An observational study by Reblin et al. [35] looked at the association between caregiver and patient well-being ($n = 61$ patient-caregiver dyads). They collected both self and patient symptom reports from the caregiver and found that when patients' symptoms were more poorly controlled, caregivers reported worse symptoms themselves. Caregivers for patients with advanced cancer are most often a female spouse or adult child, aged 50 to 65. Half of caregivers continue to work outside of the home but most eventually need to reduce hours or stop working altogether. CoPCH mental health falls below the 30th percentile of the national average, with moderate to severe levels of depression and anxiety seen in about 40% and 45%, respectively [36, 37]. CoPCHs have higher rates of depression than hospice caregivers for patients without cancer [38].

While some people find benefit in the caregiver role, many feel unprepared, both emotionally and physically. The final weeks of the patient's life are often the most difficult. While hospice provides a significant amount of support for patients at home, most of the caregiving falls to family, friends, and hired caregivers. For hospice to robustly support caregivers, it requires multiple in-person or telephone interventions, which can be difficult and costly. Mooney et al. [39] carried out an RCT assessing the impact of an automated digital caregiver coaching intervention (n = 159) vs. usual hospice care (n = 173) on caregiver burden for PCH across 13 hospice agencies in four states. The intervention resulted in a 30% reduction in caregiver burden at 8 weeks. There were higher levels of moderate to severe caregiving symptoms in the usual hospice care group.

Feelings of depression and anxiety are more common in caregivers who view their support systems as weak. Washington et al. [40] used a secondary qualitative data analysis to look at factors contributing to caregivers' willingness to participate in an online support group for CoPCH (n = 58). They found that emotional isolation and more caregiving downtime positively affect engagement, while reluctance to share personal information was a detractor. Information on pain and the dying process was most engaging for caregivers. Groups with a positive tone and taking place in a private setting on Facebook were more favorably viewed.

Given the burden of caregiving, self-care and health maintenance are thought to be an important component of maintaining caregivers' well-being. A secondary data analysis by Djin et al. found that of 86 CoPCH, approximately half felt that they did not have enough time to do self-care activities such as rest when ill or exercise. A quarter reported not having enough time to go to the doctor, and a third reported missing a doctor's appointment in the past 6 months [41].

The timing of hospice referral can affect the caregiving experience. One study used a survey to assess the correlation between caregivers' perception of the timing of hospice initiation and satisfaction with the care received. They found that one in seven bereaved CoPCH felt that referral to hospice happened too late. About half of those cited physicians as barriers to timely enrollment. The authors postulated that this may be due to overly positive prognostication and the effect this can have on pursuing aggressive care toward the end of life. Caregivers who felt like referral happened too late also reported higher rates of unmet needs in coordination of care and self-efficacy, lower rates of confidence in providing care, emotional support, recieving information regarding patient condition, and satisfaction with hospice services overall [42].

The plan of care for hospice at home is established by the interdisciplinary team (IDT) and largely communicated to CoPCH by the hospice nurse. The CoPCHs are carrying out the plan of care and look to the hospice nurse for education and support. This line of communication is particularly important to ensure good patient-centered care at EOL. Kane et al. [43] attempted to quantify effective communication between home hospice nurses and CoPCH by using semantic analysis of recorded conversations. This was a descriptive secondary analysis of self-reported nurse data and 31 audio-recorded hospice nursing visits. Communication similarity between the nurse and CoPCH was thought to signify effective communication. The similarity scores were much higher than those found in an outpatient clinical setting (0.14 versus 0.83), where visits are often significantly shorter. Nurses with higher scores tended to speak less during visits and have a high preference for caregiver-centered communication.

Conclusion

Death and suffering are a part of the current cancer experience, and while reducing deaths from cancer is often the spotlight of cancer research, reducing suffering is just as important to understand and ameliorate. We have shown that access to hospice improves symptom control and decreases caregiver morbidity, but there is so much more to learn and work to be done to provide equitable, high-quality care. End-of-life cancer research rarely examines biologic cell signaling pathways, the physics calculations of radiotherapy, or chemical development of new pharmaceuticals that undergird cancer research. At the end of life, cancer research can feel less discrete compared to bench research because the end of life involves people making difficult choices within convoluted health systems governed by labyrinthine policies. There is so much undiscovered in these messy complexities, and that is exciting. Understanding this important phase of life and investing in high-quality research to improve end-of-life care impacts all of us because we all die.

References

1. NHPCO-Facts-Figures-2024.pdf [Internet]. [Cited 27 Jan 2025]. Available from: https://www.nhpco.org/wp-content/uploads/NHPCO-Facts-Figures-2024.pdf.
2. Medicare Benefit Policy Manual. Chapter 9 – Coverage of Hospice Services Under Hospital Insurance. Available from: https://www.cms.gov/Regulations-and-Guidance/Guidance/Manuals/Downloads/bp102c09.pdf.
3. LCD – Hospice – Determining Terminal Status (L33393) [Internet]. [Cited 27 Jan 2025]. Available from: https://www.cms.gov/medicare-coverage database/view/lcd.aspx?LCDId=33393&ContrId=272&ContrVer=1&CntrctrSelected=272*1&Cntrctr=272&DocType=2.
4. White N, Reid F, Harris A, Harries P, Stone P. A systematic review of predictions of survival in palliative care: how accurate are clinicians and who are the experts? PLoS One. 2016;11(8):e0161407.
5. Spooner C, Vivat B, White N, Bruun A, Rohde G, Kwek PX, et al. What outcomes do studies use to measure the impact of prognostication on people with advanced cancer? Findings from a systematic review of quantitative and qualitative studies. Palliat Med. 2023;37(9):1345–64.
6. Williams CJ, Shuster JL, Clay OJ, Burgio KL. Interest in research participation among hospice patients, caregivers, and ambulatory senior citizens: practical barriers or ethical constraints? J Palliat Med. 2006;9(4):968–74.
7. El-Jawahri A, Traeger L, Greer JA, Vanbenschoten O, Markovitz N, Cashavelly B, et al. Randomized trial of a hospice video educational tool for patients with advanced cancer and their caregivers. Cancer. 2020;126(15):3569–78.

8. Abbas A, Madison Hyer J, Pawlik TM. Race/ethnicity and county-level social vulnerability impact hospice utilization among patients undergoing cancer surgery. Ann Surg Oncol. 2021;28(4):1918–26.
9. Barragan-Carrillo R, Pabon CM, Chavarri-Guerra Y, Soto-Perez-de-Celis E, Duma N. End-of-life care and advanced directives in Hispanic/Latinx patients: challenges and solutions for the practicing oncologist. Oncologist. 2022;27(12):1074.
10. Dressler G, Cicolello K, Anandarajah G. "Are They Saying It How I'm Saying It?" a qualitative study of language barriers and disparities in hospice enrollment. J Pain Symptom Manag. 2021;61(3):504–12.
11. Ramkumar N, Wang Q, Brooks GA, Tosteson ANA, Wong SL, Loehrer AP. Association of rurality with utilization of palliative care and hospice among Medicare beneficiaries who died from pancreatic cancer: a cohort study. J Rural Health Off J Am Rural Health Assoc Natl Rural Health Care Assoc. 2023;39(3):557–64.
12. Wan S, Lorenz KA, Fischer SM, Liao S, Lee MC, Kutner JS. Local area hospice capacity and rural disparities in hospice use among older adults with metastatic breast cancer. J Palliat Med. 2023;26(2):182.
13. Jones T, Luth EA, Lin SY, Brody AA. Advance care planning, palliative care, and end-of-life care interventions for racial and ethnic underrepresented groups: a systematic review. J Pain Symptom Manag. 2021;62(3):e248–60.
14. Mrig EH, Spencer KL. Political economy of hope as a cultural facet of biomedicalization: a qualitative examination of constraints to hospice utilization among U.S. end-stage cancer patients. Soc Sci Med. 2018;200:107–13.
15. Howell DA, Roman E, Cox H, Smith AG, Patmore R, Garry AC, et al. Destined to die in hospital? Systematic review and meta-analysis of place of death in haematological malignancy. BMC Palliat Care. 2010;9:9.
16. LeBlanc TW, Egan PC, Olszewski AJ. Transfusion dependence, use of hospice services, and quality of end-of-life care in leukemia. Blood. 2018;132(7):717–26.
17. Mor V, Wagner TH, Levy C, Ersek M, Miller SC, Gidwani-Marszowski R, et al. Association of expanded VA hospice care with aggressive care and cost for veterans with advanced lung cancer. JAMA Oncol. 2019;5(6):810–6.
18. mccm-fourth-annrpt.pdf [Internet]. [Cited 16 Dec 2024]. Available from: https://www.cms.gov/priorities/innovation/data-and-reports/2022/mccm-fourth-annrpt.
19. Washington KT, Knight A, Pitzer KA, Oliver DP, Devlin SM, Benson JJ, et al. Cancer-related fatigue in hospice: a nudge to action? J Pain Symptom Manage. 2023;65(5):e511.
20. Seow H, Barbera L, Sutradhar R, Howell D, Dudgeon D, Atzema C, et al. Trajectory of performance status and symptom scores for patients with cancer during the last six months of life. J Clin Oncol. 2011;29(9):1151–8.
21. Tayeb BO, Winegarden JA, Alashari RA, Alasmari M, Winegarden J, Boker F, et al. Scoping review of off-label topical analgesia in palliative, hospice and cancer care: towards flexibility in evidence-based medicine. J Pain Res. 2021;14:3003.
22. Chong PH, Yeo ZZ. Parenteral lidocaine for complex cancer pain in the home or inpatient hospice setting: a review and synthesis of the evidence. J Palliat Med. 2021;24(8):1154.
23. Hawley P, Fyles G, Jefferys SG. Subcutaneous lidocaine for cancer-related pain. J Palliat Med. 2020;23(10):1357–64.
24. Podgorski Iii E, Driver L, Gulati A, Abdi S. Catheter-based techniques for terminal cancer pain: a review of Nonneuraxial interventions with clinical implications for end-of-life pain management. Pain Physician. 2021;24(7):E1137–46.
25. Kutner JS, Smith MC, Corbin L, Hemphill L, Benton K, Mellis BK, et al. Massage therapy vs. simple touch to improve pain and mood in patients with advanced cancer: a randomized trial. Ann Intern Med. 2008;149(6):369.
26. Moosvi K, Schoppee TM, Xavier S, Henderson K, Suarez ML, Yao Y, et al. Feasibility and burden of lay caregivers providing daily massages to patients with cancer receiving hospice and palliative care. Am J Hosp Palliat Care. 2022;39(12):1475.
27. Mori M, Yamaguchi T, Matsuda Y, Suzuki K, Watanabe H, Matsunuma R, et al. Unanswered questions and future direction in the management of terminal breathlessness in patients with cancer. ESMO Open. 2020;5(Suppl 1):e000603.
28. Aabom B, Laier G, Christensen PL, Karlsson T, Jensen MB, Hedal B. Oral morphine drops for prompt relief of breathlessness in patients with advanced cancer—a randomized, double blinded, crossover trial of morphine sulfate oral drops vs. morphine hydrochloride drops with ethanol (red morphine drops). Support Care Cancer. 2020;28(7):3421–8.
29. Navigante AH, Cerchietti LCA, Castro MA, Lutteral MA, Cabalar ME. Midazolam as adjunct therapy to morphine in the alleviation of severe dyspnea perception in patients with advanced cancer. J Pain Symptom Manag. 2006;31(1):38–47.
30. Kako J, Morita T, Yamaguchi T, Kobayashi M, Sekimoto A, Kinoshita H, et al. Fan therapy is effective in relieving dyspnea in patients with terminally ill cancer: a parallel-arm, randomized controlled trial. J Pain Symptom Manag. 2018;56(4):493–500.
31. van der Vorst MJ, Neefjes EC, Boddaert MS, Verdegaal BA, Beeker A, Teunissen SC, et al. Olanzapine versus haloperidol for treatment of delirium in patients with advanced cancer: a phase III randomized clinical trial. Oncologist. 2019;25(3):e570.
32. Agar MR, Lawlor PG, Quinn S, Draper B, Caplan GA, Rowett D, et al. Efficacy of oral risperidone, haloperidol, or placebo for symptoms of delirium among patients in palliative care: a randomized clinical trial. JAMA Intern Med. 2017;177(1):34–42.
33. Davies A, Waghorn M, Skene S. Clinical features of audible upper airway secretions ("death rattle") in patients with cancer in the last days of life. Support Care Cancer. 2024;32(7):423.
34. van Esch HJ, van Zuylen L, Geijteman ECT, Oomen-de Hoop E, Huisman BAA, Noordzij-Nooteboom HS, et al. Effect of prophylactic subcutaneous scopolamine Butylbromide on death rattle in patients at the end of life: the SILENCE randomized clinical trial. JAMA. 2021;326(13):1268–76.
35. Reblin M, Iacob E, Tay DL, Li H, Thomas Hebdon MC, Beck A, et al. Family caregiver reports of their own and patient symptoms in cancer home hospice approaching end-of-life. Am J Hosp Palliat Med. 2023;40(5):508–16.
36. Wadhwa D, Burman D, Swami N, Rodin G, Lo C, Zimmermann C. Quality of life and mental health in caregivers of outpatients with advanced cancer. Psychooncology. 2013;22(2):403–10.
37. Oliver DP, Demiris G, Benson JJ, White P, Wallace AS, Pitzer K, et al. Family caregiving experiences with hospice lung cancer patients compared to other cancer types. J Psychosoc Oncol. 2022;41(2):210.
38. Oliver DP, Washington KT, Benson J, Mayhara M, Pitzer K, White P, et al. Depressive symptoms in caregivers of hospice cancer patients. Am J Hosp Palliat Care. 2024;41(7):786–91.
39. Mooney KH, Coombs LA, Whisenant MS, Wilson CM, Moraitis AM, Steinbach MN, et al. Impact of an automated, remote monitoring and coaching intervention in reducing hospice cancer family

caregiving burden: a multisite randomized controlled trial. Cancer. 2024;130(7):1171–82.

40. Washington KT, Oliver DP, Benson JJ, Rolbiecki AJ, Jorgensen LA, Cruz-Oliver DM, et al. Factors influencing engagement in an online support group for family caregivers of individuals with advanced cancer. J Psychosoc Oncol. 2019;38(3):235.
41. Tay DL, Reblin M, Iacob E, Cloyes KG, Hebdon MCT, Reynaga M, et al. Cancer hospice caregivers' self-care behaviors: the role of caregiving tasks, burden, and mental health. J Hosp Palliat Nurs JHPN Off J Hosp Palliat Nurses Assoc. 2023;25(5):286.
42. Schockett ER, Teno JM, Miller SC, Stuart B. Late referral to hospice and bereaved family member perception of quality of end-of-life care. J Pain Symptom Manag. 2005;30(5):400–7.
43. Kane L, Clayton MF, Baucom BR, Ellington L, Reblin M. Measuring communication similarity between hospice nurses and cancer caregivers using latent semantic analysis. Cancer Nurs. 2020;43(6):506.

Social Work and Cancer Research

32

Sean Powell, Matthew Floriani, and Briana Kraus Joyce

Introduction

Individuals diagnosed with cancer face a multitude of psychosocial challenges following a diagnosis. These issues range from logistical, such as transportation, lodging, and financial assistance, to existential, including thoughts of death, redefining their purpose, or reprioritizing based on changes to their life expectancy. Individuals are at increased risk for the development of anxious or depressive symptoms as well as suicidal ideation [1, 2]. As the primary providers of behavioral health services, oncology social workers are essential members of the treatment team and uniquely qualified to address these concerns.

Oncology social workers are highly trained individuals with comprehensive knowledge and a specialized skill set regarding the psychosocial impacts of illness, appropriate interventions, and treatment modalities to improve patient outcomes. The extensive scope and standards of practice are outlined in the Oncology Social Work Certification practice domains [3]. To ensure the most effective services are provided to individuals and their families, oncology social workers utilize evidence-informed practice to guide their clinical decision-making. Evidence-informed practice is the process of analyzing applicable research with clinical knowledge when making treatment decisions [4]. Given the expansive knowledge base of oncology social workers, this chapter focuses on screening protocols—informed by research and clinical needs—to identify and assist individuals in need of social work assessment and intervention. Specific attention is paid to screenings related to distress, suicide risk mitigation, and social determinants of health interventions.

S. Powell (✉) · M. Floriani · B. K. Joyce
H. Lee Moffitt Cancer Center, Tampa, FL, USA
e-mail: Sean.Powell@Moffitt.org

Suicide Risk Screening and Mitigation

An expansive body of peer-reviewed literature exists regarding risk for suicide mortality and suicidal ideation, both in the general population and the unique oncology patient population. According to the US Centers for Disease Control and Prevention, over 49,000 people died by suicide in 2022, which equates to one suicide death every 11 min [5]. Many more than this number experience thoughts or make plans to end their lives, a process sometimes referred to as suicidal ideation. In the USA during 2022, 13.2 million people seriously thought about suicide, 3.8 million people made a plan for suicide, and 1.6 million people attempted suicide [5]. People with cancer experience an even higher risk for suicidal thoughts and actions. A meta-analysis by Heinrich et al. found the suicide mortality rate in patients with cancer to be 85% higher than the general population [2], and a 2020 cross-sectional study by Abdel-Rahman, based on the National Health and Nutrition Examination Survey conducted for 2005–2016, similarly found suicidal ideation to be more prevalent in patients with cancer [6]. The use of evidence-informed practice is considered essential to effective and ethical oncology social work practice, and thus, continual review of the literature on these topics is the job of all oncology social workers, including patient-facing clinicians, administrators, and policymakers. Research displaying the prevalence of suicidality in cancer patients informs oncology social work practice by establishing suicide screening and assessment as paramount functions of frontline oncology social workers. Ongoing education on research findings maintains the knowledge of patient-facing clinicians in the form of identifying risk and protective factors. Research findings have led to continually more formalized and effective practices by means of validating the instruments used with patients on a daily basis and informing risk screening and mitigation policies at the institutional level.

Research informs oncology social work clinical knowledge on the individual clinician level by helping clinicians

J. Huang, H. S.L. Jim (eds.), *Cancer Research Guidance for Clinicians and Researchers*,
https://doi.org/10.1007/978-3-032-19175-5_32

understand risk factors and how they may present, both in the population at large and the oncology population. For example, the relationship between firearm ownership and suicide has been established for decades, and details continue to be studied, but relevant to the oncology social work clinician is the knowledge that suicide by any method is higher among individual handgun owners, and by all others in their household, than the general population [7, 8]. It has thus become a routine practice to ask about access to firearms when assessing patients for suicide risk and to suggest that a family member remove them from the patient's access if their risk for suicidal behavior is assessed to be high. Studies specific to the cancer patient population provide even more targeted information for oncology social workers. For instance, the retrospective population-based study by Zarosky et al. using data on 8,651,569 cancer patients from the Surveillance, Epidemiology, and End Results program from 1973–2014 revealed that cancer patients who die by suicide are roughly twice as likely to identify as male as they are to identify as female [9]. Further demographic factors associated with higher suicide mortality rates in cancer patients include identifying as White, being unmarried, being diagnosed before 50 years of age, and having cancer of the lung, head and neck, testes, or Hodgkin's lymphoma [9]. Those with poor-prognosis cancers have been found at a heightened risk within the first 2 years of diagnosis, while cancers that typically subject patients to long-term quality-of-life impairments display heightened risk after 2 years [10]. The aforementioned study by Zarosky et al. also suggests that the relative risk of suicide for cancer patients vs. the population at large may begin to decrease when a patient has been followed for their cancer diagnosis for more than 5 years [9]. Additional suicide mortality risk factors relevant specifically to the oncology patient population include being insured with Medicaid, having Medicare under age 64, suggesting disability status, or being uninsured as opposed to other insurance statuses [9]. Familial suicide history is also a risk factor among patients with cancer, but the relationship type is found to impact the level of risk, with spouses at the highest risk, followed by mothers who lost a child, children who lost a parent, siblings who lost a sibling, and fathers who lost a child, respectively [11]. A 2024 meta-analysis by Chen et al. identified risk factors for suicidal ideation, which overlap partially with those identified for suicide mortality and include being unmarried, living alone, having a lower education level, living in rural areas, having financial problems, and the presence of pain, panic disorder, post-traumatic stress disorder, vomiting, or demoralization [12]. Social workers are tasked with being lifelong learners and remaining up to date on such research findings. Indeed, each of these bits of knowledge may impact the individual oncology social worker's impression of the risk a patient presents for suicidal ideation or dying by suicide if the ideation is already present, and the intervention the social worker offers based on that impression may be life-saving.

Continuing education (CE) on research findings is key in keeping the oncology social work workforce up to date, so they may integrate the knowledge into their evidence-informed practice. This is typically achieved through attending professional or scholarly presentations. In most states, clinical social work practice requires licensure through a state agency, and oncology social workers are encouraged to maintain Oncology Social Work Certification (OSW-C) through the Board of Oncology Social Work (BOSW), Moffitt Cancer Center, in Tampa, Florida, for example, is a Florida Department of Health registered Education Provider for Clinical Social Work, Marriage and Family Therapy, and Mental Health Counseling. Moffitt provides an ongoing Multidisciplinary Psychosocial Oncology Conference program, enlisting subject matter experts as speakers for monthly educational presentations that not only qualify for the relevant CE credits but are also focused on the practice areas relevant to oncology social workers in the institution. For instance, a recent presentation *Importance of Suicide Risk Assessment in Oncology Care* authored by D. DiClementi was offered at Moffitt Cancer Center. It was open to the public, attended by other oncology social workers throughout the state, and provided a literature update on suicide prevalence in patients with cancer, risk factors, and practice recommendations for oncology social workers [13].

Ongoing education is essential to inform individual social workers' clinical judgement. However given the innumerable risk and protective factors for suicide mortality and suicidal ideation, it is not independently adequate to ensure a workforce is prepared for the task of assessing and taking appropriate steps to mitigate risk in real-life situations. It is widely accepted that there is no single predictor or cause for suicide. Even with a confluence of risk or protective factors, the outcome is impossible to predict with perfect accuracy. Many oncology institutions have thus created robust, research-informed processes for routine screening of all patients at clinic visits or hospital admission, and deeper assessment for those screened at higher risk. These institution-level policies most often employ one or more instruments with psychometric support for validity and reliability, such as the Beck Hopelessness Scale, Hamilton Depression Scale, Patient Health Questionnaire-9, or Columbia Suicide Severity Rating Scale (C-SSRS). A single item from one of the above instruments, or a distress scale, is often used for routine screening of all patients, with a positive screening result prompting the use of the full instrument [14]. Use of such instruments to screen and assess suicide risk may ensure details are not missed by individual clinicians in unstructured interviews, which can be emotionally charged conversations. They also ensure impressions are evidence-informed, leading to a more reliable assessment policy. It is essential to select an instrument that is not only respected but also a good fit for the practice setting, making this an important decision for administrators. In addition to assigning a level of risk to the individual being assessed, some, like the US Substance Abuse and Mental Health Services Administration's SAFE-T Suicide Assessment, also offer potential intervention recommendations, including emergency psychiatric treatment in a secure setting, hospital admission, outpatient referral with warm handoff, or psychoeducation on resources [15]. Widescale adoption of these practices represents improvement in psychosocial care for cancer patients, and there is evidence to suggest that cancer-related suicide may be slowing along with these improvements. Findings from Liu et al. in their 2024 large cohort study analyzed data from the Surveillance, Epidemiology, and End Results database including 4,870,410 patients diagnosed with cancer from 1975–2017, that cancer related suicides rose from 1975–1989, slowly decreased from 1989 to 2013, and began to markedly decreased from 2013 to 2017, a period of heightened industry level focus on risk screening and mitigation [16].

Distress Screening and Counseling

Anxiety and depression are highly prevalent in the oncology population and are heavily studied in this context. One frequently cited study by Brintzenhofe-Szoc et al. using cross-sectional anxiety and depression symptom data collected from 8,265 patients presenting to a tertiary cancer center found overall depression symptoms in 18%, overall anxiety symptoms in 24%, and mixed anxiety/depression symptoms in 12% of cancer patients [17]. The construct of distress has been defined from numerous perspectives. A basic definition provided by the National Institute of Health's National Cancer Institute is "Emotional, social, spiritual, or physical pain or suffering that may cause a person to feel sad, afraid, depressed, anxious, or lonely. People in distress may also feel that they are not able to manage or cope with changes caused by normal life activities or by having a disease such as cancer [18]. Cancer patients may have trouble coping with their diagnosis, physical symptoms, or treatment." Prevalence of distress in cancer patients at any time is well researched. A recent study by Sutton et al., utilizing longitudinal distress screening data from cancer patients treated or surveilled at their institution, found high levels of distress in 52% of patients [19]. Distress was found to be highest at diagnosis, with roughly 70% reporting anxiety, 50% reporting depressive symptoms, and roughly half reporting distress related to financial or insurance concerns, and often improved within 12 months, but in 20–30% of patients, it continued to worsen through the continuum of care [19]. In 2014, the American College of Surgeons introduced Standard 5.2 Psychosocial Distress Screening, which requires distress screening in cancer programs and referral to appropriate psychosocial care [20]. Clinical social workers are the primary frontline mental health professionals in the oncology setting nationwide [21]. With the prevalence of these constructs in the oncology patient population, social workers have been tasked with implementing evidence-informed practices for identifying those in distress and offering interventions to help improve patients' quality of life and ability to engage in and access care.

The first task in positively impacting oncology patient distress is identifying those experiencing it, which begins with screening as recommended by the American College of Surgeons [20]. One commonly used distress screening tool is the NCCN Distress Thermometer, which has been extensively validated and is straightforward to administer [22]. The next task is how to support patients once identified. Hundreds of randomized controlled trials have been conducted on this question. A meta-analysis displayed that common interventions include individual psychotherapy, group psychotherapy, couples psychotherapy, relaxation training, psychoeducation, and information, with individual psychotherapy, group psychotherapy, and psychoeducation producing sustained small to medium effects on emotional distress, anxiety, depression, and health-related quality of life, and relaxation training producing small to medium short-term effects [23]. A more recent meta-analysis of cognitive behavioral interventions and mindfulness-based interventions found small effects supporting the use of both methodologies equally in oncology patients with distress, as opposed to suggesting one of these practices over the other [24]. While identifying a single most effective approach to supporting patients who experience distress is difficult, this reflects the general understanding in the counseling field that a single method cannot be applied to every patient in every situation, as there is no catch-all to psychotherapy. The most effective policy is to ensure clinicians are trained in a range of techniques and ready to meet patients where they are at the time of need. For this reason, many oncology social workers become versed in a wide range of the aforementioned interventions and employ the tactic most relevant to the situation at hand. For example, a patient suffering some degree of acute pain in combination with distress may not be focused enough to engage in cognitive behavioral interventions, and the short-lived impact of relaxation techniques evidenced by the aforementioned study from Faller et al. may be the most benefit that can be offered at the moment [23]. Other patients who are more inclined or capable of engaging may benefit from cognitive behavioral and mindfulness techniques evaluated in other studies. The Board of Oncology Social Work

Certification has outlined specific core competencies and domains of practice for the certified oncology social worker, which include utilizing a broad range of theories of clinical practice and evidence-informed interventions, including but not limited to psychoeducation, cognitive behavioral therapies, narrative therapies, dialectical behavioral therapies, play therapy, and motivational interviewing [3]. The commonly understood idea that cancer can impact anyone, and different people have different capacities and needs at different times, supports ongoing use of this broad range of interventions that the clinical social worker may adapt to the patient scenario at hand.

Social Determinants of Health

Social determinants of health (SDOHs) are nonmedical factors that impact an individual's health. These include difficulty accessing transportation, healthy food, stable housing, and general financial stressors like the ability to pay utility bills, prescriptions, and co-pays. Growing research supports the connection between these potential barriers and reduced health outcomes [25, 26]. In response to these research results, clinical knowledge of direct care health workers, and support from policymakers, momentum exists to integrate SDOH screening and intervention into medical care. The next challenge is how to identify best practices and standardize screening and intervention [27]. Given social workers' knowledge base and specialized skill set, the profession can provide key clinical knowledge and leadership in the development of truly evidence-informed practices [26, 28, 29].

Centers for Medicare and Medicaid Services (CMS), the largest health insurance provider in the United States, demonstrates support of integration by including social determinants of health in the Framework for Health Equity 2022–2032 [30]. CMS has also released new reimbursement codes related to patient navigation and SDOH assessment [31]. Patient navigation plays an important role in connecting individuals to resources and assisting with obtaining access to the health care system. By providing financial support for patient navigation services and SDOH assessment services, CMS highlights the value of these interventions, a barrier often addressed in the research [25, 26]. Similarly, the Joint Commission, an accrediting organization for many health care organizations, released a new standard in 2022. Standard LD.04.03.08 requires organizations to reduce health care disparities, further demonstrating the priority paid to social determinants of health screening [32]. All this momentum illustrates the current support at the national level for SDOH screening and intervention.

The next step is integrating the research and national support into evidence-informed patient care. There currently exist several screening tools to identify individuals in need of assistance. These include Protocol for Responding to and Assessing Patients' Assets, Risks and Experiences (PREPARE), the Accountable Health Communities (AHC), and HealthBegins [25, 27]. However, none were designed for the oncology population, which leaves many health care organizations to either modify an existing tool or create their own. The development of a specialized tool and frequency protocol would greatly contribute to the standardization of screening and the development of best practices [25, 27]. One organization working on this project is the Association of Cancer Care Centers (ACCC) social drivers of health educational initiative [31]. This initiative is another example of social workers collaborating with researchers and other stakeholders to create evidence-informed practice.

Social workers are the ideal professionals to address SDOH. One of the fundamental theories of social work practice is person in environment (PIE). This foundational framework advocates for conceptualizing individuals within the context of their communities and is an excellent fit for SDOH screening and intervention. Social workers are also highly trained in engagement, psychosocial assessments, and care coordination. These skills are vital when addressing health-related social needs. However, many health care settings have caseloads that do not accommodate the long-term follow-up needed to adequately address SDOH. The CMS patient navigation and SDOH assessment reimbursement codes are an excellent step in the right direction. These codes have the potential to expand social workers' ability to positively impact patient outcomes. However, since these codes are still new, more research is needed to determine their full impact and how they are best implemented.

Another major challenge is the lack of resources—such as concrete transportation needs, affordable housing, and access to healthy foods—that are impacting health outcomes. Despite the existence of numerous databases to organize and collect information, the system to access assistance can be challenging, and the resources available are limited [26]. The apparent gap between need and capacity is a major limitation and illustrates the massive scope of the issue. The health care system cannot address social determinants of health without wider support from the community at large. However, with a standardized screening and intervention protocol, steps can be taken to identify individuals in need of assistance. The impact of health-related social needs on individual outcomes is well documented. Evidence supports the importance of more integration of SDOH screening. However, more research and collaboration are needed to ensure individuals screened have access to the concrete resources needed to be successful. Given social workers' skill set, they are uniquely positioned to provide leadership on the successful development and integration of SDOH standards.

Summary

Oncology social workers are vital members of the treatment team. The ability to utilize evidence-informed practice in selecting clinical intervention makes the profession uniquely qualified to address both the concrete and behavioral health needs of individuals seeking cancer treatment. From the established screening and interventions like suicide risk mitigation and distress to the new opportunities addressing social determinants of health, social workers can provide leadership and expertise in improving quality of life.

References

1. Hartung TJ, Brähler E, Faller H, Härter M, Hinz A, Johansen C, Keller M, Koch U, Schulz H, Weis J, Mehnert A. The risk of being depressed is significantly higher in cancer patients than in the general population: prevalence and severity of depressive symptoms across major cancer types. Eur J Cancer. 2017;72:46–53. https://doi.org/10.1016/j.ejca.2016.11.017.
2. Heinrich M, Hofmann L, Baurecht H, Kreuzer PM, Knüttel H, Leitzmann MF, Seliger C. Suicide risk and mortality among patients with cancer. Nat Med. 2022;28(4):852–9. https://doi.org/10.1038/s41591-022-01745-y.
3. Board of Oncology Social Work. OSW-C Core competencies domains for the certified oncology social worker credential. 2022. https://oswcert.org/wp-content/uploads/2023/06/OSW-C-Core-Competencies-and-Domains_Sept2022b.pdf.
4. Oktay JS. Integrating research and evidence-based practice with clinical knowledge. In: Christ G, Messner C, Behar L, editors. Handbook of oncology social work psychosocial care for people with cancer. Oxford University Press; 2015. p. 15–9.
5. U.S. Centers for Disease Control and Prevention, NCIPC Suicide Fact Sheet. 2024. Retrieved 19 Feb 2025, from https://www.cdc.gov/suicide/pdf/NCIPC-Suicide-FactSheet-508_FINAL.pdf.
6. Abdel-Rahman O. Depression and suicidal ideation among patients with cancer in the United States: a population-based study. JCO Oncol Pract. 2020;16(7):e601–9. https://doi.org/10.1200/jop.19.00497.
7. Miller M, Azrael D, Hemenway D. Household firearm ownership and suicide rates in the United States. Epidemiology. 2002;13(5):517–24. https://doi.org/10.1097/00001648-200209000-00006.
8. Studdert DM, Zhang Y, Swanson SA, Prince L, Rodden JA, Holsinger EE, Spittal MJ, Wintemute GJ, Miller M. Handgun ownership and suicide in California. N Engl J Med. 2020;382(23):2220–9. https://doi.org/10.1056/nejmsa1916744.
9. Zaorsky NG, Zhang Y, Tuanquin L, Bluethmann SM, Park HS, Chinchilli VM. Suicide among cancer patients. Nat Commun. 2019;10(1):207. https://doi.org/10.1038/s41467-018-08170-1.
10. Hu X, Ma J, Jemal A, Zhao J, Nogueira L, Ji X, Yabroff KR, Han X. Suicide risk among individuals diagnosed with cancer in the US, 2000-2016. JAMA Netw Open. 2023;6(1):e2251863. https://doi.org/10.1001/jamanetworkopen.2022.51863.
11. Jang J, Park SY, Kim YY, Kim EJ, Lee G, Seo J, Na EJ, Park J-Y, Jeon HJ. Risks of suicide among family members of suicide victims: a nationwide sample of South Korea. Front Psych. 2022;13:995834. https://doi.org/10.3389/fpsyt.2022.995834.
12. Chen J, Ping Z, Hu D, Wang J, Liu Y. Risk factors associated with suicidal ideation among cancer patients: a systematic review and meta-analysis. Front Psychol. 2024;14 https://doi.org/10.3389/fpsyg.2023.1287290.
13. DiClementi D. Importance of suicide risk assessment in oncology care [conference presentation]. In: Moffitt Cancer Center multidisciplinary psychosocial oncology conference. Tampa; 2024.
14. Hlubocky FJ, Dokucu ME. Addressing suicidal ideation in patients with cancer: recommendations for the oncology clinician on how to optimize routine screening in the outpatient setting. JCO Oncol Pract. 2023;19(7):387–8. https://doi.org/10.1200/op.23.00124.
15. SAMHSA. Safe-T suicide assessment five step evaluation and triage. 2024. SAMHSA.gov. https://library.samhsa.gov/product/safe-t-suicide-assessment-five-step-evaluation-and-triage/pep24-01-036.
16. Liu Q, Qu Z, Dong H, Qi Y, Wu J, Zhang W, Wang X, Wang Z, Fang Y, Wang J. Trends in cancer-related suicide in the United States: a population-based epidemiology study spanning 40 years of data. Transl Psychiatry. 2024;14(1):213. https://doi.org/10.1038/s41398-024-02917-9.
17. Brintzenhofe-Szoc KM, Levin TT, Li Y, Kissane DW, Zabora JR. Mixed anxiety/depression symptoms in a large cancer cohort: prevalence by cancer type. Psychosomatics. 2009;50(4):383–91. https://doi.org/10.1176/appi.psy.50.4.383.
18. National Institutes of Health. NCI dictionary of cancer terms. Comprehensive Cancer Information – NCI. 2025. https://www.cancer.gov/publications/dictionaries/cancer-terms/def/distress.
19. Sutton TL, Koprowski MA, Grossblatt-Wait A, Brown S, McCarthy G, Liu B, Gross A, Macuiba C, Hedlund S, Brody JR, Sheppard BC. Psychosocial distress is dynamic across the spectrum of cancer care and requires longitudinal screening for patient-centered care. Support Care Cancer. 2022;30(5):4255–64. https://doi.org/10.1007/s00520-022-06814-z.
20. 2020 standards and Resources. American College of Surgeons Commission on Cancer. 2020. https://www.facs.org/quality-programs/cancer-programs/commission-on-cancer/standards-and-resources/2020/.
21. Deshields T, Zebrack B, Kennedy V. The state of psychosocial services in cancer care in the United States. Psycho-Oncology. 2012;22(3):699–703. https://doi.org/10.1002/pon.3057.
22. Ownby K. Use of the distress thermometer in clinical practice. J Adv Pract Oncol. 2019;10(2):175–9. https://doi.org/10.6004/jadpro.2019.10.2.7.
23. Faller H, Schuler M, Richard M, Heckl U, Weis J, Küffner R. Effects of psycho-oncologic interventions on emotional distress and quality of life in adult patients with cancer: systematic review and meta-analysis. J Clin Oncol. 2013;31(6):782–93. https://doi.org/10.1200/jco.2011.40.8922.
24. Krueger E, Secinti E, Stewart JC, Rand KL, Mosher CE. Cognitive-behavioral and mindfulness-based interventions for distress in patients with advanced cancer: a meta-analysis. Psychooncology. 2023;33(1):e6259. https://doi.org/10.1002/pon.6259.
25. Novilla M, Goates M, Leffler T, Novilla N, Wu C, Dall A, Hansen C. Integrating social care into healthcare: a review on applying the social determinants of health in clinical settings. Int J Environ Res Public Health. 2023;20(19):6873. https://doi.org/10.3390/ijerph20196873.
26. Petruzzi L, Milano N, Chen Q, Noel L, Golden R, Jones B. Social workers are key to addressing social determinants of health in integrated care settings. Soc Work Health Care. 2024;63(2):89–101. https://doi.org/10.1080/00981389.2023.2292565.
27. Moen M, Storr C, German D, Friedmann E, Johantgen M. A review of tools to screen for social determinants of health in the United States: a practice brief. Popul Health Manag. 2020;23(6):422–9. https://doi.org/10.1089/pop.2019.0158.
28. Zebrack B, Schapmire T, Otis-Green S, Nelson K, Miller N, Donna D, Grignon M. Establishing core competencies, opportunities, roles and expertise for oncology social work. J Soc Work. 2022;22(4):1085–104. https://doi.org/10.1177/14680173211051983.

29. Zebrack B, Schapmire T, Damaskos P, Grignon M, Smith SK. The essential and evolving nature of oncology social work: accomplishments and impact, 2010– present. J Psychosoc Oncol. 2024;42(6):739–68. https://doi.org/10.1080/07347332.2024.2404577.
30. U.S Department of Health and Human Services. CMS Framework for Health Equity 2022–2032. 2024. https://www.cms.gov/files/document/cms-framework-health-equity-2022.pdf
31. Bedard T. CHI & SDOH Risk Assessment Documentation, Coding, and Billing for Oncology Providers and Administrators & Series Wrap-up. {PowerPoint slides} Association of Cancer Care Centers. 2024. https://www.accc-cancer.org/docs/documents/advocacy/billing-and-coding/accc-chi-sdoh-for-oncology-providers-and-series-wrap-up.pdf?sfvrsn=88bdb89f_2.
32. Joint Commission. New requirements to reduce health care disparities. R^3 report: requirement, rationale, reference, 36. 2022.

Medical Students and Cancer Research

33

Evan Huang

Part I: Introduction

Cancer Research Advanced Cancer Care

In 2021, cancer accounted for 17% of all deaths, the second-leading cause of all death in the United States of all ages, and the leading cause of death among people under the age of 85 years old [1]. Historically, the term "cancer" has carried the connotation of shortened survival and poor quality of life. With this connotation, cancer has invoked large amounts of research around the world in investigating not just the different types of cancer and their prognosis, but more importantly, the different treatment options that seek to prevent its metastasis and eliminate cancer completely. These efforts have led to a 5-year survival rate average for all cancers from just 49% during the mid-1970s to 69% from 2013–2019, a staggering 20% increase in the past half century [1]. This success is due in part to the array of new therapies that have been vital in managing metastatic melanoma, like first- and second-generation immunotherapy, BRAF, and MEK inhibitors. Research has also focused on cancer prevention. For example, due to increased public awareness of the causal role of smoking in many cases of lung cancer, reductions in smoking from 1991 to 2001 have translated to around 4.1 million fewer cancer deaths [1]. Further, earlier detection for different types of prostate and breast cancer, improved treatment, and recent development in targeted therapies and immunotherapy can also contribute to the mortality from cancer itself.

It is therefore evident that cancer research and advancements in the field play a crucial role in driving progress in cancer prevention and treatment. Globally, improvements in treatment and diagnosis of cancer have already proven to directly improve patient survival from 50% to around 60% [2–4]. Further research has directly linked oncologic research to better health outcomes. Treatment trials, or different studies that consist of an active patient population, have proven to be effective, with around 3.34 million life-years gained in the USA at a cost of just $125 on average for each life-year. This correlates to a 25% reduction in cancer mortality since 1991 [3]. In other words, different research-informed treatment plans or interventions on trial have proven to benefit most patients in most cases, further emphasizing the importance of generating new treatment plans or ideas in regard to cancer research on the different areas of treatment: diagnosis, quality of life, and life expectancy [4]. Specifically, these studies have proven that it is worth it to try and test these different hypotheses in treatment with the pretense that it is research-informed. Statistically, research-based treatment plans have shown to increase survival rate and reduce postoperative mortality compared to non-trial participants [5, 6]. In colorectal cancer patients, increased participation in interventional studies showed a 5-year improved survival rate of 3.8% and reduced 30 day postoperative mortality by 1.5% [5].

Obstacles to Cancer Research: Shortage of Oncological Physicians and Scientists, Insufficient Research Exposure in Medical Education

With the importance of cancer research clear, another problem has seemingly arisen: an increased demand for biomedical researchers and health science professionals in the field of cancer [7–10]. Advances in genetic sequencing technology, molecular analysis of cancer cells, and improved understanding of the immune system have created many new diagnostic and therapeutic approaches. However, there is a shortage of physicians and scientists in the field of oncology to properly address these needs. In fact, by 2025, the need for oncologists is predicted to outpace the number of clinicians

E. Huang (✉)
University of Missouri - Kansas City, School of Medicine,
Kansas City, MO, USA

J. Huang, H. S.L. Jim (eds.), *Cancer Research Guidance for Clinicians and Researchers*,
https://doi.org/10.1007/978-3-032-19175-5_33

trained, causing alarm toward the future of research-based intervention in cancer treatment [7]. Even more concerning is the decreasing number of medical students interested in research. Gathered from various studies, just 31% were interested in a career involving research [11], and participation in research for medical student research projects ranges from just 5% to 40% [12]. Further, a survey found that one in every three medical students completes medical school without significant exposure to any kind of research, presenting a significant gap in medical education [13]. As patients live longer with more chronic conditions, the need for physicians and scientists will increase [8]. Increased engagement of medical students in research may help to ameliorate these problems. In 2013, a little over a decade ago, the involvement of medical students globally in research was next to none. In fact, around 90% of reported students reported no research experience in medical school. Those who do participate in research are typically involved in data collecting and computer work, which students may have difficulty connecting with better patient care [9]. In the United States, while there is an increase in participation in medical school enrollment in recent years, their contributions could provide vital support toward benefiting the field of oncology and the different types of research surrounding it. In a research-based program in oncology that was developed to train medical students in cancer research while also exposing them to the field of clinical oncology, the students' understanding of oncology as a clinical and as a research discipline both improved [14]. As such, this chapter explores not just the benefits of cancer research for medical students but also the typical process entailed by student involvement in research. It will highlight the different ways for students to become involved in cancer research through different historical studies. Further, the chapter explores the current state of medical student participation in cancer research as a vital part in improving the field of oncological treatment and prevention.

Part II: Benefits of Research for Medical Students

Research Experience Contributes to the Development of Better Physicians

While the importance of medical research in improving healthcare has been established for decades, research is also an ever-evolving process that requires constant participation from all areas of the field of medicine [15]. However, while the benefits of research to the medical field are clear, its impact on the development of medical students is just as important. The ability to understand and integrate new knowledge in this ever-changing field into clinical practice has become a necessary skill for physicians. Especially in the field of oncology, constantly reviewing medical literature and applying it are vital to the potential well-being of patients [16]. One clear benefit that has been linked with conducting research as a medical student is improved clinicians' understanding and interpretation of clinical test data [17, 18]. Students reported more confidence in identifying and utilizing trustworthy scientific results. They also found research to be a meaningful introduction into the world of academia, which could serve as a strong motivator for a higher degree. One other benefit of medical research is that it could help address the high rate of burnout among current physicians, serving as an opportunity to take a break from the practice to explore an individual's interests [18]. This could serve as a unique opportunity to create not only more knowledge, but also more motivated students, as research creates a task outside of the general routine of medicine that could add variety to the potentially repetitive cycle physicians find themselves in. By exposing future physicians to research early, not only is their interest in the field of academia widened, but also, they could create the stepping stones to become more confident in their research and expand to other research topics. In addition, conducting research during medical school has been linked to aiding in clinical decisions and thus improving the lives of the patients that future physicians directly work with [12, 19–24]. Research provides unique opportunities for students as it not only allows them to distinguish themselves from other applicants but also can create a network of connections, expose them to different specialties they might be interested in, and, most importantly, create opportunities to publish the work they create [21]. Further, research involving review articles or other forms that require reading of journal articles can serve a strong, beneficial role in the practice of evidence-based medicine, as students learn how to read different types of articles from different journals and how to properly critique them. Through this work, students learn how to properly utilize and evaluate an article [25, 26]. Moreover, medical students can offer unique insight and input into a project as they have the time and energy to complete some of the possibly more labor-intensive elements of a project. Their contributions could also aid in the publication output of the medical school in itself, supporting institutional research goals [26]. Initially, medical students may need consistent mentorship from physicians and residents. With good mentoring, students may be able to, over time, work with increasing independence on various aspects of research [27]. Further, participating in research during medical school also serves as a strong indicator of potential career outlook in academia. Medical students engaged in research demonstrated a strong association with long-term academic achievement, characterized by a higher probability of securing faculty appointments and contributing to scholarly literature through authoring or co-authoring peer-reviewed publications [11].

Research Enhances Medical Students' Competitiveness for Desired Specialties and Training Programs

Conducting research during medical school can help students be competitive in matching to a residency of their choice and may also further establish their interest in the specialty of their choice. Many medical students who decide to undergo research typically do so in the interest of a specific specialty [12]. In fact, scholastic performance paired with research experience during medical school serves as a good predictor of future achievements in their respective fields 20 years in the future [28, 29]. The correlation between research experience and matching into competitive specialties has started to become a strong trend in medicine residency programs. For example, for matching into integrated plastic surgery, a significantly larger proportion (97%) of respondents who participated in research matched into a program compared to those who did not (81%). While a research fellowship may not serve as a complete indicator of a medical student's resume of research, it acts as a metric of measurement for confidently comparing those who have done research against those who have not [30]. This trend is also seen in otolaryngology match outcomes in applicants seeking to secure an OHNS residency position, citing a dedicated research year or fellowship as a strong boost to their application from the research produced [31]. On the other side of the application portal, studies report that an average of 41% of residency program directors value an applicant's involvement and interest in research strongly, indicating research as a strong motivator for students seeking to match not just into highly competitive residencies, but residencies as a whole [27]. Statistically, a study conducted by the National Resident Matching Program in 2016 and 2018 found that medical students with significantly more research accomplishments than their peers matched into their preferred specialties more on average. Not only does research experience add a strong boost to an application, but the student may also acquire key research skills like literature review and hypothesis generation that can have direct implication toward the setting of clinical practice [20]. On top of this, with the move of the United States Medical Licensing Exam Step 1 toward a pass/fail exam, it is evident that extracurricular research could become more valued when creating a strong residency application [32]. Further, conducting research aids in students' career progression by helping them define their career path or, more specifically, the specialty they find themselves interested in. In a study conducted at Mayo Clinics, third-year medical students reported that research in their area of interest increased their confidence about their application to residency positions [21]. Medical school research projects significantly influenced students' career choices, with a 2.7 times higher probability of specializing in the same clinical area as their research focus [11].

One potential negative of this participation in research is student motives for doing so. Of the applicants that underwent a research fellowship for integrated plastic surgery, 63% stated that they performed the research fellowship to strengthen their application, while just 37% reported doing so out of general interest [30]. When research is done not for the general curiosity and intellectual challenge it brings, but instead because of academic pressures to publish, it could sway students away from research in the future rather than attract them to it [33].

Due to the decrease in the number of physician-scientists in the USA in recent years [24], medical school and future fellowships after represents an important time or "turn-on" period for students to consider careers in academic medicine and research early on in their professional training [34]. One study reported on the integration of mandatory research training into the curricula of the University of Tennessee College of Medicine (public institution) and Vanderbilt School of Medicine (private institution). Results indicated that the research experience allowed students to evaluate their fit with conducting biomedical research, appreciate the effort it takes to research novel information in the field of medicine, and made them more likely to pursue careers in academic medicine overall [34]. Another study performed across three public universities, Pennsylvania State University College of Medicine, University of Connecticut School of Medicine, and University of Massachusetts Medical School, showed similar results. They compared students who had performed research against those who did not, showing that, regardless of medical school, performing medical research in medical school was strongly associated with postgraduate research involvement [17]. Overall, introducing medical students to research could not only encourage them to pursue academic medicine and aid in the shortage of physician-scientists [12, 24] but also create physicians who appreciate the research enterprise within medicine in itself, a vital trait to the progression of healthcare in the future.

Part III: How to Get Involved

Understand the Barriers to Medical Students' Ability to Engage in Research

Several barriers hinder research participation by medical students, including limited access to research opportunities, scarcity of available mentors, and insufficient knowledge about how to effectively pursue research endeavors [13, 21, 35]. For medical students seeking research opportunities, a study found that while 53% of students approached a mentor for extracurricular research, only 38% gained a successful research experience from it, indicating that the process of finding a mentor is a strong barrier in itself. Further, because of the level of their medical experience, many students have the perception that there is a lack of support to publish their work to the academic community. Even when the opportunity to publish is available, there runs a possibility that the credit students receive does not correlate to the amount of work that they put in. For example, a student might do a lot of work on a major paper yet receive the same amount of credit as a student who contributed less to a less significant paper. In essence, when a medical student is recognized for their work, it often leaves out the authorship position of the medical student and the impact of the paper itself [35].

Medical Schools Should Establish Required and Targeted Research Programs for Medical Students

One potential idea that has been incorporated in various institutions around the world is the idea of establishing a required or integrated research portion into the curriculum of medical schools. The Albert Einstein School of Medicine implemented a requirement that fourth-year medical students undergo a 6-month-long research project to replace an elective course. The result was that 85% of applicants reported that it positively impacted their career in medicine, and 97% found it useful as a replacement for an elective [36]. Similarly, at Queen's University Faculty of Health Sciences, students were required to take a course on medical research, where a significant increase in the number of students interested in pursuing a research year following the class was seen [22]. This trend of the benefits of establishing a mandatory research experience linked with positive outcomes in interest and publications in research is a common trend found in other medical schools around the world [12]. A study from the University of Calgary found a significant increase from 11% to 59% in manuscript submissions after a formal research program was established [25]. Another idea is the establishment of an honors year in different specialties focused on research within that specialty, which has been shown to encourage entry into research and academic careers [37]. In terms of programs that include a mandatory research project, on average, one in four medical students is able to publish their findings in a peer-reviewed paper, mostly as a first or second author [24]. These studies further indicate the link between establishing or creating an option of a research elective and a medical student's increased interest in research following that elective. The option or requirement to conduct research in medical school could serve as a vital solution, as, in general, there is no consistent method for easily integrating medical students into research across all institutions. Currently, in the United States, these students find opportunities in summer research electives, extracurricular activities, or various external options [11].

A clear research infrastructure is key to motivating medical students to engage in some form of research, as long as resources can be provided to identify and support research opportunities. These programs act as a strong introduction to research and may serve as a gateway toward helping the decline in physician-scientists [21]. The perception of a supportive supervisor can be the biggest factor in a successful research experience and allows them to acquire the necessary training and support provided by the mentors to achieve a publication [35].

Mentorship Is Key for the Success of Medical Student Research

When choosing to do medical research, two components are vital for the student to identify: their field of interest and the mentor who will guide them along the way. First, it is important to narrow down a wide range of potential topics to just a few focused ones of interest to the study. Committing oneself to a research project of one's interest will greatly increase the student's willingness to enhance their knowledge on a specialty further in the research field, serving as a powerful motivator to do the research in itself [23]. Next, ensuring that the student is paired with the right mentor is equally as important in the development of not just the research project, but the medical student's research career in itself. Good mentors are enthusiastic, have strong records of research productivity, and have the time and interest to work with the student directly. Good mentors must also understand students' constraints and set appropriate expectations. As such, the first meeting with the mentor is vital in determining the potential fit between student and mentor [13, 23]. A study conducted at Queen's University found that faculty interaction was a motivating factor for 75% of its students who conducted research, indicating a mentor's influence on a student's medical research [21]. It is important that the student communicates clearly with the mentor in terms of the skills and knowledge they hope to gain from the experience while also being realistic about their time commitment [38]. Typically, finding a mentor can be done through a medical university's established system or application process or through directly contacting clinicians and researchers as an alternative. One important factor to note when contacting potential mentors is to ensure there is consistency in the rate of publishing publications while also ensuring that they are willing to help [23]. The application process in itself can vary depending on institution to institution and, if applying to a program, across various programs. Nevertheless, it is important to establish and prepare a well-written curriculum vitae (CV) and personal statement. The CV functions as a way to describe one's educational and professional background while also showing how the applicant can meet the expectations of the required research. Preparatory and introductory courses in statistics and dataset enquire can demonstrate that a student has the skills and background to complete the task. The personal statement acts as a reinforcement of the applicant's interest in the specialty and the research area [23].

Because of the constraints of their time schedule, medical students are typically only given a few months to dedicate to research. As such, mentors should be aware of these constraints, and target dates should be set to aid in the process [13]. Staying up to date and active with the research project or commitment is vital not only to ensure continuous progression of the project, but also the relationship between the mentor and medical student. While a student's schedule cannot be controlled, it is the responsibility of the medical student to provide updates on these restrictions with clear communication [23, 33].

Medical Students' Publications

Translating the research into a publication or presentation is often in the student's best interest in terms of career advancement [39]. As such, good writing skills are needed for the proposal, publication, and/or poster. While constant reading of various journal articles can aid in developing these skills, medical students should continuously work on their writing style. When reading, it is important to note the different formats and categories used in different journals. One approach called the "reverse approach" is to do the writing process in reverse. First, a journal is chosen to be published in. Then, the specialty or topic of the publication is chosen, where, soon after, the editor is contacted, and a due date is set. Overall, experiences in writing can aid development in the future as there is an increasing expectation for new physicians to publish as a sign of their career progression and training [40]. Letter to the editor, opinion pieces, and systematic reviews can serve as publications that are suitable for new medical students and within their ability to produce [23]. In terms of submitting a conference abstract, it is important to ensure the abstracts are submitted with the proper components. If the abstract is graded highly based on the scoring criteria given, then they are selected to present as posters at the conference, another accomplishment for not just the research, but the student presenting the poster [32]. Regardless, the process toward publication or creating a poster can vary depending on the type of research and the pace of the project. Historically, for medical students seeking publication in a peer-reviewed journal, the process took around 1.63 years on average [39].

Part IV: Addressing Cancer Research for Medical Students

The increasing demand for clinical researchers in oncology [41–43] requires interventions to increase interest in oncologic research geared toward medical students. Further, with the increasingly changing field of different cancers projected over the course of the next few decades, a medical student's engagement with cancer research is vital to exposing them to the array of different specialties involved with patient care [42]. Globally, studies indicate that medical school curricula offer limited exposure to oncology, with students commonly reporting an overall lack of confidence in providing oncology care [43].

To address these issues, institutions have recently established oncology-focused research programs in medical schools, targeted at not just increasing students' exposure to the different fields of oncology but also promoting the idea of research within the field. Further, cancer research is distinctly different from other forms of clinical research, emphasizing the need to create specific programs targeted toward oncologic research education, creating a more focused research experience individualized to the field of oncology [42]. One program named Scholars in Oncology-Associated Research (SOAR) was developed to directly train medical students in clinical cancer research while also exposing them to clinical oncology across an 11-week span that resulted in an oral presentation and internal manuscript submission. Participants reported that the program not only gave them firsthand research experience, but also allowed them to understand how different facets of cancer care intersect [42]. Another example that originated at the University of Alabama at Birmingham (UAB) in 1999, called the Cancer Research Experience for Students (CaRES), involves a paid summer cancer research internship with similar results as the SOAR program. Specifically, students reported an increased understanding and expanded views on cancer research. From this program, 13.6% of participants were able to generate a presentation or publication, and 110 out of 499 alumni of the program published a total of 238 cancer-related, peer-reviewed papers [41]. Similar programs exhibited similar results with reported significant improvements in the students' understanding of the role of medical oncologist as well as cancer research [43, 44]. One important aspect reported by students was the presence of strong mentorship, which they believed was foundational to their success in research [43, 44].

Another opportunity for improving medical students' exposure to cancer research is the presence of student interest groups or societies. The Student Oncology Society provides opportunities for interested students to gain exposure to oncology, identifying potential research mentors [45]. Finally, it is important to note that the structure of the program itself is also an important factor in the student experience. For example, the Radiation Oncology Mentorship Initiative (ROMI) includes a research project that connects senior medical students with junior ones paired with a mentor that work toward an eventual publication. The results showed that 75% of students became more interested in research, and 85% better understood the methodology behind the research through the program. Further, the program produced 106 abstracts among 58 students, with 76 having the student as first author [46].

Conclusion

Cancer research has significantly improved cancer care, extending lives and enhancing quality of life. However, a looming shortage of oncologists and cancer researchers threatens these advancements. Insufficient research exposure in medical education exacerbates this crisis. Recognizing this, many medical schools have implemented required and targeted research programs for students. These initiatives have shown promise in motivating future researchers. As a medical student, engaging in a research project can foster a deeper understanding of a chosen specialty and cultivate the skills of a more effective physician. The success of this endeavor hinges on the quality of mentorship. Ideal mentors are passionate, accomplished researchers who actively guide students, considering their individual needs and research aspirations.

References

1. Siegel RL, Giaquinto AN, Jemal A. Cancer statistics. CA Cancer J Clin. 2024;74(1):12–49.
2. Lawler M, Banks I, Law K, et al. The European cancer patient's bill of rights, update and implementation. ESMO Open. 2016;1:e000127.
3. Unger JM, LeBlanc M, Blanke CD. The effect of positive SWOG treatment trials on survival of patients with cancer in the US population. JAMA Oncol. 2017;3:1345–51.
4. Selby P, Kaplan R, Cameron D, Cooper M, Seymour M. Clinical research networks and the benefits of intensive healthcare systems. Clin Med. 2012;12:446–52.
5. Downing EJ, Morris N, Corrigan D, Sebag-Montefiore PJ, Finan JD, Thomas M, Chapman R, Hamilton H, Campbell D, Cameron R, Kaplan M, Parmar R, Stephens M, Seymour W, Gregory P. Selby, High hospital research participation and improved colorectal cancer survival outcomes: a population-based study. Gut. 2017;66:89–96.
6. Liu L, Giusti F, Schaapveld M, Aleman B, Lugtenburg P, Meijnders P, Hutchings M, Lemmens V, Bogaerts J, Visser O. Survival differences between patients with Hodgkin lymphoma treated inside and outside clinical trials. A study based on the EORTC-Netherlands cancer registry linked data with 20 years of follow-up. Br J Haematol. 2017;176:65–75.
7. Ezelle HJ, Geiman T, Schnaper LA, Cullen KJ, Lapidus RS, Hassel BA. A translational approach to cancer research, education and training. J Cancer Educ 2021;36(3):621–629.
8. Goldstein Michael Workforce Advisory Group Report. Future supply of and demand for oncologists. J Oncol Pract. 2008;4:300.
9. Jimmy R, Palatty PL, D'Silva P, Baliga MS, Singh A. Are medical students inclined to do research? J Clin Diagn Res. 2013;7:2892–5.
10. Heimburger DC, Waterbor J, Fish L, Brooks CM. An interdisciplinary program in nutrition sciences and cancer. J Cancer Educ. 2000;15:130–3.
11. Amgad M, Man Kin Tsui M, Liptrott SJ, et al. Medical student research: an integrated mixed-methods systematic review and meta-analysis. PLoS One. 2015;10:e0127470.
12. Al-Busaidi IS, Tarr GP. Dissemination of results from medical student public health research training and factors associated with publication. Postgrad Med J. 2018;94:330–4.
13. Young BK, Cai F, Tandon VJ, George P, Greenberg PB. Promoting medical student research productivity: the student perspective. R I Med J (2013). 2014;97(6):50–2.
14. Vayani OR, Asif H, Klein A, Hahn OM, Pearson AT, Arora VM, Olopade OI, Golden DW. Adapting a medical school cancer research education program to the virtual environment: a mixed-methods study. J Cancer Educ. 2023;38(5):1501–8.
15. Global Forum for Health Research. 10/90 Report on health research 2003–2004. Geneva: Global forum for Health research; 2004. Accessed 12 Dec 2024. Available from http://www.globalforumhealth.org/Media-Publications/Publications/10-90-Report-2003-2004
16. Parsonnet J, Gruppuso PA, Kanter SL, et al. Required vs. elective research and in-depth scholarship programs in the medical student curriculum. Acad Med. 2010;85:405–8.
17. Segal S, Lloyd T, Houts PS, Stillman PL, Jungas RL, Greer RB 3rd. The association between students' research involvement in medical school and their postgraduate medical activities. Acad Med. 1990;65:530–3.
18. Ashcroft J, Yousefpour C. Medical student research: it is necessary and beneficial! Postgrad Med J. 2018;94:539.
19. Gonzalez-Blasco P, Wong R, St. George, I. The role of research in undergraduate medical education: building capacity for the changing medical environment. BMC Med Educ. 2019;19(1):91.
20. Hamby T, Wilson DP, Bui P, Lowery J, Basha R. Medical student research opportunities: a survey of osteopathic medical schools in the United States. J Osteopath Med. 2022;122(6):289–95.
21. Chang Y, Ramnanan CJ. A review of literature on medical students and scholarly research: experiences, attitudes, and outcomes. Acad Med. 2015;90(8):1162–73.
22. Houlden RL, Raja JB, Collier CP, Clark AF, Wuagh JM. Medical students' perceptions of an undergraduate research elective. Med Teach. 2004;26:659–61.
23. Vasilica AM, Kumar NS. Twelve tips for successfully getting involved in research as a medical student. Med Teach. 2022;44(9):962–6.
24. den Bakker CR, Ommering BW, van Leeuwen TN, Dekker FW, De Beaufort AJ. Assessing publication rates from medical students' mandatory research projects in The Netherlands: a follow-up study of 10 cohorts of medical students. BMJ Open. 2022;12(4):e056053.
25. Griffin MF, Hindocha S. Publication practices of medical students at British medical schools: experience, attitudes and barriers to publish. Med Teach. 2011;33(1):e1–8.
26. Metcalfe D. Involving medical students in research. J R Soc Med. 2008;101(3):102–3.
27. Ward B, Schultz JJ, Halsey JN, Hoppe IC, Lee ES, Granick MS. Mentorship through research: a novel approach to increasing resident and medical student research competency through an institutional database. J Surg Educ. 2020;77(6):1331–3.
28. Brancati FL, Mead LA, Levine DM, Martin D, Margolis S, Klag MJ. Early predictors of career achievement in academic medicine. JAMA. 1992;267:1372–6.
29. Reinders JJ, Kropmans TJ, Cohen-Schotanus J. Extracurricular research experience of medical students and their scientific output after graduation. Med Educ. 2005;39:237.
30. Mehta K, Sinno S, Thanik V, Weichman K, Janis JE, Patel A. Matching into integrated plastic surgery: the value of research fellowships. Plast Reconstr Surg. 2019;143(2):640–5.
31. Dorismond C, Shah RN, Ebert CS Jr, Buckmire RA. Impact of medical student research fellowships on otolaryngology match outcomes. Laryngoscope. 2021;131(9):E2506–12.
32. Santhumayor BA, Chen A, Pelcher I, Cater E, Mishra A, Ward M, White TG, Schulder M, Sciubba DM, Tracey KJ, Baum GR. Organizing a regional in-person medical student symposium in neuroscience and neurosurgery research: a how-to guide. World Neurosurg. 2024;189:249–55.

33. Cheung BMY. Medical student research: is it necessary and beneficial? Postgrad Med J. 2018;94:317.
34. Solomon SS, Tom SC, Pichert J, et al. Impact of medical student research in the development of physician-scientists. J Investig Med. 2003;51:149–56.
35. Mahalingam J, Khatri C, Fitzgerald JE. Pressure of academic publishing for medical students: a student's perspective. Postgrad Med J. 2018;94(1113):397.
36. Frishman WH. Student research projects and theses: should they be a requirement for medical school graduation. Heart Dis. 2001;3:140–4.
37. Nguyen-Van-Tam JS, Logan RF, Logan SA, et al. What happens to medical students who complete an honours year in public health and epidemiology? Med Educ. 2001;35:134–6.
38. Alexander L. How can I get involved in research as a medical student? BMJ. 2020;370:m2586.
39. Volodarskaya M, Tucker AB, Tseng J. Medical student research in surgery: from abstract presentation to publication. J Surg Educ. 2020;77(6):1450–3.
40. George S, Moreira K. Publishing non-research papers as a trainee: a recipe for beginners. Singapore Med J. 2009;50:756–8.
41. Desmond RA, Padilla LA, Daniel CL, et al. Career outcomes of graduates of R25E short-term cancer research training programs. J Cancer Educ. 2016;31(1):93–100.
42. Vayani OR, Asif H, Klein A, et al. Adapting a medical school cancer research education program to the virtual environment: a mixed-methods study. J Cancer Educ. 2023;38(5):1501–8.
43. Rallis KS, Wozniak A, Hui S, et al. Mentoring medical students towards oncology: results from a pilot multi-institutional mentorship Programme. J Cancer Educ. 2022;37(4):1053–65.
44. Ben-David K, Lin JJ, Ferrara JLM, Gabrilove JL. Tisch cancer institute scholars program: mentored cancer research training pipeline for medical students. J Cancer Educ. 2022;37(4):1166–71.
45. Huang D, Childs E, Uppalapati AV, Tai EC, Hirsch AE. Medical student leadership in the student oncology society: evaluation of a student-run interest group. J Cancer Educ. 2022;37(6):1629–33.
46. Huang D, Qureshi MM, Sarfaty S, et al. Longitudinal outcomes of medical student research mentorship: a 15-year analysis of the radiation oncology mentorship initiative. J Cancer Educ. 2023;38(1):153–60.

Oncology Nurses and Cancer Research

34

Brandon Dyer, Joel Kallarackal, and Jeffrey Huang

Role of the Oncology Nurse in Patient Care

Oncology nurses are on the front lines of delivering therapy to patients, with one study finding that each patient requires an average of 3.3 h of nursing staff time for a chemotherapy protocol, comprising 1.7 h of direct contact time and 1.6 h of non-contact time [1]. Thus, nurses are usually the first to ascertain if the patient is having any adverse responses from treatment-related toxicity or suffering from cancer-related symptoms that require additional treatment, such as nausea/vomiting, fatigue, or pain. Furthermore, when oncologists become focused on evolving treatment evidence or innovative therapies, nurses hold a prime position to advocate effectively for the patient's current and immediate needs [2].

Beyond advocating for patients directly, oncology nurses empower patients to self-advocate and take an active role in their care. Nurses facilitate patient empowerment by directing individuals to resources and tools, shifting the locus of control back to patients themselves. Enhancing patients' sense of autonomy can lead to improved adherence to treatment regimens and stronger self-efficacy in expressing their needs and concerns to the broader healthcare team [3]. Ultimately, empowering patients to become self-advocates helps to mitigate feelings of helplessness and anxiety, resulting in improved psychological resilience throughout treatment.

Patient education represents another critical component of oncology nursing. Given the extensive time nurses spend interacting with patients, they are most likely to build the trust and rapport that enable tailored patient education for specific learning styles [4]. Oncology nurses ensure patients fully comprehend their diagnoses, understand treatment decisions and potential side effects, and are aware of resources available. This level of education becomes increasingly significant as outpatient chemotherapy treatments rise, placing greater responsibilities on patients to self-manage their symptoms and treatment schedules [5].

Multidisciplinary collaboration also underscores the critical role of oncology nurses. As cancer care has evolved into complex multidisciplinary team–based approaches, oncology nurses serve as vital coordinators among healthcare providers. A multidisciplinary tumor board may have up to 14 different members, yet this model still excludes dietitians, physical therapists, and holistic care professionals [6]. Oncology nurses help to fill coordination gaps to ensure comprehensive communication both between team members and the patient. Thus, maintaining continuity and consistency of care is essential. Nurses' holistic understanding of both medical and psychosocial aspects of care makes them particularly suited to integrating these diverse perspectives into a coherent care plan.

Lastly, outcomes for cancer patients are dependent on factors far beyond the treatment regimen selected. Quality of life and patient-reported outcomes (PROs) are increasingly recognized as central to successful cancer management. Oncology nurses are pivotal in monitoring and evaluating PROs, which provide insight into symptom burden, physical functioning, emotional well-being, and overall patient satisfaction [7]. PROs offer valuable data that enable healthcare providers to adjust treatment plans proactively, potentially improving adherence and reducing symptom burden. Moreover, nurses provide essential emotional and psychological support, which is paramount for improving quality of life through rigorous treatments [8, 9].

Areas for Oncology Nursing Research

Oncology nurses' engagement in direct patient care, patient education, and advocacy creates multiple avenues for impactful nurse-driven research. Areas ripe for nursing investiga-

B. Dyer · J. Kallarackal
University of South Florida Morsani College of Medicine, Tampa, FL, USA

J. Huang (✉)
Anesthesiology and Critical Care, Moffitt Cancer Center, Tampa, FL, USA
e-mail: Jeffrey.huang@moffitt.org

J. Huang, H. S.L. Jim (eds.), *Cancer Research Guidance for Clinicians and Researchers*,
https://doi.org/10.1007/978-3-032-19175-5_34

tion include symptom management, survivorship care, health equity, telehealth, and digital health innovations. Numerous nurse-led interventions have demonstrated efficacy in improving patient outcomes, such as communication-based strategies, coping skills training, multicomponent interventions, and stress-reduction techniques. These interventions have shown promise in alleviating patient distress, anxiety, and depression and improving overall quality of life, self-efficacy, and coping mechanisms [9].

Symptom management remains a pivotal research priority, addressing persistent issues such as chemotherapy-induced nausea, fatigue, neuropathy, and cognitive dysfunction. Oncology nursing research can evaluate the effectiveness of targeted interventions to mitigate these symptoms, examining both pharmacological and non-pharmacological strategies to enhance patient comfort and improve treatment outcomes [10].

Long-term effects of cancer therapies, especially with emerging treatments such as immunotherapies and targeted therapies, represent another significant gap in current research. Clinical trials have traditionally prioritized overall survival or progression-free survival as primary endpoints, often neglecting the critical patient experience and long-term quality of life. Oncology nurses, who closely monitor patients over extended periods, are well positioned to lead research initiatives that track patient-reported outcomes (PROs), thus informing survivorship care plans and rehabilitation protocols tailored to the long-term needs of patients [11].

Health equity and addressing social determinants of health (SDOH) also play a significant role in oncology, making them solid areas for nursing research to prioritize. Factors such as socioeconomic status, education level, geographical location, and minority status are significantly associated with cancer outcomes. They influence diagnosis delays, access to treatment, and treatment adherence [12]. Nurse-led research can offer valuable insights into developing culturally sensitive interventions, targeted education programs, and advocacy strategies to reduce disparities and enhance equitable cancer care delivery.

Alongside health equity, telehealth and digital health innovations represent novel avenues for nursing research. Particularly, these can be used to address geographical barriers and enhance patient support. The use of telehealth has increased substantially, partly necessitated by the COVID-19 pandemic, revealing significant potential to improve access, symptom monitoring, and ongoing patient education. Research evaluating the effectiveness of telehealth, patient and provider satisfaction, barriers to implementation, and long-term outcomes can further establish telehealth as a core component of comprehensive oncology care [13].

Additionally, nursing research into big data analytics and artificial intelligence (AI) can optimize oncology care delivery by identifying patterns predictive of adverse events, therefore enhancing personalized treatment regimens and streamlining clinical workflows. Oncology nurses can critically assess these innovations from a patient-centered perspective, ensuring that safety, privacy, ethics, and equitable access remain at the forefront of technology implementation [14].

In summary, oncology nurses' unique roles in patient care, education, advocacy, and now research position them at the nexus of innovation and patient-centered practice. Nurse-led research initiatives are crucial for continually improving the quality of cancer care, patient satisfaction, and clinical outcomes.

Role of Nurses in Current Oncology Clinical Trials and Research

Nurses involved in oncology clinical research play multiple roles throughout the trial's progression. Oftentimes, this starts with the recruitment and enrollment of patients for the research. During this process, nurses play a crucial role in screening potential participants using inclusionary and exclusionary criteria. This involves reviewing medical records, pathology reports, imaging, and laboratory results to assess initial eligibility. At this stage of the research process, clinical judgment from the nurses helps reduce screen failure rates and facilitates the efficient identification of eligible participants [15]. As previously mentioned, patient education is a key aspect of the nurse's role in oncology clinical trials and research. This process begins by educating patients on the purpose of the trial, including its potential benefits and risks. Patients have reported greater satisfaction and a better understanding of the trials when clinical staff, such as nurses, conveyed the information rather than relying solely on written consent forms [16]. This education is closely related to the nurse's role of obtaining informed consent. The nurse must ensure the participant truly understands the content of the informed consent and clarify any possible misconceptions [17].

Strict adherence to the study protocol is critical to ensuring both patient safety and the integrity of the research being conducted. Oncology nurses play a pivotal role in ensuring the appropriate implementation of protocols and determining compliance. Oncology clinical trials often employ treatment regimens that differ significantly from standard-of-care therapies. As such, nurses must be well versed in the handling, dosing, and timing protocols for the investigational treatment [18]. Further, since many investigational treatments come with minimal safety data, nurses must adapt and recognize the signs of adverse reactions while adhering to the protocol [19]. In the case of deviations from protocol, the nurse should be the first to identify and address them. Frequent communication with other members of the clinical team, such as physicians and pharmacists, can enhance compliance with protocol. In a review of oncology trials, consistent nurse engagement and clearly defined protocols were found to diminish deviations and improve the quality of the trial. A prominent role of the oncology nurse is to document patient status and side effects using standardized criteria, such as the Common Terminology Criteria for Adverse Events (CTCAE), to reduce variability in adverse event reporting [20, 21]. This documentation is crucial for gathering information regarding the efficacy and safety of the investigational treatment for future use.

Accurate data management and reporting are crucial to oncology clinical research. In this realm, nurses link clinical care to research data. Oncology nurses are often tasked with collecting and reporting clinical data through both electronic and paper systems. This requires a nuanced understanding of the research methodology and meticulous attention to detail [22]. This aspect of the oncology nurse reinforces their role in quality data oversight. With the advancement of electronic systems, such as Clinical Trial Management Systems (CTMS) and EMR-integrated platforms, data management has shifted primarily to online systems [23]. Nurses should utilize these systems and establish clear workflows with consistent audits to ensure accurate data collection [24]. Through their oversight roles, oncology clinical nurses must uphold secure data handling, monitor protocol adherence, and assist with auditing.

Another key role of the oncology clinical nurse is patient advocacy. While trials may focus on patient survival and poor outcomes, nurses can address the patient's concerns. This includes treatment burden, quality of life, and other needs. Oncology nurses should develop the ability to identify distress in a patient, promote shared decision-making, and support self-advocacy [25]. In this role, nurses should be able to identify barriers to trial participation and address these issues accordingly. This can range from having a level of cultural competency and tailoring communication to address any challenges in that area to providing patient navigation services [26]. Forming these relationships with trial participants enables patient-centered outcomes while maintaining adherence to the protocol.

The role of oncology nurses does not end after the patient treatment period. Nurses continue their responsibilities by disseminating and translating research findings from the trial. This includes publishing articles, presenting at conferences, and sharing findings with the community to promote change and inform decision-making in the field [27]. Oncology nurses play a vital role in initiating change to clinical practice guidelines through the integration of research findings. Evidence-based practice should be implemented in oncology settings to advance overall quality of care, decrease healthcare costs, and improve patient outcomes [28].

Conclusion

The role of the oncology nurse has become increasingly significant in recent years. As the frontline in the clinical team, oncology nurses find themselves in a unique position to effectively address patients' concerns while also integrating research and clinical practice. As oncology research evolves, nurses are increasingly involved in both the design and implementation of clinical trials, offering a unique and vital perspective for patient care. Their advocacy for evidence-based practice improves patient outcomes and overall quality of care. As the autonomy of this role increases, oncology nurses may need to develop additional competencies in the related field, including data literacy and knowledge of emerging technologies such as artificial intelligence.

References

1. de Raad J, van Gool K, Haas M, et al. Nursing takes time: workload associated with administering cancer protocols - PubMed. Clin J Oncol Nurs. 2010;14(6) https://doi.org/10.1188/10.CJON.735-741.
2. Vaartio-Rajalin H, Leino-Kilpi H. Nurses as patient advocates in oncology care: activities based on literature - PubMed. Clin J Oncol Nurs. 2011;15(5) https://doi.org/10.1188/11.CJON.526-532.
3. Alsbrook KE, Donovan HS, Wesmiller SW, Thomas TH. Oncology nurses' role in promoting patient self-advocacy. Clin J Oncol Nurs. 2022;26(3) https://doi.org/10.1188/22.CJON.239-243.
4. Padberg RMPL, Yarbro CH, Frogge MH, Goodman M. Cancer nursing: principles and practice. 5th ed. Jones and Bartlett; 2000.
5. Rieger PTYC, Kufe DW, Pollock RE, Weichselbaum RR, et al. Cancer medicine. 6th ed; 2003.
6. Berardi R, Morgese F, Rinaldi S, et al. Benefits and limitations of a multidisciplinary approach in cancer patient management. Cancer Manag Res. 2020;12 https://doi.org/10.2147/CMAR.S220976.
7. Caminiti C, Maglietta G, Diodati F, et al. The effects of patient-reported outcome screening on the survival of people with cancer: a systematic review and meta-analysis. Cancer. 2022;14(21) https://doi.org/10.3390/cancers14215470.
8. Lyu X-C, Jiang H-J, Lee L-H, Yang C-I, Sun X-Y. Oncology nurses' experiences of providing emotional support for cancer patients: a qualitative study. BMC Nurs. 2024;23(1) https://doi.org/10.1186/s12912-024-01718-1.
9. Kedia SK, Collins A, Dillon PJ, Akkus C, Ward KD, Jackson BM. Psychosocial interventions for informal caregivers of lung cancer patients: a systematic review. Psycho-Oncol. 2020;29(2) https://doi.org/10.1002/pon.5271.
10. Kwekkeboom KL. Cancer symptom cluster management - PubMed. Semin Oncol Nurs. 2016;32(4) https://doi.org/10.1016/j.soncn.2016.08.004.
11. Rosenzweig M, Belcher SM, Braithwaite LE, et al. Research priorities of the Oncology Nursing Society: 2024–2027 – PubMed. Oncol Nurs Forum. 2024;51(6) https://doi.org/10.1188/24.ONF.502-515.
12. Tucker-Seeley R, Abu-Khalaf M, Bona K, et al. Social determinants of health and cancer care: an ASCO policy statement. JCO Oncol Pract. 2024;20(5) https://doi.org/10.1200/OP.23.00810.
13. Kamei T. Telenursing and artificial intelligence for oncology nursing. Asia-Pac J Oncol Nurs. 2022;9(12) https://doi.org/10.1016/j.apjon.2022.100119.

14. Zhou T, Luo Y, Li J, et al. Application of artificial intelligence in oncology nursing: a scoping review – PubMed. Cancer Nurs. 2024;47(6) https://doi.org/10.1097/NCC.0000000000001254.
15. Isaacman DJ, Reynolds EA. Effect of a research nurse on patient enrollment in a clinical study. Pediatr Emerg Care. 1996;12(5):340–2.
16. Forbes Shepherd R, Bradford A, Lieschke M, Shackleton K, Hyatt A. Patient communication and experiences in cancer clinical drug trials: a mixed-method study at a specialist clinical trials unit. Trials. 2023;24(1):400.
17. White B. Ethical issues surrounding informed consent: part III. The crucial role of nursing in ensuring valid consent. Urol Nurs. 1989;9(5):6–9.
18. Portier WS. Cancer clinical trials: implications for oncology nurses. Elsevier; 2020. p. 150998.
19. Komatsu H, Hara A, Koyama F, Komatsu Y. Enhancing high reliability in oncology care: the critical role of nurses—a systematic review and thematic analysis. MDPI; 2025:283, Healthcare, 13.
20. Liu L, Liu Z, Ma C, et al. Exploring differences in symptomatic adverse events assessment between nurses and physicians in the clinical trial setting. Sci Rep. 2023;13(1):4917.
21. Miller TP, Marx MZ, Henchen C, et al. Challenges and barriers to adverse event reporting in clinical trials: a children's oncology group report. J Patient Saf. 2022;18(3):e672–9.
22. Cassidy J. The role of the data manager in clinical cancer research: an opportunity for nurses. Cancer Nurs. 1993;16(2):131–8.
23. Lee M, Kim K, Shin Y, Lee Y, Kim T-J. Advancements in electronic medical Records for Clinical Trials: enhancing data management and research efficiency. Cancer. 2025;17(9):1552.
24. Jedwab RM, Franco M, Owen D, Ingram A, Redley B, Dobroff N. Improving the quality of electronic medical record documentation: development of a compliance and quality program. Appl Clin Inform. 2022;13(04):836–44.
25. Neves FB, Vargas MAO, Zilli F, Trentin D, Huhn A, LCDF B. Health advocacy in oncology nursing: an integrative literature review. Esc Anna Nery. 2020;25:e20200106.
26. Meropol NJ, Buzaglo JS, Millard J, et al. Barriers to clinical trial participation as perceived by oncologists and patients. J Natl Compr Canc Netw. 2007;5(8):753–62.
27. Van Hecke A, Decoene E, Courtens A, Coolbrandt A, Decadt I, Pape E. The role of researcher for advanced practice nurses in oncology: challenges and lessons learned. Elsevier; 2024:151634, Semin Oncol Nurs, 40.
28. Ginex PK, Dickman E, Thomas B, Tucker S, Gallagher-Ford L. Evidence-based practice in oncology nursing: Oncology Nursing Society survey results. Clin J Oncol Nurs. 2021;25(3):282.

Correction to: Research on GI Cancer (Hepato-Pancreato-Biliary (HPB) Cancers)

Shane Zhang, Arnav Chavda, and Ji Fan

Correction to:
Chapter 19 in: J. Huang, H. S. L. Jim (eds.), *Cancer Research Guidance for Clinicians and Researchers*, https://doi.org/10.1007/978-3-032-19175-5_19

In Chapter 19 "Research on GI Cancer (Hepato-Pancreato-Biliary (HPB) Cancers)," the author's name was incorrectly printed as Arnarv Chavda. This has been corrected to Arnav Chavda in Chapter 19 (page 203) and Table of Contents (page X).

The updated version of this chapter can be found at
https://doi.org/10.1007/978-3-032-19175-5_19

J. Huang, H. S.L. Jim (eds.), *Cancer Research Guidance for Clinicians and Researchers*,
https://doi.org/10.1007/978-3-032-19175-5_35

Index

J. Huang, H. S.L. Jim (eds.), *Cancer Research Guidance for Clinicians and Researchers*,
https://doi.org/10.1007/978-3-032-19175-5

D

T

GPSR Compliance

The European Union's (EU) General Product Safety Regulation (GPSR) is a set of rules that requires consumer products to be safe and our obligations to ensure this.

If you have any concerns about our products, you can contact us on ProductSafety@springernature.com

In case Publisher is established outside the EU, the EU authorized representative is:

Springer Nature Customer Service Center GmbH
Europaplatz 3
69115 Heidelberg, Germany

Batch number: 10731667

Printed by Printforce, the Netherlands